The Dietitian's Guide to
Vegetarian Diets

Issues and Applications

Third Edition

Reed Mangels, PhD, RD, LDN
The Vegetarian Resource Group, Baltimore, Maryland
University of Massachusetts, Amherst, Massachusetts

Virginia Messina, MPH, RD
Nutrition Matters, Inc., Port Townsend, Washington
Loma Linda University, Loma Linda, California

Mark Messina, PhD
Nutrition Matters, Inc., Port Townsend, Washington
Loma Linda University, Loma Linda, California

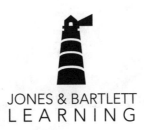

JONES & BARTLETT
LEARNING

World Headquarters

Jones & Bartlett Learning
40 Tall Pine Drive
Sudbury, MA 01776
978-443-5000
info@jblearning.com
www.jblearning.com

Jones & Bartlett Learning Canada
6339 Ormindale Way
Mississauga, Ontario L5V 1J2
Canada

Jones & Bartlett Learning International
Barb House, Barb Mews
London W6 7PA
United Kingdom

Jones & Bartlett Learning books and products are available through most bookstores and online booksellers. To contact Jones & Bartlett Learning directly, call 800-832-0034, fax 978-443-8000, or visit our website, www.jblearning.com.

Substantial discounts on bulk quantities of Jones & Bartlett Learning publications are available to corporations, professional associations, and other qualified organizations. For details and specific discount information, contact the special sales department at Jones & Bartlett Learning via the above contact information or send an email to specialsales@jblearning.com.

The authors, editor, and publisher have made every effort to provide accurate information. However, they are not responsible for errors, omissions, or for any outcomes related to the use of the contents of this book and take no responsibility for the use of the products and procedures described. Treatments and side effects described in this book may not be applicable to all people; likewise, some people may require a dose or experience a side effect that is not described herein. Drugs and medical devices are discussed that may have limited availability controlled by the Food and Drug Administration (FDA) for use only in a research study or clinical trial. Research, clinical practice, and government regulations often change the accepted standard in this field. When consideration is being given to use of any drug in the clinical setting, the health care provider or reader is responsible for determining FDA status of the drug, reading the package insert, and reviewing prescribing information for the most up-to-date recommendations on dose, precautions, and contraindications, and determining the appropriate usage for the product. This is especially important in the case of drugs that are new or seldom used.

Production Credits

Publisher, Higher Education: Cathleen Sether
Senior Acquisitions Editor: Shoshanna Goldberg
Senior Associate Editor: Amy L. Bloom
Editorial Assistant: Prima Bartlett
Production Manager: Julie Champagne Bolduc
Production Editor: Jessica Steele Newfell
Associate Marketing Manager: Jody Sullivan
V.P., Manufacturing and Inventory Control: Therese Connell

Composition: Dedicated Business Solutions, Inc.
Project Management: Thistle Hill Publishing Services, LLC
Cover Design: Kate Ternullo
Cover Image: © shyshak roman/ShutterStock, Inc.
Printing and Binding: Malloy, Inc.
Cover Printing: Malloy, Inc.

Library of Congress Cataloging-in-Publication Data

Mangels, Reed.
The dietitian's guide to vegetarian diets / Reed Mangels, Virginia Messina, Mark Messina. — 3rd ed.
   p. ; cm.
Includes bibliographical references and index.
ISBN-13: 978-0-7637-7976-4 (pbk.)
ISBN-10: 0-7637-7976-8 (pbk.)
1. Vegetarianism. 2. Diet. I. Messina, Virginia. II. Messina, Mark. III. Title.
   [DNLM: 1. Diet, Vegetarian. WB 430 M277d 2011]
   RM236.M444 2011
   613.2'62—dc22
                    2010024218

6048
Printed in the United States of America
14 13 12 11 10   10 9 8 7 6 5 4 3 2 1

Contents

Preface

Nutrition is an ever-changing field, and vegetarian nutrition is no exception. During the past 14 years since the *First Edition* of *The Dietitian's Guide to Vegetarian Diets* was published, much new research has been conducted in areas related to vegetarian nutrition. Of course, vegetarian nutrition is not limited to studies of the nutritional status of vegetarians. Vegetarian nutrition also examines the nutrient needs and sources of nutrients for those following vegetarian diets, the use of vegetarian diets in the prevention and treatment of disease, and the impact on health of vegetarian diets.

This *Third Edition* of *The Dietitian's Guide to Vegetarian Diets* is an update and expansion of the information presented in the 1996 and 2004 volumes. Since the last edition of *The Dietitian's Guide to Vegetarian Diets*, new discoveries have been made in a number of areas related to vegetarian nutrition. These are the result of several large-scale studies of vegetarians, increased interest in vegetarian diets in the treatment of chronic diseases and in athletes, and new research into several key nutrients. In addition, changes have been made in federal food programs that affect vegetarians.

Like its predecessors, this edition of *The Dietitian's Guide to Vegetarian Diets* is written for dietitians and other healthcare professionals and is meant to be used as an aid for counseling vegetarian clients and those interested in becoming vegetarian. It can also serve as a textbook for classroom study for students who have completed introductory coursework in nutrition. Finally, investigators will find it a useful review of the literature on vegetarian diets.

All chapters have been updated to include the latest research on vegetarian diets as well as newer recommendations and findings regarding general nutrition. Several chapters have undergone particularly extensive revision.

- Chapter 2 provides an update on the latest research related to the role of vegetarian diets in disease including cardiovascular disease, hypertension, cancers, diabetes, and obesity.
- Chapter 4 addresses fatty acid needs of vegetarians with particular attention to questions about the ability of vegetarian diets to meet requirements for omega-3 fatty acids.

- Chapter 7 supplies much new information on vitamin D, which is receiving increasing attention for its potential health effects and the possibility of benefits from higher intakes than current recommendations. This chapter also provides an update on the B vitamins and their role in homocysteine metabolism.
- Chapter 9 addresses the role of soyfoods in diets. Soyfoods present an increasingly popular topic in general nutrition, and they play an important role in the diets of many vegetarians. A growing body of data—reviewed in this book—suggests important links between soyfood consumption and disease risk.
- Chapter 14 examines the proposed link between eating disorders and vegetarian diets and presents an update on nutritional needs of adolescent athletes.
- Chapter 16 introduces material on the role of macronutrient distribution in healthy diets. This chapter includes recommendations for modifying vegetarian diets to manage chronic conditions including diabetes, obesity, cardiovascular disease, and the metabolic syndrome.

To make this text a more practical tool for dietetics practice, many chapters include expanded counseling points to help professionals translate the material into simple messages for clients. Many chapters also include case studies that allow practitioners and students to test their understanding of the material presented.

As before, the book is divided into five parts. Part I provides an overview of the vegetarian population and health status of this group. Chapters address demographics of vegetarianism and vegetarian health status including chronic disease rates. Part II examines nutritional needs within the context of a vegetarian diet with chapters devoted to protein, fatty acids, calcium, other minerals, vitamins, soyfoods, and phytochemicals. This part also includes a chapter on meal-planning guidance for vegetarians. Part III of the book addresses vegetarian diets throughout the life cycle with chapters devoted to pregnancy and lactation, infants, children, adolescents, and the elderly. Part IV summarizes practical issues for vegetarians with a chapter devoted to the role of macronutrients in planning diets for weight control, and for treatment of diabetes and heart disease. This section also contains material on food preparation with particular emphasis on foods that play important roles in vegetarian diets. The final part of the book includes a glossary of vegetarian foods as well as a resource list for both professionals and clients. The appendixes present data on vegetarian and nonvegetarian micronutrient and macronutrient intakes, serum lipid levels, blood pressure, and anthropometry, all in tabular form.

It is our hope that this updated and expanded review of the vegetarian literature combined with practical recommendations will help dietitians and other health professionals to continue to serve the needs of their vegetarian clients.

Acknowledgments

We are greatly indebted to a number of dietitians who have been instrumental in educating consumers and health professionals on vegetarian issues. Their efforts have had a great impact on our own work and on this book. We offer warm thanks to Suzanne Havala, Winston Craig, Jack Norris, Dina Aronson, Brenda Davis, Vesanto Melina, and the late Cyndi Reeser. In addition, we are grateful to Charles Stahler and Debra Wasserman of the Vegetarian Resource Group for their support.

As always, we are thankful for the love, support, and encouragement of our families.

PART I

An Overview of Vegetarian Diet

CHAPTER 1

Demographics and Definitions

HISTORY OF VEGETARIANISM

The term *vegetarian* was not coined until the mid-1800s. The concept dates back to at least the 6th century BC, however, when the Greek philosopher Pythagoras, considered the father of vegetarianism, encouraged meatless eating among his followers as the diet that was considered to be most natural and healthful.[1] Other early philosophers, including Socrates, Plato, Horace, Ovid, and Virgil, all favored the idea of meatless diets.

It was many centuries before the Western world showed an interest in vegetarianism. The 19th century saw the birth of a true vegetarian movement that was largely church related. In 1800, the Reverend William Cowherd, a minister of the Church of England, established the Bible Christians, a sect with Bible literalism as its foundation that embraced a vegetarian diet as the one prescribed by God in the book of Genesis.[2] Later Bible Christians traveled to Philadelphia and established a church there. Among the converts to the dietary philosophy of this group was Sylvester Graham, who toured the United States lecturing on the evils of meat, refined white bread, alcohol, coffee, extramarital sex, and tight pants. Although Graham was an advocate of meatless eating, his most important legacy was in encouraging the use of whole wheat flour, which came to be called graham flour. In the mid-1840s, Bible Christians in England established the Vegetarian Society of Great Britain, and the American church quickly followed suit by initiating the formation of the American Vegetarian Society.[2]

Another church group that had an extensive impact on the rise in vegetarianism in this country was the Seventh-day Adventist (SDA) Church, founded by Ellen White in the 1840s. Mrs. White produced copious teachings on the relationship of physical health to religious life and encouraged church members to eat a vegetarian diet.[3] Today, approximately 40% of SDAs are vegetarians, and the church is active in health education, producing materials on nutrition and teaching classes on vegetarianism.

One church member was especially instrumental in establishing the popularity of vegetarianism in the late 19th and early 20th centuries. John Harvey Kellogg headed the SDA-run Battle Creek Sanitarium in Battle Creek, Michigan, and was a protégé of Ellen White. Among Kellogg's greatest achievements was the production of some of the first breakfast cereals—corn flakes and granola—to provide his patients with healthy breakfast options. He also invented nuttose, the first meat analog made from peanuts and flour; produced the first peanut butter; and was an early enthusiast of soymilk.[4]

Kellogg's sanitarium regimen, which he called biologic living and included a vegetarian diet; total abstinence from alcohol, caffeine, sugar, and strong spices; and emphasized exercise, hydrotherapy, fresh air, sunshine, good posture, simple dress, and good mental health, was popular with some of the most powerful personalities of the day. His sanitarium was visited by William Howard Taft, William Jennings Bryan, John D. Rockefeller, Alfred Dupont, J. C. Penney, Montgomery Ward, Thomas Edison, Henry Ford, George Bernard Shaw, and Admiral Richard Byrd.

As a result of the efforts of the diet reformers, interest in vegetarian diet was at a peak from the mid-19th century through the early part of the 20th century. Vegetarian sanitariums and eateries opened throughout the country. A popular vegetarian restaurant in New York City at the turn of the century was the Physical Culture and Strength Food Restaurant. Vegetarian organizations existed in Kansas City, St. Louis, Minneapolis, Boston, Pittsburgh, Chicago, Washington, D.C., and many European countries.[5]

By the middle of the 20th century, however, with the discovery of vitamins and the production of government-sponsored food guides, meat-based diets were touted as the healthiest ways to eat. All food guides developed at the time encouraged generous consumption of both meat and dairy products. Nevertheless, the results of a 1943 Gallup poll showed that between 2.5 and 3.0 million Americans were vegetarians, representing 2% of the total population.[6] In 1944, the term *vegan* was coined for vegetarians who consumed no dairy or egg products, and the Vegan Society was formed in Great Britain in that year.[7]

Vegetarianism enjoyed a resurgence in popularity again in the 1960s and 1970s as a natural choice of the new health-conscious members of the counterculture. An important influence was macrobiotic teacher Michio Kushi. Even though vegetarianism was popular with young people, it had little mainstream appeal at that time.

Surprisingly, two influences that had little to do with health concerns served to popularize vegetarian diet among more diverse groups and led the way for a more mainstream view of meatless eating. The publication of Frances Moore Lappé's *Diet for a Small Planet* linked diet to global concerns and focused attention on the adverse effects of meat production on the environment.[8] Her book became an important influence on the way people viewed food choices. Second, the birth of the modern animal rights movement, heralded by the publication in 1975 of *Animal Liberation* by Peter Singer and the formation of the animal rights group People for the Ethical Treatment of Animals, focused new attention on the treatment of animals by the factory farming industry. Research suggests that ethical and health concerns are most commonly cited as reasons for adopting a vegetarian diet.[9]

Over the past two decades, interest in vegetarian diets has remained strong. The number of vegetarians in the United States doubled between 1985 and 1992 when a Gallup poll found that 12 million American adults called themselves vegetarian.[10] A Zogby poll conducted for the Vegetarian Resource Group (VRG) in 2000 found there were about 4.8 million vegetarian adults in the United States or about 2.5% of the population.[11] A similar survey conducted for VRG in 2003 showed that 2.8% of Americans never ate meat, fish, or poultry, and 1.8% were vegans.[12]

These numbers were smaller than those from the Gallup poll presumably because of the way the questions were asked. The Zogby poll, which surveyed actual eating habits, probably gives a more accurate picture of rates of vegetarianism in the United States and may slightly underestimate these rates, whereas other surveys may considerably overestimate the number of people who don't eat meat, fish, or poultry. Using data from the Continuing Survey of Food Intake by Individuals 1994–1996, Haddad and Tanzman found that two thirds of those who identified themselves as vegetarians reported consuming meat, fish, or poultry on either or both of the 2-day dietary recall collected in the survey.[13] More recently, a survey conducted in Finland found that 80% of self-identified vegetarians consumed meat.[14] According to the Zogby poll, vegetarians are most likely to live on the East or West Coast in large cities and are more likely to be women who work outside of the home. Slightly fewer than 1% of the 968 people polled were vegans. In a Roper poll conducted in 2000 of 6- to 17-year-olds, nearly 1% of 6- to 7-year olds were vegetarians and 2% of 8- to 17-year olds were vegetarian.[15] Harris Interactive polls taken in 2006 and 2009 showed that vegetarians and vegans continue to make up 3% and 1% of the U.S. population, respectively. Among women between the ages of 18 and 34 years, approximately 5% are vegetarian.[16,17]

It is likely that interest in vegetarian diet will continue, especially because diet-related problems such as heart disease and cancer continue to be pressing concerns today and because their link to diet is firmly established. Interest in the effects of diet on climate change is also affecting diet choices. An additional factor that may impact the number of vegetarians in the United States is the arrival of immigrants from countries where vegetarianism is commonly practiced.[18]

PROFILE OF VEGETARIANS

Early views among health professionals of the vegetarian population were usually unfavorable. In the early 1970s, those who reported on vegetarians often linked meatless diets with drug use (an observation that may have been accurate in some cases), and vegetarian communities were described as cults.[19-22] Food habits of vegetarians were not viewed positively. For example, the eating habits of young American vegetarians, which included avoidance of processed foods and extensive use of natural foods, were pronounced as bizarre in one 1971 article in the medical journal *Lancet*.[19] In 1979, a study of simulated counseling sessions revealed that many dietitians encouraged meat consumption among their vegetarian clients.[23]

Growing professional interest in vegetarianism is evident, however, from the increase in the number of articles in the scientific literature related to vegetarianism, from fewer than 10 articles per year in the late 1960s to an average of 76 articles per year in the 1990s.[24] The focus of articles has changed as well from articles that primarily had themes questioning the nutritional adequacy of vegetarian diets to those evaluating the use of vegetarian diets in the prevention and treatment of disease. There has also been a shift toward more epidemiologic studies and fewer case reports.

Vegetarian food preferences are of interest to anyone who works in a food- or medical-related capacity. Increasing interest in vegetarian foods is having a significant impact on food choices in the marketplace. A 1999 Zogby poll found that 5.5% of those surveyed said they always order a vegetarian dish when eating out.[25] Most school systems, particularly in urban areas, are likely to have vegetarian students in their cafeteria, and vegetarianism is growing in popularity on college campuses. A survey conducted by food service provider Aramak in 2005 found that nearly one in four college students said that access to vegan meals on campus was important to them.[26] Some schools and businesses also participate in Meatless Monday campaigns, serving vegetarian meals 1 day a week in response to climate change.[27] Caterers, airlines, school food services, and hospitals need to be prepared to serve the vegetarian client.

The growth of vegetarian foods, such as meat analogs, nondairy milks, and vegetarian entrees, is another indicator of growing interest in this way of eating. The market for these products was estimated to be $1.5 billion in 2002, an increase from $310 million in 1996.[28] This market is expected to reach $2.8 billion by 2006. Sales of soyfoods, often used to replace meat and dairy products on menus, increased from $300 million in 1992 to $4 billion in 2008.[29] According to a 2009 survey conducted for the United Soybean Board, nearly 25% of consumers drink soymilk regularly.[30] Soymilk and tofu, as alternatives to dairy products, are also available now for families enrolled in the Women, Infants, and Children (WIC) program. About half of vegetarian foods volume is sold through supermarkets and half through natural foods stores. Seventy-five percent of soymilk sales are through supermarkets.

TYPES OF VEGETARIAN DIETS

In working with vegetarian clients, it is important to understand what a vegetarian diet is and to realize that several different styles of eating fall under this umbrella. At its broadest, a vegetarian diet is one that includes no meat, poultry, or fish. Beyond that, however, there are many variations on the vegetarian theme (Exhibits 1-1 and 1-2).

Lacto-Ovo Vegetarian Diets

Most self-proclaimed vegetarians fall into this category. A lacto-ovo vegetarian diet includes dairy products and eggs but no animal flesh. Meat, poultry, and fish are avoided. A smaller subset of this group avoids eggs and are more accurately termed *lacto-vegetarians*. Likewise, some vegetarians may eat an ovo-vegetarian diet if they avoid dairy products but consume eggs.

One cause for concern in lacto-ovo vegetarian diets can be overreliance on cheese, milk, and eggs. Particularly new vegetarians, those who are making the transition to this new pattern of eating and therefore may have limited skills in planning meals or may have concerns about protein intake, may base many meals on these animal products. Dairy products, particularly whole milk products and cheese, and eggs can contribute excessive saturated fat and cholesterol to meals and can displace the healthier fiber-rich plant foods in vegetarian menus. Counseling clients about the ease with which protein needs are met on vegetarian diets, helping them explore the use of nonfat dairy foods in their diet, and providing information about alternative sources of calcium can be ways to help them limit the use of fattier dairy foods and eggs. Calcium intakes of lacto-ovo vegetarians suggest that many do not consume more dairy foods than meat eaters, however, which may be due to increased availability of meat and dairy substitutes (Appendix G).

The health profile of lacto-ovo vegetarians, as well as their higher intake of fiber and certain nutrients, suggests that this group, overall, consumes fewer animal products than nonvegetarians. Nearly 80% of SDA vegetarians, the most widely studied group of vegetarians in the United States, consume a lacto-ovo vegetarian diet.[31] This population exhibits low rates of heart disease, obesity, diabetes, hypertension, and certain cancers compared with the general population.[32]

Exhibit 1-1 Types of Vegetarian Diets

Types of Vegetarians	Foods Consumed	Foods Avoided	Comments
Lacto-ovo	Grains, legumes, vegetables, nuts, seeds, dairy, eggs	Meat, poultry, fish	Diet can be high in total fat if full-fat dairy products and eggs are used
Vegan	Grains, legumes, vegetables, fruits, nuts, seeds	Meat, poultry, fish, dairy, eggs; foods with small amounts of added animal products, such as casein or whey, are also generally avoided, as are foods that involve animal processing, such as white sugar, beer, and vinegar	Requires vitamin B_{12}-fortified foods or supplements; may also require vitamin D–fortified foods if sun exposure is inadequate
Macrobiotic	Grains, legumes, vegetables (nuts, seeds, fruits to a lesser extent); makes wide use of sea vegetables, soy products, and Asian condiments; seafood may be consumed	Meat, poultry, sometimes fish, dairy products, eggs, vegetables of nightshade family, tropical fruits, processed sweeteners	Guidelines for this diet may need to be adjusted to make it suitable for children. Requires vitamin B_{12}-fortified foods if sun exposure is inadequate
Fruitarian	Fruits, vegetables that are botanically fruits (tomatoes, eggplant, peppers, avocado, squash), nuts, seeds	Meat, fish, poultry, dairy foods, eggs, grains, legumes, most vegetables	Some modified versions of this pattern may allow grains and/or legumes; difficult to plan nutritionally adequate diets on strict fruitarian plans; not suitable for children
Raw foods	Vegetables, fruits, nuts, seeds, sprouted grains, sprouted beans, all consumed in the raw state; some adherents may use raw dairy products	Meat, fish, poultry, any cooked plant foods	Percentage of raw foods in the diet may actually vary among adherents from as little as 50–100%; completely raw foods diet not appropriate for children
Natural hygiene	Emphasis on raw vegetables and fruits; includes whole grains, legumes, nuts, sprouted grains, seeds, legumes	Varies; some regimens prohibit meat consumption, dairy, eggs	Emphasis on eating or avoiding certain combinations of foods

Exhibit 1-2 Sample Meal Plans for Different Types of Vegetarian Diets

Type of Diet	Breakfast	Lunch	Dinner
Lacto-ovo	Cheerios with low-fat milk Whole wheat toast with fruit spread Sliced bananas Coffee	Veggie burger on whole wheat roll with lettuce, tomato, ketchup Carrot sticks Apple juice Oatmeal cookies	Vegetable fajitas with zucchini, carrots, peppers, onions in soft corn tortillas Refried beans Tossed salad Fresh fruit cocktail
Vegan	Scrambled tofu Rye bread toast with fruit spread Fresh fruit salad	Vegetable soup Whole wheat rolls Tossed salad with low-fat dressing Cantaloupe chunks	Pasta primavera with broccoli, carrots, pea pods Steamed kale French bread
Macrobiotic	Miso soup with tofu, daikon, carrots Oatmeal	Udon noodles seasoned with miso Steamed Brussels sprouts Peas and mushrooms	Miso soup with kombu and shitake mushrooms Brown rice seasoned with umeboshi plum Steamed kale Baked winter squash
Fruitarian*	Granola with raisins, almonds Sliced bananas Fresh pineapple and orange juice	Steamed eggplant and zucchini in tomato sauce Fruit salad with bananas, chopped figs, apples, chopped Brazil nuts Almond milk	Zucchini stuffed with sprouted wheat berries, raisins, walnuts and tahini dressing Apple slices spread with almond butter Sliced fresh papaya Fresh figs
Raw foods	Granola with homemade almond milk Fresh fruit salad	Gazpacho soup Salad of fresh greens Almond-fig-oat bars (ground oats soaked in fruit juice, mixed with pureed figs and ground almonds, pressed into bars)	Salad of raw vegetables, sprouted lentils, and sprouted wheat berries, oil and lemon juice dressing, fresh herbs Fresh squeezed carrot juice Apple slices and celery spread with tahini
*Modified, with limited amounts of grain.			

Vegan Diets

Although only a small percentage of self-identified vegetarians follow a vegan diet, surveys of eating habits suggest that a third or more of the *actual* vegetarian population avoids all dietary animal products.[17] Although the word *vegan* was coined in 1944 to describe avoidance of all animal products for ethical reasons, including those used in clothing, medications, and personal care products, the term is typically used for those who subscribe to an ethical vegan lifestyle as well as those who consume a vegan diet for health reasons. Evidence indicates that vegans have a lower risk of heart disease than lacto-ovo vegetarians.[33] Vegans may also have lower body mass indexes than either meat eaters or lacto-ovo vegetarians.[34] Vegan diets are likely to be lower in fat and higher in fiber than both nonvegetarian and lacto-ovo vegetarian diets (Appendix A).

Vegans avoid meat, fish, poultry, dairy, and eggs. Many other foods may not be acceptable to vegans, however. Foods that involve animal processing to any degree are often avoided. These may include honey, refined sugar, vinegar, wine, and beer.

Some avoid foods with small amounts of added whey or casein or additives of nonspecific origin, such as monoglycerides or so-called natural flavorings. Many foods that are marketed directly to vegetarians are not acceptable to vegans. Veggie burgers may use egg whites as a binder, for example. Many soy cheeses contain casein, a milk protein.

A dietitian who is counseling a vegan client needs to listen carefully to the client's own description of which foods are acceptable. Vegan meal plans may make frequent use of ethnic cuisine, and many vegans are willing and eager to explore new foods and eating styles. As a result, an eating pattern that seems confining to some may actually be viewed as one with particularly expansive menu choices and culinary opportunities.

The nutrient of concern in vegan diets is vitamin B_{12}, which, for all practical purposes, is found only in foods of animal origin. All vegans need to identify a source of vitamin B_{12} in their diet, however. For vegans who do not use fortified foods, a supplement is the best choice, and dietitians should be able to identify locally available brands of B_{12} that are not derived from animal foods.

Vegan diets are often low in vitamin D. This is not a problem if vegans have adequate sun exposure, but it can be an unreliable means of maintaining normal vitamin D levels. Vegans can also obtain this vitamin from fortified foods. Many breakfast cereals are fortified, as are many brands of soymilk.

Because milk products are the most common source of calcium in the American diet, concern about the calcium content of vegan diets has been raised. Vegans can meet the recommended dietary allowance for calcium, however, especially when fortified products such as calcium-fortified soymilks or orange juice are used.

Finally, zinc intake of vegans may be low, and zinc bioavailability is poorer from plant foods than in animal foods. Vegans need to give some attention to using zinc-rich foods in their menu planning.

Raw Foods Diet

Adherents to a raw foods diet believe it most closely resembles the natural eating pattern of humans and that this diet preserves the integrity of food constituents such as enzymes. Followers of this diet consume vegetables, fruits, nuts, seeds, and sprouted grains and beans, all in their raw state. The diet actually varies among adherents, who may consume anywhere from 50% to 100% of their foods as raw foods.

Although cooking can destroy significant amounts of nutrients in foods, heat also improves the digestibility of most foods and destroys antinutritional factors. The premise for consuming a raw foods diet is not scientifically supported, but the diet can be safe if sprouted grains and beans are used. Diets that are 100% raw take considerable planning to meet nutrient needs. In particular, it is not clear that those consuming a completely raw diet can meet needs for the essential amino acid lysine. Research also suggests that those following a raw foods diet have lower blood levels of the antioxidant lycopene.[35] Koebnick et al found that long-term consumption of a raw foods diet was associated with favorable serum low-density lipoprotein (LDL) cholesterol and triglyceride levels, but also with elevated homocysteine and low serum high-density lipoprotein (HDL) cholesterol as well as low protein intakes.[36] A raw foods diet is not recommended for children.

Macrobiotic Diets

Observations of macrobiotic communities in the 1970s revealed serious nutrition deficiencies in infants and young children.[36–39] These were directly attributed to macrobiotic feeding practices that were not nutritionally adequate for children. Some of these practices are discussed in Chapters 12 and 13. For adults, however, a macrobiotic diet can be a safe and healthy approach to eating. With some modifications, described in Chapters 12 and 13, macrobiotics can also be an acceptable choice for children.

The macrobiotic philosophy is loosely linked to Buddhism and more strongly linked to the ancient Taoist principle of yin and yang. The foods that are central to macrobiotic cuisine reflect Asian influences. The diet makes extensive use of rice; sea vegetables; Asian condiments such as tamari, miso, and umeboshi plum; and root vegetables such as daikon and lotus root.

The macrobiotic lifestyle focuses on principles of balance and harmony with nature and the universe. Foods consumed should be in season and locally produced if possible, so that climate and geography dictate the makeup of a macrobiotic diet to a large extent. People living in most of North America, Europe, Asia, parts of Latin America, and parts of Australia, however, all considered temperate zones, eat roughly the same diet.

Macrobiotic meals are based largely on grains, which make up between 50% and 60% of the diet. Vegetables, especially sea vegetables, play a central role in meals, and soups (especially miso soup) and beans are served in smaller amounts. Fruits, nuts, seeds, and breads are used in moderation and not consumed every day. Foods that are avoided on a macrobiotic diet are vegetables of the nightshade family (potatoes, tomatoes, eggplant, and peppers), tropical fruits, and processed sweeteners. Some macrobiotics use limited amounts of fish.

Many people choose a macrobiotic diet because they believe it is the healthiest way of eating. It has also been widely promoted as a diet with curative powers, particularly for diseases such as cancer. Support for protective effects of macrobiotic diets remains limited.[40,41]

Semivegetarian or Flexitarian Diet

As interest in healthy vegetarian diets and optimal eating patterns grows, particularly in regard to environmental issues, many people are limiting meat in their diet and calling themselves semivegetarians or flexitarians. The term *semivegetarian* can actually cover a wide range of eating practices. It includes individuals who may eat a variety of meat products but use them as condiments or consume them just a few times a week. It may include those who eat only certain animal products, such as fish or chicken, but eat them frequently. In counseling, it is important to ascertain the true extent of meat, fish, and poultry consumption because the nutrient composition of these diets can vary considerably from true vegetarian plans. Although the inclusion of small amounts of meat in diets can increase nutrient intake, data from the Adventist Health Study show that semivegetarians—defined as those who consumed no red meat and ate fish and chicken less than once per week—had higher rates of diabetes and hypertension.[42]

REFERENCES

1. Roe DA. History of promotion of vegetable cereal diets. *J Nutr.* 1986;116(7):1355–1363.
2. Spencer C. *The Heretics Feast.* London, England: Fourth Estate; 1993.
3. White EG. *Counsels on Diet and Foods: A Compilation from the Writings of Ellen G. White.* Hagerstown, MD: Review and Herald; 1938.
4. Shurtleff W, Aoyagi A. *History of Soybeans and Soyfoods* [unpublished]. Lafayette, CA: Soyfoods Center; n.d.
5. Unti B. *The Bible Christians and the Origins of Vegetarianism in North America* [unpublished manuscript].
6. Hardinge MG, Crooks H. Non-flesh dietaries. *J Am Diet Assoc.* 1963;43:545–549.
7. Long A. The well nourished vegetarian. *New Sci.* 1981;89:330–333.
8. Lappe FM. *Diet for a Small Planet.* New York, NY: Ballantine; 1971.
9. Fox N, Ward K. Health, ethics and environment: a qualitative study of vegetarian motivations. *Appetite.* 2008;50:422–429.
10. Yankelovich, Skelly, White/Clancy, Shulman, Inc. *The American vegetarian: Coming of age in the 90s (A study of the vegetarian marketplace conducted by Vegetarian Times, Inc.).* Oak Park, IL; 1992.
11. Vegetarian Resource Group. How many vegetarians are there? http://www.vrg.org/nutshell/poll2000.htm.
12. Vegetarian Resource Group. How many vegetarians are there? http://www.vrg.org/journal/vj2003issue3/vj2003issue3poll.htm.
13. Haddad EH, Tanzman JS. What do vegetarians in the United States eat? *Am J Clin Nutr.* 2003;78(suppl):626S–636S.
14. Vinnari M, Montonen J, Harkaene T, Mannisto S. Identifying vegetarians and their food consumption according to self-identification and operationalized definition in Finland. *Public Health Nutr.* 2009;12:481–488.
15. Vegetarian Resource Group. How many teens are vegetarian? How many kids don't eat meat? http://www.vrg.org/journal/vj2001jan/2001janteen.htm.
16. Vegetarian Resource Group. How many adults are vegetarian? http://www.vrg.org/journal/vj2006issue4/vj2006issue4poll.htm.
17. Vegetarian Resource Group. How many vegetarians are there? http://www.vrg.org/press/2009poll.htm.
18. Raj S, Ganganna P, Bowering J. Dietary habits of Asian Indians in relation to length of residence in the United States. *J Am Diet Assoc.* 1999;99(9):1106–1108.
19. Dwyer JT, Mayer J. Vegetarianism in drug users. *Lancet.* 1971;2(7739):1429–1430.
20. Dwyer JT, Mayer LD, Dowd K, Kandel RF, Mayer J. The new vegetarians: the natural high? *J Am Diet Assoc.* 1974;65(5):529–536.
21. Dwyer JT, Mayer LD, Kandel RF, Mayer J. The new vegetarians. *J Am Diet Assoc.*1973;62(5):503–509.
22. Erhard D. The new vegetarians. Part two: Zen macrobiotic movement and other cults based on vegetarianism. *Nutr Today.* 1974;9:20–27.
23. Strobl CM, Groll L. Professional knowledge and attitudes on vegetarianism: implications for practice. *J Am Diet Assoc.* 1981;79(5):568–574.
24. Sabate J, Duk A, Lee CL. Publication trends of vegetarian nutrition articles in biomedical literature, 1966–1995. *Am J Clin Nutr.* 1999;70(3 suppl):601S–607S.
25. Vegetarian Resource Group. Dining out. *Vegetarian J.* 1999 (Sept/Oct):11.
26. Aramak. http://www.businesswire.com/portal/site/google/?ndmViewId=news_view&newsId=20050621005207&newsLang=en.
27. http://www.jhsph.edu/publichealthnews/press_releases/2009/clf_event_farm.

28. Mintel International Group. *The Vegetarian Food Market US Report.* Chicago, IL: Mintel International Group; 2001.
29. Soyatech, Inc. *Soyfoods: The U.S. Market 2009.* http://www.spins.com.
30. http://www.soyconnection.com/health_nutrition/pdf/ConsumerAttitudes2009.pdf.
31. Butler TL, Fraser GE, Beeson WL, et al. Cohort profile: The Adventist Health Study-2 (AHS-2). *Int J Epidemiol.* 2008;37(2):260–265.
32. Craig WJ, Mangels AR. Position of the American Dietetic Association: vegetarian diets. *J Am Diet Assoc.* 2009; 109:1266–1282.
33. Appleby PN, Davey GK, Key TJ. Hypertension and blood pressure among meat eaters, fish eaters, vegetarians and vegans in EPIC-Oxford. *Public Health Nutr.* 2002;5:645–654.
34. Spencer EA, Appleby PN, Davey GK, Key TJ. Diet and body-mass index in 38000 EPIC-Oxford meat-eaters, fish-eaters, vegetarians, and vegans. *Int J Obes Relat Metab Disord.* 2003;27:728–734.
35. Garcia AL, Koebnick C, Dagnelie PC, et al. Long-term strict raw food diet is associated with favourable plasma beta-carotene and low plasma lycopene concentrations in Germans. *Br J Nutr.* 2008;99:1293–1300.
36. Koebnick C, Garcia AL, Dagnelie PC, et al. Long-term consumption of a raw food diet is associated with favorable serum LDL cholesterol and triglycerides but also with elevated plasma homocysteine and low serum HDL cholesterol in humans. *J Nutr.* 2005;135:2372–2378.
37. Dwyer JT, Palombo R, Valadian I, Reed RB. Preschoolers on alternate life-style diets. Associations between size and dietary indexes with diets limited in types of animal foods. *J Am Diet Assoc.* 1978;72(3):264–270.
38. Dagnelie PC, van Staveren WA, Vergote FJ, et al. Nutritional status of infants aged 4 to 18 months on macrobiotic diets and matched omnivorous control infants: a population-based mixed-longitudinal study. II. Growth and psychomotor development. *Eur J Clin Nutr.* 1989;43(5):325–338.
39. Dagnelie PC, van Staveren WA, Verschuren SA, Hautvast JG. Nutritional status of infants aged 4 to 18 months on macrobiotic diets and matched omnivorous control infants: a population-based mixed-longitudinal study. I. Weaning pattern, energy and nutrient intake. *Eur J Clin Nutr.* 1989;43(5):311–323.
40. Carter JP, Saxe GP, Newbold V, Peres CE, Campeau RJ, Bernal-Green L. Hypothesis: dietary management may improve survival from nutritionally linked cancers based on analysis of representative cases. *J Am Coll Nutr.* 1993;12(3):209–226.
41. Weisburger JH. Guest editorial: a new nutritional approach in cancer therapy in light of mechanistic understanding of cancer causation and development. *J Am Coll Nutr.* 1993;12:205–208.
42. Phillips RL, Garfinkel L, Kuzma JW, et al. Mortality among California Seventh-day Adventists for selected cancer sites. *J Natl Cancer Inst.* 1980;65:1097–1107.

CHAPTER 2

Health Consequences of Vegetarian Diets

Populations consuming vegetarian and semi-vegetarian diets have lower rates of several chronic diseases that typically plague Western countries, including heart disease, hypertension, diabetes, and certain cancers. This is true of vegetarians living in Western countries and of populations consuming plant-based diets in developing countries. Migration studies indicate these differences are due to environmental factors. The incidence of heart disease and many cancers increases when people from countries where plant-based diets are consumed relocate to countries with diets predominantly based on animal products. Similarly, when people in developing countries become more affluent and begin to add more animal products to their diet, rates of chronic disease increase.[1,2]

Much of the available information about health effects of vegetarian diets comes from two large prospective epidemiologic studies. The Adventist Health Study (AHS)-1 is a cohort of 34,192 California Seventh-day Adventists (SDAs) that began in 1974–1976. The European Prospective Investigation into Cancer and Nutrition-Oxford (EPIC-Oxford) in the United Kingdom has 65,429 participants and oversampled for vegetarians. In addition, a second study of Adventists, the AHS-2, began in 2002 and had enrolled 96,194 participants as of 2007. It includes subjects from all 50 states and Canada and has provided some preliminary cross-sectional data based on enrollment questionnaires.

Smaller cohorts that also enrolled vegetarians were the Health Food Shoppers Study, the Oxford Vegetarian Study, both in the United Kingdom, and the Heidelberg Vegetarian Study in Germany.

Data from the AHS-1 showed that SDAs had longer life expectancies compared to the general population, which was attributable to a healthy lifestyle that includes exercise, tobacco avoidance, and healthful diet, and also that among the study participants, Adventist vegetarians had even greater life expectancy than nonvegetarians.[3] However, results from the EPIC-Oxford and the Oxford Vegetarian Study showed that, although British vegetarians were found to have low mortality rates compared to the general population, there was no difference in mortality between vegetarians and other study participants who had healthful lifestyles, although mortality from ischemic heart disease was 19% lower among the vegetarians.[4] Identifying precisely which dietary factors affect disease rates of vegetarians is difficult because so many differences exist between vegetarians and nonvegetarians. It is therefore instructive to consider some of these dietary differences within the context of what is known about the relationship between specific dietary components and disease risk.

DIFFERENCES IN DIETARY COMPONENTS OF VEGETARIAN AND NONVEGETARIAN DIETS

Dietary Fat and Cholesterol

Differences in fat intake between vegetarians and nonvegetarians are not as striking as commonly thought. In the United States, fat intake has declined and now averages about 34% of caloric intake.[5,6] By comparison, lacto-ovo vegetarians and vegans consume diets that are 28–34% and 25–30% fat, respectively, although there is considerable variation among studies (Appendix A).

From studies involving direct comparisons (Appendix A; Table 2-1), it is clear that omnivores consume considerably more saturated fat than vegetarians, although both lacto-ovo vegetarians and omnivores consume more saturated fat than polyunsaturated fat. In contrast, vegans consume more polyunsaturated fat than saturated fat. Their lower saturated fat content is likely part of the explanation for the reduced rates of coronary heart disease (CHD) seen in some vegetarians and vegans, although recent research has raised some uncertainty about the relationship between saturated fat intake and CHD risk.[7]

Cholesterol intake is also lower among vegetarians. Data from the National Health and Nutrition Examination (NHANES)-III indicate average U.S. cholesterol intake is about 300 mg/d.[5] Lacto-ovo vegetarian cholesterol intake is typically between 150 and 300 mg/d, and strict vegan diets contain no cholesterol.

Dietary Fiber and Carbohydrate Intake

Fiber intake differs markedly between vegetarians and nonvegetarians. Older dietary surveys indicated that Americans consumed as little as 10 to 12 g of fiber/d,[8] but more recent data suggest fiber intake may be as high as 17 g/d for men and 16 g/d for women; these figures are more

Table 2-1 Comparison of Vegetarian and Nonvegetarian Intakes of Protein, Fat, Carbohydrate, Cholesterol, and Fiber

Nutrient	Nonvegetarian	Lacto-Ovo Vegetarian	Vegan
Fat (% total calories)	34	28–34	25–30
Cholesterol (total grams)	300	150–300	0
Carbohydrate (% total calories)	<50	50–55	50–65
Dietary fiber (total grams)	15–20	20–35	25–50
Protein (% total calories)	14–18	12–14	10–12
Animal protein (% total protein)	60–70	40–60	0

consistent with the data in Appendix A.[9,10] Nevertheless, lacto-ovo vegetarians generally consume between 50% and 100% more fiber than nonvegetarians, and vegans consume more fiber than lacto-ovo vegetarians. The U.S. Dietary Guidelines recommend 14 g fiber/1000 kcal.[11]

Not surprisingly, vegetarian diets are higher in carbohydrate than omnivore patterns. Vegans consume roughly 50–65% of their calories in the form of carbohydrate, lacto-ovo vegetarians about 50–55%, and omnivores generally <50% (Appendix A).

Protein

Protein accounts for approximately 15% of calories in the diet of Western omnivores. Americans typically consume 50–100% more than the adult protein recommended dietary allowance (0.8 g/kg body weight). Lacto-ovo vegetarians consume diets containing between 12% and 14% protein, and vegan diets are between 10% and 12% protein (Appendix A). Clearly, the type of protein consumed also differs. American omnivores derive about two thirds of their protein from animal foods; this has changed from the early 20th century when only half of dietary protein was derived from animal sources.[12] In contrast to the omnivore diet, about 40–60% of the protein in lacto-ovo vegetarian diets is derived from animal products, whereas vegans consume plant protein only.[13-15] In a sample of >6000 individuals who participated in the NHANES-III survey, Smith et al found that animal protein intake was directly associated with higher serum cholesterol levels even after controlling for saturated fat, fiber, and cholesterol intake, although it is extremely difficult to determine specific effects when variables are strongly collinear.[5]

Phytochemicals and Antioxidants

Antioxidants may reduce risk of a wide array of diseases, including arthritis, cancer, and heart disease,[16,17] although in recent years the importance of antioxidants has been called into question. Vegetarians consume higher levels of the three primary vitamin antioxidants: β-carotene and vitamins C and E. In addition, vegetarian diets are higher in phytochemicals (discussed later and in Chapter 8), many of which are potent antioxidants and may be protective against chronic diseases such as cancer and heart disease.

CARDIOVASCULAR DISEASE

In 1925, British physician Sir John McNee described to his colleagues two cases of atherosclerosis, a "rare disease" that he had observed while visiting the United States.[18,19] Today, slightly more than a third (34%) of Americans die of cardiovascular disease, although mortality rates have come down significantly since the mid-1960s. There are a number of reasons for this decline; lifestyle changes have contributed, but the widespread use of cardiopulmonary resuscitation and improved medical procedures are also very important factors.

Blood cholesterol levels in Americans have dropped somewhat in recent years and now average about 199 mg/dl.[20] Analysis of NHANES III data suggests that cholesterol levels have continued to decline, although the rate of decline has slowed in recent years.[21] Nevertheless, about 17% of the population have blood cholesterol levels that place them at high risk for heart disease (≥240 mg/dl), and another 30% have levels >200 mg/dl.[19] The biologically normal or desirable level of blood cholesterol may be as low as 100 to 150 mg/dl.[22] Populations consuming traditional plant-based diets often have levels within this range.

Mortality rates from heart disease differ markedly throughout the world; in fact, the death rate due to heart attack is 10 times higher in some countries than in others. For example, in Shanghai, China, just 1 of every 15 deaths is due to heart disease.[23] Although genetic factors affect heart disease risk, they are unlikely to account for a substantial portion of this worldwide variation. Even within countries, differences in mortality rates clearly suggest an environmental influence; for example, rural Chinese have only half the rate of heart disease of urban Chinese.[24]

In a systematic review of cohort studies and randomized controlled trials (RCTs), Mente et al found that dietary factors strongly protective against CHD included vegetables, nuts, monounsaturated fat, and a Mediterranean-style diet, whereas factors that were strongly associated with increased risk were trans fats, high glycemic index, and a Western dietary pattern.[7]

Vegetarians and Heart Disease Risk

Nearly all studies in countries throughout the world show SDA and non-SDA vegetarian men have approximately half the risk of death due to ischemic heart disease in comparison to the general population.[25–33] Among SDAs, nonvegetarian men have a twofold to threefold increase in risk for CHD in comparison with vegetarian men.[33,34]

In an analysis of five prospective studies involving >76,000 individuals, death due to ischemic heart disease was 32% lower among vegetarian compared to nonvegetarian men. Protective effects were greater in vegetarians who had followed their diet for at least 5 years and, interestingly, were greater at younger ages.[35] However, not all data are supportive of a protective effect of a vegetarian diet against CHD. In the Oxford Vegetarian Study, although heart disease rates were reduced >50% when compared to the general British population, meat eaters in this study had a lower risk than vegetarians.[29] Similarly, in a later analysis of this study, vegetarian diet was also not associated with a significantly reduced risk.[36]

A vegetarian diet also appears to be less protective against heart disease in women. In the combined prospective analysis just cited, death rates due to CHD were only 20% lower for female vegetarians versus 32% for men.[35] Consistent with this finding, in the AHS, beef consumption was associated with a more than twofold increased risk of fatal ischemic heart disease in men but was unrelated to risk in women.[37] Finally, in the AHS, vegetarianism was associated with a greatly reduced risk for heart disease among men but not among women.

Because smoking increases cardiovascular disease risk by approximately two- to threefold, the lower rates of heart disease seen in some studies may be due, in part, to avoidance of tobacco products. (Fewer than 5% of SDAs smoke.[38]) Even after controlling for smoking, however, several studies have found heart disease rates are still much lower among vegetarians.[26,28,32]

The lower incidence of hypertension among vegetarians, as discussed later, probably contributes to their reduced incidence of heart disease. Smokers who are hypertensive and hypercholesterolemic have 20 times the risk of heart disease of nonsmoking normocholesterolemic, normotensive men.[39]

It is well established that dietary pattern influences blood cholesterol levels and that high blood cholesterol increases risk for heart disease (Figure 2-1). As long ago as the early 1960s,

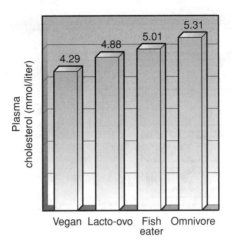

Figure 2-1 Effects of eating patterns on plasma cholesterol. Cholesterol values in vegans ($N = 114$), lacto-ovo vegetarians ($N = 1550$), fish eaters (lacto-ovo vegetarians who ate fish, $N = 415$), and omnivores ($N = 1198$). All groups included both men and women, but values were adjusted for age and gender. Average ages for each group ranged from 36 to 40 years. Cholesterol values for omnivores were significantly higher than for the other groups; values for fish eaters and lacto-ovo vegetarians were not significantly different from each other but were higher than those for vegans. *Source*: Data from Thorogood M, Carter R, Benfield L, et al. Plasma lipids and lipoprotein cholesterol concentrations in people with different diets in Britain. *BMJ*. 1978;295:351–353.

---

investigators observed that a vegan diet was effective in reducing angina in heart disease patients.[40] The lower heart disease rate and the lower blood cholesterol levels of vegetarians have prompted several investigators to examine the effects on blood cholesterol in subjects changing from a meat-based diet to a vegetarian diet. Not surprisingly, these studies have shown that adoption of a vegetarian diet lowers total cholesterol (TC).[41–48]

In 1991, the American Health Foundation in Valhalla, New York, concluded that a vegan diet could help both children and adults maintain low cholesterol levels.[49] The report found that, in comparison with omnivores, lacto-ovo vegetarians and vegans had blood cholesterol levels that were 14% and 35% lower, respectively. These findings were based on a review of only nine studies but are similar to those from the larger group of studies presented in Appendix B. More recently, a review of the health effects of 27 studies found significantly lower blood lipid concentrations among those following plant-based diets.[50] Vegetarians also had fewer and smaller age-related increases in circulating lipid levels.

In RCTs, plant-based and lacto-ovo vegetarian dietary interventions produce decreases in TC and low-density lipoprotein cholesterol (LDL-C) of about 10–15% compared to 15–25% for vegan diets.[50] Estimates suggest that a 1% decrease in cholesterol levels results in as much as a 2–4% decrease in risk[51,52] (Figure 2-2). Although vegetarians are leaner than omnivores and leanness results in lower TC levels, this is not the primary factor responsible for the lower cholesterol levels seen in vegetarians. In fact, Sacks et al found that, even when vegetarian subjects were

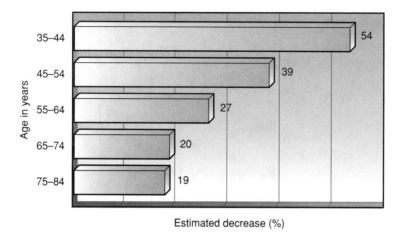

Figure 2-2 Percentage reduction in heart disease risk in men according to age associated with 10% decrease in blood cholesterol levels. The estimated decreased risk shown here for ischemic heart disease associated with a 0.6 mmol/liter (about 10%) decrease in serum cholesterol is based on findings of 10 prospective studies that involved approximately 500,000 men and 18,000 ischemic heart disease events. *Source*: Data from Cooper RS, Goldberg RB, Trevisan M, et al. The selective lipid-lowering effect of vegetarianism on low density lipoproteins in a cross-over experiment. *Atherosclerosis* 1982;44(3):293–305.

heavier than a similar group of omnivores, plasma lipoprotein levels were still markedly lower among the vegetarians.[53]

Some studies, although not most, reported lower high-density lipoprotein cholesterol (HDL-C) levels in vegetarians in comparison with omnivores (Appendix B). In a review of the relationship between diet and lipoproteins, Knuiman et al concluded that replacing fat in the diet with carbohydrate lowers HDL-C levels.[54] In a study of 43 free-living men and women in England, switching from an omnivore diet to a self-selected vegetarian diet for 6 months caused HDL-C levels to decrease by an average of 21%.[55] However, Jenkins et al found that when carbohydrates were replaced with higher protein plant foods such as soy and nuts, the ratio of LDL to HDL cholesterol improved.[56]

Whether low HDL-C levels in vegetarians represent an increased risk for heart disease is the subject of debate.[57–59] Fraser noted that if low-fat diets equally decrease both LDL-C and HDL-C, this may explain why vegetarian diet is not protective, or is only modestly protective, against CHD in women, because on a percentage basis, HDL-C is more protective against CHD in women than LDL-C is harmful.[60]

As discussed in Chapter 16, lower fat diets are often associated with higher serum triglyceride levels, which may increase CHD risk. However, in one intervention study using a very low-fat (10% of energy) vegan diet based on whole unprocessed plant foods, triglyceride levels decreased from a mean of 148.1 ± 16.1 to 120.02 ± 10.2 mg/dl.[61] Overall, though, studies indicate there is little if any difference in triglyceride levels between vegetarians and nonvegetarians. However, in many of those studies, total fat intake differed little between these two groups (Appendix B).

Other Factors Affecting Heart Disease Risk in Vegetarians

Protein

The higher polyunsaturated fat to saturated fat ratio of vegetarian diets compared to nonvegetarian diets primarily explains the decreased cholesterol level in habitual vegetarians and in omnivores adopting a vegetarian diet.[62,63] Nevertheless, there is some evidence, albeit weak, that meat protein, independent of dietary fat, may increase cholesterol levels. For example, subjects who consumed a 30% fat diet that included lean meat experienced only half the reduction in TC compared with subjects who consumed a lacto-ovo vegetarian diet and similar amounts of total fat, saturated fat, and cholesterol.[64] Also, data from the NHANES-III show animal protein intake is directly associated with higher serum cholesterol levels even after controlling for several other dietary factors known to affect blood cholesterol.[5,65]

However, most studies that have found animal products to be associated with an increase in blood cholesterol have concluded that the elevated cholesterol results from their fat and cholesterol content and not protein content.[62,66,67] In general the effects, if any, of protein type on cholesterol levels are probably minor, although there are important exceptions. Even soy protein, which was granted a health claim by the U.S. Food and Drug Administration in 1999, lowers LDL-C by only 3% or 4%[68] (Chapter 9). However, Jenkins et al have shown that a low-carbohydrate, high vegetable-protein diet was more effective than a similar diet using animal protein in reducing LDL-C and apolipoprotein-B.[56] In addition, these investigators have shown that a comprehensive dietary approach to lowering cholesterol can result in reductions of LDL-C by as much as 30%.[69]

Fiber

Soluble fiber has been shown to lower blood cholesterol levels. A pooled analysis of data from 10 prospective cohort studies found that higher fiber intake was associated with reduced risk of all coronary events.[70] And, in the EURODIAB IDDM Complications Study, which involved nearly 2000 participants, higher fiber intakes were independently related to beneficial alterations in serum cholesterol levels in both men and women with type 1 diabetes.[71]

Glore et al found that in 68 of 77 studies reviewed, soluble fiber decreased blood cholesterol by an average of about 10%.[72] However, other estimates suggest that the effects of fiber on cholesterol are more modest. For example, a meta-analysis that included 67 controlled trials found that whereas insoluble fiber had little effect, soluble fiber at levels that can reasonably be consumed (3 g/d) lowered LDL-C by about 5 mg/dl.[71,73] In addition to lowering cholesterol, increasing dietary fiber has been shown to inhibit the rise in triglyceride levels that often occurs with low-fat diets.[74,75]

In regard to fiber and CHD rates, in the Alpha-Tocopherol, Beta-Carotene Cancer Prevention Study, for men in the highest quintile of total dietary fiber intake (median, 34.8 g/d), the relative risk (RR) for coronary death was 0.69 (95% confidence interval (CI), 0.54 to 0.88; $P < 0.001$ for trend) compared with men in the lowest quintile of intake (median, 16.1 g/d) after controlling for a host of cardiovascular risk factors. Soluble fiber was slightly more strongly associated with reduced coronary death than insoluble fiber.[76] In agreement, a prospective study involving male health professionals found that a 10 g increase in total dietary fiber corresponded to an RR for total myocardial infarction of 0.81 (95% CI, 0.70 to 0.93).[77] Furthermore, cereal fiber was most strongly associated with a reduced risk of total myocardial infarction (RR, 0.71; 95% CI, 0.55 to 0.91 for each 10 g/d increase in cereal fiber).[77] And finally, based on data from four studies, high intakes of whole grains were associated with a significant 26% reduction of risk for ischemic strokes.[10] The higher amounts of fiber consumed in these prospective and cross-sectional studies are similar to those consumed by vegetarians.

Phytochemicals

As discussed in Chapter 8, phytochemicals may exert a multitude of biologic effects, although much of the support for the beneficial effects of phytochemicals is based on in vitro and animal data or on the beneficial effects associated with fruit and vegetable consumption in epidemiologic studies.

In regard to cholesterol reduction, several phytochemicals have been investigated, but phytosterols, in particular, have received much attention during the past 15 years. A health claim for the cholesterol-lowering effects of phytosterols was approved by the U.S. Food and Drug Administration in 2000. Phytosterols, when consumed in amounts ranging from 1 to 2 g/d, lower serum cholesterol levels approximately 10%, even in normocholesterolemic subjects.[78] Vegetarians and people consuming plant-based diets consume considerably more phytosterols than omnivores, but intake is still no more than 500 mg/d.[79–82] Interestingly, Howell et al concluded that the higher phytosterol content of polyunsaturated oils partially explains the ability of these oils to lower serum cholesterol to a greater extent than olive oil, which is low in phytosterols.[83] Also, in a controlled feeding study, Racette et al found that approximately 500 mg of phytosterols lowered LDL-C about 5%, although the results were not quite statistically significant.[84]

Antioxidants and Pro-oxidants

The high antioxidant content of vegetarian diets may reduce heart disease risk, although this is quite speculative. Clearly many heart attacks occur in people with normal or only mildly elevated cholesterol. In fact, although smoking, high blood cholesterol, and high blood pressure are major risk factors for heart disease, these three risk factors may predict only about 30% of all cardiovascular events.[85] The role of antioxidants in preventing atherosclerosis remains unclear,[86] but the oxidation of serum lipoproteins appears to be a factor in atherosclerosis. Some findings suggest that only oxidized LDL-C is taken up by macrophages that are found within the intima, the innermost layer of the arteries.[87] Also, only nonoxidized HDL-C is thought to remove cholesterol from deposits along the walls of the arteries.[88]

The primary antioxidant nutrient thought to protect LDL-C from oxidation is vitamin E, but vitamin C may also have an important role by helping regenerate the reduced form of vitamin E.[89–92] Vegetarians have higher blood levels of both vitamins E and C, and, not surprisingly, the molar ratio of vitamin E to cholesterol in LDL-C is higher among vegetarians than omnivores.[93–96] Serum levels of β-carotene are also higher in vegetarians, and limited data suggest carotenoids may reduce CHD risk.[97,98] In one study, vegetarians ($n = 31$) had approximately 15% higher levels of plasma carotenoids compared to omnivores ($n = 58$), including lutein, α-cryptoxanthin, lycopene, α-carotene, and β-carotene.[99] However, among vegetarians in Slovakia, differences in levels of antioxidants were seen in older but not younger vegetarians.[100] Despite initial promise, recent clinical studies evaluating the coronary benefits of vitamin E have proven disappointing.[101,102] Although results of RCTs have been unsupportive of a role for either vitamin E or β-carotene, large prospective cohort studies provide evidence for a protective effect of a diet high in carotenoid-rich fruits and vegetables.[103]

In vitro, β-carotene has been shown to inhibit the oxidation of lipoprotein(a) (LPA) a modified form of LDL-C.[104] LPA is an independent risk factor for CHD.[105] In one study, serum LPA levels in female vegetarians were 45% lower than in a similarly matched group of omnivores.[106] The lower saturated fat and cholesterol intake of vegetarians may also act to reduce LDL-C oxidation.[107] Finally, and of particular interest, is the finding that dietary cholesterol increases LDL-C oxidation; therefore, it may be through this mechanism that dietary cholesterol increases CHD rather than by increasing serum cholesterol levels.[108]

In addition to nutrients, there is a wealth of information indicating that many of the main dietary phytochemicals (discussed in Chapter 8) are potent antioxidants, in some cases, much more so than vitamins C or E. Phytochemicals, even more so than nutrients, may play a protective role against CHD.[109] Several studies have found that flavonoid intake is associated with a reduced risk of CHD.[110–114] Flavonoids are potent antioxidants and widely distributed among fruits and vegetables, and they are also found in wine. In fact, the flavonoid content of red wine may play a role in the French paradox, the relatively low rate of heart disease in France compared with other Western countries with similar intakes of saturated fat,[115] although the concept of the French paradox has been challenged.[116]

Antioxidant Status

Evidence that the antioxidant status of vegetarians is superior to that of their nonvegetarian counterparts is somewhat equivocal. For example, although Nagyová et al failed to find in vitro conjugated diene (a measure of oxidation) formation in LDL-C isolated from vegetarians differed from that of nonvegetarians, they did find that vegetarians' LDL-C was more resistant to oxidation on the basis of thiobarbituric acid–reacting substances and also that the total antioxidant status of vegetarians was greater than in nonvegetarians.[94] The latter finding agrees with many, but not all, studies.[95] Vegetarians also have higher blood catalase activity and lower levels of conjugated dienes in comparison with omnivores.[117] In regard to intervention studies, the consumption of a vegan diet (in combination with walking) was shown to markedly reduce serum peroxide levels[118] and to lower concentrations of lipid peroxides.[119,120]

Some evidence suggests that iron may increase heart disease risk because it can act as a prooxidant, thereby increasing LDL-C oxidation.[121,122] Therefore, the lower iron stores seen in vegetarians (Chapter 6) may be an additional factor in reducing heart disease risk. Harvard University researchers found that the intake of heme iron, but not nonheme iron, was associated with a marked increase in heart disease risk.[123] However, they found that blood donation, which would result in lower iron stores, was not associated with a lower risk of CHD in men.[124] Furthermore, in a systematic review of prospective studies, Danesh and Appleby concluded there was no association between iron status and CHD risk.[125] Controlled feeding studies have also failed to support this relationship.[126] Therefore, it is not clear if the combination of the higher intake of antioxidants and the lower iron stores of vegetarians work to inhibit LDL-C oxidation and to reduce heart disease risk. Interestingly, higher iron stores have been associated with increased insulin resistance,[127] which could increase risk of developing diabetes and thereby indirectly increase risk of heart disease.

Homocysteine

Some research has suggested that increased serum levels of the amino acid homocysteine are an independent risk factor for vascular disease.[128,129] In 1995, Boushey et al, on the basis of a meta-analysis that included 27 studies, concluded that about 10% of coronary artery disease was attributable to elevated homocysteine levels and that a 5 mmol/liter homocysteine increment elevates coronary artery disease risk as much as an increase in cholesterol of 20 mg/dl.[129] However, several recently conducted RCTs using homocysteine-lowering therapies failed to show any benefit in patients with prior stroke or coronary artery disease[130,131–133] or in patients without preexisting cardiovascular disease.[134] Thus the link between circulating homocysteine levels and risk of CHD has been called into question.

Low serum levels of folate, vitamin B_{12}, vitamin B_6, and riboflavin are associated with high homocysteine levels. When folate intake is adequate, vitamin B_{12} appears to be an important determinant of homocysteine levels. The connection between vitamin B_{12} and homocysteine may explain why several studies,[135–142] but not all[143,144] have found that serum homocysteine levels are higher in vegetarians than nonvegetarians (Figure 2-3). Furthermore, vitamin B_{12} injections were shown to lower serum homocysteine levels in a group of vegetarians, many of whom had abnormally low vitamin B_{12} and high homocysteine levels at baseline.[145] Thus the poorer vitamin B_{12} status of many vegetarians appears to increase homocysteine levels, countering the possible homocysteine-lowering effects of the higher folate intake. As previously noted, the clinical implications if any of these possibly higher levels are unclear. However, among Taiwanese postmenopausal women, low LDL-C levels in the vegetarians were not associated with differences in carotid atherosclerosis, a finding that may have been attributable to their higher levels of homocysteine.[146]

Factors Affecting Platelet Aggregation

Many CHD risk factors, aside from the most discussed ones such as elevated blood pressure and cholesterol, are affected by diet and may affect CHD in vegetarians. These include high fibrinogen levels,[147] increased platelet aggregation,[148,149] and elevated serum and tissue concentrations of certain prostaglandins. Dietary fat, and saturated fat in particular, increases factor VII levels, which increases platelet aggregation[150–152] Thus vegetarian diets may favorably affect these processes because they are lower in both total and saturated fat.

No clear picture emerges in regard to vegetarian diet and platelet aggregation, however. In a study of fibrositis/fibromyalgia patients placed on a vegetarian diet, fibrinogen levels decreased after 3 weeks.[153] However, although Ernst et al[154] found that vegetarians had reduced blood viscosity, vegetarians in this study and in other studies[155–158] did not have lower fibrinogen levels. Furthermore, in several studies no differences in platelet aggregation were noted between vegetarians and omnivores.[156,157,159,160] In fact, one study found that, contrary to expectation, vegetarians

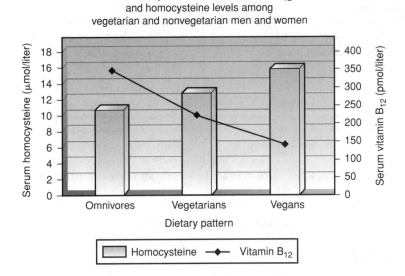

Relationship between serum vitamin B$_{12}$
and homocysteine levels among
vegetarian and nonvegetarian men and women

Figure 2-3 Inverse relationship between serum vitamin B$_{12}$ and homocysteine levels: $N = 59$ omnivores, 54 vegetarians, and 32 vegans.

had a significantly higher platelet aggregation in comparison to meat eaters,[158] although this study disagrees with that from another group of researchers.[145]

Specific Fatty Acids and Heart Disease

Unsupplemented vegetarian diets generally do not contain the long-chain polyunsaturated n-3 (omega 3) fatty acids EPA and DHA or may contain only small amounts if sea vegetables and eggs are regularly consumed. The plasma concentrations of EPA and DHA have been found to be lower in vegetarians than in omnivores in some studies.[106,136,161,162] These fatty acids, which are found predominantly in certain types of fish, may have a role in reducing chronic diseases such as heart disease, via their conversion into the n-3 series prostacyclins and thromboxanes, which can favorably affect physiologic processes such as platelet aggregation. In contrast, vegetarian diets can be high in the essential fatty acid, linoleic acid, an n-6 fatty acid that can serve (via arachidonic acid) as a precursor to the n-2 series prostacyclins and thromboxanes. Also, linoleic acid competitively inhibits the conversion of the n-3 fatty acid, α-linolenic acid, which vegetarians do consume, into EPA and DHA, thereby decreasing the synthesis of the n-3 series prostacyclins and thromboxanes. The relationship of fatty acids to heart disease is discussed in detail in Chapter 4.

Specific Foods

Certain foods that are commonly consumed by vegetarians may play a role in reducing risk for heart disease. Soyfoods are believed to reduce cholesterol levels due to both their protein and

Exhibit 2-1 Factors Common to Vegetarians That Are Thought to Reduce Coronary Heart Disease Risk

• Lower saturated fat intake	• Higher phytochemical intake
• Lower cholesterol intake	• Higher folate intake
• Lower heme iron intake	• Lower iron stores
• Higher fiber intake	• Lower body mass index
• Higher antioxidant intake	• Lower blood pressure

isoflavone contents (Chapter 9). Tree nuts are frequently an important part of vegetarian diets, particularly those of SDA vegetarians, and have been shown to reduce serum cholesterol levels with decreases greater than predicted from their fatty acid content.[163–166] Exhibit 2-1 summarizes the factors in vegetarian diets that may reduce heart disease risk.

HYPERTENSION

In the United States, nearly 30% of adults have hypertension.[167] There are striking differences in blood pressure among populations worldwide. In industrialized societies, blood pressure typically increases with advancing age, and the prevalence of hypertension is high. Migrant studies demonstrate an environmental influence on blood pressure in that blood pressure rises in children and adults after they move from indigenous cultures to areas having a diet and lifestyle more characteristic of economically developed societies. Also, in some agrarian societies, sizable age-related blood pressure changes do not occur in most adults, and the prevalence of hypertension among the elderly remains low.[168]

Interest in the possible blood pressure–lowering effect of a vegetarian diet dates back to 1917 when Hamman concluded that meat was harmful for patients with hypertension.[169] Subsequently, in 1926, Donaldson reported that blood pressures of vegetarian college students increased significantly within 2 weeks of adding meat to their diet.[170] Four years later, Saile reported that German vegetarian monks had lower blood pressures at all ages than monks who ate meat.[171] About that same time, Heun observed a mean decline in systolic blood pressure of 60 mm Hg and a decrease in diastolic blood pressure of 28 mm Hg in 14 severely hypertensive patients who were treated with a fruit and vegetable diet.[172] These observations are consistent with studies showing that vegetarian Buddhist monks did not experience the rise in blood pressure with age seen in omnivore controls matched for age, sex, and body mass index (BMI) and that the duration of vegetarianism was inversely related to blood pressure.[173,174]

Appendix C lists studies in which blood pressure in vegetarians was compared with that in omnivores (see also Figure 2-4). In many of these studies vegetarians had both lower systolic and diastolic blood pressure. Although differences between vegetarians and omnivores were generally between 5 and 10 mm Hg, this degree of difference may have a significant impact on morbidity or mortality. In 55- to 59-year-old men, a reduction in systolic blood pressure of only 5 mm Hg has been estimated to result in a 7% reduction in major coronary events.[175] Similarly, a reduction

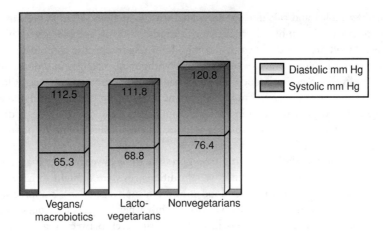

Figure 2-4 Differences in blood pressure between vegetarians and meat eaters. There were 226 vegans (macrobiotics), 63 lacto vegetarians, and 458 nonvegetarians. The vegans and lacto vegetarians had adhered to their dietary patterns for approximately 2 and 3 years, respectively. The systolic and diastolic blood pressures of both groups of vegetarians were significantly lower than those of the omnivores ($P < 0.0001$), and the diastolic pressure of vegans was significantly lower than that of the lacto vegetarians ($P < 0.02$). Significant differences between vegetarians and nonvegetarians existed after controlling for body weight. *Source*: Data from Sacks FM, Svetkey LP, Vollmer WM, et al. Effects on blood pressure of reduced dietary sodium and the Dietary Approaches to Stop Hypertension (DASH) diet. DASH-Sodium Collaborative Research Group. *N Engl J Med* 2001;344(1):3–10.

in blood pressure of only 4 mm Hg was found to cause a marked reduction in mortality from all causes in the Hypertension Detection and Follow-Up Program.[176] Also, differences in blood pressure between vegetarians and nonvegetarians were likely minimized because of the selection criteria for study subjects.

Not only is average blood pressure lower in vegetarians, but the extent of actual hypertension appears to be lower as well. In the AHS-1, nonvegetarian men and women, and semi-vegetarian men and women, were more than twice, and about 50% more likely, respectively, to be hypertensive than vegetarians.[37] Preliminary results from the AHS-2 show lower rates of hypertension among vegetarians and show that vegans have less hypertension than other vegetarians.[177]

An analysis of a prospective epidemiologic study that included 11,004 British subjects showed that omnivore men were >2.5 times as likely as vegan men to have hypertension.[178] Ophir et al reported that 42% of the nonvegetarians studied had hypertension (140 mm Hg/90 mm Hg) compared with only 13% of the vegetarians.[179] The prevalence of blood pressure >160/95 was 13 times higher in the nonvegetarians (26% vs 2%).[179] In another study, 37% of the nonvegetarians but only 14% of the vegetarians had a history of physician-diagnosed hypertension.[180] Similarly, the prevalence of hypertension requiring current medication use was 44% and 22% among African American and white nonvegetarian subjects, respectively, but only 18% and 7% among African American and white vegetarians.[181]

There is conclusive evidence that dietary changes can significantly lower blood pressure.[182] For example, in the Dietary Approaches to Stop Hypertension (DASH) trial, a low-fat diet that was high in fruits, vegetables, and calcium was associated with reductions in blood pressure that were similar to those expected from blood pressure medication.[183,184] Even in subjects with high normal blood pressure, blood pressure declined by 3.5 mg Hg in response to the combination diet. Furthermore, reductions in blood pressure were achieved without any changes in sodium intake.

Obesity is positively related to blood pressure, whereas regular exercise and weight loss tend to lower it.[185–189] In the Nurses' Health Study, obesity and weight gain during adulthood were both related to higher blood pressure. Gaining just 20 pounds since the age of 18 years doubled the chances of having high blood pressure during midlife, whereas losing about 20 pounds reduced the risk of having high blood pressure by about 25%.[190]

Nevertheless, in most studies that found blood pressure to be lower in vegetarians, weight was controlled for, and in two where it was not, weight differences were thought to have little if any impact.[191,192] Ophir et al found that the blood pressure of nonvegetarians is appreciably higher than that of vegetarians with similar body weights.[179] Only when subjects were obese (i.e., >20% of the average weight) were no differences in blood pressure seen between vegetarians and nonvegetarians. However, the results of these studies contrast with those from the EPIC-Oxford Study, which showed that most of the difference in blood pressure between vegans and omnivores was explained by differences in BMI.[178]

Although exercise helps reduce blood pressure, Rouse et al found that Mormon women had higher blood pressures than SDA women, even though the Mormons exercised more.[193] For men, there were no differences in the frequency of activity among Mormon omnivores, Adventist omnivores, and Adventist vegetarians, but the vegetarians had the lowest systolic blood pressure.

Rouse et al were the first to clinically evaluate the effects of a vegetarian diet on blood pressure.[42] They found that systolic and diastolic blood pressures decreased by about 6 and 2 mm Hg, respectively, when normotensive omnivore subjects were placed on a lacto-ovo vegetarian diet. In a later study involving a similar design, mean systolic and diastolic blood pressures decreased 6.8 and 2.7 mm Hg, respectively, on a lacto-ovo vegetarian diet.[194] Other studies have also reported hypotensive effects of a vegetarian diet in normotensive subjects,[195] mildly hypertensive subjects,[196] and hypertensive subjects.[43]

Several studies have tried to determine the dietary component of vegetarian diets that is responsible for their hypotensive effect, but the absence of neither meat[197,198] nor milk protein[199] appears to be a contributing factor. However, studies suggest that increased plant protein intake may be associated with lower blood pressure[200,201] and that replacing carbohydrate with either protein or monounsaturated fat could reduce blood pressure as well. Furthermore, in a prospective study of 2895 adults, a lower intake of nonheme iron at baseline was associated with higher systolic blood pressure and pulse pressure at 5.4-year follow-up.[202] Among French adults, higher fiber consumption was associated with lower blood pressure.[203] Differences in potassium, magnesium, and calcium[42] or vitamin C appear to be too small to account for the observed blood pressure differences.[204] Although blood pressure in agrarian societies with primarily vegetarian diets and low sodium intakes is lower than in industrialized nations, the sodium intake of vegetarians in industrialized countries is similar to, or only modestly lower than, that of omnivores (Appendix G). Thus sodium intake does not appear to be the explanation for blood pressure differences between omnivores and vegetarians.

The lower glycemic index typical of vegetarian diets has been suggested as one possible explanation for lower blood pressure in vegetarians.[205] The lower blood pressure of vegetarians may be partly affected through a blood glucose-insulin sympathoadrenal mechanism, as postulated by Landsberg and Young.[206] They suggested that the lower blood pressures of vegetarians may be related to the slower delivery of glucose to the blood as a result of an increased consumption of complex carbohydrates and a decreased sucrose intake. Sacks and Kass suggested that modest intake of animal products may be a marker for a large intake of other potentially beneficial nutrients from vegetable products that collectively have a hypotensive effect.[207] It is almost certain that it is the combination of dietary changes incurred when changing to a vegetarian diet that elicits the blood pressure–lowering response, rather than just one or two dietary factors.[189,204,208–210]

CANCER

There are striking dissimilarities in cancer rates among countries and geographic regions. Although genetic differences among populations may contribute to international variations in cancer rates, the evidence that lifestyle-related factors are important is persuasive and is based on migration studies, intracountry variations, and trends within countries. Migration data also suggest that, at least for some cancers, events that occur late in life markedly influence cancer mortality.[211] Thus dietary interventions in adulthood hold the potential to reduce cancer risk.

In most respects, vegetarian diets, because of their lower fat and higher fiber content, are closer to matching the dietary guidelines issued by the World Cancer Research Fund/American Institute for Cancer Research (WCRF/AICR) than typical American eating patterns. Vegetarians may also achieve the cornerstone of dietary guidelines aimed at reducing cancer risk—to increase fruit and vegetable consumption. Epidemiologic data support the anticancer effects of fruits and vegetables, although not all studies support this relationship.[212,213] The proposed biologic mechanisms for these protective effects include enhanced antioxidant activity, increased levels of detoxification enzymes, regulation of cellular growth factors,[214,215] and modulation of steroid hormones and metabolism.[216]

Only limited data are available, however, on vegetarian fruit and vegetable intake, although data from the Continuing Survey of Food Intake by Individuals confirmed that vegetarians had higher intakes of fruit and vegetables than nonvegetarians,[217] as did a study of dietary habits of Swedish vegans.[218] Also, a study of 35,367 British women taking part in the UK Women's Cohort Study found that being a vegetarian was among the strongest predictors of a high fruit and vegetable intake.[219] Nevertheless, the simple elimination of meat and/or dairy products from the diet does not necessarily lead to greater fruit and vegetable intake because these foods are typically not used as replacements for animal foods. It is more likely that the greater health awareness of vegetarians results in their higher fruit and vegetable intake.[220–225]

Furthermore, in recent years, evidence in support of the protective effects of plant-based diets has arguably not been as strong as was anticipated. For example, in their comprehensive review of the diet and cancer literature, published in 2007, the WCRF/AICR concluded that the evidence that fruit and vegetable intake reduces cancer risk is not as strong as it was a decade earlier.[226] However, they also emphasized consumption of more plant foods and less meat, especially processed meat, as a means of decreasing cancer risk.

Establishing the relationship of diet to cancer is difficult because of the lack of noninvasive or minimally invasive intermediary markers for cancer risk. In contrast, serum cholesterol and blood pressure are confidently viewed as indicators of CHD risk, and both respond fairly rapidly to dietary change and can be easily measured in humans. Some cancer markers do exist, such as prostate-specific antigen levels for prostate cancer and breast tissue density for breast cancer, but each of these carries with it important limitations. Another limitation is that early life events (even those that occur in utero) may play a particularly important role in the etiology of certain cancers.[211] This may especially be the case for breast cancer.[211,227] For example, there is substantial evidence that modest soy consumption during childhood and/or adolescence markedly reduces adult breast cancer risk (Chapter 9).[228] Because epidemiologic studies typically obtain recent dietary intake data from older adults, they may miss important links between diet and cancer risk.

The cancer process is extremely complex and likely affected by a multitude of factors; therefore, dietary impact on risk may result from the effect of interactions among foods and food constituents that are difficult to identify from epidemiologic observations. For example, a case-control study in Shanghai found the relative risk of breast cancer in women who excreted large amounts of both phenols and isoflavonoids was only 0.14 (95% CI, 0.02 to 0.88), whereas the excretion of phenols was by itself not protective.[229] Finally, genetic differences, such as those that result in differences in the metabolism of carcinogens, may determine whether a given individual is sensitive to dietary influences.

Cancer Rates in Vegetarians

Vegetarians have an overall lower cancer rate than the general population. What is not clear is to what extent, if any, diet is responsible for this difference. Vegetarians are generally more health conscious, smoke less, drink less alcohol, are often more highly educated, and are leaner than the general population. Consequently, differences in cancer rates between vegetarians and nonvegetarians are probably the result of a multitude of factors. After controlling for nondietary cancer risk factors, differences in cancer rates between vegetarians and nonvegetarians are not striking.

In a collaborative analysis of five prospective studies involving vegetarians that included over 76,172 men and women (27,808 vegetarians), Key et al found that after adjustment for age, sex, and smoking status, vegetarian diet was not associated with a reduced mortality risk for stomach, colorectal, lung, breast, or prostate cancer.[35] Similarly, no protective effect of vegetarian diet was found when comparing subjects who had been vegetarians for at least 5 years to more recent vegetarians or to nonvegetarians.[35] It should be noted, however, that the reference group in this analysis included subjects who ate meat as infrequently as one time per week and, in many cases, had cancer mortality rates that were lower than the general population.

Much of our understanding about vegetarian cancer rates comes from studies involving SDAs. Approximately half of the SDAs in the cancer age range (>40 years) are adult converts to the church, with the remaining half either being born into an Adventist home or joining the church before 20 years of age.[230] Initial reports that SDAs (including both vegetarians and nonvegetarians) had lower overall cancer mortality rates, and specifically lower rates for cancers of the lung, esophagus, bladder, stomach, colon-rectum, pancreas, breast, cervix, and ovary, as well as leukemia, were not adjusted for socioeconomic status (SES).[34] This is important because the church members tend to be of above-average SES, and people of higher SES in the United States are generally at a lower cancer risk.

Based on information collected from participants in the AHS-2, about 36% of SDA church members are vegetarians, and approximately 88% of these are lacto-ovo vegetarians.[231] Historically, however, a higher percentage of vegetarian Adventists have followed a lacto-ovo vegetarian diet, and, consequently, there is relatively little information about the cancer rates of vegans from the first AHS.

In an analysis of the AHS, after adjustment for age, sex, and smoking status, nonvegetarian SDAs had a 54% increased risk for prostate cancer and an 88% increased risk for colorectal cancer in comparison to vegetarians, but incidence rates were similar for lung, breast, uterine, and stomach cancer.[37] The lower colon cancer incidence is consistent with the lower rate of colon cell proliferation in vegetarians,[232] and the prostate cancer data are consistent with results from a study showing that mean serum insulin-like growth factor (IGF)-1 levels were 9% lower in 233 vegan men in comparison to 226 meat eaters and 237 vegetarians ($p = 0.002$).[233] Because of its proliferative effects, higher serum levels of IGF-1 are thought to be involved in the etiology of several cancers.[234-236]

Lower risk of prostate cancer in the AHS-1 was associated with the consumption of dried fruit and possibly tomato and fish.[237] The intake of both red and white meat was independently associated with the higher incidence of colon cancer among nonvegetarians. One of the more intriguing observations from the AHS was that legume consumption was associated with a marked reduction in the incidence of colon cancer ($\geq$3 times/week vs <1 time per week; RR, 0.33; 95% CI, 0.13 to 0.83) but only among those who ate red meat. And the positive association between colon cancer and red meat was seen only in those who consumed legumes infrequently. In addition, the consumption of legumes, dried fruits, and meat analogs were each associated with a lower risk of pancreatic cancer, and fruit consumption, after adjustment for smoking, was associated with a lower risk of lung cancer.

In contrast, no significant difference in incidence in colorectal cancer was found among vegetarians in the Oxford Vegetarian Study. And in the EPIC-Oxford, a surprising finding was a higher risk for colorectal cancer among vegetarians, although rates for all cancers combined were lower.[238] In a pooled analysis of data from the EPIC-Oxford study and the Oxford Vegetarian Study, the incidence of all cancers combined was lower among both fish eaters and vegetarians compared to omnivores.[239]

Finally, in a cohort of 37,643 British women in EPIC-Oxford, there was no evidence of an association between vegetarian diet and risk for breast cancer.[240] In contrast, in the UK Women's Cohort Study, women who did not eat any meat had a lower risk for breast cancer,[241] and both red meat and iron intake were positively associated with risk for invasive postmenopausal breast cancer in a prospective study of 52,158 women.[242]

Factors in Vegetarian Diets That May Affect Cancer Risk

Despite the rather modest differences between vegetarians and nonvegetarians in regard to cancer mortality, and even incidence, there are a variety of ways in which vegetarian diet, at least when consumed over the course of a lifetime, may be protective.

Several studies have reported that vegetarians have lower serum or urinary estrogen levels, perhaps because dietary fat and fiber intakes are associated with increases and decreases, respectively, in estrogen levels. Higher lifetime exposure to estrogen is thought to increase breast cancer risk, and differences in lifelong exposure to estrogen have been suggested as the partial or complete explanation for the variation in breast cancer mortality among countries.[243–252]

Pike et al has estimated that later menses and earlier menopause may explain as much as 80% of the difference in breast cancer mortality rates between Japan and the United States.[243] Vegetarians may begin menstruation at a later age than omnivores.[253,254] In addition to lower estrogen levels, breast cancer risk may be affected by the way in which estrogen is metabolized. Evidence suggests that foods such as cruciferous vegetables and soy alter estrogen metabolism in a way that reduces breast cancer risk.[221,255–258]

In addition to their higher fiber intake, the environment of the colon in vegetarians differs significantly from nonvegetarians in ways that could favorably affect colon cancer risk. For example, vegetarians have a lower concentration of potentially carcinogenic bile acids[259–263] and possibly also lower amounts of bacteria that convert the primary bile acids into the more carcinogenic secondary bile acids.[264–268] Furthemore, colon pH is lower, which would tend to decrease the activity of enzymes responsible for converting primary bile acids into secondary bile acids.[269,270] Vegetarians also have larger and heavier feces and experience more frequent elimination,[263,271,272] which may limit contact between potential carcinogens and the lining of the colon.[273] Fecal weight is related to fiber intake and is inversely related to the incidence of colon cancer among countries[274] (Figure 2-5).

Vegetarians also have lower levels of enzymes that hydrolyze conjugated xenobiotics, thereby enhancing the elimination of potential colon carcinogens.[244,259] Finally, most studies indicate that vegetarians have lower levels of fecal mutagens.[275–278]

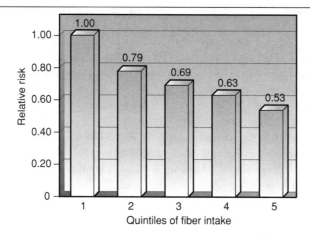

Figure 2-5 Relationship between fiber intake and risk of colon and rectal cancer. Data are based on 13 studies involving 5225 cases and 10,349 controls. The inverse trend between fiber intake and colorectal cancer risk was statistically significant ($P < 0.001$). If causality is assumed, these data suggest that increasing fiber intake by approximately 13 g/d could reduce risk of colorectal cancer by approximately 31% in the United States. Dietary fiber intake in the highest quintile was approximately 31 g/d. *Source*: Data from Smith-Warner SA, Spiegelman D, Yaun SS, et al. Intake of fruits and vegetables and risk of breast cancer: a pooled analysis of cohort studies. *JAMA* 2001;285(6):769–776.

Diet may contribute to the large differences in prostate cancer rates among countries. In Japan and other Asian countries, the incidence of histologic prostate cancer is similar to that in the United States, but the incidence of clinical prostate cancer is much lower, suggesting that some factor common to the Japanese culture delays the onset and/or slows the growth of prostate tumors.[279] Interestingly, the size of the prostate gland does not increase with age among Japanese men as it does in white men.[280]

Some studies have found that high-fiber intake decreases, whereas high-fat intake increases, risk of prostate cancer.[279,281–283] Animal fat in particular may raise risk.[284] There is also some evidence, although the data are inconsistent, that vegetarian diet may affect hormone levels in a way that lowers prostate cancer risk.[285–288] In animals, low-fat diets have been shown to slow the growth of tumors established from human prostatic adenocarcinoma cells.[289] Soybean isoflavones have been shown to inhibit the growth of chemically induced tumors and inhibit the metastasis of existing tumors.[290,291] (See Chapter 9 for a discussion of soy and prostate cancer.)

There has been much enthusiasm for the protective effects of lycopene,[292] selenium,[293] and vitamin E[294] against prostate cancer. However, the results of the Selenium and Vitamin E Cancer Prevention Trial (SELECT), which included 35,533 men, showed neither vitamin E nor selenium alone or in combination helped to prevent prostate cancer in healthy men.[295] In the Physicians Health Study, neither vitamin E nor vitamin C was associated with reduced risk.[296] Finally, high serum vitamin D levels may be protective against prostate cancer, which, according to one school of thought, accounts for the positive association between dairy consumption and prostate cancer risk, as discussed later.[297]

Animal Products and Cancer

International studies show that meat- and dairy-based diets are associated with an increased incidence of breast, colon, prostate, renal, and endometrial cancer.[298] Whether animal products specifically increase cancer risk or whether animal-based diets are associated with a higher risk of certain cancers because they are lower in protective plant components, such as fiber, phytochemicals, and antioxidants, is unknown.

An expert panel commissioned by the WCRF/AICR authored one of the most comprehensive reviews on the subject of diet and cancer, categorizing evidence of risk into four different categories: convincing, probable, possible, and insufficient. The evidence that meat increased colorectal cancer risk was rated as convincing in the 2007 report. Red meat intake was also associated with increased risk for colorectal cancer in a subsequently published large prospective study.[299] In a qualitative overview of the epidemiologic evidence, Huxley et al found high meat intake was associated with a 20% higher risk of colorectal cancer.[300] In the EPIC study, red and processed meat intake was also positively associated with risk for some types of stomach cancer[301] and possibly bladder cancer[302] but not ovarian[303] or breast cancer.[304]

O'Keefe et al found that the low rate of colon cancer mortality among South African blacks was likely a result of their low animal product intake, not their high fiber intake, as had been proposed by Burkitt et al 40 years ago.[305] Their research showed that colon cell proliferation, an indicator of risk, was lower among blacks than white South Africans, which is consistent with the lower colon cancer rates among blacks, but the intake of fiber by these two groups was similar, whereas the intake of meat was much higher among whites. In support of this finding are four case-control studies, three in Asian countries, which found red meat consumption to be associated with increased colon cancer risk.[306–309] However, other analyses have concluded that meat does not directly cause colorectal cancer, or any other form of cancer, but rather is only coincidentally related to cancer risk.[310–311] Most importantly in this regard, in a 2009 meta-analysis that included six prospective studies, no support for an independent association between either animal fat intake or animal protein intake and colorectal cancer was found.[312]

The relationship between meat intake and breast cancer risk is also unclear. Although a case-control study in southern France found that breast cancer risk increased by 50–60% for each additional 100 g of meat consumed daily,[313] several other studies have not confirmed this type of relationship.[304, 314–318] One theory is that meat intake increases risk primarily if consumed during adolescence.[319] Red meat intake has also been linked to prostate[283] and lung[320] cancer.

Although the data on the relationship between animal food intake and cancer are conflicting, there are a number of proposed explanations for the hypothesized carcinogenic effects of meat. For example, heterocyclic amines (HCAs), which are potent mutagens, are formed when meat is cooked at high temperatures, especially when it has been grilled.[321] In experimental models, HCAs have been shown to increase risk for a wide array of cancers, including cancer of the liver, lung, breast, and small and large intestines.[322] Higher temperatures increase HCA formation, whereas microwaving foods produces only small amounts of mutagens. HCAs are also present in pan scrapings and fat drippings.[322] As noted previously, some evidence suggests the association between meat and cancer is particularly pronounced in people who rapidly metabolize certain putative carcinogens.[323] High levels of meat also increase fecal ammonia and N-nitroso compound concentration, which could increase colon cancer risk.[324]

Although quite speculative, the cholesterol in meat, by increasing the level of cholesterol in the large intestinal lumen that is then subject to extensive oxidation, could lead to mutagenic metabolites.[325] And finally, dietary heme may lead to the formation of highly cytotoxic factors in the colonic lumen, which may damage the colonic mucosa resulting in hyperproliferation and an increased colon cancer risk.[326]

One of the more intriguing observations about the relationship between animal product intake and cancer risk is that high dairy consumption increases risk of prostate cancer. A comparison of food intake in 42 countries found milk consumption to be the dietary factor most closely associated with prostate cancer risk.[327] High calcium and dairy intake were found to increase risk for prostate cancer in a Swedish case-control study[328] and in the Health Professional's Follow-Up Study, a prospective study of 20,885 men. In the latter study, calcium from both foods and supplements were linked to increased risk.[329] Among 142,251 men in the EPIC study, a 35 g/d increase in dairy protein was associated with a 32% increased risk in prostate cancer. Calcium from dairy products was also associated with risk but not calcium from other foods.[330]

High intakes of calcium and phosphorus, largely from dairy products, are believed to lower circulating $1,25(OH)_2D$ levels, which may increase prostate cancer risk.[297] In addition, sulfur-containing amino acids from animal products, because they lower blood pH which suppresses $1,25(OH)2D$ production, will also increase prostate cancer risk. However, the evidence is too preliminary to draw any firm conclusions about this hypothesis. In contrast to findings regarding calcium and prostate cancer risk, calcium may be protective against colorectal cancer.[331]

DIABETES

The prevalence of diabetes is reaching epidemic proportions throughout the world as rates increase in both developed and developing countries. Type 2 diabetes is now common even among children. Differences in disease rates among countries and regions within countries, in combination with migration data, indicate that lifestyle plays a critical role in the etiology of this disease.[332,333] Obesity is clearly the single most important risk factor for type 2 diabetes,[334] and weight loss in overweight diabetics is the most effective treatment. International comparisons generally show that the prevalence of diabetes correlates positively with serum cholesterol levels and with intake of fat, animal fat, protein, animal protein, and sugar and correlates negatively with intakes of carbohydrates and vegetable fat.[335] A Western dietary pattern high in processed meats has been associated with greater risk for diabetes.[336]

There is some evidence that vegetarians are less likely to develop diabetes. Rates of diabetes among SDAs are less than half (47% for men, 45% for women) those of the general population. Within the Adventist population, vegetarians have lower rates of diabetes than nonvegetarians. In the AHS, the prevalence of diagnosed diabetes at the outset, after adjusting for age and weight, was 1.9 and 1.4 times higher in nonvegetarian men and women, respectively, than in vegetarian men and women.[337] During the 21-year follow-up of individuals without a history of diabetes, the age-adjusted risk of diabetes appearing on a death certificate for nonvegetarians compared with vegetarians was 2.2 fold and 1.4 fold for men and women, respectively. After adjusting for weight, however, risk was still 80% higher in nonvegetarian men but was no longer elevated in women. In a later analysis of the AHS, the age-adjusted risk of developing diabetes for vegetarian, semi-vegetarian, and nonvegetarian men was 1.00, 1.35, and 1.97, and for women was 1.00, 1.08, and 1.93, respectively.[60] And analyses based on cross-sectional data obtained at baseline from participants in the AHS-2 suggest that risk for diabetes is lower by nearly half for vegetarians compared to nonvegetarians after adjusting for lifestyle factors and BMI.[338] In this study, even occasional meat or fish consumption increased risk.

In Adventist men, meat consumption was directly associated with an increased risk of diabetes. Relative risks for men consuming meat 1 to 2 days per week, 3 to 5 days per week, and $\geq$6 days per week were 1.3, 1.5, and 2.4, respectively, compared with vegetarian men.[337] Among women, only those consuming meat six times or more per week were at an increased risk relative to vegetarian women. In this study, nonvegetarian men and women were 1.9 and 1.6 times as likely to be overweight compared with vegetarian men and women. However, in a recent prospective cohort study of 8401 subjects from the Adventist Mortality Study and the Adventist Health Study, weekly consumers of all meats were 29% more likely to develop diabetes. Long-term adherence (over a 17-year interval) to a diet that included at least weekly meat intake was associated with a 74% increased risk for diabetes relative to long-term adherence to a vegetarian diet.[339] Red meat intake was also associated with increased risk of diabetes in the Women's Health Study.[340]

Hua et al found that in a comparison of 30 lacto-ovo vegetarians and 30 meat eaters, the vegetarians were more insulin sensitive and also had lower body iron stores. Interestingly, when iron stores of the meat eaters were reduced by phlebotomy to levels comparable to those of the vegetarians, insulin sensitivity improved.[341] And in agreement, in a study of 98 healthy Taiwanese women, lacto-ovo vegetarians had significantly lower levels of fasting insulin and plasma glucose and also lower insulin resistance.[342] Insulin sensitivity was also better in a group of Chinese vegetarians compared to omnivores and correlated with years on a vegetarian diet.[343]

One reason for the lower diabetes risk among vegetarians may be that vegetarian, particularly vegan, diets have been found to have a lower glycemic index,[344] and they include foods that may reduce risk of diabetes including nuts,[345] legumes,[346] and fruits and vegetables.[347]

The metabolic consequences of vegetarian diets as they relate to diabetes and insulin sensitivity are discussed in Chapter 16. Clearly, though, the protective effects of vegetarian diets against heart disease offer an important advantage to diabetics given that their risk of CHD is increased more than threefold compared to nondiabetics.[348] Intervention studies have shown benefits of low-fat vegan diets for reducing both LDL-C levels and glycosylated hemoglobin.[61]

OBESITY

Obesity is becoming the number-one health problem in the United States as its prevalence continues to increase. Currently, nearly two thirds of Americans are overweight. The prevalence of obesity (generally defined as ≥20% overweight) reaches 50% in some populations, particularly Native American, African American, and Hispanic women.[349,350] Obesity is much more common in American women below the poverty line, whereas in men it is more common above the poverty line.

Research on the BMI and body fat content of vegetarians compared with nonvegetarians is summarized in Appendixes D and E. Collectively, these studies indicate that vegetarians are either similar to nonvegetarians or have lower BMIs and/or less body fat. Differences between vegetarians and nonvegetarians were likely minimized in many studies, however, because of the selection criteria for study subjects (i.e., obese people were often ineligible). In the EPIC-Oxford Study, Spencer et al found that on average, vegetarians have a BMI about 1 kg/m² lower than that of nonvegetarians, which leads to obesity rates that are only about half those of vegetarians, with vegans having lower rates than other vegetarians.[351] During 5 years of follow-up, small differences in weight gain were observed among meat eaters, fish eaters, vegetarians, and vegans, and the lowest weight was seen among those who reduced their animal food intake during the follow-up period.[352] In the AHS, BMI increased as frequency of meat consumption increased.[37] And among Adventists in Barbados, those who had been vegetarian for <5 years had BMIs similar to nonvegetarians; those who had been vegetarian for at least 5 years were 70% less likely to be obese compared to nonvegetarians.[353] The lower BMI of vegans in comparison to lacto-ovo vegetarians in an analysis by Spencer et al is consistent with the findings from several smaller studies.[351,354,355]

Differences in levels of physical activity do not appear to contribute to the lower BMI/body fat of vegetarians because several studies indicated little if any difference between the two groups in this regard.[42,356-359] In the Oxford Vegetarian study, the lower BMI of non-meat eaters was associated in part, with a higher intake of fiber, and a lower intake of animal fat, and in men only, a lower intake of alcohol, but this explained only a third of the difference in BMI.

The effect of calcium and dairy products on weight management is an area of ongoing research. One pilot study showed that fortified soymilk was as effective as skim milk in promoting weight loss.[360] In fact, a comprehensive analysis of the data published in 2008 concluded that soyfoods are as effective as other protein sources for promoting weight loss and found a suggestive body of evidence that soyfoods may confer additional benefits.[361]

Interestingly, vegetarians may have a higher metabolic rate than nonvegetarians. In a study of lacto-ovo vegetarians and vegans in their mid-20s, resting metabolic rate (RMR) was 11% higher in vegetarians than in nonvegetarians. This was at least partly due to a higher level of plasma norepinephrine, which could result from the higher carbohydrate and lower fat intake of vegetarians.[362] Previous studies found a trend toward a higher RMR in male[363] but not female[364] vegetarians. Also, based on differences in urinary amino acid excretion, Hubbard et al speculated that vegans had higher amino acid metabolic activity.[365] Vegetarian diet per se, however, may be no more effective in producing weight loss than other dietary patterns that emphasize low fat and high carbohydrate intake.[366,367]

KIDNEY DISEASE

In 1982, Brenner et al first hypothesized that glomerular capillary hypertension, which is associated with increased glomerular filtration rates, results from an unrestricted intake of protein-rich foods and can lead to the progressive decrease of renal function seen in aging.[368] The relationship between protein intake and renal function is not without uncertainty,[369] but one school of thought is that high dietary protein may exacerbate existing kidney disease and increase the risk for developing renal disease.[370,371] Because vegetarian protein intake is adequate but lower than omnivore intake, vegetarian diets may have a role in the prevention and/or management of kidney disease. In fact, the glomerular filtration rate (GFR) of healthy vegetarians is lower than that of healthy nonvegetarians (based on creatinine clearance), and vegans have an even lower GFR than lacto-ovo vegetarians.[372]

Dietary protein increases the GFR in healthy individuals.[373] Furthermore, in healthy people without kidney disease, factors that increase the GFR may negatively affect kidney health, especially in those who are susceptible to developing kidney disease and in the elderly because kidney function declines with age. Support for the Brenner et al hypothesis comes from a study of 2500 older subjects who reported previous kidney problems. Consuming an additional 15 g of protein was associated with a 25% increase in overall mortality during the 14-year follow-up period.[374]

Findings indicate that the type of protein consumed may also affect kidney function. For example, GFR was shown to be 16% higher in healthy subjects after eating a meal containing animal protein in comparison with a meal containing soy protein (Figure 2-6).[375] Similarly, challenging the kidneys of healthy subjects with a high dose of meat protein adversely affected a variety of kidney function parameters in comparison with a challenge with soy protein.[376] Kontessis et al found that in normotensive, nonproteinuric subjects with type 1 diabetes, consuming a diet in which all of the protein was derived from plant foods resulted in more favorable effects on renal function than consuming a diet in which 70% of protein was derived from animal products.[377] In the Nurses' Health Study, animal protein but not overall protein intake was associated with continued loss of renal function in women who had some degree of renal impairment at

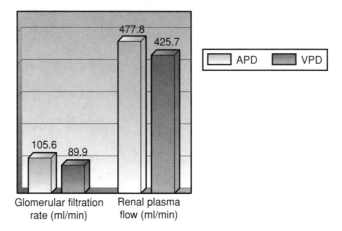

Figure 2-6 Effects of vegetarian diet on kidney function in diabetic subjects. Kidney function was studied in nine normotensive, nonproteinuric individuals with non-insulin-dependent diabetes mellitus fed in random order for 4 weeks either an animal protein diet (APD; protein intake 1.1 g/kg per day) or a vegetable protein diet (VPD; 0.95 g/kg per day) with similar caloric densities. Differences in glomerular filtration rate and renal plasma flow between the two dietary periods were notably significant ($P < 0.05$, Wilcoxon's signed rank test). *Source*: Data from Linos E, Willett WC, Cho E, Colditz G, Frazier LA. Red meat consumption during adolescence among premenopausal women and risk of breast cancer. *Cancer Epidemiol Biomarkers Prev* 2008;17(8):2146–2151.

baseline.[371] And in one study, removing red meat from the diet while keeping protein intake constant, reduced urinary protein losses in patients with diabetes.[378]

Among healthy Thai women, urinary protein levels were significantly lower in vegans compared to nonvegetarians.[379] The consumption of a vegetarian diet that included soy protein was shown to reduce urinary protein excretion in nephrotic patients.[380] The protective effect of protein restriction is most apparent in diabetic nephropathy[381] and advanced renal disease.[382]

However, not all studies have found that plant proteins have favorable effects on renal function. Soroka et al fed a low-protein, soy-based vegetarian diet or an animal-based diet to 15 patients with chronic renal failure and found that after 6 months, both diets were equally effective in retarding the progression of renal failure.[383] They suggested that these findings may have differed from much of the literature because subjects in their study had interstitial types of renal disease, rather than glomerular diseases associated with marked proteinuria. However, they did find that compliance with the vegetarian diet was better than the animal-based diet, and that phosphorous intake and urinary phosphate excretion were lower on the vegetarian diet, which could be an advantage for predialysis and dialysis patients.[384]

Finally, because the pathology of kidney disease is now thought to be similar to that of atherosclerosis, reducing high serum cholesterol levels and inhibiting cholesterol oxidation are thought to be important for reducing risk of developing kidney disease and for preventing the deterioration of kidney function in patients with existing kidney disease.[385,386] Consequently, vegetarian diets may offer additional protection against kidney disease because cholesterol levels are lower in vegetarians and because their intake of antioxidants is higher than that of omnivores, as discussed previously. The combination of reduced intakes of saturated fat, protein, and animal protein and higher intake of antioxidants suggests that vegetarian diets may be useful in both prevention and treatment of kidney disease. Because soy protein may favorably affect renal function and lower serum cholesterol, substituting soy protein for animal protein may be particularly helpful for those with renal problems.[387]

RENAL STONES

Renal stones affect 10–15% of Americans and are more common in men than women.[388,389] Renal stones may be 10 times more common today than they were at the beginning of the 20th century[390] and are a public health problem particularly in affluent countries.[391] About 80% of all renal stones are composed of calcium oxalate, sometimes with a nucleus of calcium phosphate. Oxalate is present in foods and is also synthesized endogenously. Contrary to a long-held belief, consuming diets high in calcium does not appear to increase risk for renal stones; rather, calcium seems to reduce risk (although calcium supplements may increase risk).[392,393] The reason may be that calcium binds oxalates in foods and in the intestines, making less oxalate available for renal stone formation.

As discussed in Chapter 3, protein in general, and animal protein in particular, may enhance urinary calcium excretion.[394] This may explain why people who have recurrent bouts of kidney stones tend to eat diets high in animal protein.[395–398] One large prospective study involving 45,000 men found a 30% increased risk of renal stone formation associated with above-average protein intakes.[392] In support of this observation is the finding that vegetarians appear to have a lower incidence of renal stone formation. A survey of approximately 2500 British vegetarians, 73% of whom were lacto-ovo vegetarians, found that the prevalence of urinary stone formation was roughly half that of the general population.[399] Brockis et al found that increased intake of animal protein was associated with an increase in the urinary output of compounds that raised risk of renal stone formation by 250%.[395] Based on such evidence, Robertson et al suggested a more vegetarian diet as a means of reducing the risk of stone recurrence.[397] On the basis of a review of the data, Zuckerman et al recently recommended a diet high in fluid and citrus fruits, with normal calcium, and restricted sodium, oxalates, and animal protein for the prevention of kidney stones.[400] Meat protein in particular appears to cause an imbalance between promoters and inhibitors of urinary crystallization by at least five mechanisms.[401] Some research suggests that patients with chronic renal stones are more likely to consume high-sodium diets that tend to be moderate or low in potassium.[402]

Although most kidney stones are comprised primarily of calcium oxalate, they may also be formed of uric acid. Uric acid is derived primarily from the metabolism of purines, which are highly concentrated in meat, although some plant foods (e.g., lentils) are also high. Breslau et al found that when subjects switched from a vegetarian diet, in which most of the protein came from soy and some cheese, to a mixed diet containing both animal and plant protein, to one in which protein came predominantly from animal sources, dietary purine intake increased from 1 to 2 to 72 mg/d, respectively.[403] Others have found that a diet rich in animal protein causes a doubling of urinary excretion of urate.[404–406] Citrate, an organic acid that is abundant in plant foods, interferes with kidney stone formation.[407] Urinary pH also influences stone formation.

Animal proteins tend to decrease urinary pH, and a low pH is thought to increase the risk of forming both types of kidney stones.[408] For these reasons, vegetarian diets may offer additional protection against renal stone formation.

Inadequate fluid intake raises risk for kidney stones, which may explain a higher incidence in warm climates. The American Urological Association projects that global warming will lead to increased prevalence of kidney stones.

GALLSTONES

Gallstones, one of the main components of which is cholesterol, are the major cause of gall-bladder disease in the United States, affecting approximately 10% of the population. They are as much as three times more common in women as in men. In Japan, the incidence of gallstones increased by a factor of 5 between 1950 and 1975.[409] During this time the intake of animal protein and fat increased by 129% and 190%, respectively. In contrast, rural Africans, who consume a largely vegan diet, rarely if ever develop gallstones.[410] Similarly, vegetarians are much less likely to develop gallstones than meat eaters.

In a study of >800 women between the ages of 40 and 69 years, Pixley et al found that only 12% of the vegetarians but 25% of the nonvegetarians had gallstones.[411] Many factors have long been thought to be risk factors for gallstones, but of these only obesity, gender, and aging have been confirmed.[412] Even after controlling for these factors, however, vegetarians were still only half as likely to develop gallstones as meat eaters.[411]

Why vegetarians have a reduced risk is uncertain. Some studies have found that higher intakes of calories, saturated fat, and simple sugars increase risk, whereas moderate alcohol consumption and fiber decrease risk.[413] Legume intake[414] and the intake of lecithin-containing foods may also help prevent gallstones.[415] An anthropometric advantage for vegetarians may be their leanness because obesity increases risk for gallstones. Although speculative, vegetable protein, in particular soy protein, may also have some advantages for reducing the risk of developing gallstones.[416,417]

Finally, there is evidence that sedentary lifestyle, a diet rich in animal fats and low in fiber,[418] folate, calcium, vitamin C, and magnesium has also been associated with increased risk.[419,420]

DIVERTICULAR DISEASE

Diverticular disease has been referred to as a deficiency disease of Western civilization, referring to the lack of fiber in Western diets.[421] It is characterized by pouching and inflammation of the wall of the bowel. This defect is common in Western industrialized nations and is estimated to occur in 60% of people at least 60 years of age in the United States. Symptomatic diverticular disease results in 200,000 hospitalizations in this country annually.[422] As recently as 1916, however, the disease was not prevalent enough to merit a mention in medical textbooks. Research indicates that diverticulitis is less common in vegetarians.[423]

In a study conducted by Gear et al, both male and female vegetarians 45 to 59 years of age were only 50% as likely to have diverticulitis as nonvegetarians.[423] The effects of vegetarian diets on diverticular disease are probably due to their increased fiber content, especially the insoluble cereal fibers, such as wheat bran. Bran has been shown to be useful in the treatment of diverticular disease,[424] although research also suggests that fiber from fruits and vegetables is helpful.[425] In the study by Gear et al, vegetarians consumed 41.5 g of fiber per day, whereas meat eaters consumed only 21.4 g/d. Fiber increases fecal bulk and presumably decreases colon pressure, so that the products of digestion are more easily propelled through the colon.[426] Stool weights of vegetarians were shown to be two to three times those of omnivores and of individuals with diverticular disease in one study.[427]

Other factors common to Western diets may also play a role in promoting diverticulitis. In a prospective study involving >40,000 U.S. health professionals, high-fat diets increased risk of diverticulitis independent of fiber intake.[428] Men on a high-fat, low-fiber diet were more than twice as likely to develop the disease. Findings also suggest that the insoluble component of fiber, especially cellulose, is significantly associated with a decreased risk of diverticular disease.[428] Even more striking, men on a high-red meat, low-fiber diet, were more than three times as likely to develop diverticulitis, suggesting that meat may increase risk.[425] A Taiwanese case-control study that included 192 subjects found an association between past meat consumption and diverticulosis.[429] These findings support a previous observation that red meat intake may promote the growth of bacteria that produce a toxic metabolite or a spasmogen that weakens the wall of the colon and favors the formation of diverticula.[430] In an analysis of U.S. health professionals, vigorous activity, such as running and jogging, was also very protective; in fact, sedentary men who consumed low-fiber diets were 2.5 times more likely to develop diverticulitis than men who ran or jogged for exercise and consumed high-fiber diets.[431] Contrary to popular belief, the evidence does not support restriction of seeds and nuts for those with diverticular disease.[432,433]

OTHER CONDITIONS

Vegetarians may be less likely to suffer from a number of other conditions, although the evidence is not nearly as strong as for those diseases previously discussed.

Rheumatoid Arthritis (RA)

Arthritis is a general term for inflammation of the joints. Rheumatoid arthritis (RA) is the most common form of arthritis, affecting 0.3–1% of the general population. Approximately 150 studies have found dietary influences on RA, but poor methodology was used in most of these studies.[434] Several studies, primarily from one group of researchers in Finland, have suggested some relief from a vegan diet that includes substantial amounts of raw foods.[435–443] In a comprehensive review on this subject, Grant found that fat from meat, based on food disappearance data, was found to have the highest association with the incidence of RA among countries, and concluded that rather than fat, the nitrite contributed by meat intake might be the responsible agent.[444]

Some evidence indicates that RA is less common among those who adhere to a Mediterranean-type diet[445] and that the diet could be beneficial in treatment of symptoms.[446] However, in a review of RCTs, Hagen et al concluded that effects of dietary manipulation, including vegetarian, vegan, Mediterranean, and elimination diets on RA remain uncertain due to study weaknesses.[447]

Gout

The formation of crystals in the joints results in an inflammatory disease known as gout. These crystals contain uric acid, a breakdown product of purines. Only about 15% of the urate formed each day comes from dietary sources. Most comes from the normal turnover of nucleic acids. Alcohol appears to be the main dietary component associated with gout, but a diet restricted in purines can also be of some help. High-purine foods include fish, liver, and kidneys. All meats are moderately high in purines, as are some legumes. A diet high in meat and seafood has been associated with greater risk for gout.[448] Weight loss, and possibly a diet that increases insulin sensitivity, may have some advantages for the management of gout.[449] Vitamin C intake may also reduce risk for gout.[450]

Dementia and Alzheimer's Disease

Dementia is an increasing economic and public health problem. In 1997, 2.32 million people had Alzheimer's disease (AD), 68% of whom were women. More striking, the prevalence of AD in the United States is expected to triple by 2050.[451] Rates of dementia vary throughout the world, even when adjusted for age, but comparisons are difficult because of differences in diagnostic criteria.[452] Nevertheless, rates appear to be lower in Asia, and, the most common type of dementia among white populations is AD, whereas in Asia, it is vascular dementia.[452] In both cases, though, the incidence of dementia rises exponentially with age. The annual incidence rate at 70 to 74 years of age is only 0.506, but by age 85 to 90 years, it is 3.858.[453] Because of the age-related nature of this disease, interventions that can delay the onset of AD by as little as 5 years could decrease prevalence by 1 million cases after 10 years.[454]

Preliminary data suggest that diet may impact AD and dementia. One report indicated that vegetarian diets may offer some benefits in regard to cognitive function because among SDAs, those who ate meat were found to be more than twice as likely to develop dementia.[455] If they had been eating meat for many years, they were more than three times as likely to show symptoms. One theory is that free radicals might be involved in the onset of dementia.[456] There is observational support for the benefits of diets high in antioxidants and that antioxidant supplements may retard age-related dementia,[457–459] although not all studies are supportive.[460] More specifically, the intake of flavonoids was found to be associated with a reduced risk of developing dementia.[461] Interestingly, serum vitamin C levels are lower in AD patients despite an adequate intake.[462] Because vegetarian diets are higher in the antioxidants that protect against free radical damage, this might also contribute to a reduced risk of senile dementia among vegetarians.

There are also data indicating that prior stroke and hypertension are related to dementia, so the lower blood pressure of vegetarians should be an advantage in this regard.[463–465] Furthermore, prevalence of probable AD was reduced by 60–73% in patients taking statins, suggesting cholesterol reduction may be an effective means to prevent AD and dementia.[466,467]

Estrogen therapy was initially postulated to reduce risk of AD and age-related cognitive impairment, but more recent data have shown equivocal results in regard to benefits. There may be a particular window of time during which estrogen therapy is protective in postmenopausal women. Because of the interest in estrogen, the relationship between phytoestrogens and cognition has received attention (see Chapter 9 for discussion of this issue).[468–471]

Finally, there is considerable interest in the relationship among the intake of folate and vitamin B_{12}, homocysteine levels, and dementia.[472–476] The possibly protective effects of higher serum folate levels might work to the advantage of vegetarians, but as discussed previously, vegetarian homocysteine levels are similar to or higher than levels in omnivores, a likely result of the poorer vitamin B_{12} status of vegetarians.

Constipation and Hemorrhoids

A specific definition of constipation is likely to vary from person to person, but technically constipation is characterized by hard stools and elimination fewer than three times per week. Constipation affects approximately 5 million Americans, but surveys show that up to 10% of children suffer from chronic constipation.[477] The consumption of adequate liquids and fiber is the best approach to avoiding constipation. Hippocrates observed that certain food items of plant origin (fruit, vegetables, bran) resulted in soft stools.[478] Insoluble fiber, such as that found in wheat bran, is especially helpful.[479] Lack of fiber was recently suggested as a causative factor in chronic idiopathic constipation in children,[480] and fiber was shown to alleviate constipation in a

Exhibit 2-2 Factors Common to Vegetarian Diets that Have Been Associated with Reduced Risk for Chronic Disease

Factor	May protect against
Lower saturated fat intake	Heart disease, gallstones
Lower cholesterol intake	Cancer
Lower animal protein intake	Renal disease, renal stones
Higher plant protein intake	Hypertension
Higher fiber intake	Heart disease, colon cancer, diverticular disease, hypertension, gallstones
Higher fruit and vegetable intake	Hypertension, cancer
Higher antioxidant intake	Heart disease, cancer, renal disease
Higher nut intake	Heart disease, diabetes
Lower glycemic load	Hypertension, diabetes
Higher nonheme iron intake	Hypertension
Absence of dairy (vegans)	Prostate cancer
Absence of red meat	Colon cancer, breast cancer, bladder cancer, diabetes
Higher soy intake	Breast cancer, prostate cancer
Higher legume intake	Gallstones

group of children.[481] Constipation may have serious consequences because frequent constipation may be an important risk factor for colon cancer.[482]

Straining due to constipation can result in hemorrhoids, which are clusters of enlarged veins near the rectum. Because vegetarians consume 50–100% more fiber than meat eaters, they are less likely to suffer from either constipation or hemorrhoids.[483–491]

Conclusion

Vegetarians have lower rates of cancer (particularly colon and lung cancer), heart disease, hypertension, diabetes, gallstones, kidney disease, and colon disease. The extent to which vegetarian diet plays a role in the better health of vegetarians is not easy to determine, but the evidence

---

Case Study

Harold is a 63-year-old man with a history of elevated blood cholesterol and hypertension. He has a strong family history of heart disease. Since adopting a lacto-ovo vegetarian diet 2 years ago, he has lost 15 pounds and is close to his goal weight, and both his cholesterol and blood pressure have dropped, but not to his goal levels. He works full time as an accountant and buys his lunch most days from a cafeteria or restaurant. He sometimes brings snacks to work or else buys them from a vending machine.

24-hour recall

Breakfast
    2 oz Kellogg's Corn Flakes
    1 cup skim milk
    ½ English muffin with 1 tbsp strawberry jam
    6 ounces orange juice
    Black coffee

Snack
    Coffee
    Low-fat granola bar

Lunch
    Hummus wrap with chopped tomato and lettuce
    Small tossed salad with oil and vinegar dressing

Snack
    ½ cup unsalted pretzels

Dinner
    1½ cups black bean chili
    1 cup zucchini sautéed in olive oil and topped with 1 tbsp low-fat parmesan cheese
    2 whole wheat dinner rolls with 2 tsp reduced fat margarine
    12 oz beer

What changes would you suggest to lower Harold's blood pressure further and to reduce his risk for coronary heart disease?

indicates it is an important factor in many instances. Vegetarian diets differ in many ways from omnivore diets. They are lower in fat (particularly saturated fat), protein, and animal protein and are higher in fiber, complex carbohydrates, antioxidants, and phytochemicals. All these factors may contribute to the health-promoting effects of vegetarian diets. Animal product intake per se may also directly increase risk of some chronic diseases. It is clear that vegetarian eating patterns adhere more closely to guidelines for optimal diet and are similar to the diets of populations with reduced chronic disease risk. Exhibit 2-2 (see page 41) summarizes factors common to vegetarian diets that have been associated with reduced risk for chronic disease.

REFERENCES

1. World Health Organization Study Group on Diet NaPoND. Diet, nutrition and the prevention of chronic diseases. *Nutr Rev.* 1991;49:291–301.
2. Allen NE, Appleby PN, Davey GK, Kaaks R, Rinaldi S, Key TJ. The associations of diet with serum insulin-like growth factor I and Its main binding proteins in 292 women meat-eaters, vegetarians, and vegans. *Cancer Epidemiol Biomarkers Prev.* 2002;11(11):1441–1148.
3. Fraser LR, Adeoya-Osiguwa SA. Fertilization promoting peptide—a possible regulator of sperm function in vivo. *Vitam Horm.* 2001;63:1–28.
4. Key TJ, Appleby PN, Spencer EA, Travis RC, Roddam AW, Allen NE. Mortality in British vegetarians: results from the European Prospective Investigation into Cancer and Nutrition (EPIC-Oxford). *Am J Clin Nutr.* 2009;89(5): 1613S–1619S.
5. Smit E, Nieto FJ, Crespo CJ. Blood cholesterol and apolipoprotein B levels in relation to intakes of animal and plant proteins in US adults. *Br J Nutr.* 1999;82(3):193–201.
6. Freedman LS, Guenther PM, Dodd KW, Krebs-Smith SM, Midthune D. The population distribution of ratios of usual intakes of dietary components that are consumed every day can be estimated from repeated 24-hour recalls. *J Nutr.* 2010;140(1):111–116.
7. Mente A, de Koning L, Shannon HS, Anand SS. A systematic review of the evidence supporting a causal link between dietary factors and coronary heart disease. *Arch Intern Med.* 2009;169(7):659–669.
8. Lanza E, Jones DY, Block G, Kessler L. Dietary fiber intake in the US population. *Am J Clin Nutr.* 1987;46(5):790–797.
9. Alaimo K, McDowell MA, Briefel RR, et al. Dietary intake of vitamins, minerals, and fiber of persons ages 2 months and over in the United States: Third National Health and Nutrition Examination Survey, Phase 1, 1988–91. *Adv Data.* 1994(258):1–28.
10. Anderson JW, Baird P, Davis RH, Jr., et al. Health benefits of dietary fiber. *Nutr Rev* 2009;67(4):188–205.
11. Services DoHaH. Dietary Guidelines for Americans. http://www.health.gov/dietaryguidelines/dga2005/document/html/chapter7.htm.
12. Committee on Diet and Health FaNB, Commission on Life Sciences, National Research Council. *Diet and Health, Implications for Reducing Chronic Disease Risk.* Washington, DC: National Academy Press; 1989.
13. Shickle D, Lewis PA, Charny M, Farrow S. Differences in health, knowledge and attitudes between vegetarians and meat eaters in a random population sample. *J R Soc Med.* 1989;82(1):18–20.
14. Nieman DC, Sherman KM, Arabatzis K, et al. Hematological, anthropometric, and metabolic comparisons between vegetarian and nonvegetarian elderly women. *Int J Sports Med.* 1989;10(4):243–251.
15. Nieman DC, Underwood BC, Sherman KM, et al. Dietary status of Seventh-Day Adventist vegetarian and non-vegetarian elderly women. *J Am Diet Assoc* 1989;89(12):1763–1769.
16. Weisburger JH. Mechanisms of action of antioxidants as exemplified in vegetables, tomatoes and tea. *Food Chem Toxicol.* 1999;37(9–10):943–948.
17. Cross CE. Oxygen radicals and human disease. *Ann Intern Med.* 1987;107:526–545.

18. Burkitt DP, Walker AR, Painter NS. Dietary fiber and disease. *JAMA.* 1974;229(8):1068–1074.

19. American Heart Association. *Heart and Stroke Facts: 1999 Statistical Supplement.* Dallas, TX: American Heart Association National Center; 1999.

20. Schober SE, Carroll MD, Lacher DA, Hirsch R. High serum total cholesterol—an indicator for monitoring cholesterol lowering efforts: U.S. adults, 2005–2006. *NCHS Data Brief.* 2007(2):1–8.

21. Ford ES, Mokdad AH, Giles WH, Mensah GA. Serum total cholesterol concentrations and awareness, treatment, and control of hypercholesterolemia among US adults: findings from the National Health and Nutrition Examination Survey, 1999 to 2000. *Circulation.* 2003;107(17):2185–2189.

22. Brown MS, Goldstein JL. A receptor-mediated pathway for cholesterol homeostasis. *Science.* 1986;232:34–47.

23. Chen Z, Peto R, Collins R, MacMahon S, Lu J, Li W. Serum cholesterol concentration and coronary heart disease in population with low cholesterol concentrations [see comments]. *BMJ.* 1991;303(6797):276–282.

24. Ministry of Public Health. *Health Statistics Information in China 1949–1988.* People's Republic of China: Ministry of Public Health; 1990.

25. Kinlen LJ, Hermon C, Smith PG. A proportionate study of cancer mortality among members of a vegetarian society. *Br J Cancer.* 1983;48(3):355–361.

26. Phillips RL, Lemon FR, Beeson WL, Kuzma JW. Coronary heart disease mortality among Seventh-Day Adventists with differing dietary habits: a preliminary report. *Am J Clin Nutr.* 1978;31(10 suppl):S191–S198.

27. Burr ML, Butland BK. Heart disease in British vegetarians. *Am J Clin Nutr.* 1988;48(3 suppl):830–832.

28. Burr ML, Sweetnam PM. Vegetarianism, dietary fiber, and mortality. *Am J Clin Nutr.* 1982;36(5):873–877.

29. Thorogood M, Mann J, Appleby P, McPherson K. Risk of death from cancer and ischaemic heart disease in meat and non-meat eaters [see comments]. *BMJ.* 1994;308(6945):1667–1670.

30. Berkel J, de Waard F. Mortality pattern and life expectancy of Seventh-Day Adventists in the Netherlands. *Int J Epidemiol.* 1983;12(4):455–459.

31. Chang-Claude J, Frentzel-Beyne R, Eilber U. Mortality pattern of German vegetarians after 11 years of follow-up. *Epidemiology.* 1992;3:395–401.

32. Hirayama T. Mortality in Japanese with life-styles similar to Seventh-day Adventists: strategy for risk reduction by life-style modification. *Natl Cancer Inst Monogr.* 1985;69:143–153.

33. Snowdon DA, Phillips RL, Fraser GE. Meat consumption and fatal ischemic heart disease. *Prev Med.* 1984; 13(5):490–500.

34. Phillips RL. Role of life-style and dietary habits in risk of cancer among Seventh-day Adventists. *Cancer Res.* 1975; 35(11 Pt. 2):3513–3522.

35. Key TJ, Fraser GE, Thorogood M, et al. Mortality in vegetarians and nonvegetarians: detailed findings from a collaborative analysis of 5 prospective studies. *Am J Clin Nutr.* 1999;70(3 suppl):516S–524S.

36. Key TJ, Thorogood M, Appleby PN, Burr ML. Dietary habits and mortality in 11,000 vegetarians and health conscious people: results of a 17-year follow-up [see comments]. *BMJ.* 1996;313(7060):775–779.

37. Fraser GE. Associations between diet and cancer, ischemic heart disease, and all-cause mortality in non-Hispanic white California Seventh-day Adventists. *Am J Clin Nutr.* 1999;70(3 suppl):532S–538S.

38. Phillips RL, Kuzma JW, Beeson WL, Lotz T. Influence of selection versus lifestyle on risk of fatal cancer and cardiovascular disease among Seventh-day Adventists. *Am J Epidemiol.* 1980;112(2):296–314.

39. Neaton JD, Wentworth D. Serum cholesterol, blood pressure, cigarette smoking, and death from coronary heart disease. *Arch Intern Med.* 1992;152:56–64.

40. Ellis FR, Sander TAB. Angina and vegan diet. *Am Heart J.* 1977;93:803–807.

41. Cooper RS, Goldberg RB, Trevisan M, et al. The selective lipid-lowering effect of vegetarianism on low density lipoproteins in a cross-over experiment. *Atherosclerosis.* 1982;44(3):293–305.

42. Rouse IL, Beilin LJ, Armstrong BK, Vandongen R. Blood-pressure-lowering effect of a vegetarian diet: controlled trial in normotensive subjects. *Lancet.* 1983;1(8314–5):5–10.

43. Masarei JR, Rouse IL, Lynch WJ, Robertson K, Vandongen R, Beilin LJ. Effects of a lacto-ovo vegetarian diet on serum concentrations of cholesterol, triglyceride, HDL-C, HDL2-C, HDL3-C, apoprotein-B, and Lp(a). *Am J Clin Nutr.* 1984;40(3):468–478.

44. Lindahl O, Lindwall L, Spangberg A, Stenram A, Ockerman PA. A vegan regimen with reduced medication in the treatment of hypertension. *Br J Nutr.* 1984;52(1):11–20.

45. Fernandes J, Dijkhuis-Stoffelsma R, Groot PH, Grose WF, Ambagtsheer JJ. The effect of a virtually cholesterol-free, high-linoleic-acid vegetarian diet on serum lipoproteins of children with familial hypercholesterolemia (type II-A). *Acta Paediatr Scand*. 1981;70(5):677–682.

46. Ornish D, Brown SE, Scherwitz LW, et al. Can lifestyle changes reverse coronary heart disease? The Lifestyle Heart Trial. *Lancet*. 1990;336(8708):129–133.

47. Arntzenius AC, Kromhout D, Barth JD, et al. Diet, lipoproteins, and the progression of coronary atherosclerosis. The Leiden Intervention Trial. *N Engl J Med*. 1985;312(13):805–811.

48. Barnard ND, Cohen J, Jenkins DJ, et al. A low-fat vegan diet improves glycemic control and cardiovascular risk factors in a randomized clinical trial in individuals with type 2 diabetes. *Diabetes Care*. 2006;29(8):1777–1783.

49. Resnicow K, Barone J, Engle A, et al. Diet and serum lipids in vegan vegetarians: a model for risk reduction [published erratum appears in *J Am Diet Assoc*. 1991;91(6):655]. *J Am Diet Assoc*. 1991;91(4):447–453.

50. Ferdowsian HR, Barnard ND. Effects of plant-based diets on plasma lipids. *Am J Cardiol*. 2009;104(7):947–956.

51. Law MR, Wald NJ, Wu T, Hackshaw A, Bailey A. Systematic underestimation of association between serum cholesterol concentration and ischaemic heart disease in observational studies: data from the BUPA study. *BMJ*. 1994;308(6925):363–366.

52. Holme I. An analysis of randomized trials evaluating the effect of cholesterol reduction on total mortality and coronary heart disease incidence. *Circulation*. 1990;82(6):1916–1924.

53. Sacks FM, Castelli WP, Donner A, Kass EH. Plasma lipids and lipoproteins in vegetarians and controls. *N Engl J Med*. 1975;292(22):1148–1151.

54. Knuiman JT, West CE, Katan MB, Hautvast JG. Total cholesterol and high density lipoprotein cholesterol levels in populations differing in fat and carbohydrate intake. *Arteriosclerosis*. 1987;7(6):612–619.

55. Robinson F, Hackett AF, Billington D, Stratton G. Changing from a mixed to self-selected vegetarian diet—influence on blood lipids. *J Hum Nutr Diet*. 2002;15(5):323–329.

56. Jenkins DJ, Wong JM, Kendall CW, et al. The effect of a plant-based low-carbohydrate ("Eco-Atkins") diet on body weight and blood lipid concentrations in hyperlipidemic subjects. *Arch Intern Med*. 2009;169(11):1046–1054.

57. Masarei JR, Rouse IL, Lynch WJ, Robertson K, Vandongen R, Beilin LJ. Vegetarian diets, lipids and cardiovascular risk. *Aust N Z J Med*. 1984;14(4):400–404.

58. Rader DJ, Ikewaki K, Duverger N, et al. Very low high-density lipoproteins without coronary atherosclerosis. *Lancet*. 1993;342(8885):1455–1458.

59. Kukita H, Imamura Y, Hamada M, Joh T, Kokubu T. Plasma lipids and lipoproteins in Japanese male patients with coronary artery disease and in their relatives. *Atherosclerosis*. 1982;42(1):21–29.

60. Fraser GE. Diet as primordial prevention in Seventh-Day Adventists. *Prev Med*. 1999;29(6 Pt 2):S18–23.

61. Barnard ND, Cohen J, Jenkins DJ, et al. A low-fat vegan diet and a conventional diabetes diet in the treatment of type 2 diabetes: a randomized, controlled, 74-wk clinical trial. *Am J Clin Nutr*. 2009;89(5):1588S–1596S.

62. Sacks FM, Handysides GH, Marais GE, Rosner B, Kass EH. Effects of a low-fat diet on plasma lipoprotein levels. *Arch Intern Med*. 1986;146(8):1573–1577.

63. Roshanai F, Sanders TA. Assessment of fatty acid intakes in vegans and omnivores. *Hum Nutr Appl Nutr*. 1984;38(5):345–354.

64. Kestin M, Rouse IL, Correll RA, Nestel PJ. Cardiovascular disease risk factors in free-living men: comparison of two prudent diets, one based on lactoovovegetarianism and the other allowing lean meat. *Am J Clin Nutr*. 1989;50(2):280–287.

65. Carroll KK. Dietary protein in relation to plasma cholesterol levels and atherosclerosis. *Nutr Rev*. 1978;36:1–5.

66. Sacks FM, Donner A, Castelli WP, et al. Effect of ingestion of meat on plasma cholesterol of vegetarians. *JAMA*. 1981;246(6):640–644.

67. Sacks FM, Ornish D, Rosner B, McLanahan S, Castelli WP, Kass EH. Plasma lipoprotein levels in vegetarians. The effect of ingestion of fats from dairy products. *JAMA*. 1985;254(10):1337–1341.

68. Anderson JW, Johnstone BM, Cook-Newell ME. Meta-analysis of the effects of soy protein intake on serum lipids. *N Engl J Med*. 1995;333(5):276–282.

69. Jenkins DJ, Kendall CW, Marchie A, et al. Direct comparison of a dietary portfolio of cholesterol-lowering foods with a statin in hypercholesterolemic participants. *Am J Clin Nutr*. 2005;81(2):380–387.

70. Pereira MA, O'Reilly E, Augustsson K, et al. Dietary fiber and risk of coronary heart disease: a pooled analysis of cohort studies. *Arch Intern Med.* 2004;164(4):370–376.

71. Toeller M, Buyken AE, Heitkamp G, de Pergola G, Giorgino F, Fuller JH. Fiber intake, serum cholesterol levels, and cardiovascular disease in European individuals with type 1 diabetes. EURODIAB IDDM Complications Study Group. *Diabetes Care.* 1999;22 (suppl 2):B21–28.

72. Glore SR, Van Treeck D, Knehans AW, Guild M. Soluble fiber and serum lipids: a literature review. *J Am Diet Assoc.* 1994;94(4):425–436.

73. Brown L, Rosner B, Willett WW, Sacks FM. Cholesterol-lowering effects of dietary fiber: a meta-analysis. *Am J Clin Nutr.* 1999;69(1):30–42.

74. Lichtenstein AH, Ausman LM, Jalbert SM, et al. Efficacy of a Therapeutic Lifestyle Change/Step 2 diet in moderately hypercholesterolemic middle-aged and elderly female and male subjects. *J Lipid Res.* 2002;43(2):264–273.

75. Chandalia M, Garg A, Lutjohann D, von Bergmann K, Grundy SM, Brinkley LJ. Beneficial effects of high dietary fiber intake in patients with type 2 diabetes mellitus [see comments]. *N Engl J Med.* 2000;342(19):1392–1398.

76. Pietinen P, Rimm EB, Korhonen P, et al. Intake of dietary fiber and risk of coronary heart disease in a cohort of Finnish men. The Alpha-Tocopherol, Beta-Carotene Cancer Prevention Study [see comments]. *Circulation.* 1996; 94(11):2720–2727.

77. Rimm EB, Ascherio A, Giovannucci E, Spiegelman D, Stampfer MJ, Willett WC. Vegetable, fruit, and cereal fiber intake and risk of coronary heart disease among men [see comments]. *JAMA.* 1996;275(6):447–451.

78. Law M. Plant sterol and stanol margarines and health. *BMJ.* 2000;320(7238):861–864.

79. Connor WE, Cerqueira MT, Connor RW, Wallace RB, Malinow MR, Casdorph HR. The plasma lipids, lipoproteins, and diet of the Tarahumara indians of Mexico. *Am J Clin Nutr.* 1978;31(7):1131–1142.

80. Hirai K, Shimazu C, Takezoe R, Ozeki Y. Cholesterol, phytosterol and polyunsaturated fatty acid levels in 1982 and 1957 Japanese diets. *J Nutr Sci Vitaminol (Tokyo).* 1986;32(4):363–372.

81. Nair PP, Turjman N, Kessie G, et al. Diet, nutrition intake, and metabolism in populations at high and low risk for colon cancer. Dietary cholesterol, beta-sitosterol, and stigmasterol. *Am J Clin Nutr.* 1984;40(4 suppl):927–930.

82. Abdulla M, Andersson I, Asp NG, et al. Nutrient intake and health status of vegans. Chemical analyses of diets using the duplicate portion sampling technique. *Am J Clin Nutr.* 1981;34(11):2464–2477.

83. Howell WH, McNamara DJ, Tosca MA, Smith BT, Gaines JA. Plasma lipid and lipoprotein responses to dietary fat and cholesterol: a meta-analysis [see comments]. *Am J Clin Nutr.* 1997;65(6):1747–1764.

84. Racette SB, Lin X, Lefevre M, et al. Dose effects of dietary phytosterols on cholesterol metabolism: a controlled feeding study. *Am J Clin Nutr.* 2010;91(1):32–38.

85. Heller RF, Chinn S, Pedoe HD, Rose G. How well can we predict coronary heart disease? Findings in the United Kingdom Heart Disease Prevention Project. *BMJ (Clin Res Ed).* 1984;288(6428):1409–1411.

86. Kaliora AC, Dedoussis GV, Schmidt H. Dietary antioxidants in preventing atherogenesis. *Atherosclerosis.* 2006; 187(1):1–17.

87. Steinberg D, Witztum JL. Lipoproteins and atherogenesis. Current concepts. *JAMA.* 1990;264(23):3047–3052.

88. Nagano Y, Arai H, Kita T. High density lipoprotein loses its effect to stimulate efflux of cholesterol from foam cells after oxidative modification. *Proc Natl Acad Sci U S A.* 1991;88(15):6457–6461.

89. Jackson RL, Ku G, Thomas CE. Antioxidants: a biological defense mechanism for the prevention of atherosclerosis. *Med Res Rev.* 1993;13:161–182.

90. Retsky KL, Freeman MW, Frei B. Ascorbic acid oxidation product(s) protect human low density lipoprotein against atherogenic modification. *J Biol Chem.* 1993;268:1304–1309.

91. Hamilton IM, Gilmore WS, Benzie IF, Mulholland CW, Strain JJ. Interactions between vitamins C and E in human subjects. *Br J Nutr.* 2000;84(3):261–267.

92. Tribble DL. AHA Science Advisory. Antioxidant consumption and risk of coronary heart disease: emphasis on vitamin C, vitamin E, and beta-carotene: a statement for healthcare professionals from the American Heart Association. *Circulation.* 1999;99(4):591–595.

93. Richter V, Purschwitz K, Bohusch A, et al. Lipoproteins and other clinical-chemistry parameters under the conditions of lacto-ovo-vegetarian nutrition. *Nutr Res.* 1999;19:545–554.

94. Nagyová A, Kudláčková M, Grancičová E, Magálová T. LDL oxidizability and antioxidative status of plasma in vegetarians. *Ann Nutr Metab.* 1998;42(6):328–332.

95. Rauma AL, Mykkanen H. Antioxidant status in vegetarians versus omnivores [see comments]. *Nutrition.* 2000; 16(2):111–119.

96. Waldmann A, Koschizke JW, Leitzmann C, Hahn A. Dietary intakes and blood concentrations of antioxidant vitamins in German vegans. *Int J Vitam Nutr Res.* 2005;75(1):28–36.

97. Tribble DL. Further evidence of the cardiovascular benefits of diets enriched in carotenoids [editorial; comment]. *Am J Clin Nutr.* 1998;68(3):521–522.

98. Kardinaal AF, Aro A, Kark JD, et al. Association between beta-carotene and acute myocardial infarction depends on polyunsaturated fatty acid status. The EURAMIC Study. European Study on Antioxidants, Myocardial Infarction, and Cancer of the Breast. *Arterioscler Thromb Vasc Biol.* 1995;15(6):726–732.

99. Haldar S, Rowland IR, Barnett YA, et al. Influence of habitual diet on antioxidant status: a study in a population of vegetarians and omnivores. *Eur J Clin Nutr.* 2007;61(8):1011–1122.

100. Krajcovicova-Kudlackova M, Valachovicova M, Paukova V, Dusinska M. Effects of diet and age on oxidative damage products in healthy subjects. *Physiol Res.* 2008;57(4):647–651.

101. Lonn E, Bosch J, Yusuf S, et al. Effects of long-term vitamin E supplementation on cardiovascular events and cancer: a randomized controlled trial. *JAMA.* 2005;293(11):1338–1347.

102. Sesso HD, Buring JE, Christen WG, et al. Vitamins E and C in the prevention of cardiovascular disease in men: the Physicians' Health Study II randomized controlled trial. *JAMA.* 2008;300(18):2123–2133.

103. He FJ, Nowson CA, Lucas M, MacGregor GA. Increased consumption of fruit and vegetables is related to a reduced risk of coronary heart disease: meta-analysis of cohort studies. *J Hum Hypertens.* 2007;21(9):717–728.

104. Naruszewicz M, Selinger E, Davignon J. Oxidative modification of lipoprotein(a) and the effect of beta-carotene. *Metabolism.* 1992;41(11):1215–1224.

105. Stein JH, Rosenson RS. Lipoprotein Lp(a) excess and coronary heart disease [see comments]. *Arch Intern Med.* 1997;157(11):1170–1176.

106. Li D, Ball M, Bartlett M, Sinclair A. Lipoprotein(a), essential fatty acid status and lipoprotein lipids in female Australian vegetarians. *Clin Sci (Colch).* 1999;97(2):175–181.

107. Yu-Poth S, Etherton TD, Reddy CC, et al. Lowering dietary saturated fat and total fat reduces the oxidative susceptibility of LDL in healthy men and women. *J Nutr.* 2000;130(9):2228–2237.

108. Schwab US, Ausman LM, Vogel S, et al. Dietary cholesterol increases the susceptibility of low density lipoprotein to oxidative modification. *Atherosclerosis.* 2000;149(1):83–90.

109. Visioli F, Borsani L, Galli C. Diet and prevention of coronary heart disease: the potential role of phytochemicals. *Cardiovasc Res.* 2000;47(3):419–425.

110. Yochum L, Kushi LH, Meyer K, Folsom AR. Dietary flavonoid intake and risk of cardiovascular disease in postmenopausal women [published erratum appears in *Am J Epidemiol.* 1999;150(4):432] [see comments]. *Am J Epidemiol.* 1999;149(10):943–949.

111. Hertog MG, Kromhout D, Aravanis C, et al. Flavonoid intake and long-term risk of coronary heart disease and cancer in the seven countries study [published erratum appears in *Arch Intern Med.* 1995;155(11):1184]. *Arch Intern Med.* 1995;155(4):381–386.

112. Huxley RR, Neil HA. The relation between dietary flavonol intake and coronary heart disease mortality: a meta-analysis of prospective cohort studies. *Eur J Clin Nutr.* 2003;57(8):904–908.

113. Perez-Vizcaino F, Duarte J, Andriantsitohaina R. Endothelial function and cardiovascular disease: effects of quercetin and wine polyphenols. *Free Radic Res.* 2006;40(10):1054–1065.

114. Mursu J, Nurmi T, Tuomainen TP, Ruusunen A, Salonen JT, Voutilainen S. The intake of flavonoids and carotid atherosclerosis: the Kuopio Ischaemic Heart Disease Risk Factor Study. *Br J Nutr.* 2007;98(4):814–818.

115. Fuhrman B, Lavy A, Aviram M. Consumption of red wine with meals reduces the susceptibility of human plasma and low-density lipoprotein to lipid peroxidation [see comments]. *Am J Clin Nutr.* 1995;61(3):549–554.

116. Law M, Wald N. Why heart disease mortality is low in France: the time lag explanation [see comments]. *BMJ.* 1999;318(7196):1471–1476.

117. Krajcovicova-Kudlackova M, Spustova V, Paukova V. Lipid peroxidation and nutrition. *Physiol Res.* 2004;53:219–224.

118. Hostmark AT, Lystad E, Vellar OD, Hovi K, Berg JE. Reduced plasma fibrinogen, serum peroxides, lipids, and apolipoproteins after a 3-week vegetarian diet. *Plant Foods Hum Nutr.* 1993;43(1):55–61.

119. Haugen MA, Kjeldsen-Kragh J, Bjerve KS, Hostmark AT, Forre O. Changes in plasma phospholipid fatty acids and their relationship to disease activity in rheumatoid arthritis patients treated with a vegetarian diet. *Br J Nutr.* 1994;72(4):555–566.

120. Krajcovicova-Kudlackova M, Simoncic R, Bederova A, Ondreicka R, Klvanova J. Selected parameters of lipid metabolism in young vegetarians. *Ann Nutr Metab.* 1994;38(6):331–335.

121. Beard JL. Are we at risk for heart disease because of normal iron status? *Nutr Rev.* 1993;51:112–115.

122. de Valk B, Marx JJ. Iron, atherosclerosis, and ischemic heart disease [see comments]. *Arch Intern Med.* 1999; 159(14):1542–1548.

123. Ascherio A, Willett WC, Rimm EB, Giovannucci EL, Stampfer MJ. Dietary iron intake and risk of coronary disease among men [see comments]. *Circulation.* 1994;89(3):969–974.

124. Ascherio A, Rimm EB, Giovannucci E, Willett WC, Stampfer MJ. Blood donations and risk of coronary heart disease in men. *Circulation.* 2001;103(1):52–57.

125. Danesh J, Appleby P. Coronary heart disease and iron status: meta-analyses of prospective studies. *Circulation.* 1999;99(7):852–854.

126. Derstine JL, Murray-Kolb LE, Yu-Poth S, Hargrove RL, Kris-Etherton PM, Beard JL. Iron status in association with cardiovascular disease risk in 3 controlled feeding studies. *Am J Clin Nutr.* 2003;77(1):56–62.

127. Syrovatka P, Kraml P, Potockova J, et al. Relationship between increased body iron stores, oxidative stress and insulin resistance in healthy men. *Ann Nutr Metab.* 2009;54(4):268–274.

128. Taylor BV, Oudit GY, Evans M. Homocysteine, vitamins, and coronary artery disease. Comprehensive review of the literature. *Can Fam Physician* 2000;46:2236–2245.

129. Boushey CJ, Beresford SA, Omenn GS, Motulsky AG. A quantitative assessment of plasma homocysteine as a risk factor for vascular disease. Probable benefits of increasing folic acid intakes. *JAMA.* 1995;274(13):1049–1057.

130. Albert CM, Cook NR, Gaziano JM, et al. Effect of folic acid and B vitamins on risk of cardiovascular events and total mortality among women at high risk for cardiovascular disease: a randomized trial. *JAMA.* 2008;299(17):2027–2036.

131. Toole JF, Malinow MR, Chambless LE, et al. Lowering homocysteine in patients with ischemic stroke to prevent recurrent stroke, myocardial infarction, and death: the Vitamin Intervention for Stroke Prevention (VISP) randomized controlled trial. *JAMA.* 2004;291(5):565–575.

132. Lonn E, Yusuf S, Arnold MJ, et al. Homocysteine lowering with folic acid and B vitamins in vascular disease. *N Engl J Med.* 2006;354(15):1567–1577.

133. Bazzano LA, Reynolds K, Holder KN, He J. Effect of folic acid supplementation on risk of cardiovascular diseases: a meta-analysis of randomized controlled trials. *JAMA.* 2006;296(22):2720–2726.

134. Hodis HN, Mack WJ, Dustin L, et al. High-dose B vitamin supplementation and progression of subclinical atherosclerosis: a randomized controlled trial. *Stroke.* 2009;40(3):730–736.

135. Mann NJ, Li D, Sinclair AJ, et al. The effect of diet on plasma homocysteine concentrations in healthy male subjects. *Eur J Clin Nutr.* 1999;53(11):895–899.

136. Mezzano D, Munoz X, Martinez C, et al. Vegetarians and cardiovascular risk factors: hemostasis, inflammatory markers and plasma homocysteine. *Thromb Haemost.* 1999;81(6):913–917.

137. Krajcovicova-Kudlackova M, Blazicek P, Kopcova J, Bederova A, Babinska K. Homocysteine levels in vegetarians versus omnivores. *Ann Nutr Metab.* 2000;44(3):135–138.

138. Hung CJ, Huang PC, Lu SC, et al. Plasma homocysteine levels in Taiwanese vegetarians are higher than those of omnivores. *J Nutr.* 2002;132(2):152–158.

139. Karabudak E, Kiziltan G, Cigerim N. A comparison of some of the cardiovascular risk factors in vegetarian and omnivorous Turkish females. *J Hum Nutr Diet.* 2007;21:13–22.

140. Koebnick C, Garcia AL, Dagnelie PC, et al. Long-term consumption of a raw food diet is associated with favorable serum LDL cholesterol and triglycerides but also with elevated plasma homocysteine and low serum HDL cholesterol in humans. *J Nutr.* 2005;135(10):2372–2378.

141. Waldmann A, Koschizke JW, Leitzmann C, Hahn A. German vegan study: diet, life-style factors, and cardiovascular risk profile. *Ann Nutr Metab.* 2005;49(6):366–372.

142. Waldmann A, Koschizke JW, Leitzmann C, Hahn A. Homocysteine and cobalamin status in German vegans. *Public Health Nutr.* 2004;7(3):467–472.

143. Houghton LA, Green TJ, Donovan UM, Gibson RS, Stephen AM, O'Connor DL. Association between dietary fiber intake and the folate status of a group of female adolescents. *Am J Clin Nutr.* 1997;66(6):1414–1421.

144. Haddad EH, Berk LS, Kettering JD, Hubbard RW, Peters WR. Dietary intake and biochemical, hematologic, and immune status of vegans compared with nonvegetarians. *Am J Clin Nutr.* 1999;70(3 suppl):586S–593S.

145. Mezzano D, Kosiel K, Martinez C, et al. Cardiovascular risk factors in vegetarians. Normalization of hyperhomocysteinemia with vitamin B(12) and reduction of platelet aggregation with n-3 fatty acids. *Thromb Res.* 2000; 100(3):153–160.

146. Su TC, Jeng JS, Wang JD, et al. Homocysteine, circulating vascular cell adhesion molecule and carotid atherosclerosis in postmenopausal vegetarian women and omnivores. *Atherosclerosis.* 2006;184(2):356–362.

147. Mehta J, Mehta P. Role of blood platelets and prostaglandins in coronary artery disease. *Am J Cardiol.* 1981; 48(2):366–373.

148. Weksler BB, Nachman RL. Platelets and atherosclerosis. *Am J Med.* 1981;71(3):331–333.

149. Kinsella JE, Lokesh B, Stone RA. Dietary n-3 polyunsaturated fatty acids and amelioration of cardiovascular disease: possible mechanisms [see comments]. *Am J Clin Nutr.* 1990;52(1):1–28.

150. Marckmann P, Sandstrom B, Jespersen J. Favorable long-term effect of a low-fat/high-fiber diet on human blood coagulation and fibrinolysis. *Arterioscler Thromb.* 1993;13(4):505–511.

151. Renaud S, Godsey F, Dumont E, Thevenon C, Ortchanian E, Martin JL. Influence of long-term diet modification on platelet function and composition in Moselle farmers. *Am J Clin Nutr.* 1986;43(1):136–150.

152. Renaud S, de Lorgeril M. Dietary lipids and their relation to ischaemic heart disease: from epidemiology to prevention. *J Intern Med Suppl.* 1989;225(731):39–46.

153. Barsotti G, Morelli E, Cupisti A, Bertoncini P, Giovannetti S. A special, supplemented 'vegan' diet for nephrotic patients. *Am J Nephrol.* 1991;11(5):380–385.

154. Ernst E, Pietsch L, Matrai A, Eisenberg J. Blood rheology in vegetarians. *Br J Nutr.* 1986;56:555–560.

155. Haines AP, Chakrabarti R, Fisher D, Meade TW, North WR, Stirling Y. Haemostatic variables in vegetarians and non-vegetarians. *Thromb Res.* 1980;19(1–2):139–148.

156. Sanders TA, Roshanai F. Platelet phospholipid fatty acid composition and function in vegans compared with age- and sex-matched omnivore controls. *Eur J Clin Nutr.* 1992;46(11):823–831.

157. Pan WH, Chin CJ, Sheu CT, Lee MH. Hemostatic factors and blood lipids in young Buddhist vegetarians and omnivores. *Am J Clin Nutr.* 1993;58(3):354–359.

158. Li D, Sinclair A, Mann N, et al. The association of diet and thrombotic risk factors in healthy male vegetarians and meat-eaters. *Eur J Clin Nutr.* 1999;53(8):612–619.

159. Fisher M, Levine PH, Weiner B, et al. The effect of vegetarian diets on plasma lipid and platelet levels. *Arch Intern Med.* 1986;146(6):1193–1197.

160. Chetty N, Bradlow BA. The effects of a vegetarian diet on platelet function and fatty acids. *Thromb Res.* 1983;30(6):619–624.

161. Dickerson JWT, Sanders TAB, Ellis FR. The effects of a vegetarian and vegan diet on plasma and erythrocyte lipids. *Qual Plant Fds Hum Nutr.* 1979;49:85–94.

162. Agren JJ, Tormala ML, Nenonen MT, Hanninen OO. Fatty acid composition of erythrocyte, platelet, and serum lipids in strict vegans. *Lipids.* 1995;30(4):365–369.

163. Spiller GA, Miller A, Olivera K, et al. Effects of plant-based diets high in raw or roasted almonds, or roasted almond butter on serum lipoproteins in humans. *J Am Coll Nutr.* 2003;22(3):195–200.

164. Sabate J. Nut consumption, vegetarian diets, ischemic heart disease risk, and all-cause mortality: evidence from epidemiologic studies. *Am J Clin Nutr.* 1999;70(3 suppl):500S–503S.

165. Kris-Etherton PM, Yu-Poth S, Sabate J, Ratcliffe HE, Zhao G, Etherton TD. Nuts and their bioactive constituents: effects on serum lipids and other factors that affect disease risk. *Am J Clin Nutr.* 1999;70(3 suppl):504S–511S.

166. Kelly JH Jr, Sabate J. Nuts and coronary heart disease: an epidemiological perspective. *Br J Nutr.* 2006;96(suppl 2):S61–S67.

167. Hajjar I, Kotchen TA. Trends in prevalence, awareness, treatment, and control of hypertension in the United States, 1988–2000. *JAMA.* 2003;290(2):199–206.

168. King H, Collins A, King LF, et al. Blood pressure in Papua New Guinea: a survey of two highland villages in the Asaro Valley. *J Epidemiol Community Health.* 1985;39(3):215–219.

169. Hamman L. Hypertension. Its clinical aspects. *Med Clin North Am.* 1917;1:155–176.

170. Donaldson AN. The relation of protein foods to hypertension. *Calif West Med.* 1926;24:328–331.

171. Saile F. Uber den Einfluss der vegetarischen Ernahrung auf den Blutdruck. *Med Klin.* 1930;26:929–931.

172. Heun E. Vegetarian fruit juices in therapy in obesity and hypertension. *Forsch Ther.* 1936;12:403–411.

173. Ko YC. Blood pressure in Buddhist vegetarians. *Nutr Rep Int.* 1983;28:1375–1383.

174. Melby CL, Goldflies DG, Toohey ML. Blood pressure differences in older black and white long-term vegetarians and nonvegetarians [published erratum appears in *J Am Coll Nutr.* 1993;12(6):following table of contents]. *J Am Coll Nutr.* 1993;12(3):262–269.

175. Wilkins JR, Calabrese EJ. Health implications of a 5 mm Hg increase in blood pressure. In: Calabrese EJ, Tuthill RW, Condie L, eds. *Inorganics in Drinking Water and Cardiovascular Disease.* Princeton, NJ: Princeton Scientific; 1985:85–100.

176. Five-year findings of the hypertension detection and follow-up program. I. Reduction in mortality of persons with high blood pressure, including mild hypertension. Hypertension Detection and Follow-up Program Cooperative Group. *JAMA.*1979;242(23):2562–2571.

177. Fraser GE. Vegetarian diets: what do we know of their effects on common chronic diseases? *Am J Clin Nutr.* 2009; 89(5):1607S–1612S.

178. Appleby PN, Davey GK, Key TJ. Hypertension and blood pressure among meat eaters, fish eaters, vegetarians and vegans in EPIC-Oxford. *Public Health Nutr.* 2002;5(5):645–654.

179. Ophir O, Peer G, Gilad J, Blum M, Aviram A. Low blood pressure in vegetarians: the possible role of potassium. *Am J Clin Nutr.* 1983;37(5):755–762.

180. Melby CL, Hyner GC, Zoog B. Blood pressure in vegetarians and non-vegetarians: A cross-sectional analysis. *Nutr Res.* 1985;5:1077–1082.

181. Melby CL, Goldflies DG, Hyner GC, Lyle RM. Relation between vegetarian/nonvegetarian diets and blood pressure in black and white adults. *Am J Public Health.* 1989;79(9):1283–1288.

182. Appel LJ, Moore TJ, Obarzanek E, et al. A clinical trial of the effects of dietary patterns on blood pressure. DASH Collaborative Research Group. *N Engl J Med.* 1997;336(16):1117–1124.

183. Svetkey LP, Simons-Morton D, Vollmer WM, et al. Effects of dietary patterns on blood pressure: subgroup analysis of the Dietary Approaches to Stop Hypertension (DASH) randomized clinical trial. *Arch Intern Med.* 1999;159(3): 285–293.

184. Sacks FM, Svetkey LP, Vollmer WM, et al. Effects on blood pressure of reduced dietary sodium and the Dietary Approaches to Stop Hypertension (DASH) diet. DASH-Sodium Collaborative Research Group. *N Engl J Med.* 2001;344(1):3–10.

185. Wadsworth ME, Cripps HA, Midwinter RE, Colley JR. Blood pressure in a national birth cohort at the age of 36 related to social and familial factors, smoking, and body mass. *Br Med J (Clin Res Ed).* 1985;291(6508):1534–1538.

186. Nelson L, Jennings GL, Esler MD, Korner PI. Effect of changing levels of physical activity on blood-pressure and haemodynamics in essential hypertension. *Lancet.* 1986;2(8505):473–476.

187. Juhaeri, Stevens J, Chambless LE, et al. Associations of weight loss and changes in fat distribution with the remission of hypertension in a bi-ethnic cohort: the Atherosclerosis Risk in Communities Study. *Prev Med.* 2003;36(3): 330–339.

188. Wilson PW, D'Agostino RB, Sullivan L, Parise H, Kannel WB. Overweight and obesity as determinants of cardiovascular risk: the Framingham experience. *Arch Intern Med.* 2002;162(16):1867–1872.

189. Beilin LJ. Lifestyle and hypertension—an overview. *Clin Exp Hypertens.* 1999;21(5–6):749–762.

190. Huang Z, Willett WC, Manson JE, et al. Body weight, weight change, and risk for hypertension in women [see comments]. *Ann Intern Med.* 1998;128(2):81–88.

191. Gear JS, Mann JI, Thorogood M, Carter R, Jelfs R. Biochemical and haematological variables in vegetarians. *Br Med J.* 1980;280(6229):1415.

192. Anholm AC. The relationship of a vegetarian diet to blood pressure [abstract]. *Prev Med.* 1978;7:35.

193. Rouse IL, Armstrong BK, Beilin LJ. The relationship of blood pressure to diet and lifestyle in two religious populations. *J Hypertens.* 1983;1(1):65–71.

194. Margetts BM, Beilin LJ, Vandongen R, Armstrong BK. Vegetarian diet in mild hypertension: a randomised controlled trial. *Br Med J (Clin Res Ed).* 1986;293(6560):1468–1471.

195. Sciarrone SE, Strahan MT, Beilin LJ, Burke V, Rogers P, Rouse IL. Biochemical and neurohormonal responses to the introduction of a lacto- ovovegetarian diet. *J Hypertens.* 1993;11(8):849–860.

196. Rouse IL, Beilin LJ, Mahoney DP, et al. Nutrient intake, blood pressure, serum and urinary prostaglandins and serum thromboxane B2 in a controlled trial with a lacto-ovo-vegetarian diet. *J Hypertens.* 1986;4(2):241–250.

197. Prescott SL, Jenner DA, Beilin LJ, Margetts BM, Vandongen R. A randomized controlled trial of the effect on blood pressure of dietary non-meat protein versus meat protein in normotensive omnivores. *Clin Sci.* 1988;74(6):665–672.

198. Prescott SL, Jenner DA, Beilin LJ, Margetts BM, Vandongen R. Controlled study of the effects of dietary protein on blood pressure in normotensive humans. *Clin Exp Pharmacol Physiol.* 1987;14(3):159–162.

199. Brussaard JH, van Raaij JM, Stasse-Wolthuis M, Katan MB, Hautvast JG. Blood pressure and diet in normotensive volunteers: absence of an effect of dietary fiber, protein, or fat. *Am J Clin Nutr.* 1981;34(10):2023–2029.

200. Wang YF, Yancy WS, Jr., Yu D, Champagne C, Appel LJ, Lin PH. The relationship between dietary protein intake and blood pressure: results from the PREMIER study. *J Hum Hypertens.* 2008;22(11):745–754.

201. He J, Gu D, Wu X, Chen J, Duan X, Whelton PK. Effect of soybean protein on blood pressure: a randomized, controlled trial. *Ann Intern Med.* 2005;143(1):1–9.

202. Galan P, Vergnaud AC, Tzoulaki I, et al. Low total and nonheme iron intakes are associated with a greater risk of hypertension. *J Nutr.* 2010;140(1):75–80.

203. Lairon D, Arnault N, Bertrais S, et al. Dietary fiber intake and risk factors for cardiovascular disease in French adults. *Am J Clin Nutr.* 2005;82(6):1185–1194.

204. Appel LJ, Miller ER. Editorial commentary: bbs and bullets: the impact of dietary factors on blood pressure. *Hypertension.* 2001;37(2):268–269.

205. Sciarrone SE, Strahan MT, Beilin LJ, Burke V, Rogers P, Rouse IR. Ambulatory blood pressure and heart rate responses to vegetarian meals. *J Hypertens.* 1993;11(3):277–285.

206. Landsberg L, Young JB. The role of the sympathetic nervous system and catecholamines in the regulation of energy metabolism. *Am J Clin Nutr.* 1983;38(6):1018–1024.

207. Sacks FM, Kass EH. Low blood pressure in vegetarians: effects of specific foods and nutrients. *Am J Clin Nutr.* 1988;48(3 suppl):795–800.

208. Beilin LJ, Burke V. Vegetarian diet components, protein and blood pressure: which nutrients are important? *Clin Exp Pharmacol Physiol.* 1995;22(3):195–198.

209. Beilin LJ, Margetts BM. Vegetarian diet and blood pressure. *Bibl Cardiol.* 1987;41:85–105.

210. Beilin LJ. Vegetarian and other complex diets, fats, fiber, and hypertension. *Am J Clin Nutr.* 1994;59(5 suppl): 1130S–1135S.

211. Shimizu H, Ross RK, Bernstein L, Yatani R, Henderson BE, Mack TM. Cancers of the prostate and breast among Japanese and white immigrants in Los Angeles County. *Br J Cancer.* 1991;63(6):963–966.

212. Zhang CX, Ho SC, Chen YM, Fu JH, Cheng SZ, Lin FY. Greater vegetable and fruit intake is associated with a lower risk of breast cancer among Chinese women. *Int J Cancer.* 2009;125(1):181–188.

213. Nomura AM, Wilkens LR, Murphy SP, et al. Association of vegetable, fruit, and grain intakes with colorectal cancer: the Multiethnic Cohort Study. *Am J Clin Nutr.* 2008;88(3):730–737.

214. George SM, Park Y, Leitzmann MF, et al. Fruit and vegetable intake and risk of cancer: a prospective cohort study. *Am J Clin Nutr.* 2009;89(1):347–353.

215. Takachi R, Inoue M, Ishihara J, et al. Fruit and vegetable intake and risk of total cancer and cardiovascular disease: Japan Public Health Center-Based Prospective Study. *Am J Epidemiol.* 2008;167(1):59–70.

216. Lampe JW. Health effects of vegetables and fruit: assessing mechanisms of action in human experimental studies. *Am J Clin Nutr.* 1999;70(3 suppl):475S–490S.

217. Haddad EH, Tanzman JS. What do vegetarians in the United States eat? *Am J Clin Nutr.* 2003;78(3 suppl):626S–632S.

218. Larsson CL, Johansson GK. Dietary intake and nutritional status of young vegans and omnivores in Sweden. *Am J Clin Nutr.* 2002;76(1):100–106.

219. Pollard J, Greenwood D, Kirk S, Cade J. Lifestyle factors affecting fruit and vegetable consumption in the UK Women's Cohort Study. *Appetite.* 2001;37(1):71–79.

220. Johnston CS, Taylor CA, Hampl JS. More Americans are eating "5 A Day" but intakes of dark green and cruciferous vegetables remain low. *J Nutr.* 2000;130(12):3063–3067.

221. Schatzkin A, Lanza E, Corle D, et al. Lack of effect of a low-fat, high-fiber diet on the recurrence of colorectal ade-nomas. Polyp Prevention Trial Study Group. *N Engl J Med.* 2000;342(16):1149–1155.
222. Alberts DS, Martinez ME, Roe DJ, et al. Lack of effect of a high-fiber cereal supplement on the recurrence of col-orectal adenomas. Phoenix Colon Cancer Prevention Physicians' Network. *N Engl J Med.* 2000;342(16):1156–1162.
223. Flood A, Schatzkin A. Colorectal cancer: does it matter if you eat your fruits and vegetables? *J Natl Cancer Inst.* 2000;92(21):1706–1707.
224. Michels KB, Edward G, Joshipura KJ, et al. Prospective study of fruit and vegetable consumption and incidence of colon and rectal cancers. *J Natl Cancer Inst.* 2000;92(21):1740–1752.
225. Smith-Warner SA, Spiegelman D, Yaun SS, et al. Intake of fruits and vegetables and risk of breast cancer: a pooled analysis of cohort studies. *JAMA.* 2001;285(6):769–776.
226. World Cancer Research Fund/American Institute for Cancer Research. *Food, Nutrition, Physical Activity, and the prevention of Cancer: A Global Perspective.* Washington, DC: AICR; 2007.
227. Hilakivi-Clarke L, Cho E, deAssiss S, et al. Maternal and prepubertal diet, mammary development and breast can-cer risk. *J Nutr.* 2001;131:154S–157S.
228. Lamartiniere CA. Protection against breast cancer with genistein: a component of soy. *Am J Clin Nutr.* 2000;71(6 suppl):1705S–1707S; discussion 8S–9S.
229. Zheng W, Dai Q, Custer LJ, et al. Urinary excretion of isoflavonoids and the risk of breast cancer. *Cancer Epidemiol Biomarkers Prev.* 1999;8(1):35–40.
230. Phillips RL, Garfinkel L, Kuzma JW, Beeson WL, Lotz T, Brin B. Mortality among California Seventh-day Adven-tists for selected cancer sites. *J Natl Cancer Inst.* 1980;65(5):1097–1107.
231. Butler TL, Fraser GE, Beeson WL, et al. Cohort profile: The Adventist Health Study-2 (AHS-2). *Int J Epidemiol.* 2008;37(2):260–265.
232. Lipkin M, Uehara K, Winawer S, et al. Seventh-Day Adventist vegetarians have a quiescent proliferative activity in colonic mucosa. *Cancer Lett.* 1985;26(2):139–144.
233. Allen NE, Appleby PN, Davey GK, Key TJ. Hormones and diet: low insulin-like growth factor-I but normal bio-available androgens in vegan men. *Br J Cancer.* 2000;83(1):95–97.
234. Burroughs KD, Dunn SE, Barrett JC, Taylor JA. Insulin-like growth factor-I: a key regulator of human cancer risk? [editorial; comment] [see comments]. *J Natl Cancer Inst.* 1999;91(7):579–581.
235. Khosravi J, Diamandi A, Mistry J, Scorilas A. Insulin-like growth factor I (IGF-I) and IGF-binding protein-3 in benign prostatic hyperplasia and prostate cancer. *J Clin Endocrinol Metab.* 2001;86(2):694–699.
236. Roberts CT Jr. IGF-1 and prostate cancer. *Novartis Found Symp.* 2004;262:193–199; discussion 199–204, 265–268.
237. Mills PK, Beeson WL, Phillips RL, Fraser GE. Cohort study of diet, lifestyle, and prostate cancer in Adventist men. *Cancer.* 1989;64(3):598–604.
238. Key TJ, Appleby PN, Spencer EA, Travis RC, Roddam AW, Allen NE. Cancer incidence in vegetarians: results from the European Prospective Investigation into Cancer and Nutrition (EPIC-Oxford). *Am J Clin Nutr.* 2009; 89(5):1620S–1626S.
239. Key TJ, Appleby PN, Spencer EA, et al. Cancer incidence in British vegetarians. *Br J Cancer.* 2009;101(1):192–197.
240. Travis RC, Allen NE, Appleby PN, Spencer EA, Roddam AW, Key TJ. A prospective study of vegetarianism and isoflavone intake in relation to breast cancer risk in British women. *Int J Cancer.* 2008;122(3):705–710.
241. Taylor EF, Burley VJ, Greenwood DC, Cade JE. Meat consumption and risk of breast cancer in the UK Women's Cohort Study. *Br J Cancer.* 2007;96(7):1139–1146.
242. Ferrucci LM, Cross AJ, Graubard BI, et al. Intake of meat, meat mutagens, and iron and the risk of breast cancer in the Prostate, Lung, Colorectal, and Ovarian Cancer Screening Trial. *Br J Cancer.* 2009;101(1):178–184.
243. Pike MC, Spicer DV, Dahmoush L, Press MF. Estrogens, progestogens, normal breast cell proliferation, and breast cancer risk. *Epidemiol Rev.* 1993;15(1):17–35.
244. Goldin BR, Adlercreutz H, Gorbach SL, et al. Estrogen excretion patterns and plasma levels in vegetarian and omnivorous women. *N Engl J Med.* 1982;307(25):1542–1547.
245. Adlercreutz H, Fotsis T, Bannwart C, Hamalainen E, Bloigu S, Ollus A. Urinary estrogen profile determination in young Finnish vegetarian and omnivorous women. *J Steroid Biochem.* 1986;24(1):289–296.

246. Barbosa JC, Shultz TD, Filley SJ, Nieman DC. The relationship among adiposity, diet, and hormone concentrations in vegetarian and nonvegetarian postmenopausal women[see comments]. *Am J Clin Nutr.* 1990;51(5):798–803.

247. Prentice R, Thompson D, Clifford C, Gorbach S, Goldin B, Byar D. Dietary fat reduction and plasma estradiol concentration in healthy postmenopausal women. The Women's Health Trial Study Group. *J Natl Cancer Inst.* 1990;82(2):129–134.

248. Goldin BR, Woods MN, Spiegelman DL, et al. The effect of dietary fat and fiber on serum estrogen concentrations in premenopausal women under controlled dietary conditions. *Cancer.* 1994;74(3 suppl):1125–1131.

249. Adlercreutz H, Gorbach SL, Goldin BR, Woods MN, Dwyer JT, Hamalainen E. Estrogen metabolism and excretion in Oriental and Caucasian women [see comments] [published erratum appears in *J Natl Cancer Inst.* 1995;87(2):147]. *J Natl Cancer Inst.* 1994;86(14):1076–1082.

250. Rose DP, Goldman M, Connolly JM, Strong LE. High-fiber diet reduces serum estrogen concentrations in premenopausal women. *Am J Clin Nutr.* 1991;54(3):520–525.

251. Wu AH, Pike MC, Stram DO. Meta-analysis: dietary fat intake, serum estrogen levels, and the risk of breast cancer. *J Natl Cancer Inst.* 1999;91(6):529–534.

252. Shultz TD, Howie BJ. In vitro binding of steroid hormones by natural and purified fibers. *Nutr Cancer.* 1986;8(2):141–147.

253. Sanchez A, Kissinger DG, Phillips RI. A hypothesis on the etiological role of diet on age of menarche. *Med Hypotheses.* 1981;7(11):1339–1345.

254. Kissinger DG, Sanchez A. The association of dietary factors with the age of menarche. *Nutr Res.* 1987;7:471–479.

255. Lu LJ, Cree M, Josyula S, Nagamani M, Grady JJ, Anderson KE. Increased urinary excretion of 2-hydroxyestrone but not 16alpha-hydroxyestrone in premenopausal women during a soya diet containing isoflavones. *Cancer Res.* 2000;60(5):1299–1305.

256. Xu X, Duncan AM, Wangen KE, Kurzer MS. Soy consumption alters endogenous estrogen metabolism in postmenopausal women. *Cancer Epidemiol Biomarkers Prev.* 2000;9(8):781–786.

257. Fowke JH, Longcope C, Hebert JR. Brassica vegetable consumption shifts estrogen metabolism in healthy postmenopausal women. *Cancer Epidemiol Biomarkers Prev.* 2000;9(8):773–779.

258. Howe GR, Benito E, Castelleto R, et al. Dietary intake of fiber and decreased risk of cancers of the colon and rectum: evidence from the combined analysis of 13 case-control studies [see comments]. *J Natl Cancer Inst.* 1992;84(24):1887–1896.

259. Reddy BS, Wynder EL. Large-bowel carcinogenesis: fecal constituents of populations with diverse incidence rates of colon cancer. *J Natl Cancer Inst.* 1973;50(6):1437–1442.

260. Nair PP, Turjman N, Goodman GT, Guidry C, Calkins BM. Diet, nutrition intake, and metabolism in populations at high and low risk for colon cancer. Metabolism of neutral sterols. *Am J Clin Nutr.* 1984;40(4 suppl):931–936.

261. Turjman N, Goodman GT, Jaeger B, Nair PP. Diet, nutrition intake, and metabolism in populations at high and low risk for colon cancer. Metabolism of bile acids. *Am J Clin Nutr.* 1984;40(4 suppl):937–941.

262. Korpela JT, Adlercreutz H, Turunen MJ. Fecal free and conjugated bile acids and neutral sterols in vegetarians, omnivores, and patients with colorectal cancer. *Scand J Gastroenterol.* 1988;23(3):277–283.

263. van Faassen A, Hazen MJ, van den Brandt PA, van den Bogaard AE, Hermus RJ, Janknegt RA. Bile acids and pH values in total feces and in fecal water from habitually omnivorous and vegetarian subjects. *Am J Clin Nutr.* 1993;58(6):917–922.

264. Aries VG, Crowther JS, Drasar BS, Hill MJ, Ellis FR. The effect of a strict vegetarian diet on the faecal flora and faecal steroid concentration. *J Pathol.* 1972;103:54–56.

265. Hill MJ, Aries VG. Faecal steroid composition and its relationship to cancer of the large bowel. *J Pathol.* 1971;104:129–139.

266. Finegold SM, Sutter VL, Sugihara PT, Elder HA, Lehmann SM, Phillips RL. Fecal microbial flora in Seventh Day Adventist populations and control subjects. *Am J Clin Nutr.* 1977;30(11):1781–1192.

267. Finegold SM, Attebery HR, Sutter VL. Effect of diet on human fecal flora: Comparison of Japanese and American diets. *Am J Clin Nutr.* 1974;27:1456–1469.

268. Finegold SM, Flora DJ, Attebery HR, Sutter VL. Fecal bacteriology of colonic polyp patients and control patients. *Cancer Res.* 1975;35:3407–3417.

269. Thornton JR. High colonic pH promotes colorectal cancer. *Lancet.* 1981;1(8229):1081–1083.

270. van Dokkum W, de Boer BC, van Faassen A, Pikaar NA, Hermus RJ. Diet, faecal pH and colorectal cancer. *Br J Cancer.* 1983;48(1):109–110.

271. Davies GJ, Crowder M, Reid B, Dickerson JW. Bowel function measurements of individuals with different eating patterns. *Gut.* 1986;27(2):164–169.

272. Burkitt DP, Walker ARP, Painter NS. Effect of dietary fibre on stools and transit times, and its role in the causation of disease. *Lancet.* 1972;2:1408–1411.

273. Glober GA, Kamiyama S, Nomura A, Shimada A, Abba BC. Bowel transit-time and stool weight in populations with different colon- cancer risks. *Lancet.* 1977;2(8029):110–111.

274. Cummings JH, Bingham SA, Heaton KW, Eastwood MA. Fecal weight, colon cancer risk, and dietary intake of nonstarch polysaccharides (dietary fiber) [see comments]. *Gastroenterology.* 1992;103(6):1783–1789.

275. Reddy BS, Sharma C, Wynder E. Fecal factors which modify the formation of fecal co-mutagens in high- and low-risk population for colon cancer. *Cancer Lett.* 1980;10(2):123–132.

276. Reddy BS, Sharma C, Darby L, Laakso K, Wynder EL. Metabolic epidemiology of large bowel cancer. Fecal mutagens in high- and low-risk population for colon cancer. A preliminary report. *Mutat Res.* 1980;72(3):511–522.

277. Kuhnlein U, Bergstrom D, Kuhnlein H. Mutagens in feces from vegetarians and nonvegetarians. *Mutat Res.* 1981;85:1–12.

278. Nader CJ, Potter JD, Weller RA. Diet and DNA-modifying activity in human fecal extracts. *Nutr Rep Int.* 1981;23:113–117.

279. Nomura AMY, Kolonel LN. Prostate cancer: a current perspective. *Am J Epidemiol.* 1991;13:200–227.

280. Masumori N, Tsukamoto T, Kumamoto Y, et al. Japanese men have smaller prostate volumes but comparable urinary flow rates relative to American men: results of community based studies in 2 countries. *J Urol.* 1996;155(4): 1324–1327.

281. Slattery ML, Schumacher MC, West DW, Robison LM, French TK. Food-consumption trends between adolescent and adult years and subsequent risk of prostate cancer. *Am J Clin Nutr.* 1990;52(4):752–757.

282. Snowdon DA, Phillips RL, Choi W. Diet, obesity, and risk of fatal prostate cancer. *Am J Epidemiol.* 1984; 120(2):244–250.

283. Lophatananon A, Archer J, Easton D, et al. Dietary fat and early-onset prostate cancer risk. *Br J Nutr.* 2010:1–6.

284. Rose DP, Boyar AP, Wynder EL. International comparisons of mortality rates for cancer of the breast, ovary, prostate, and colon, and per capita food consumption. *Cancer.* 1986;58(11):2363–2371.

285. Hill PB, Wynder EL. Effect of a vegetarian diet and dexamethasone on plasma prolactin, testosterone and dehydroepiandrosterone in men and women. *Cancer Lett.* 1979;7(5):273–282.

286. Howie BJ, Shultz TD. Dietary and hormonal interrelationships among vegetarian Seventh-Day Adventists and nonvegetarian men. *Am J Clin Nutr.* 1985;42(1):127–134.

287. Ross JK, Pusateri DJ, Shultz TD. Dietary and hormonal evaluation of men at different risks for prostate cancer: fiber intake, excretion, and composition, with in vitro evidence for an association between steroid hormones and specific fiber components. *Am J Clin Nutr.* 1990;51(3):365–370.

288. Pusateri DJ, Roth WT, Ross JK, Shultz TD. Dietary and hormonal evaluation of men at different risks for prostate cancer: plasma and fecal hormone-nutrient interrelationships. *Am J Clin Nutr.* 1990;51(3):371–377.

289. Wang Y, Corr JG, Thaler HT, Tao Y, Fair WR, Heston WD. Decreased growth of established human prostate LNCaP tumors in nude mice fed a low-fat diet [see comments]. *J Natl Cancer Inst.* 1995;87(19):1456–1462.

290. Zhou JR, Gugger ET, Tanaka T, Guo Y, Blackburn GL, Clinton SK. Soybean phytochemicals inhibit the growth of transplantable human prostate carcinoma and tumor angiogenesis in mice. *J Nutr.* 1999;129(9):1628–1635.

291. Makela SI, Pylkkanen LH, Santti RS, Adlercreutz H. Dietary soybean may be antiestrogenic in male mice. *J Nutr.* 1995;125(3):437–445.

292. Kristal AR, Cohen JH. Invited commentary: tomatoes, lycopene, and prostate cancer. How strong is the evidence? [comment]. *Am J Epidemiol.* 2000;151(2):124–127; discussion 8–30.

293. Alaejos MS, Diaz Romero FJ, Diaz Romero C. Selenium and cancer: some nutritional aspects. *Nutrition.* 2000; 16(5):376–383.

294. Helzlsouer KJ, Huang HY, Alberg AJ, et al. Association Between alpha-tocopherol, gamma-tocopherol, selenium, and subsequent prostate cancer. *J Natl Cancer Inst.* 2000;92(24):2018–2023.

295. Lippman SM, Klein EA, Goodman PJ, et al. Effect of selenium and vitamin E on risk of prostate cancer and other cancers: the Selenium and Vitamin E Cancer Prevention Trial (SELECT). *JAMA*. 2009;301(1):39–51.

296. Gaziano JM, Glynn RJ, Christen WG, et al. Vitamins E and C in the prevention of prostate and total cancer in men: the Physicians' Health Study II randomized controlled trial. *JAMA*. 2009;301(1):52–62.

297. Giovannucci E. Dietary influences of 1,25(OH)2 vitamin D in relation to prostate cancer: a hypothesis [see comments]. *Cancer Causes Control.* 1998;9(6):567–582.

298. Armstrong B, Doll R. Environmental factors and cancer incidence and mortality in different countries, with special reference to dietary practices. *Int J Cancer.* 1975;15(4):617–631.

299. Cross AJ, Leitzmann MF, Gail MH, Hollenbeck AR, Schatzkin A, Sinha R. A prospective study of red and processed meat intake in relation to cancer risk. *PLoS Med.* 2007;4(12):e325.

300. Huxley RR, Ansary-Moghaddam A, Clifton P, Czernichow S, Parr CL, Woodward M. The impact of dietary and lifestyle risk factors on risk of colorectal cancer: a quantitative overview of the epidemiological evidence. *Int J Cancer.* 2009;125(1):171–180.

301. Gonzalez CA, Jakszyn P, Pera G, et al. Meat intake and risk of stomach and esophageal adenocarcinoma within the European Prospective Investigation Into Cancer and Nutrition (EPIC). *J Natl Cancer Inst.* 2006;98(5):345–354.

302. Lumbreras B, Garte S, Overvad K, et al. Meat intake and bladder cancer in a prospective study: a role for heterocyclic aromatic amines? *Cancer Causes Control.* 2008;19(6):649–656.

303. Schulz M, Nothlings U, Allen N, et al. No association of consumption of animal foods with risk of ovarian cancer. *Cancer Epidemiol Biomarkers Prev.* 2007;16(4):852–855.

304. Pala V, Krogh V, Berrino F, et al. Meat, eggs, dairy products, and risk of breast cancer in the European Prospective Investigation into Cancer and Nutrition (EPIC) cohort. *Am J Clin Nutr.* 2009;90(3):602–612.

305. O'Keefe SJ, Kidd M, Espitalier-Noel G, Owira P. Rarity of colon cancer in Africans is associated with low animal product consumption, not fiber. *Am J Gastroenterol.* 1999;94(5):1373–1380.

306. Butler LM, Sinha R, Millikan RC, et al. Heterocyclic amines, meat intake, and association with colon cancer in a population-based study. *Am J Epidemiol.* 2003;157(5):434–445.

307. Chiu BC, Ji BT, Dai Q, et al. Dietary factors and risk of colon cancer in Shanghai, China. *Cancer Epidemiol Biomarkers Prev.* 2003;12(3):201–208.

308. Seow A, Quah SR, Nyam D, Straughan PT, Chua T, Aw TC. Food groups and the risk of colorectal carcinoma in an Asian population. *Cancer.* 2002;95(11):2390–2396.

309. Yeh CC, Hsieh LL, Tang R, Chang-Chieh CR, Sung FC. Risk factors for colorectal cancer in Taiwan: a hospital-based case-control study. *J Formos Med Assoc.* 2003;102(5):305–312.

310. Klurfeld DM. Human nutrition and health. Implications of meat with more muscle and less fat. In: Hafs HD, Zimbelman RG, eds. *Low-Fat Meats.* Orlando, FL: Academic Press; 1994:35–51.

311. Phillips RL, Snowdon DA, Brin BN. Cancer in vegetarians. In: Wynder EL, Leville GA, Weisburger JH, Livingston GE, eds. *Environmental Aspects of Cancer: The Role of Macro and Micro Components of Foods.* Westport, CT: Food and Nutrition Press; 1983:53–72.

312. Alexander DD, Cushing CA, Lowe KA, Sceurman B, Roberts MA. Meta-analysis of animal fat or animal protein intake and colorectal cancer. *Am J Clin Nutr.* 2009;89(5):1402–1409.

313. Bessaoud F, Daures JP, Gerber M. Dietary factors and breast cancer risk: a case control study among a population in Southern France. *Nutr Cancer.* 2008;60(2):177–187.

314. Holmes MD, Colditz GA, Hunter DJ, et al. Meat, fish and egg intake and risk of breast cancer. *Int J Cancer.* 2003;104(2):221–227.

315. Shannon J, Cook LS, Stanford JL. Dietary intake and risk of postmenopausal breast cancer (United States). *Cancer Causes Control.* 2003;14(1):19–27.

316. Hermann S, Linseisen J, Chang-Claude J. Nutrition and breast cancer risk by age 50: a population-based case-control study in Germany. *Nutr Cancer.* 2002;44(1):23–34.

317. Larsson SC, Bergkvist L, Wolk A. Long-term meat intake and risk of breast cancer by oestrogen and progesterone receptor status in a cohort of Swedish women. *Eur J Cancer.* 2009;45(17):3042–3046.

318. Taylor VH, Misra M, Mukherjee SD. Is red meat intake a risk factor for breast cancer among premenopausal women? *Breast Cancer Res Treat.* 2009;117(1):1–8.

319. Linos E, Willett WC, Cho E, Colditz G, Frazier LA. Red meat consumption during adolescence among premenopausal women and risk of breast cancer. *Cancer Epidemiol Biomarkers Prev.* 2008;17(8):2146–2151.
320. De Stefani E, Boffetta P, Deneo-Pellegrini H, et al. Meat intake, meat mutagens and risk of lung cancer in Uruguayan men. *Cancer Causes Control.* 2009;20(9):1635–1643.
321. Hatch FT, Knize MG, Moore DHI, Felton JS. Quantitative correlation of mutagenic and carcinogenic potencies for heterocyclic amines from cooked foods and additional aromatic amines. *Mutat Res.* 1992;271:269–287.
322. Wakabayashi K, Nagao M, Esumi H, Sugimura T. Food-derived mutagens and carcinogens. *Cancer Res.* 1992; 52(suppl):2092s–2098s.
323. Deitz AC, Zheng W, Leff MA, et al. N-Acetyltransferase-2 genetic polymorphism, well-done meat intake, and breast cancer risk among postmenopausal women. *Cancer Epidemiol Biomarkers Prev.* 2000;9(9):905–910.
324. Bingham S. Meat, starch and non-starch polysaccharides: are epidemiological and experimental findings consistent with acquired genetic alterations in sporadic colorectal cancer? *Cancer Lett.* 1997;114(1–2):25–34.
325. Kendall CW, Koo M, Sokoloff E, Rao AV. Effect of dietary oxidized cholesterol on azoxymethane-induced colonic preneoplasia in mice. *Cancer Lett.* 1992;66(3):241–248.
326. Sesink AL, Termont DS, Kleibeuker JH, Van der Meer R. Red meat and colon cancer: the cytotoxic and hyperproliferative effects of dietary heme. *Cancer Res.* 1999;59(22):5704–5709.
327. Ganmaa D, Li XM, Wang J, Qin LQ, Wang PY, Sato A. Incidence and mortality of testicular and prostatic cancers in relation to world dietary practices. *Int J Cancer.* 2002;98(2):262–267.
328. 3rd International Symposium on the Role of Soy in Preventing and Treating Chronic Disease. Washington DC, USA. October 31–November 3, 1999. Proceedings and abstracts. *J Nutr* 2000;130(3):653S–711S.
329. Chan JM, Stampfer MJ, Ma J, Gann PH, Gaziano JM, Giovannucci EL. Dairy products, calcium, and prostate cancer risk in the Physicians' Health Study. *Am J Clin Nutr.* 2001;74(4):549–554.
330. Allen NE, Key TJ, Appleby PN, et al. Animal foods, protein, calcium and prostate cancer risk: the European Prospective Investigation into Cancer and Nutrition. *Br J Cancer.* 2008;98(9):1574–1581.
331. Park Y, Leitzmann MF, Subar AF, Hollenbeck A, Schatzkin A. Dairy food, calcium, and risk of cancer in the NIH-AARP Diet and Health Study. *Arch Intern Med.* 2009;169(4):391–401.
332. Harris MI, Flegal KM, Cowie CC, et al. Prevalence of diabetes, impaired fasting glucose, and impaired glucose tolerance in U.S. adults. The Third National Health and Nutrition Examination Survey, 1988–1994 [see comments]. *Diabetes Care.* 1998;21(4):518–524.
333. King H, Aubert RE, Herman WH. Global burden of diabetes, 1995–2025: prevalence, numerical estimates, and projections. *Diabetes Care.* 1998;21(9):1414–1431.
334. Thompson D, Edelsberg J, Colditz GA, Bird AP, Oster G. Lifetime health and economic consequences of obesity. *Arch Intern Med.* 1999;159(18):2177–2183.
335. West KM, Kalbfleisch JM. Influence of nutritional factors on prevalence of diabetes. *Diabetes.* 1971;20:99–108.
336. Fung TT, Schulze M, Manson JE, Willett WC, Hu FB. Dietary patterns, meat intake, and the risk of type 2 diabetes in women. *Arch Intern Med.* 2004;164(20):2235–2240.
337. Snowdon DA, Phillips RL. Does a vegetarian diet reduce the occurrence of diabetes? *Am J Public Health.* 1985;75(5):507–512.
338. Tonstad S, Butler T, Yan R, Fraser GE. Type of vegetarian diet, body weight, and prevalence of type 2 diabetes. *Diabetes Care.* 2009;32(5):791–796.
339. Vang A, Singh PN, Lee JW, Haddad EH, Brinegar CH. Meats, processed meats, obesity, weight gain and occurrence of diabetes among adults: findings from Adventist Health Studies. *Ann Nutr Metab.* 2008;52(2):96–104.
340. Song Y, Manson JE, Buring JE, Liu S. A prospective study of red meat consumption and type 2 diabetes in middle-aged and elderly women: the women's health study. *Diabetes Care.* 2004;27(9):2108–2115.
341. Hua NW, Stoohs RA, Facchini FS. Low iron status and enhanced insulin sensitivity in lacto-ovo vegetarians. *Br J Nutr.* 2001;86(4):515–519.
342. Hung CJ, Huang PC, Li YH, Lu SC, Ho LT, Chou HF. Taiwanese vegetarians have higher insulin sensitivity than omnivores. *Br J Nutr.* 2006;95(1):129–135.
343. Kuo CS, Lai NS, Ho LT, Lin CL. Insulin sensitivity in Chinese ovo-lactovegetarians compared with omnivores. *Eur J Clin Nutr.* 2004;58(2):312–316.

344. Waldmann A, Strohle A, Koschizke JW, Leitzmann C, Hahn A. Overall glycemic index and glycemic load of vegan diets in relation to plasma lipoproteins and triacylglycerols. *Ann Nutr Metab.* 2007;51(4):335–344.

345. Jiang R, Manson JE, Stampfer MJ, Liu S, Willett WC, Hu FB. Nut and peanut butter consumption and risk of type 2 diabetes in women. *JAMA.* 2002;288(20):2554–2560.

346. Villegas R, Gao YT, Yang G, et al. Legume and soy food intake and the incidence of type 2 diabetes in the Shanghai Women's Health Study. *Am J Clin Nutr.* 2008;87(1):162–167.

347. Bazzano LA, Li TY, Joshipura KJ, Hu FB. Intake of fruit, vegetables, and fruit juices and risk of diabetes in women. *Diabetes Care.* 2008;31(7):1311–1317.

348. Lotufo PA, Gaziano JM, Chae CU, et al. Diabetes and all-cause and coronary heart disease mortality among US male physicians. *Arch Intern Med.* 2001;161(2):242–247.

349. Williamson DF, Kahn HS, Remington PL, Anda RF. The 10-year incidence of overweight and major weight gain in US adults. *Arch Intern Med.* 1990;150(3):665–672.

350. Flegal KM, Carroll MD, Ogden CL, Curtin LR. Prevalence and trends in obesity among US adults, 1999–2008. *JAMA.* 2010;303(3):235–241.

351. Spencer EA, Appleby PN, Davey GK, Key TJ. Diet and body mass index in 38000 EPIC-Oxford meat-eaters, fish-eaters, vegetarians and vegans. *Int J Obes Relat Metab Disord.* 2003;27(6):728–734.

352. Rosell M, Appleby P, Spencer E, Key T. Weight gain over 5 years in 21,966 meat-eating, fish-eating, vegetarian, and vegan men and women in EPIC-Oxford. *Int J Obes (Lond).* 2006;30(9):1389–1396.

353. Braithwaite N, Fraser H, Modeste N, Broome H, King R. Obesity, diabetes, hypertension and vegetarian status among Seventh-day Adventists in Barbados: Preliminary results. *Eth Dis.* 2003;13:34–39.

354. Freeland-Graves JH, Bodzy PW, Eppright MA. Zinc status of vegetarians. *J Am Diet Assoc.* 1980;77(6):655–661.

355. Hardinge MG, Stare FJ. Nutritional studies of vegetarians. *Am J Clin Nutr.* 1954;2:73–82.

356. McKenzie J. Profile on vegans. *Plant Foods Hum Nutr.* 1971;2:79–88.

357. Armstrong B, van Merwyk AJ, Coates H. Blood pressure in Seventh-day Adventist vegetarians. *Am J Epidemiol.* 1977;105(5):444–449.

358. Slattery ML, Jacobs DR, Jr., Hilner JE, et al. Meat consumption and its associations with other diet and health factors in young adults: the CARDIA study [published erratum appears in *Am J Clin Nutr.* 1992;55(1):iv]. *Am J Clin Nutr.* 1991;54(5):930–935.

359. Janelle KC, Barr SI. Nutrient intakes and eating behavior scores of vegetarian and nonvegetarian women. *J Am Diet Assoc.* 1995;95(2):180–186, 189; quiz 7–8.

360. Lukaszuk JM, Luebbers P, Gordon BA. Preliminary study: soy milk as effective as skim milk in promoting weight loss. *J Am Diet Assoc.* 2007;107(10):1811–1814.

361. Cope MB, Erdman JW, Jr., Allison DB. The potential role of soyfoods in weight and adiposity reduction: an evidence-based review. *Obes Rev.* 2008;9(3):219–235.

362. Toth MJ, Poehlman ET. Sympathetic nervous system activity and resting metabolic rate in vegetarians. *Metabolism.* 1994;43(5):621–665.

363. Poehlman ET, Arciero PJ, Melby CL, Badylak SF. Resting metabolic rate and postprandial thermogenesis in vegetarians and nonvegetarians. *Am J Clin Nutr.* 1988;48(2):209–213.

364. Oberlin P, Melby CL, Poehlman ET. Resting energy expenditures in young vegetarian and nonvegetarian women. *Nutr Res.* 1990;10:39–49.

365. Hubbard R, Haddad E, Berk L, Peters W, Tan S. Urinary amino acid level differences between adult human omnivores and vegans [abstract]. *FASEB J.* 1994;8 (suppl):A464.

366. Hakala P, Karvetti R-L. Weight reduction on lactovegetarian and mixed diets. *Eur J Clin Nutr.* 1988;43:421–430.

367. Caswell K, Linet OJ, Metzler C, Vantassel M. Effect of lacto-ovo-vegetarian diet on compliance and success of weight reduction program [abstract]. *J Am Diet Assoc.* 1991;87:1718.

368. Brenner BM, Meyer TW, Hostetter TH. Dietary protein intake and the progressive nature of kidney disease: the role of hemodynamically mediated glomerular injury in the pathogenesis of progressive glomerular sclerosis in aging, renal ablation, and intrinsic renal disease. *N Engl J Med.* 1982;307(11):652–659.

369. Levey AS, Adler S, Caggiula AW, et al. Effects of dietary protein restriction on the progression of advanced renal disease in the Modification of Diet in Renal Disease Study. *Am J Kidney Dis.* 1996;27(5):652–663.

370. Toeller M, Buyken AE. Protein intake—new evidence for its role in diabetic nephropathy [editorial]. *Nephrol Dial Transplant.* 1998;13(8):1926–1927.

371. Knight EL, Stampfer MJ, Hankinson SE, Spiegelman D, Curhan GC. The impact of protein intake on renal function decline in women with normal renal function or mild renal insufficiency. *Ann Intern Med.* 2003;138(6):460–467.

372. Wiseman MJ, Hunt R, Goodwin A, Gross JL, Keen H, Viberti GC. Dietary composition and renal function in healthy subjects. *Nephron.* 1987;46(1):37–42.

373. Bosch JP, Saccaggi A, Lauer A, Ronco C, Belledonne M, Glabman S. Renal functional reserve in humans. Effect of protein intake on glomerular filtration rate. *Am J Med.* 1983;75(6):943–950.

374. Dwyer JT, Madans JH, Turnbull B, et al. Diet, indicators of kidney disease, and later mortality among older persons in the NHANES I Epidemiologic Follow-Up Study. *Am J Public Health.* 1994;84(8):1299–1303.

375. Kontessis P, Jones S, Dodds R, et al. Renal, metabolic and hormonal responses to ingestion of animal and vegetable proteins. *Kidney Int.* 1990;38(1):136–144.

376. Dhaene M, Sabot JP, Philippart Y, Doutrelepont JM, Vanherweghem JL. Effects of acute protein loads of different sources on glomerular filtration rate. *Kidney Int Suppl.* 1987;22:S25–S28.

377. Kontessis PA, Bossinakou I, Sarika L, et al. Renal, metabolic, and hormonal responses to proteins of different origin in normotensive, nonproteinuric type I diabetic patients. *Diabetes Care.* 1995;18(9):1233.

378. de Mello VD, Zelmanovitz T, Perassolo MS, Azevedo MJ, Gross JL. Withdrawal of red meat from the usual diet reduces albuminuria and improves serum fatty acid profile in type 2 diabetes patients with macroalbuminuria. *Am J Clin Nutr.* 2006;83(5):1032–1038.

379. Wiwanitkit V. Renal function parameters of Thai vegans compared with non-vegans. *Ren Fail.* 2007;29(2):219–220.

380. D'Amico G, Gentile MG, Manna G, et al. Effect of vegetarian soy diet on hyperlipidaemia in nephrotic syndrome. *Lancet.* 1992;339(8802):1131–1134.

381. Zeller K, Whittaker E, Sullivan L, Raskin P, Jacobson HR. Effect of restricting dietary protein on the progression of renal failure in patients with insulin-dependent diabetes mellitus [see comments]. *N Engl J Med.* 1991;324(2):78–84.

382. Ihle BU, Becker GJ, Whitworth JA, Charlwood RA, Kincaid-Smith PS. The effect of protein restriction on the progression of renal insufficiency [see comments]. *N Engl J Med.* 1989;321(26):1773–1777.

383. Soroka N, Silverberg DS, Greemland M, et al. Comparison of a vegetable-based (soya) and an animal-based low-protein diet in predialysis chronic renal failure patients. *Nephron.* 1998;79(2):173–180.

384. Ritz E, Hergesell O. Oral phosphate binders without aluminium and calcium—a pipe-dream? [editorial]. *Nephrol Dial Transplant.* 1996;11(5):766–768.

385. Grone EF, Walli AK, Grone HJ, Miller B, Seidel D. The role of lipids in nephrosclerosis and glomerulosclerosis. *Atherosclerosis.* 1994;107(1):1–13.

386. Fried LF, Orchard TJ, Kasiske BL. Effect of lipid reduction on the progression of renal disease: a meta-analysis. *Kidney Int.* 2001;59(1):260–269.

387. Anderson JW, Smith BM, Washnock CS. Cardiovascular and renal benefits of dry bean and soybean intake. *Am J Clin Nutr.* 1999;70(3 suppl):464S–474S.

388. Johnson CM, Wilson DM, O'Fallon WM, Malek RS, Kurland LT. Renal stone epidemiology: a 25-year study in Rochester, Minnesota. *Kidney Int.* 1979;16(5):624–631.

389. Stamatelou KK, Francis ME, Jones CA, Nyberg LM, Curhan GC. Time trends in reported prevalence of kidney stones in the United States: 1976–1994. *Kidney Int.* 2003;63(5):1817–1823.

390. Danileson BG. Renal stones—current viewpoints on etiology and management. *Scand J Urol Nephrol Suppl.* 1985;19:1–5.

391. Goldfarb S. Diet and nephrolithiasis. *Annu Rev Med.* 1994;45:235–243.

392. Curhan GC, Willett WC, Rimm EB, Stampfer MJ. A prospective study of dietary calcium and other nutrients and the risk of symptomatic kidney stones. *N Engl J Med.* 1993;328(12):833–838.

393. Heaney RP. Calcium supplementation and incident kidney stone risk: a systematic review. *J Am Coll Nutr.* 2008;27(5):519–527.

394. Kerstetter JE, Allen LH. Dietary protein increases urinary calcium. *J Nutr.* 1990;120(1):134–136.

395. Brockis JG, Levitt AJ, Cruthers SM. The effects of vegetable and animal protein diets on calcium, urate and oxalate excretion. *Br J Urol.* 1982;54(6):590–593.

396. Martini LA, Heilberg IP, Cuppari L. Dietary habits of calcium stone formers. *Braz J Med Biol Res.* 1993;26:805–812.

397. Robertson WG, Peacock M, Heyburn PJ, et al. Should recurrent calcium oxalate stone formers become vegetarians? *Br J Urol.* 1979;51(6):427–431.

398. Jibani MM, Bloodworth LL, Foden E, Griffiths KD, Galpin OP. Predominantly vegetarian diet in patients with incipient and early clinical diabetic nephropathy: effects on albumin excretion rate and nutritional status. *Diabet Med.* 1991;8(10):949–953.

399. Robertson WG, Peacock M, Marshall DH. Prevalence of urinary stone disease in vegetarians. *Eur Urol.* 1982; 8(6):334–339.

400. Zuckerman JM, Assimos DG. Hypocitraturia: pathophysiology and medical management. *Rev Urol.* 2009; 11(3):134–144.

401. Jaeger P. Prevention of recurrent calcium stones: diet versus drugs. *Miner Electrolyte Metab.* 1994;20(6):410–413.

402. Martini LA, Cuppari L, Cunha MA, Schor N, Heilberg IP. Potassium and sodium intake and excretion in calcium stone forming patients. *J Ren Nutr.* 1998;8(3):127–131.

403. Breslau NA, Brinkley L, Hill KD, Pak CY. Relationship of animal protein-rich diet to kidney stone formation and calcium metabolism. *J Clin Endocrinol Metab.* 1988;66(1):140–146.

404. Fellstrom B, Danielson BG, Karlstrom B, et al. Effects of high intake of dietary animal protein on mineral metabolism and urinary supersaturation of calcium oxalate in renal stone formers. *Br J Urol.* 1984;56(3):263–269.

405. Fellstrom B, Danielson BG, Karlstrom B, Lithell H, Ljunghall S, Vessby B. The influence of a high dietary intake of purine-rich animal protein on urinary urate excretion and supersaturation in renal stone disease. *Clin Sci.* 1983;64(4):399–405.

406. Fellstrom B, Danielson BG, Karlstrom B, Lithell H, Ljunghall S, Vessby B. Dietary animal protein and urinary supersaturation in renal stone disease. *Proc Eur Dial Transplant Assoc.* 1983;20:411–416.

407. Nikkila M, Koivula T, Jokela H. Urinary citrate excretion in patients with urolithiasis and normal subjects. *Eur Urol.* 1989;16(5):382–385.

408. Dwyer J, Foulkes E, Evans M, Ausman L. Acid/alkaline ash diets: time for assessment and change. *J Am Diet Assoc.* 1985;85(7):841–845.

409. Kameda H, Ishihara F, Shibata K, Tsukie E. Clinical and nutritional study on gallstone disease in Japan. *Jpn J Med.* 1984;23:109–113.

410. Burkitt DP, Tunstall M. Gallstones: geographical and chronological features. *J Trop Med Hyg.* 1975;78:140–144.

411. Pixley F, Wilson D, McPherson K, Mann J. Effect of vegetarianism on development of gall stones in women. *Br Med J (Clin Res Ed).* 1985;291(6487):11–12.

412. Bennion LJ, Grundy SM. Risk factors for the development of cholelithiasis in man. *N Engl J Med.* 1978;299:1161–1167.

413. Smith DA, Gee MI. A dietary survey to determine the relationship between diet and cholelithiasis. *Am J Clin Nutr.* 1979;32:1519–1526.

414. Thijs C, Knipschild P. Legume intake and gallstone risk: results from a case-control study. *Int J Epidemiol.* 1990; 19:660–663.

415. Tompkins RK, Burke LG, Zollinger RM, Cornwell DG. Relationship of biliary phospholipid and cholesterol concentrations to the occurrence and dissolution of human gallstones. *Ann Surg.* 1970;172:936–945.

416. Ozben T. Biliary lipid composition and gallstone formation in rabbits fed on soy protein, cholesterol, casein and modified casein. *Biochem J.* 1989;263:293–296.

417. Tomotake H, Shimaoka I, Kayashita J, Yokoyama F, Nakajoh M, Kato N. A buckwheat protein product suppresses gallstone formation and plasma cholesterol more strongly than soy protein isolate in hamsters. *J Nutr.* 2000; 130(7):1670–1674.

418. Misciagna G, Centonze S, Leoci C, et al. Diet, physical activity, and gallstones—a population-based, case-control study in southern Italy. *Am J Clin Nutr.* 1999;69(1):120–126.

419. Ortega RM, Fernandez-Azuela M, Encinas-Sotillos A, Andres P, Lopez-Sobaler AM. Differences in diet and food habits between patients with gallstones and controls. *J Am Coll Nutr.* 1997;16(1):88–95.

420. Tseng M, Everhart JE, Sandler RS. Dietary intake and gallbladder disease: a review. *Public Health Nutr.* 1999;2(2):161–172.
421. Painter NS, Burkitt DP. Diverticular disease of the colon: a deficiency disease of Western civilization. *Br Med J.* 1971;2(759):450–454.
422. Thompson WG, Patel DG. Clinical picture of diverticular disease of the colon. *Clin Gastroenterol.* 1986;15(4):903–916.
423. Gear JS, Ware A, Fursdon P, et al. Symptomless diverticular disease and intake of dietary fibre. *Lancet.* 1979;1(8115):511–514.
424. Painter NS, Almeida AZ, Colebourne KW. Unprocessed bran in treatment of diverticular disease of the colon. *Br Med J.* 1972;2(806):137–140.
425. Aldoori WH, Giovannucci EL, Rimm EB, Wing AL, Trichopoulos DV, Willett WC. A prospective study of diet and the risk of symptomatic diverticular disease in men. *Am J Clin Nutr.* 1994;60(5):757–764.
426. Manousos O, Day NE, Tzonou A, et al. Diet and other factors in the aetiology of diverticulosis: an epidemiological study in Greece. *Gut.* 1985;26(6):544–549.
427. Segal I, Solomon A, Hunt JA. Emergence of diverticular disease in the urban South African black. *Gastroenterology.* 1977;72(2):215–219.
428. Aldoori WH, Giovannucci EL, Rockett HR, Sampson L, Rimm EB, Willett WC. A prospective study of dietary fiber types and symptomatic diverticular disease in men. *J Nutr.* 1998;128(4):714–719.
429. Lin OS, Soon MS, Wu SS, Chen YY, Hwang KL, Triadafilopoulos G. Dietary habits and right-sided colonic diverticulosis. *Dis Colon Rectum.* 2000;43(10):1412–1418.
430. Heaton KW. Diet and diverticulosis—new leads [editorial]. *Gut.* 1985;26(6):541–543.
431. Aldoori WH, Giovannucci EL, Rimm EB, et al. Prospective study of physical activity and the risk of symptomatic diverticular disease in men [see comments]. *Gut.* 1995;36(2):276–282.
432. Eglash A, Lane CH, Schneider DM. Clinical inquiries. What is the most beneficial diet for patients with diverticulosis? *J Fam Pract.* 2006;55(9):813–815.
433. Wess L, Eastwood M, Busuttil A, Edwards C, Miller A. An association between maternal diet and colonic diverticulosis in an animal model [see comments]. *Gut.* 1996;39(3):423–427.
434. Henderson CJ, Panush RS. Diets, dietary supplements, and nutritional therapies in rheumatic diseases. *Rheum Dis Clin North Am.* 1999;25(4):937–968, ix.
435. Hamberg VJ, Lindahl O, Lindwall L, Ockerman PA. Fasting and vegetarian diet in the treatment of rheumatoid arthritis—a controlled study. *Rheuma.* 1982;4:9–14.
436. Lithell H, Bruce A, Gustafsson IB, et al. A fasting and vegetarian diet treatment trial on chronic inflammatory disorders. *Acta Derm Venereol.* 1983;63(5):397–403.
437. Skoldstam L. Fasting and vegan diet in rheumatoid arthritis. *Scand J Rheumatol.* 1986;15:219–221.
438. Kjeldsen-Kragh J, Haugen M, Borchgrevink CF, et al. Controlled trial of fasting and one-year vegetarian diet in rheumatoid arthritis [see comments]. *Lancet.* 1991;338(8772):899–902.
439. Kjeldsen-Kragh J. Rheumatoid arthritis treated with vegetarian diets [see comments]. *Am J Clin Nutr.* 1999;70(3 suppl):594S–600S.
440. Hafstrom I, Ringertz B, Spangberg A, et al. A vegan diet free of gluten improves the signs and symptoms of rheumatoid arthritis: the effects on arthritis correlate with a reduction in antibodies to food antigens. *Rheumatology (Oxford).* 2001;40(10):1175–1179.
441. Abuzakouk M, O'Farrelly C. Diet, fasting, and rheumatoid arthritis. *Lancet.* 1992;339:68.
442. Panavi GS. Diet, fasting, and rheumatoid arthritis. *Lancet.* 1992;339:69.
443. Muller H, de Toledo FW, Resch KL. Fasting followed by vegetarian diet in patients with rheumatoid arthritis: a systematic review. *Scand J Rheumatol.* 2001;30(1):1–10.
444. Grant WB. The role of meat in the expression of rheumatoid arthritis. *Br J Nutr.* 2000;84:589–595.
445. Perez-Lopez FR, Chedraui P, Haya J, Cuadros JL. Effects of the Mediterranean diet on longevity and age-related morbid conditions. *Maturitas.* 2009;64(2):67–79.
446. McKellar G, Morrison E, McEntegart A, et al. A pilot study of a Mediterranean-type diet intervention in female patients with rheumatoid arthritis living in areas of social deprivation in Glasgow. *Ann Rheum Dis.* 2007;66(9):1239–1243.

447. Hagen KB, Byfuglien MG, Falzon L, Olsen SU, Smedslund G. Dietary interventions for rheumatoid arthritis. *Cochrane Database Syst Rev* 2009(1):CD006400.
448. Choi HK, Liu S, Curhan G. Intake of purine-rich foods, protein, and dairy products and relationship to serum levels of uric acid: the Third National Health and Nutrition Examination Survey. *Arthritis Rheum.* 2005;52(1): 283–289.
449. Dessein PH, Shipton EA, Stanwix AE, Joffe BI, Ramokgadi J. Beneficial effects of weight loss associated with moderate calorie/carbohydrate restriction, and increased proportional intake of protein and unsaturated fat on serum urate and lipoprotein levels in gout: a pilot study. *Ann Rheum Dis.* 2000;59(7):539–543.
450. Choi HK, Gao X, Curhan G. Vitamin C intake and the risk of gout in men: a prospective study. *Arch Intern Med.* 2009;169(5):502–507.
451. Middleton LE, Yaffe K. Promising strategies for the prevention of dementia. *Arch Neurol.* 2009;66(10):1210–1215.
452. Jorm AF, Jolley D. The incidence of dementia: a meta-analysis. *Neurology.* 1998;51(3):728–733.
453. Gao S, Hendrie HC, Hall KS, Hui S. The relationships between age, sex, and the incidence of dementia and Alzheimer disease: a meta-analysis. *Arch Gen Psychiatry.* 1998;55(9):809–815.
454. Brookmeyer R, Gray S, Kawas C. Projections of Alzheimer's disease in the United States and the public health impact of delaying disease onset. *Am J Public Health.* 1998;88(9):1337–1342.
455. Glem P, Beeson WL, Fraser GE. The incidence of dementia and intake of animal products: preliminary findings from the Adventist Health Study. *Neuroepidemiology.* 1993;12:28–36.
456. Harman D. Free radical theory of aging: a hypothesis on pathogenesis of senile dementia of the Alzheimer's type. *Age Ageing.* 1993;16:23–30.
457. Riedel WJ, Jorissen BL. Nutrients, age and cognitive function. *Curr Opin Clin Nutr Metab Care.* 1998;1(6):579–585.
458. Olson DA, Masaki KH, White LR, et al. Association of vitamin E and C supplement use with cognitive function and dementia in elderly men. *Neurology.* 2000;55(6):901–902.
459. Ross GW, Petrovitch H, White LR, et al. Characterization of risk factors for vascular dementia: the Honolulu-Asia Aging Study. *Neurology.* 1999;53(2):337–343.
460. Kang JH, Cook NR, Manson JE, Buring JE, Albert CM, Grodstein F. Vitamin E, vitamin C, beta-carotene, and cognitive function among women with or at risk of cardiovascular disease: The Women's Antioxidant and Cardiovascular Study. *Circulation.* 2009;119(21):2772–2780.
461. Commenges D, Scotet V, Renaud S, Jacqmin-Gadda H, Barberger-Gateau P, Dartigues JF. Intake of flavonoids and risk of dementia. *Eur J Epidemiol.* 2000;16(4):357–363.
462. Riviere S, Birlouez-Aragon I, Nourhashemi F, Vellas B. Low plasma vitamin C in Alzheimer patients despite an adequate diet. *Int J Geriatr Psychiatry.* 1998;13(11):749–754.
463. Farkas E, De Vos RA, Jansen Steur EN, Luiten PG. Are Alzheimer's disease, hypertension, and cerebrocapillary damage related? *Neurobiol Aging.* 2000;21(2):235–243.
464. Rigaud AS, Seux ML, Staessen JA, Birkenhager WH, Forette F. Cerebral complications of hypertension. *J Hum Hypertens.* 2000;14(10/11):605–616.
465. Pohjasvaara T, Mantyla R, Salonen O, et al. MRI correlates of dementia after first clinical ischemic stroke. *J Neurol Sci.* 2000;181(1–2):111–117.
466. Wolozin B, Kellman W, Ruosseau P, Celesia GG, Siegel G. Decreased prevalence of Alzheimer disease associated with 3-hydroxy-3-methyglutaryl coenzyme A reductase inhibitors. *Arch Neurol.* 2000;57(10):1439–1443.
467. Fonseca AC, Resende R, Oliveira CR, Pereira CM. Cholesterol and statins in Alzheimer's disease: Current controversies. *Exp Neurol.* 2009; September 25 (Epub ahead of print).
468. Benson S. Hormone replacement therapy and Alzheimer's disease: an update on the issues. *Health Care Women Int.* 1999;20(6):619–638.
469. Pan Y, Anthony M, Clarkson TB. Evidence for up-regulation of brain-derived neurotrophic factor mRNA by soy phytoestrogens in the frontal cortex of retired breeder female rats. *Neurosci Lett.* 1999;261(1–2):17–20.
470. White LR, Petrovitch H, Ross GW, et al. Brain aging and midlife tofu consumption. *J Am Coll Nutr.* 2000; 19(2):242–255.
471. Rice MM, Graves AB, McCurry SM, et al. Tofu consumption and cognition in older Japanese American men and women. *J Nutr.* 2000;130:676S.

472. Snowdon DA, Tully CL, Smith CD, Riley KP, Markesbery WR. Serum folate and the severity of atrophy of the neo-cortex in Alzheimer disease: findings from the Nun study [see comments]. *Am J Clin Nutr.* 2000;71(4):993–998.

473. Nourhashemi F, Gillette-Guyonnet S, Andrieu S, et al. Alzheimer disease: protective factors. *Am J Clin Nutr.* 2000;71(2):643S–649S.

474. Nilsson K, Gustafson L, Hultberg B. The plasma homocysteine concentration is better than that of serum methyl-malonic acid as a marker for sociopsychological performance in a psychogeriatric population. *Clin Chem.* 2000; 46(5):691–696.

475. Delport R. Hyperhomocyst(e)inemia, related vitamins and dementias. *J Nutr Health Aging.* 2000;4(4):195–196.

476. Miller JW, Green R, Ramos MI, et al. Homocysteine and cognitive function in the Sacramento Area Latino Study on Aging. *Am J Clin Nutr* 2003;78(3):441–447.

477. Leung AK, Chan PY, Cho HY. Constipation in children. *Am Fam Physician.* 1996;54(2):611–618, 627.

478. Bruce JL, Watt CH. Effects of dietary fibre. *BMJ.* 1972;4:49–50.

479. Odes HS, Lazovski H, Stern I, Madar Z. Double-blind trial of a high dietary fiber, mixed grain cereal in patients with chronic constipation and hyperlipidemia. *Nutr Res.* 1993;13:979–985.

480. Roma E, Adamidis D, Nikolara R, Constantopoulos A, Messaritakis J. Diet and chronic constipation in children: the role of fiber [see comments]. *J Pediatr Gastroenterol Nutr.* 1999;28(2):169–174.

481. Tse PW, Leung SS, Chan T, Sien A, Chan AK. Dietary fibre intake and constipation in children with severe devel-opmental disabilities. *J Paediatr Child Health.* 2000;36(3):236–239.

482. Jacobs EJ, White E. Constipation, laxative use, and colon cancer among middle-aged adults [see comments]. *Epidemiology.* 1998;9(4):385–391.

483. Glass RL, Hayden J. Dental caries in Seventh-day Adventist children. *J Dent Child.* 1966;33:22–23.

484. Harris RD. Biology of children of Hopewood House. *J Dent Res.* 1963;42:1387–1398.

485. Tovey FI, Yiu YC, Husband EM, Baker L, Jayaraj AP. Helicobacter pylori and peptic ulcer recurrence [letter; comment]. *Gut.* 1992;33(9):1293.

486. Moayyedi P, Soo S, Deeks J, et al. Systematic review and economic evaluation of helicobacter pylori eradication treatment for non-ulcer dyspepsia. *BMJ.* 2000;321(7262):659–664.

487. Misciagna G, Cisternino AM, Freudenheim J. Diet and duodenal ulcer. *Dig Liver Dis.* 2000;32(6):468–472.

488. Aldoori WH, Giovannucci EL, Stampfer MJ, Rimm EB, Wing AL, Willett WC. Prospective study of diet and the risk of duodenal ulcer in men. *Am J Epidemiol.* 1997;145(1):42–50.

489. Izzo AA, Di Carlo G, Mascolo N, Capasso F, Autore G. Antiulcer effect of flavonoids. Role of endogenous PAF. *Phytother Res.* 1994;8:179–181.

490. Di Carlo G, Mascolo N, Izzo AA, Capasso F. Flavonoids: old and new aspects of a class of natural therapeutic drugs. *Life Sci.* 1999;65(4):337–353.

491. Sanchez de Medina F, Galvez J, Gonzalez M, Zarzuelo A, Barrett KE. Effects of quercetin on epithelial chloride secretion. *Life Sci.* 1997;61(20):2049–2055.

PART II

Vegetarian Nutrition

CHAPTER 3

Protein

There has been much emphasis in the past on the ability of vegetarian, and particularly vegan, diets to supply adequate protein. This misplaced emphasis is based on the misconception that vegetarian protein intake is markedly lower than that of nonvegetarians and a lack of understanding about the value of plant foods as sources of protein. However, the quality of most plant proteins is lower than that of animal proteins—with the primary exception soy protein—and vegan protein intake is lower than that of omnivores. Nevertheless, protein needs can easily be met when no animal products are consumed.

Protein has had an interesting place in the field of nutrition over the past century and continues to be a much debated macronutrient. Protein experts are still working on identifying the ideal method for evaluating protein quality and determining optimal dietary protein intake. The outcome of both of these issues may be especially relevant to vegetarians.

HISTORICAL PERSPECTIVE ON PROTEIN NEEDS

Over the years, the emphasis placed of the role of protein in the diet has waxed and waned. In part, this is because of changing understandings about physiologic requirements for amino acids and because of insights gained about the role of protein and muscle accretion in health and disease. In fact, even today, according to the World Health Organization (WHO), "the large between-study variability that is apparent in studies assessing protein needs indicates that protein utilization in humans may depend on complex extrinsic factors that influence the behavior of the organism but that have not been captured in the short-term nitrogen balance studies, as well as by the intrinsic properties of the protein, such as amino acid content."[1]

Between 1950 and 1975, the Nutrition Division of the Food and Agriculture Organization (FAO) addressed the problem of protein deficiency under the assumption that it was the most serious and widespread problem in the world.[2] However, it came to be realized that the world "protein gap" was actually a food and calorie gap. Throughout the world, protein deficiency is nearly always the result of inadequate caloric intake, not consumption of poor-quality proteins.[3]

There are several reasons why such an unwarranted emphasis was placed on protein during the period following World War II. First, early estimates of the protein needs of 6-month-old infants were greatly overestimated. Between 1948 and 1974, these estimates decreased by about two thirds, from >3 g/kg body weight (bw) to a little over 1 g/kg bw.[1] Second, there was a marked underappreciation for the value of plant proteins and their ability to meet protein needs. As late as 1939, nutritionist J. S. McLester, in his book *Nutrition and Diet in Health and Disease*, credited the consumption of large amounts of animal protein (far in excess of current recommendations) with the accomplishments of Western civilization.[4] Animal food still remains a symbol of prestige and status throughout the world. In developing countries, where many traditional diets often contained little meat and dairy foods, as the standard of living rises, so does consumption of these foods. This transition occurs despite warnings by the WHO that this trend will undoubtedly lead to the same disease patterns that plague the West.[5] Increasingly, the environmental consequences of the world moving toward an animal-based diet are also raising alarms.[6–8]

For about two decades beginning in the 1970s, Western populations were generally viewed as consuming protein in amounts incompatible with optimal health and that were environmentally unsustainable. In regard to the former, concerns arose not only because of the types of foods that provided the bulk of the protein but because the excess protein itself was thought to be harmful, possibly increasing risk of chronic diseases including osteoporosis,[9] renal disease,[10] and even certain cancers.[11] However, support for these concerns has generally not been as forthcoming as anticipated. The adverse effects on bone health thought to result from consuming diets too high in sulphur amino acids (SAA) (for commentary, see Kerstetter[12]) haven't been demonstrated in clinical studies evaluating calcium balance[13,14] or in epidemiologic studies evaluating bone mineral density[15] and fracture risk.[16] Similarly, although there is evidence that excessive dietary protein may predispose susceptible individuals, such as people with diabetes, to develop renal disease, this is likely not the case for healthy individuals.[17]

Furthermore, there is evidence not only that higher-protein diets are not harmful but that they may actually be advantageous. For example, because dietary protein appears to be more satiating than carbohydrate and fat, higher-protein diets may aid in weight loss.[18,19] Also, there is some research linking higher-protein-content diets with muscle accretion, which may have important implications beyond physical appearance because the central role of muscle in the prevention of many common pathologic conditions and chronic diseases is gaining attention.[20] Whether higher-protein intake prevents sarcopenia (age-related loss in muscle mass) is a matter of some debate, but some evidence indicates the elderly would benefit by consuming protein in excess of the recommended dietary allowance (RDA),[21] and one group of experts recently recommended that the elderly consume 30 g protein at each meal.[22] Thus, in many respects, the protein discussion over the past decade has switched from one focused on establishing the intake needed to prevent deficiency, subtle signs of which are difficult to detect, to the intake associated with optimal health.

One point is clear: humans are able to easily survive on a wide range of protein intakes. This observation is consistent with the Acceptable Macronutrient Distribution Range (AMDR) for protein set by the Institute of Medicine/Food and Nutrition Board (IOM/FNB) for adults at 10–35% of energy intake.[23] It is also consistent with a recent analysis of the diets of hunter-gatherer societies, which revealed there was a huge range of dietary plant food-to-animal food ratios,[24] although according to Eaton et al,[25] the dietary protein content of humans just before the "out of

Africa" diaspora was 30–35% of energy intake. Whether the "evolutionary" diet is best for modern humans with a dramatically longer life expectance who are plagued by heart disease, cancer, and diabetes rather than being threatened by saber-toothed tigers is an interesting question.

PROTEIN INTAKE

Most Westerners consume diets that are adequate in protein and typically exceed the RDA for total protein intake by a considerable margin. But there are subgroups within the U.S. population for whom this is not the case; for example, 30–40% of teenage girls and older women and men don't meet the RDA for protein, although this in no way implies deficiency.[26] According to data from the National Health and Nutrition Examination Survey (NHANES), 2003–2004, usual protein intake (mean $\pm$ standard deviation) averaged 56 $\pm$ 14 g/d in young children, increased to a high of approximately 91 $\pm$ 22 g/d in adults age 19 to 30 years, and decreased to approximately 66 $\pm$ 17 g/d in the elderly.[27] Approximately 7.7% of adolescent females and 7.2–8.6% of older adult women reported consuming protein levels below their estimated average requirement. The median intake of protein on a percentage of calories basis ranged from 13.4% in children age 4 to 8 years to 16.0% in men age 51 to 70 years. It has been noted by others that the expected estimate of the protein intake in the MyPyramid food patterns ranges from 44 to 126 g protein/d, depending on calorie levels, and as a percentage of calories, the expected estimated intake of protein from the MyPyramid food patterns ranged from 17% to 21% of calories.[27] Even these values are still well within the AMDR, however.

Concerns regarding the ability of plant-based diets to meet protein needs are based primarily on the quality, not the quantity, of protein consumed. The reason for this is obvious when the adult protein RDA is viewed as a percentage of calories, rather than grams of protein, According to the IOM/FNB, the recommended energy intake for an active man 30 years of age who is 73 inches tall, weighs 63.3 kg (139 pounds), and has a body mass index (kg/m^2) of 18.5 is 2883 kcal/d. To meet the protein RDA of 0.8 g/kg, this individual would require only 50.6 g of protein per day, which represents about 7% of total caloric intake. Worldwide, protein contributes approximately 10.7% of total caloric intake for all ages.[28] Although there are major differences among regions, no countries consume diets that are <8% protein. Thus no countries consume diets that are too low in protein on a percentage calorie basis even though the RDA is 25% higher than biologic requirements to account for individual variation and in reality is set at a level that surpasses the protein needs of 97.5% of the population. However, diets containing 8% protein by calories are below the AMDR guidelines.

According to the FAO (disappearance data), North American diets are composed of approximately 12.3% protein, but NHANES III data indicate U.S. protein intake represented nearly 15% of calories,[29] which is consistent with the data from NHANES 2003–2004, as noted earlier.[27] In comparison, diets among sub-Saharan and African countries are composed of 9.6% and 9.9% protein, respectively. Individual surveys (Appendix A) show that omnivore, lacto-ovo vegetarian, and vegan protein intakes are 14–18%, 12–14 %, and 10–12%, respectively. Therefore, it is clear that although total protein intake is lower among vegetarians than nonvegetarians, it is still adequate. However, protein sources differ markedly between omnivores and vegetarians and also among populations throughout the world.

Diets in different geographic regions differ markedly in their percentage of protein derived from plant and animal sources. Disappearance data indicate plants provide approximately 63% of the edible protein in the world,[28] but in Africa and the sub-Saharan countries this figure is 80%, whereas only about 37% of the protein consumed by North Americans comes from plants. In fact, NHANES-III data indicate that plants may contribute as little as a third of total protein intake in the United States.[29] On a worldwide basis, cereals provide approximately 47% of protein, and legumes, nuts, and seeds, about 8%.[30] In developing countries, the major sources of cereal protein are wheat (43%), rice (39%), and maize (12%).[31] The major sources of protein in the United States are meat, fish, and poultry (42%), and dairy products (20%), with grains providing only 18%.[29]

The small contribution of animal sources to total protein intake in many parts of the world has sometimes been considered problematic.[32] However, this concern appears unwarranted; otherwise widespread protein deficiency might be expected, but this is not the case. This having been said, there is a difference between adequate protein intakes and optimal protein intakes.

PROTEIN QUALITY

Protein quality is determined by two factors: digestibility and amino acid content. Digestibility is of far less importance in Western diets, but it does have some bearing on vegetarian protein needs.

Digestibility

In North America, protein derived from plant-based diets, consisting largely of whole grains, beans, and vegetables, is about 85% digestible, whereas the protein from mixed diets based on refined grains and meat products, typical of most omnivores, is about 95% digestible.[33] The digestibility of selected diets and foods is shown in Table 3-1. In some countries, such as India, overall protein digestibility is relatively low, about 75%, because fewer animal products and refined plant foods are consumed. The digestibility of dried beans, which are an excellent source of protein, is relatively low at about 75%.

Once plant cell wall constituents are removed, however, the inherent digestibility of plant foods in many cases may be indistinguishable from that of animal proteins, which accounts for why the digestibility of wheat gluten, wheat flour, and isolated soy protein is >90%. Whole millet, beans, and some breakfast cereals have lower digestibility, ranging from 50% to 80%. This lower digestibility reflects particularly tough plant cell walls in some foods such as millet, fiber and antinutritional factors in beans, and processing or heat treatment in breakfast cereals. According to Gilani et al,[34] naturally occurring antinutritional factors that can interfere with protein digestion include glucosinolates in mustard and rapeseed protein products, trypsin inhibitors and hemagglutinins in legumes, tannins in legumes and cereals, and phytates in cereals and oilseeds. Differences in digestibility may also arise as a result of inherent differences in the way the amino acids in a protein are linked together. In addition, a variety of processing conditions, such as heat, oxidation, and the addition of organic solvents and acids, can all adversely affect digestion.[34-37] Table 3-1 shows that ready-to-eat wheat and rice cereals are digested less well than unprocessed

Table 3-1 Digestibility of Selected Diets and Individual Foods

Type of Diet/Food	Digestibility (%)
Diet	
North American, typical mixed diet	94
North American, lacto vegetarian	88
North American, lacto-ovo vegetarian	93
Brazil (rice, beans, meat, eggs, vegetables)	78
Guatemala (black beans, corn tortillas, rice, wheat rolls, cheese, eggs, vegetables)	77
India (rice, red gram dahl, milk powder, vegetables)	75
Food	
Oats, ready-to-eat cereals	72
Dried beans (various types)	75
Rice, ready-to-eat cereals	75
Wheat, ready-to-eat cereals	77
Soybeans	78
Soybean flour	86
Wheat, whole	87
Rice, polished	89
Bread, whole wheat	92
Meat poultry, fish, eggs, milk	95
Bread, white wheat	97

Source: Data from Sarwar G. Digestibility of protein and bioavailability of amino acids in foods. *World Rev Nutr Diet.* 1987;54:26–70.

wheat and rice. Vegetarian diets in particular may be high in components, such as fiber, that tend to decrease protein digestibility.[38]

There are two important methodological considerations regarding the evaluation of protein digestibility. One is that individual amino acids may not be as available or digestible as the total protein in a food.[39] For example, 90% of the total protein in wheat is digestible, but only 80% of the lysine is.[40] In fact, the bioavailability of individual amino acids may be up to 44% lower than the digestibility of protein in the same food.[41,42] Consequently, the overall digestibility of a protein may be an overestimate of the actual digestibility of the individual amino acids. In addition, protein digestibility may typically be overestimated because the impact of bacterial metabolism in the ileum is not considered.

To understand the potential impact of intestinal bacteria on estimates of protein digestibility requires some understanding of how digestibility is determined. Traditionally, protein digestibility has been determined by comparing the amount of nitrogen consumed with the amount of nitrogen excreted in the feces after correcting for endogenous nitrogen excretion. This approach is possible because on average protein is approximately 16% nitrogen on a weight basis. However, studies have demonstrated that bacteria in the colon metabolize and use some of the nitrogen or amino acids in the intestine which will decrease the amount of nitrogen excreted and therefore overestimate the amount retained. The FAO/WHO Expert Consultation on protein quality evaluation recognized this problem, as have many other protein experts who have called for the use of ileal digestibility, rather than fecal digestibility, for determining protein digestibility.[43] Since the publication of this report, it is accurate to say that support for measuring digestibility at the ileal rather than fecal level has increased.[1,44]

According to the WHO Technical Report Series 935 (2007),

> The concept of digestibility, usually defined in terms of the balance of amino acids across the small intestine (mouth to terminal ileum: ileal digestibility), or across the entire intestine (mouth to anus: faecal digestibility), is based on the principle that the difference between intake and losses provides a measure of the extent of digestion and absorption of food protein as amino acids by the gastrointestinal tract for use by the body. In fact, such net balance across the intestine involves considerable exchange of nitrogen in terms of protein, amino acids and urea between systemic pools and the gut lumen.[1]

Interestingly, some data suggest that the intestinal bacteria can actually contribute indispensable amino acids (IAA) to the dietary supply,[45 46] whereas other data suggest on average that amino acid losses due to bacterial metabolism/use may represent 5% of the total protein consumed. However, for plant protein sources that are poorly digested in the upper intestine and increase ileal nitrogen fermentation in the colon, loss of IAAs may be higher.[37] For example, Mariotti et al[47] found that milk or milk protein had a similar ileal digestibility (95%) compared with data from previous balance studies (95 ± 3% for milk), but ileal soy protein digestibility was slightly lower (91% vs 92–98%) than that seen in previous balance studies. Similarly, cooked egg proteins present a true ileal digestibility of 91%, whereas corrected fecal digestibility has been reported to be 97 ± 3%.

Finally, one other issue related to "digestion" may affect protein quality, at least in some circumstances. Within the past several years, research has suggested that the rate at which proteins (i.e., fast and slow digested proteins) are digested may affect the degree to which the amino acids formed upon digestion can be used systemically for protein synthesis, as opposed to being metabolized by the splanchnic bed (visceral or internal organs such as intestines).[48] Whether this issue relates primarily only to the degree to which muscle accretion occurs in response to resistance exercise in a relatively acute setting or also applies to sedentary individuals over the long term has yet to be determined. In any event, neither nitrogen absorption kinetics nor ileal digestibility has been adopted as part of the official assays for evaluating protein quality. It is likely this will remain the case for a considerable time.

Amino Acid Patterns

There is no biologic requirement for protein per se; rather the requirement is for amino acids and nitrogen. Of the 20 amino acids used for protein synthesis, 9 are considered indispensable. In relatively recent years, a new category has come into use in which the dispensable amino acids are broken into two classifications, truly dispensable and conditionally dispensable, the latter referring to amino acids whose synthesis could be limited under certain pathophysiologic conditions. The quality of a protein influences dietary protein requirements; consumption of low-quality proteins can increase overall protein requirements. Vegans derive all their protein from plant foods, lacto-ovo vegetarians (LOVs) approximately half from plant foods, and omnivores approximately a third. Therefore, the RDA for protein is not necessarily applicable to vegetarians.

Plant proteins tend to be limiting in one or more IAAs (Table 3-2); cereals are low in lysine and threonine, whereas legumes are low in the SAAs. Thus, if a given plant protein served as the sole source of protein and was consumed at the RDA level (0.8 g/kg bw) for total protein intake, with few exceptions neither individual grains nor beans would provide the required amount of one or more of the IAAs.

Proteins are considered to be "complete" if they supply all the IAAs necessary to meet biologic requirements when consumed at the recommended level of total protein intake. This terminology is a bit misleading, however, because with the exception of gelatin, all proteins contain all of the IAAs. Therefore, individual plant proteins can meet protein and amino acid needs. When lower quality proteins are consumed, more of the given protein must be consumed to meet amino acid requirements.

Historically, protein quality has been determined by the protein efficiency ratio (PER), nitrogen balance studies, or by chemical or amino acid score in which the amino acid pattern of a protein is compared to that of reference protein (egg protein), or more commonly, with the theoretical biologic requirements for IAAs. For quite some time, the PER was the official U.S. procedure for evaluating protein quality and was used for regulations regarding food labeling and for the protein RDA. The PER measures the growth of laboratory animals, most often rats, in response to a given amount of protein. Rats grow at a much faster rate than infants, however, and therefore they have a much higher protein requirement. Also, rats have different requirements for individual amino acids than humans. For certain amino acids, such as methionine, the rat requirement is a full 50% higher.[49] Because the limiting amino acid in beans is methionine, the value of legume protein has been underestimated by the use of the PER.

The limitations of the PER led the FAO/WHO[50] and the Food and Drug Administration[51] to adopt an alternative method, the protein digestibility corrected amino acid score (PDCAAS) as an official assay for evaluating protein quality. The PDCAAS reflects the amino acid score using amino acid requirements for all ages from ≥ 1 year corrected for digestibility. The PDCAAS is

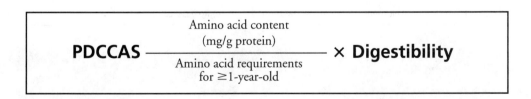

$$\text{PDCCAS} \quad \frac{\text{Amino acid content (mg/g protein)}}{\text{Amino acid requirements for } \geq 1\text{-year-old}} \times \textbf{Digestibility}$$

Table 3-2 Limiting Amino Acid Content of Legumes and Grains

Food 100 g edible portion	Lysine (mg/g protein)	Threonine (mg/g protein)	Sulfur amino acids (mg/g protein)	Database Identification number
Beans				
Adzuki beans	75.4	34.0	19.9	16002
Black beans	68.6	42.1	25.8	16015
Black-eyed peas	67.7	38.0	25.2	16063
Fava beans	63.9	35.5	20.9	16053
Garbanzo beans	66.9	37.2	26.5	16057
Great northern beans	68.7	42.1	25.9	16025
Kidney beans	70.0	36.8	22.4	16028
Lentils	69.8	35.8	21.6	16070
Lima beans	66.8	43.1	23.7	16072
Mung beans	69.8	32.7	20.8	16081
Navy beans	63.2	35.1	22.7	16038
Pinto beans	69.9	36.7	22.3	16043
Soybeans	68.6	42.1	25.9	16019
Split peas	72.2	35.5	25.4	16086
Grains				
Amaranth	55.1	41.1	30.7	20001
Barley (pearled)	37.7	34.0	41.1	2006
Buckwheat groats	50.9	38.2	30.2	2010
Bulgur	27.5	28.9	38.6	20013
Corn grits	32.5	43.9	45.5	08164
Couscous	19.2	26.4	43.3	20029
Oatmeal	53.1	37.8	56.3	08121
Quinoa	54.2	29.8	36.3	20035
Rice, brown	38.0	36.6	34.5	20041
Whole wheat bread	12.8	13.3	17.9	18075
Refined wheat flour	22.1	27.2	39.0	20080

Source: USDA National Nutrient Database for Standard Reference, Release 22, 2009.

primarily determined by the limiting amino acid because, as discussed, differences in digestibility among proteins tend to be relatively minor.

The PDCAAS has been criticized on several grounds, but it is considered to be an improvement over previous assays and is seen as a relatively accurate and quick way to determine protein quality.[52–54] One criticism is that proteins, such as egg protein, that give values or scores >100% (or 1) are truncated because they are rounded down to 100%.[1] This is because proteins are assessed for their ability to meet protein needs as the sole source of protein in the diet. In this situation, IAAs provided in excess of needs are not used for protein synthesis. However, humans consume mixed diets with proteins from different sources. Under such conditions, the ability of high-quality proteins to balance the amino acid pattern of a lower quality protein can be important.

For example, to meet the preschool age child's lysine requirement level of 52 mg/g mixed crude protein, it would take approximately 1.0 g of beef protein, 1.8 g cow's milk protein, 2.8 g of egg protein, or 6.2 g of soy protein to compensate for the low lysine content of 1 g of wheat protein. But each of these proteins receives a similar PDCAAS value. Thus truncated PDCAAS values do not provide information about the potency of a protein to balance lower quality proteins. Recommendations to reevaluate the practice of truncating scores downward to 100% have been made[55] and may be considered in the future by the WHO.[1]

The merits of the PDCAAS depend primarily on the extent to which the biologic requirements for IAAs can be accurately established. There is, however, considerable disagreement about lysine requirements in particular. These disagreements greatly impact perceptions about the ability of plant-based diets to meet protein requirements because lysine is the limiting amino acid in grains, and grains are the predominant source of protein in diets devoid of animal products.

In 1985, the FAO/WHO set the adult lysine requirement at 16 mg/g protein. However, researchers from the Massachusetts Institute of Technology (MIT) have argued for several years that the lysine requirements were far too low, recommending that the value be changed to 50 mg/g protein.[56] In 1991, the FAO/WHO decided to use the lysine value for preschool children as the standard for all age groups as an interim measure until more precise requirements could be established. Thus the lysine requirement for adults was changed from 16 mg/g to 58 mg/g protein. However, Millward et al[57] from the University of Surrey have suggested that the lysine requirement is only 31 mg/g protein, considerably less than the MIT and FAO/WHO values. They have argued that the lysine intakes of people in India, West Bengal, and even among vegetarians in the United Kingdom do not meet the higher lysine intake requirements despite any obvious problems in these populations. Nevertheless, in the 2007 report from the FAO/WHO, the lysine requirement for ages 1 to 2, 3 to 10, 11 to 14, 15 to 18, and >18 years was set at 52, 48, 48, 47, and 45, mg/g protein, respectively.[1] Recent data are supportive of these higher requirements and also indicate there is no adaptation to lysine needs in healthy men consuming diets providing markedly different amounts of lysine[58] nor by children in developing countries.[59] The longest adaptation period in the former study was only 7 days, leaving open the possibility that at least in adults some adaptation still may occur.

PLANT PROTEINS AND NITROGEN BALANCE

Until recently, nitrogen balance studies were considered the gold standard for evaluating protein quality and establishing amino acid requirements. However, methodological concerns caused these studies to fall into disfavor [60] and to be replaced by stable isotope methodologies and the indicator oxidation method in which the oxidation of an amino acid indicates when the requirement for an IAA has been met. There have been criticisms of this method,[37] but it is now very widely used.[61]

Nitrogen balance studies, not surprisingly, often show the quality of individual plant proteins to be inferior to that of animal proteins. For example, Young and colleagues from MIT found that to maintain nitrogen balance in 16 young men, twice as much wheat protein as beef protein (178 vs 96 mg of nitrogen/kg bw) was required.[62] Similarly, about 35% more rice protein than egg protein was required to achieve nitrogen balance in young men (0.87 vs 0.65 g/kg).[63] But because of the high quality of soybean protein, similar amounts of protein from soy and cow's milk[64,65] or beef[65] were required to maintain nitrogen balance.

However, in contrast to the findings of Young and colleagues, the Michigan State University Bread Study, conducted three decades ago, found that when college students were fed diets for 50 days that provided 70 g (essentially the RDA) of protein per day, 90–95% of which was derived from wheat flour, with the remaining protein coming from fruits and vegetables, subjects were in nitrogen balance.[66] Several other studies,[67–70] although not all,[71] have also found that subjects were able to achieve nitrogen balance when fed wheat protein as well as potato protein,[72,73] corn protein,[74] and rice protein[75,76] despite the fact that lysine intakes were much less than the requirement established by the IOM/FNB.[30,61,77,78]

The studies just cited suggesting that the ability of plant proteins to meet protein requirements has been underestimated may account for the lack of protein deficiency in the Middle East, where at one time bread provided 70–95% of the calories in the diet.[79,80] It has been suggested that these observations indicate there is an inherent ability of humans to adapt to low protein intakes.

Adaptation to Low Protein Intakes

Adaptation is defined as a purposive response to a new feeding circumstance that results in a functional state that is better suited to the changed situation.[81] In adults who are maintaining weight and in nitrogen balance, the need for amino acids is determined by three components: (1) net protein synthesis (repletion of postabsorptive losses and any growth), (2) irreversible amino acid conversion into essential metabolites, and (3) oxidative catabolism of amino acids at a rate that varies with habitual protein intake and occurs continually throughout the day.[82,83] Humans have an impressive ability to modulate this third component over a wide range of intakes such that there is little actual difference in protein turnover with different levels of protein intake, although maximal adaptation may take several months.

A fairly immediate physiologic response to conserve body protein when challenged with a low protein intake is to reduce the rate at which individual amino acids are catabolized.[84] In rats, splanchnic amino acid catabolism appears to be a major adaptive response to an increase in the protein content of the diet.[85,86] Of particular interest is the finding that in rats, the catabolism of lysine is decreased by as much as 50% in response to a lysine-deficient diet.[87] The ability to reuse the nitrogen from the catabolism of amino acids is also enhanced when protein is in short supply.[88] This flexibility allows the body to adapt to different levels of protein intake. It is well known that in malnourished children, protein catabolism and synthesis are slowed.[89] Noted nutrition researcher D. M. Hegsted stated, "If the requirement of any nutrient is to be defined, the subjects must be allowed the time to adapt. Otherwise one simply estimates the nutrient supply in the current diet, which has little nutritional significance."[69]

As noted previously, Millward et al[57] found that the efficiency of wheat protein utilization is much higher than would be expected if the lysine requirements used by IOM/FNB are correct. They noted that there is a large intracellular pool of lysine compared to other IAAs, which can be tapped for protein synthesis upon feeding to compensate for the lower lysine content of a food or meal[90] and that lysine is not oxidized nearly as quickly as other amino acids.[91] Interestingly, the previously referred to Michigan State University Bread Study, which found that wheat protein was able to meet protein requirements, was considerably longer (70 d) than is typical for nitrogen balance studies. Short-term studies may fail to allow for adaptation to low-protein diets and therefore may overestimate protein needs. In fact, subjects in the Michigan State Bread Study were actually in negative nitrogen balance during the first 2 weeks of the study but gradually entered into nitrogen balance by the end of the 70 days of feeding.[66]

Clearly, some form of adaptation occurs, although there is concern that chronic low protein intakes will result in subtle adverse effects; that is, the level of protein and individual amino acids in these diets may be sufficient for one to survive but not necessarily to thrive.[78] The question of whether humans can adequately adapt to low protein intakes without any ill effects is one that warrants further research according to the WHO.[1] In any event, it does appear that plant proteins support protein needs better than commonly perceived. Furthermore, because vegetarians in Western countries consume a variety of plant protein foods, requirements can be met with ease on diets that contain no animal products. According to the WHO, despite somewhat higher amino acid requirement values for adults established in 2007, "mixtures of cereal proteins with relatively modest amounts of legumes or oil seeds . . . are unlikely to be limited through their amino acid content."[1] Protein complementarity is one factor that enhances the protein quality of foods.

PROTEIN COMPLEMENTARITY

Historically, recommendations were to combine complementary proteins at each meal to ensure adequate protein intake on vegetarian diets. But since 1993, the American Dietetic Association has concluded that this practice is unnecessary.[92] According to the 2009 position paper on vegetarian diets, "Research indicates that an assortment of plant foods eaten over the course of a day can provide all essential amino acids and ensure adequate nitrogen retention and use in healthy adults; thus, complementary proteins do not need to be consumed at the same meal."[93]

Experts in protein nutrition concur with this conclusion, although recommendations for children may be less flexible.[30,84] These less restrictive guidelines take into consideration the contribution of the pool of IAAs that is maintained by the body, as noted previously.[94,95] This reserve provides free amino acids that can be used to complement dietary proteins. This pool of amino acids comes from as many as four sources.[96,98]

- Enzymes secreted into the intestine to digest proteins
- Intestinal cells sloughed off into the intestine
- Intracellular spaces of the skeletal musculature
- Synthesis of amino acids by intestinal microflora

These four sources may be quite significant. In fact, the amount of endogenous protein present in the gut may be much greater than the amount of protein ingested, but this is a matter of debate.[99] Also, it has been estimated that within 3 hours after a protein-rich meal, as much as 60% of the adult daily requirement for lysine may be deposited in the intracellular spaces of the skeletal musculature.[30,90] Consequently, if one were to consume at one sitting a meal composed primarily of beans, which are high in lysine, there would be plenty of stored lysine to be used for protein synthesis if a meal comprising primarily grains was consumed later in the day. As a result, complementary plant proteins can still combine to produce proteins of a higher quality even when they are not consumed at the same time.

Animal studies first demonstrating the benefits of protein complementarity were conducted some 60 years ago.[100,101] These studies and others[102] suggest that feeding complementary proteins between 10 hours and 1 day apart does not promote growth in comparison with feeding these proteins simultaneously, whereas complementary effects were observed when rats were fed complementary proteins (rice and mung beans) approximately 5 hours apart.[103] However, in rats fed a lysine-deficient mixture of protein and amino acids, a lysine supplement given 12 hours later was used as effectively as was lysine given with a balanced meal. In contrast, tryptophan was not utilized as well when fed 12 hours later.[104] The timing of consumption to derive the benefits of complementary amino acid patterns in humans in particular is still not well understood. In children, the benefits of adding beans to a corn diet were somewhat less when the supplement was given at intervals of >6 hours.[30]

Although many questions about combining complementary proteins remain unresolved, they may be of little practical significance. Populations consuming largely plant-based diets tend to eat complementary proteins at the same meal as part of their normal eating pattern. Examples include rice and soybean products in Asian countries, chick peas and sesame tahini in Middle Eastern countries, and pinto beans and corn tortillas in Latin American countries. Furthermore, although combining proteins can reduce the amount of dietary protein required to meet biologic requirements,[105–107] adults can meet IAA requirements by eating plant foods, even if those foods do not complement one another. Protein combining may be of significance for infants, however, but because infants eat more frequently than adults, some complementary effects are likely to occur even without conscious effort toward combining proteins at each meal.

Infants and young children do have higher protein needs on a bw basis. The average requirement for infants 6 months of age and children age 2 and 5 years, is 1.12, 0.79, and 0.69 g/kg per day, respectively. The energy requirements of infants are also higher on a bw basis. Even so, infants have very high IAA requirements relative to adults when expressed per gram of protein required; in fact, total IAA needs (mg/g protein) according to IOM/FNB decrease with age from 378 for infants 6 months old to 277 for adults.

PROTEIN NEEDS OF VEGETARIANS

Other than allowances for the somewhat lower digestibility of plant proteins, there appears to be little reason to think that protein intake should be increased on vegetarian diets.[1] In a meta-analysis published in 2003 that involved 235 individual subjects from 19 studies, the median estimated average requirement of nitrogen was found to be similar whether the dietary protein was from animal, vegetable, or mixed protein sources.[108] In most cases, the experimental diets that were characterized as vegetable included complementary mixtures of vegetable proteins such as corn and beans, and rice and beans, or good quality soy protein. There is little reason for any adjustment for LOVs who derive a substantial portion of their protein from animal sources. However, if one wants to err on the conservative side, a reasonable adjustment to the current RDA value for adults, allowing for the lower digestibility and perhaps the somewhat poorer amino acid pattern of plant proteins, would be about a 25% increase for some vegans to 1.0 g of protein per kg/bw.

Although this value is consistent with the results of some nitrogen balance studies involving plant-based diets, the higher figure is only relevant to vegans consuming plant proteins with a very low digestibility—mainly beans or harshly processed proteins—or who might not consume a diet composed of a variety of different protein sources.[109–111] This higher level of protein results in a diet that derives approximately 10% of its calories from protein. Both LOVs and vegans consume diets that typically contain at least this amount (Appendix A). Of course, protein recommendations assume an adequate caloric intake. Energy intake positively influences nitrogen retention; in fact, studies have shown that the consumption of excess calories (700 to 1000 excess calories per day) reduces the amount of protein required to achieve nitrogen balance by approximately 30% and 50% for animal and plant proteins, respectively.[63] The notion that strictly plant-based diets can adequately meet protein is not new. In 1946, based on a series of nitrogen balance studies, Hegsted et al concluded "it is most unlikely that protein deficiency will develop in apparently healthy adults on a diet in which cereals and vegetables supply adequate calories."[112]

In setting the most recent RDA for protein, no allowance for work or training was made. It was believed that the margin of safety included in the protein RDA and marked disagreements among experts about the effect of physical activity on protein requirements precluded any need to recommend increased protein intakes for athletes. However, the joint position of the Canadian and American Dietetic Associations, published in 2009, is that protein recommendations for endurance and strength-trained athletes range from 1.2 to 1.7 g/kg bw.[113] The associations noted that these recommended protein intakes can generally be met through diet alone, without the use of protein or amino acid supplements. In addition, because protein digestibility of a vegetarian diet may be reduced by 10%, they recommended increasing protein intake by that amount to 1.3 to 1.8 g/kg bw for vegetarian athletes.

In general, protein should be an issue of little concern to vegetarians. Protein needs are easily met when the diet includes a variety of plant foods and calorie intake is adequate. The protein intake of vegetarians, even with slightly elevated needs, is adequate. As noted in Table 3-3, with the exception of fruits many plant foods are high in protein when expressed on a caloric basis. In fact, because of the high fat content of animal foods, on a caloric basis, many plant foods are actually higher in protein than animal products, such as regular ground beef and whole milk.

In their position paper published in 2007, the International Society of Sports Nutrition also concluded athletes require more protein, recommending intakes of 1.4 to 2.0 g/kg bw.[114] In addition, they also acknowledged that it is possible to obtain this much protein through a varied regular diet; however, they noted that supplemental protein in various forms is a practical way of ensuring adequate and quality protein intake for athletes. Finally, they concluded that the superiority of one protein type over another in terms of optimizing recovery and/or training adaptations remains to be convincingly demonstrated but that appropriately timed protein intake is an important component of an overall exercise training program, essential for proper recovery, immune function, and the growth and maintenance of lean body mass.

Table 3-3 Protein Content of Selected Plant Foods

Food	Kcal	Protein (g) per serving	Protein (% of kcal)
Brown rice, cooked, 1 cup	216	5.0	9
White rice, cooked 1 cup	205	4.25	8
Barley, pearled, cooked, 1 cup	193	3.5	7
Quinoa, cooked, 1 cup	222	8.4	15
Garbanzo beans, cooked, 1 cup	269	14.5	21
Lentils	230	18.0	31
Lima beans, cooked, 1 cup	216	14.6	27
Tofu, firm, ½ cup	183	20.0	44
Tofu, soft, ½ cup	151	16.2	43
Soymilk, 1 cup	109	7.1	26
Peanuts, ¼ cup	214	8.6	16
Sunflower seeds, 2 tbsp	93	3.0	13
Broccoli, raw, 1 cup	31	2.6	33
Carrots, raw, 1 medium	25	0.57	9
Green beans, cooked, 1 cup	44	2.36	21
Bread, whole wheat, 1 slice	69	3.6	20
Apple, raw with skin, 1 medium	95	0.47	2

Source: USDA National Nutrient Database for Standard Reference, Release 22, 2009.

If an athlete chooses to increase protein intake, it can be done without much additional planning on a vegetarian diet. You can see this point by again using a 30-year-old man as an example. He would need only 75 g (300 kcal) protein per day assuming a requirement of 1.5 g protein/kg bw. If intense exercise led to an additional energy expenditure of 1000 kcal/day, it would be necessary to consume a diet that was only about 8% (2883 plus 1000 kcal/300) protein. Because strength athletes expend fewer calories for exercise, their diets needs to be a little higher in protein as a percentage of calories, but these needs are still easily met. For example, if the same 30-year-old man carried an additional 20 kg of muscle, and expended only an additional 750 calories per day, to meet protein requirements the diet would need (4544/500) to be 9% protein.

COUNSELING POINTS: PROTEIN

Research suggests that the protein quality of grains and beans is good and that protein needs are easily met on vegetarian and vegan diets. The following points can help vegetarians to plan diets that meet protein needs.

- Consume adequate calories to maintain a healthful weight. Vegetarians who consume low-calorie diets may need to make a conscious effort to include high protein foods, like soy-foods, in their diet to meet protein needs.
- Although vegetarians have slightly higher protein needs because plant proteins are less well digested, these needs are easily met on vegetarian diets that provide adequate calories and a variety of foods. Research shows that LOVs and vegans meet protein needs.
- The terms *complete protein* and *incomplete protein* exaggerate the differences in quality between animal and plant proteins. Plant proteins contain all of the indispensable amino acids.
- Conscious combining of foods at meals is not necessary for adults to meet protein needs. It is important to eat a variety of plant proteins throughout the day; eat whole grains and legumes every day.
- Young children may benefit from consuming grains and legumes or legumes and nuts at the same meal (Chapter 13).

REFERENCES

1. World Health Organization. Protein and amino acid requirements in human nutrition. World Technical Series 935, Report of a Joint WHO/FAO/UNU Expert Consultation, United Nations University, 2007, Geneva.
2. Carpenter KJ. The history of enthusiasm for protein. *J Nutr.* 1986;116:1364–1370.
3. Sukahatme PV. Size and nature of the protein gap. *Nutr Rev.* 1970;28:223–226.
4. McLester JS. *Nutrition and Diet in Health and Disease.* Philadelphia, PA: Saunders; 1939.
5. World Health Organization (WHO). Diet, Nutrition, and the Prevention of Chronic Diseases (Technical Report Series 797). Geneva, Switzerland: WHO; 1990.
6. Friel S, Dangour AD, Garnett T, et al. Public health benefits of strategies to reduce greenhouse-gas emissions: food and agriculture. *Lancet.* 2009;374:2016–2025.
7. Marlow HJ, Hayes WK, Soret S, Carter RL, Schwab ER, Sabate J. Diet and the environment: does what you eat matter? *Am J Clin Nutr.* 2009;89:1699S–1703S.

8. Carlsson-Kanyama A, Gonzalez AD. Potential contributions of food consumption patterns to climate change. *Am J Clin Nutr.* 2009;89:1704S–1709S.

9. Barzel US. The skeleton as an ion exchange system: implications for the role of acid-base imbalance in the genesis of osteoporosis. *J Bone Miner Res.* 1995;10:1431–1436.

10. King AJ, Levey AS. Dietary protein and renal function. *J Am Soc Nephrol.* 1993;3:1723–1737.

11. Visek WJ, Clinton SK, Truex CR. Nutrition and experimental carcinogenesis. *Cornell Vet.* 1978;68:3–39.

12. Kerstetter JE. Dietary protein and bone: a new approach to an old question. *Am J Clin Nutr.* 2009;90:1451–1452.

13. Fenton TR, Lyon AW, Eliasziw M, Tough SC, Hanley DA. Meta-analysis of the effect of the acid-ash hypothesis of osteoporosis on calcium balance. *J Bone Miner Res.* 2009;24:1835–1840.

14. Roughead ZK, Hunt JR, Johnson LK, Badger TM, Lykken GI. Controlled substitution of soy protein for meat protein: effects on calcium retention, bone, and cardiovascular health indices in postmenopausal women. *J Clin Endocrinol Metab.* 2005;90:181–189.

15. Darling AL, Millward DJ, Torgerson DJ, Hewitt CE, Lanham-New SA. Dietary protein and bone health: a systematic review and meta-analysis. *Am J Clin Nutr.* 2009;90:1674–1692.

16. Wengreen HJ, Munger RG, Cutler DR, Corcoran CD, Zhang J, Sassano NE. Dietary protein intake and risk of osteoporotic hip fracture in elderly residents of Utah. *J Bone Miner Res.* 2004;19:537–545.

17. Knight EL, Stampfer MJ, Hankinson SE, Spiegelman D, Curhan GC. The impact of protein intake on renal function decline in women with normal renal function or mild renal insufficiency. *Ann Intern Med.* 2003;138:460–467.

18. Astrup A. The satiating power of protein—a key to obesity prevention? *Am J Clin Nutr.* 2005;82:1–2.

19. Weigle DS, Breen PA, Matthys CC, et al. A high-protein diet induces sustained reductions in appetite, ad libitum caloric intake, and body weight despite compensatory changes in diurnal plasma leptin and ghrelin concentrations. *Am J Clin Nutr.* 2005;82:41–48.

20. Wolfe RR. The underappreciated role of muscle in health and disease. *Am J Clin Nutr.* 2006;84:475–482.

21. Gaffney-Stomberg E, Insogna KL, Rodriguez NR, Kerstetter JE. Increasing dietary protein requirements in elderly people for optimal muscle and bone health. *J Am Geriatr Soc.* 2009;57:1073–1079.

22. Paddon-Jones D, Rasmussen BB. Dietary protein recommendations and the prevention of sarcopenia. *Curr Opin Clin Nutr Metab Care.* 2009;12:86–90.

23. IOM/FNB (Istitute of Medicine/Food and Nutrition Board). *Dietary Reference Intakes for Energy, Carbohydrate, Fiber, Fat, Protein and Amino Acids. A Report of the Panel on Micronutrients, Subcommittee on Upper Reference Levels of Nutrients and Interpretation and Uses of Dietary Reference Intakes and the Standing Committee on the Scientific Evaluation of Dietary Reference Intakes* [uncorrected prepublication version]. Washington, DC: The National Academy Press; 2002.

24. Strohle A, Hahn A, Sebastian A. Estimation of the diet-dependent net acid load in 229 worldwide historically studied hunter-gatherer societies. *Am J Clin Nutr.* 2010;91:406–412.

25. Eaton SB, Konner MJ, Cordain L. Diet-dependent acid load, Paleolithic nutrition, and evolutionary health promotion. *Am J Clin Nutr.* 2010;91:295–297.

26. Kerstetter JE, O'Brien KO, Insogna KL. Low protein intake: the impact on calcium and bone homeostasis in humans. *J Nutr.* 2003;133:855S–861S.

27. Fulgoni VL 3rd. Current protein intake in America: analysis of the National Health and Nutrition Examination Survey, 2003–2004. *Am J Clin Nutr.* 2008;87:1554S–1557S.

28. FAO Statistical Databases—Food Balance Sheets, 2000. http://apps.fao.org/default.htm.

29. Smit E, Nieto FJ, Crespo CJ, Mitchell P. Estimates of animal and plant protein intake in US adults: results from the Third National Health and Nutrition Examination Survey, 1988–1991. *J Am Diet Assoc.* 1999;99:813–820.

30. Young VR, Pellett PL. Plant proteins in relation to human protein and amino acid nutrition. *Am J Clin Nutr.* 1994;59:1203S–1212S.

31. Rosegrant MW, Leach N, Gerpacio RV. Alternative futures for world cereal and meat consumption. *Proc Nutr Soc.* 1999;58:219–234.

32. Young VR, Pellett PL. Current concepts conerning amino acid needs in adults and their implications for international nutrition planning. *Food Nutr Bull.* 1990;12:289–300.

33. World Health Organization. Joint Food and Agricultural Organization/World Health Organization/United Nations University Expert Consultation. Geneva, Switzerland; 1985. World Health Organization Technical Report Series 724.

34. Gilani GS, Cockell KA, Sepehr E. Effects of antinutritional factors on protein digestibility and amino acid availability in foods. *J AOAC Int.* 2005;88:967–987.
35. Sarwar G, L'Abbe MR, Trick K, Botting HG, Ma CY. Influence of feeding alkaline/heat processed proteins on growth and protein and mineral status of rats. *Adv Exp Med Biol.* 1999;459:161–177.
36. Graham GG, Morales E, Placko RP, MacLean WC Jr. Nutritive value of brown and black beans for infants and small children. *Am J Clin Nutr.* 1979;32:2362–2366.
37. Millward DJ. The nutritional value of plant-based diets in relation to human amino acid and protein requirements. *Proc Nutr Soc.* 1999;58:249–260.
38. Acosta PB. Availability of essential amino acids and nitrogen in vegan diets. *Am J Clin Nutr.* 1988;48:868–874.
39. Sarwar G, Peace RW. Comparisons between true digestibility of total nitrogen and limiting amino acids in vegetable proteins fed to rats. *J Nutr.* 1986;116:1172–1184.
40. Eggum BO. Digestibility of plant proteins: animal studies. In: Finley JW, Hopkins DT, eds. *Digestibility and Amino Acid Availability of Cereals and Oilseeds.* St. Paul, MN: American Association of Cereal Chemists; 1985:275–283.
41. Sarwar G. The protein digestibility-corrected amino acid score method overestimates quality of proteins containing antinutritional factors and of poorly digestible proteins supplemented with limiting amino acids in rats. *J Nutr.* 1997;127:758–764.
42. Eggum BO, Hansen I, Larsen T. Protein quality and digestible energy of selected foods determined in balance trials with rats. *Plant Foods Hum Nutr.* 1989;39:13–21.
43. Schaafsma G. The protein digestibility-corrected amino acid score. *J Nutr.* 2000;130:1865S–1867S.
44. Deglaire A, Bos C, Tome D, Moughan PJ. Ileal digestibility of dietary protein in the growing pig and adult human. *Br J Nutr.* 2009;102:1752–1759.
45. Bingham SA. Urine nitrogen as an independent validatory measure of protein intake. *Br J Nutr.* 1997;77:144–148.
46. Gibson NR, Ah-Sing E, Badalloo A, Forrester T, Jackson A, Millward DJ. Transfer of 15N from urea to the circulating dispensible and indispensible amino acid pool in the human infant. *Proc Nutr Soc.* 1997;56:79A.
47. Mariotti F, Mahe S, Benamouzig R, et al. Nutritional value of [15N]-soy protein isolate assessed from ileal digestibility and postprandial protein utilization in humans. *J Nutr.* 1999;129:1992–1997.
48. Fouillet H, Juillet B, Gaudichon C, Mariotti F, Tome D, Bos C. Absorption kinetics are a key factor regulating postprandial protein metabolism in response to qualitative and quantitative variations in protein intake. *Am J Physiol Regul Integr Comp Physiol.* 2009;297:R1691–R1705.
49. Sarwar G, Peace RW, Botting HG. Corrected relative net protein ratio (CRNPR) method based on differences in rat and human requirements for sulfur amino acids. *J Am Oil Chem Soc.* 1985;68:68:689–693.
50. Food and Agricultural Organization (FAO). *Protein Quality Evaluation.* Rome, Italy: FAO; 1990.
51. Henley EC, Kuster JM. Protein quality evaluation by protein digestibility-corrected amino acid scoring. *Food Technol.* 1994;48:74–77.
52. Schaafsma G. The Protein Digestibility-Corrected Amino Acid Score (PDCAAS)—a concept for describing protein quality in foods and food ingredients: a critical review. *J AOAC Int.* 2005;88:988–994.
53. Sarwar G, Peace RW. The protein quality of some enteral products is inferior to that of casein as assessed by rat growth methods and digestibility-corrected amino acid scores [see comments]. *J Nutr.* 1994;124:2223–2232.
54. Sarwar G, Peace RW. Protein quality of enteral nutritionals: a response to Young. *J Nutr.* 1995;125:1365–1366.
55. Reeds P, Schaafsma G, Tome D, Young V. Criteria and significance of dietary protein sources in humans. Summary of the workshop with recommendations. *J Nutr.* 2000;130:1874S–1876S.
56. Young VR, el-Khoury AE. Can amino acid requirements for nutritional maintenance in adult humans be approximated from the amino acid composition of body mixed proteins? *Proc Natl Acad Sci U S A.* 1995;92:300–304.
57. Millward DJ, Fereday A, Gibson NR, Pacy PJ. Human adult amino acid requirements: [1–13C] leucine balance evaluation of the efficiency of utilization and apparent requirements for wheat protein and lysine compared with those for milk protein in healthy adults. *Am J Clin Nutr.* 2000;72:112–121.
58. Elango R, Humayun MA, Ball RO, Pencharz PB. Indicator amino acid oxidation is not affected by period of adaptation to a wide range of lysine intake in healthy young men. *J Nutr.* 2009;139:1082–1087.
59. Pillai RR, Elango R, Muthayya S, Ball RO, Kurpad AV, Pencharz PB. Lysine requirement of healthy, school-aged Indian children determined by the indicator amino acid oxidation technique. *J Nutr.* 2010;140:54–59.

60. Young VR. Nutritional balance studies: indicators of human requirements or of adaptive mechanisms? *J Nutr.* 1986;116:700–703.
61. Elango R, Ball RO, Pencharz PB. Indicator amino acid oxidation: concept and application. *J Nutr.* 2008;138:243–246.
62. Young VR, Fajardo L, Murray E, Rand WM, Scrimshaw NS. Protein requirements of man: comparative nitrogen balance response within the submaintenance-to-maintenance range of intakes of wheat and beef proteins. *J Nutr.* 1975;105:534–542.
63. Inoue G, Fujita Y, Niiyama Y. Studies on protein requirements of young men fed egg protein and rice protein with excess and maintenance energy intakes. *J Nutr.* 1973;103:1673–1687.
64. Scrimshaw NS, Wayler AH, Murray E, Steinke FH, Rand WM, Young VR. Nitrogen balance response in young men given one of two isolated soy proteins or milk proteins. *J Nutr.* 1983;113:2492–2497.
65. Wayler A, Queiroz E, Scrimshaw NS, Steinke FH, Rand WM, Young VR. Nitrogen balance studies in young men to assess the protein quality of an isolated soy protein in relation to meat proteins. *J Nutr.* 1983;113:2485–2491.
66. Bolourchi S, Friedemann CM, Mickelsen O. Wheat flour as a source of protein for adult human subjects. *Am J Clin Nutr.* 1968;21:827–835.
67. Edwards CH, Booker LK, Rumph CH, Wright WG, Ganapathy SN. Utilization of wheat by adult man: nitrogen metabolism, plasma amino acids and lipids. *Am J Clin Nutr.* 1971;24:181–193.
68. Begum A, Radhakrishnan AN, Pereira SM. Effect of amino acid composition of cereal-based diets on growth of pre-school children. *Am J Clin Nutr.* 1970;23:1175–1183.
69. Hegsted DM, Trulson MF, Stare FJ. Role of wheat and wheat products in human nutrition. *Physiol Rev.* 1954; 34:221–258.
70. Widdowson EM, McCance RA. *Studies on the Nutritive Value of Bread and on the Effect of Variation in the Extraction Rate of Flour on Growth of Undernourished Children* Special Report Series 287. London, UK: Medical Research Council; 1954.
71. Fujita Y, Yamamoto T, Rikimaru T, Inoue G. Effect of low protein diets on free amino acids in plasma of young men: effect of wheat gluten diet. *J Nutr Sci Vitaminol.* 1979;25:427–439.
72. Markakis P. The nutritive quality of potato protein. In: Friedman M, ed. *Protein Nutritional Quality of Foods and Feeds.* New York, NY: Dekker; 1975:471–487.
73. Kon SK, Kleen A. The value of whole potato protein in human nutrition. *Biochem J.* 1928;22:258.
74. Clark HE, Allen PE, Meyers SM, Tuckett SE, Yamamura Y. Nitrogen balances of adults consuming opaque-2 maize protein. *Am J Clin Nutr.* 1967;20:825–833.
75. Lee CJ, Howe JM, Carlson K, Clark HE. Nitrogen retention of young men fed rice with or without supplementary chicken. *Am J Clin Nutr.* 1971;24:318–323.
76. Clark HE, Howe JM, Lee CJ. Nitrogen retention of adult human subjects fed a high protein rice. *Am J Clin Nutr.* 1971;24:324–328.
77. Young VR, Bier DM, Pellett PL. A theoretical basis for increasing current estimates of the amino acid requirements in adult man, with experimental support [see comments]. *Am J Clin Nutr.* 1989;50:80–92.
78. Young VR, Marchini JS. Mechanisms and nutritional significance of metabolic responses to altered intakes of protein and amino acids, with reference to nutritional adaptation in humans. *Am J Clin Nutr.* 1990;51:270–289.
79. Browe JH, Butts JS, Youmans P. A nutrition survey of the armed forces of Iran. *Am J Clin Nutr.* 1961;9:478–514.
80. Pelshenke PF. Bread as a daily food. *Cereal Sci Today.* 1961;7:325.
81. Waterlow JC. What do we mean by adaptation? In: Baxter K, Waterlow JC, eds. *Nutritional Adaptation in Man.* London, UK: John Libbey; 1985:1–11.
82. Millward DJ. Optimal intakes of protein in the human diet. *Proc Nutr Soc.* 1999;58:403–413.
83. Millward DJ. An adaptive metabolic demand model for protein and amino acid requirements. *Br J Nutr.* 2003; 90:249–260.
84. Young VR, Pellett PL. Protein intake and requirements with reference to diet and health. *Am J Clin Nutr.* 1987; 45:1323–1343.
85. Morens C, Gaudichon C, Metges CC, et al. A high-protein meal exceeds anabolic and catabolic capacities in rats adapted to a normal protein diet. *J Nutr.* 2000;130:2312–2321.
86. Jean C, Rome S, Mathé V, et al. Metabolic evidence for adaptation to a high protein diet in rats. *J Nutr.* 2000; 131:91–98.

87. Yamashita K, Ashida K. Lysine metabolism in rats fed lysine-free diet. *J Nutr.* 1969;99:267–273.

88. Langran M, Moran BJ, Murphy JL, Jackson AA. Adaptation to a diet low in protein: effect of complex carbohydrate upon urea kinetics in normal man. *Clin Sci (Colch).* 1992;82:191–198.

89. Young VR, Scrimshaw NS. Human protein and amino acid metabolism and requirements in relation to protein quality. In: Bodwell CE, ed. *Evaluation of Proteins for Humans.* Westport, CT: AVI; 1977:11–54.

90. Bergstrom J, Furst P, Vinnars E. Effect of a test meal, without and with protein, on muscle and plasma free amino acids. *Clin Sci (Colch).* 1990;79:331–337.

91. Millward DJ, Rivers JP. The nutritional role of indispensable amino acids and the metabolic basis for their requirements. *Eur J Clin Nutr.* 1988;42:367–393.

92. Havala S, Dwyer J. Position of the American Dietetic Association: vegetarian diets [published erratum appears in *J Am Diet Assoc.* 1994;94(1):19]. *J Am Diet Assoc.* 1993;93:1317–1319.

93. Craig WJ, Mangels AR. Position of the American Dietetic Association: vegetarian diets. *J Am Diet Assoc.* 2009; 109:1266–1282.

94. Nasset ES. Amino acid homeostasis in the gut lumen and its nutritional significance. *World Rev Nutr Diet.* 1972; 14:134–153.

95. Nasset ES. Role of the digestive tract in the utilization of protein and amino acids. *JAMA.* 1957;164:172–177.

96. Fuller MF, Reeds PJ. Nitrogen cycling in the gut. *Annu Rev Nutr.* 1998;18:385–411.

97. Badaloo A, Boyne M, Reid M, et al. Dietary protein, growth and urea kinetics in severely malnourished children and during recovery. *J Nutr.* 1999;129:969–979.

98. Millward DJ, Forrester T, Ah-Sing E, et al. The transfer of 15N from urea to lysine in the human infant. *Br J Nutr.* 2000;83:505–512.

99. Nassett ES, Ju JS. Mixture of endogenous and exogenous protein in the alimentary tract. *J Nutr.* 1961;74:461–465.

100. Geiger E. The role of the time factor in feeding supplementary proteins. *J Nutr.* 1948;36:813–819.

101. Henry KM, Kon SK. The supplementary relationships between the proteins of dairy products and those of bread and potato as affected by the method of feeding. With a note on the value of soya bean protein. *J Dairy Res.* 1946;14:330–339.

102. Mills EB, Canolty NL. Role of the time factor in protein complementation. *Nutr Rep Int.* 1984;30:311–322.

103. Sanchez A, Hernado I, Shavlik GW, Register UD, Hubbard RW, Burke KI. Complementation of proteins from one meal to the next. *Nutr Res.* 1987;7:629–635.

104. Yang SP, Tilton KS, Ryland LL. Utilization of a delayed lysine or tryptophan supplement for protein repletion of rats. *J Nutr.* 1968;94:178–184.

105. Chick H. Nutritive value of a vegetable protein and its enhancement by admixture. *Br J Nutr.* 1951;5:261–265.

106. Bressani R, Elias LG, Gomez Brenes RA. Improvement of protein quality by amino acid and protein supplementation. In: Bigwood EJ, ed. *Protein and Amino Acid Functions.* Oxford, UK: Pergamon; 1972:475–540.

107. Bricker M, Mitchell HH, Kinsman GM. The protein requirements of adult human subjects in terms of the protein contained in individual foods and food combinations. *J Nutr.* 1945;30:269–283.

108. Rand WM, Pellett PL, Young VR. Meta-analysis of nitrogen balance studies for estimating protein requirements in healthy adults. *Am J Clin Nutr.* 2003;77:109–127.

109. Agarwal DK, Agarwal KN, Shankar R, Bhatia BD, Mishra KP, Tripathi BN. Determination of protein requirements of vegetarian diet in healthy female volunteers. *Indian J Med Res.* 1984;79:60–67.

110. Yanez E, Uauy R, Zacarias I, Barrera G. Long-term validation of 1 g of protein per kilogram body weight from a predominantly vegetable mixed diet to meet the requirements of young adult males. *J Nutr.* 1986;116:865–872.

111. Patwardhan VN, Mukundan R, Rama Sastri BV. Studies in protein metabolism. The influence of dietary protein on the urinary nitrogen excretion. *Indian J Med Res.* 1949;37:327–346.

112. Hegsted DM, Tsongas AG, Abbott DB, Stare FJ. Protein requirements of adults. *J Lab Clin Med.* 1946;31:261–284.

113. Rodriguez NR, Di Marco NM, Langley S. American College of Sports Medicine position stand. Nutrition and athletic performance. *Med Sci Sports Exerc.* 2009;41:709–731.

114. Campbell B, Kreider RB, Ziegenfuss T, et al. International Society of Sports Nutrition position stand: protein and Exercise. *J Int Soc Sports Nutr.* 2007;4:8.

CHAPTER 4

Fats

In comparison to nonvegetarians, on average vegetarians have lower intakes of total fat and saturated fat, and similar or higher intakes of linoleic acid (LA, 18:2n-6) and alpha-linolenic acid (ALA, 18:3n-3).[1] These dietary differences may explain the typically lower serum cholesterol levels of vegetarians. However, concerns have been raised about the lack of long-chain omega-3 polyunsaturated fatty acids (PUFA), eicosapentaenoic acid (EPA, 20:5n-3), and docosahexaenoic acid (DHA, 22:6n-3), found primarily in certain types of cold-water fatty fish, in vegetarian diets. EPA and DHA have potential protective effects against a number of conditions including sudden cardiac death, Alzheimer's disease, and osteoporosis. Studies of neuronal functioning and visual acuity suggest that consumption of DHA may provide some advantage for infants; this may be an important benefit of breastfeeding because breast milk contains more DHA than unfortified infant formula. This chapter focuses on the essential fatty acids LA and ALA, and on EPA and DHA.

LA AND ALA

Functions of LA and ALA and Dietary Recommendations

Humans are unable to synthesize omega-6 or omega-3 fatty acids, so the parent fatty compounds for each of these fatty acid categories, LA and ALA, respectively, are considered essential. They function as integral components of phospholipids and modulate cell function by acting as intracellular mediators of signal transduction or modulators of cell–cell interactions. They are required for growth, reproduction, maintenance of skin, and regulation of cholesterol metabolism. Although essential fatty acid deficiency is rarely seen in humans, in animal models deficiency produces reduced growth rate, dermatitis, infertility, depressed inflammatory responses, erythrocyte fragility, and liver and kidney abnormalities.[2] Evidence for ALA's essentiality in humans was first noted <30 years ago.[3]

Both LA and ALA appear to play roles in decreased risk of cardiovascular disease. LA consumption in place of saturated fat leads to a reduction in serum total and LDL cholesterol even beyond that which would be expected from simply reducing dietary saturated fat.[4] Higher LA intakes are associated with lower blood pressure[5] and a reduced risk of diabetes.[6] ALA intake is associated with a reduced risk of coronary artery disease,[7] myocardial infarction,[8,9] and fatal heart disease.[10,11] This risk reduction is due to multiple mechanisms including effects on platelet function, inflammation, endothelial cell function, arterial compliance, and ALA's role in reducing arrhythmia.[12] In the Nurses' Health Study, women in the highest two quintiles of ALA intake (median 0.60% and 0.74% of energy) had a 38–40% reduced risk of sudden cardiac death.[13] ALA intake may be especially important when intakes of EPA and DHA are low.[14]

Although some meta-analyses have reported an increased risk of prostate cancer with higher intakes or blood levels of ALA,[15,16] the relationship has been described as weak with heterogeneity across studies and the possibility of publication bias. Not all studies find this increased risk,[17] with one report[18] finding no greater risk of developing prostate cancer in general but an increased risk of developing advanced prostate cancer with higher ALA intake. To add to the uncertainty, a recent meta-analysis reported a significantly decreased risk of prostate cancer in those consuming >1.5 g/d of ALA compared to those consuming lower amounts.[19] This area requires more investigation, especially in those whose ALA intake is from plant sources. The source of ALA, whether from meat or from plant sources, does not appear to affect risk of prostate cancer.[18]

LA and ALA can be endogenously converted to longer carbon chain PUFA (Figure 4-1). LA, via conversion to arachidonic acid (AA), is the precursor to a variety of eicosanoids (thromboxanes, leukotrienes, prostaglandins, prostacyclins), some of which are proinflammatory, vasoconstrictive, and/or promoters of platelet aggregation,[20–22] whereas others are anti-inflammatory and

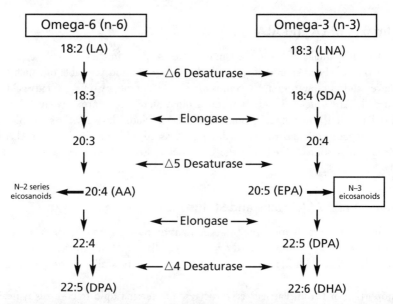

Figure 4-1 Metabolism of n-6 and n-3 fatty acids and eicosanoid production. *Source*: Adapted from Arterburn, LM, Hall, EB, Oken, H. Distribution, interconversion, and dose-response of n-3 fatty acids in humans. *Am J Clin Nutr*. 2006;83(suppl): 1467S–1476S.

inhibit platelet aggregation.[23–25] ALA, via conversion to EPA, is the precursor to the n-3 series eicosanoids, which are anti-inflammatory[24] and tend to reduce coronary heart disease (CHD) risk and prevent arrhythmias and thrombosis.[26] EPA can be further modified to produce DHA.

The Institute of Medicine (IOM) has established adequate intakes (AI) for both essential fatty acids. The AI for LA for adults is 12 g/d for women and 17 g/d for men. The AI for ALA is 1.1 g/d for women and 1.6 g/d for men.[27] The IOM has also set an acceptable macronutrient distribution range (AMDR) for LA of 5–10% of energy and for ALA of 0.6–1.2% of energy.[27] Up to 10% of the AMDR for ALA can be from EPA and/or DHA (0.06–0.12% of energy).[27] This recommendation is based on median consumption of EPA and DHA in the United States.

Because of concerns that high intakes of LA may limit conversion of ALA to EPA and DHA, contribute to overproduction of proinflammatory eicosanoids, and increase susceptibility of low-density lipoprotein cholesterol (LDL-C) to oxidation,[12,28] some groups have recommended intakes of omega-6 PUFAs that are lower than current U.S. recommendations.[29] In contrast, the American Heart Association supports an intake of at least 5–10% of energy from omega-6-PUFAs and states that "to reduce omega-6 PUFA intakes from their current levels would be more likely to increase than to decrease risk for CHD."[30] A rationale for this position is that the production of AA from LA is tightly regulated so that even wide variations in dietary LA intake would not markedly alter tissue AA levels, inflammation, or other proatherogenic effects.[31–33] In addition, questions have been raised about the extent and significance of LDL-C oxidation at higher LA intakes.[30] The effect of LA on ALA conversion to EPA is discounted because of the already limited extent of this conversion.[30] This effect, however, may be more significant in populations consuming little or no EPA or DHA.[27]

Dietary Intakes of LA and ALA

The median daily intake of LA in the United States is approximately 12 to 17 g for men and 9 to 11 g for women.[27] Food sources of LA include nuts, seeds, and vegetable oils such as soybean, corn, safflower, and sunflower oil. LA accounts for 85–90% of dietary omega-6 fatty acid intake.[30]

Median daily ALA intakes in adults in the United States are approximately 1.2 to 1.6 g for men and 0.9 to 1.1 g for women.[27] Sources of ALA include flaxseed, flaxseed oil, canola oil, hempseed oil, soybean oil, and walnuts. Although flaxseed oil is much higher in ALA than soybean oil, the largest source of ALA in the U.S. diet is soybean oil because it is consumed so extensively.[34]

Vegetarian LA and ALA Intake and Status

LA requirements are easily met even by vegetarians on relatively low-fat diets, as the LA intake of vegetarians is often at or above the AI.[1, 35–40] (Appendix F). Although there are few rich plant sources of ALA, data indicate that vegetarian intake is typically at or above the AI for ALA.[1,35,37,38,40–44]

The proportion of LA in platelets, erythrocytes, and plasma lipid fractions is typically higher in vegetarians and vegans than in nonvegetarians.[39,40,45–49] The proportion of ALA in vegetarians and vegans is higher[39,47,50] or similar to nonvegetarians.[40,49]

Meeting Recommendations for Essential Fatty Acids with Vegetarian Diets

Table 4-1 provides information on vegetarian sources of LA and ALA and the amounts of each food source that would be needed to meet the AI for ALA. By choosing a variety of foods, including plant oils, nuts, seeds, and vegetables, vegetarians can have adequate intakes of both LA and ALA. Even relatively small amounts of specific foods that are high in ALA can be used to meet the AI for this fatty acid. For example, a little more than half a teaspoon of flaxseed oil or 1¼ tablespoons of canola oil would supply the AI for ALA for an adult man.

Table 4-1 LA and ALA Content of Foods

Food	LA Content (g)	ALA Content (g)	Amount needed to provide 1.6 g ALA*	Amount needed to provide 1.1 g ALA*
Oils (1 tbsp)				
Almond oil	2.366	0		
Apricot kernel oil	3.985	0		
Avocado oil	1.754	0.134	12 tbsp	8 tbsp
Canola oil	2.61	1.279	1.25 tbsp	0.9 tbsp
Corn oil	7.239	0.158	10 tbsp	7 tbsp
Cottonseed oil	7.004	0.027	59 tbsp	41 tbsp
Flaxseed oil	1.727	7.249	0.2 tbsp	0.15 tbsp
Grapeseed oil	9.466	0.014	114 tbsp	79 tbsp
Hazelnut oil	1.374	0		
Hempseed oil	7.98	2.24	0.7 tbsp	0.5 tbsp
Mustard oil	2.146	0.826	1.9 tbsp	1.3 tbsp
Olive oil	1.318	0.103	15.5 tbsp	10.7 tbsp
Palm oil	1.238	0.027	59 tbsp	41 tbsp
Peanut oil	4.320	0		
Poppy seed oil	8.486	0		
Rice bran oil	4.542	0.218	7.3 tbsp	5 tbsp
Safflower oil	1.952	0		
Sesame oil	5.617	0.041	39 tbsp	27 tbsp
Soybean oil	6.857	0.923	1.7 tbsp	1.2 tbsp
Sunflower oil, high oleic	0.505	0.027	59 tbsp	41 tbsp
Walnut oil	7.194	1.414	1.1 tbsp	0.8 tbsp
Wheat germ oil	7.453	0.938	1.7 tbsp	1.1 tbsp
Nuts and Seeds (2 tbsp)				
Black walnuts	5.160	0.312	0.6 cup	0.4 cup
English walnuts	5.668	1.352	2.4 tbsp	1.6 tbsp

(Table 4-1 continued)

(Table 4-1 Continued)

Food	LA Content (g)	ALA Content (g)	Amount needed to provide 1.6 g ALA*	Amount needed to provide 1.1 g ALA*
Flax seeds, ground	0.826	3.194	1 tbsp	0.7 tbsp
Flax seeds, whole†	1.216	4.700	0.7 tbsp	0.5 tbsp
Pumpkin seeds	2.862	0.016	12.5 cups	8.6 cups
Fruits and Vegetables				
Avocado, ½ cup	1.248	0.080	10 cups	7 cups
Broccoli rabe, cooked, 1 cup	0.034	0.221	7,2 cups	5 cups
Broccoli, Chinese, cooked, 1 cup	0.067	0.227	7 cups	4.8 cups
Broccoli, cooked, 1 cup	0.080	0.186	8.6 cups	5.9 cups
Collards, cooked, 1 cup	0.133	0.177	9 cups	6.2 cups
Kale, cooked, 1 cup	0.103	0.134	11.9 cups	8.2 cups
Soy Products				
Soy burger, 1 patty	1.358	0.057	28 patties	19 patties
Soybeans, 1 cup	7.680	1.029	1.6 cup	1.1 cups
Soy nuts, 2 tbsp	2.610	0.350	9 tbsp	6 tbsp
Tempeh, ½ cup	2.981	0.183	4.4 cups	3 cups
Tofu, firm, ½ cup	2.013	0.228	3.5 cups	2.4 cups
Animal Products				
Egg, 1 large	0.574	0.017	94 eggs	65 eggs
Milk, 1 cup	0.066	0.010	160 cups	110 cups
Fortified Foods				
Flax cereal, ¾ cup	1.300	0.091–1.000	2–23 cups	1.5–16 cups
Margarine with flaxseed oil, 1 tbsp	1.952	0.474	3.4 tbsp	2.3 tbsp
Mayonnaise with flaxseed oil, 1 tbsp	1.1	0.500	3.2 tbsp	2.2 tbsp
Peanut butter with flaxseed oil, 1 tbsp	0.650	0.500	3.2 tbsp	2.2 tbsp

*1.6 g and 1.1 g are the AI for ALA for men and women, respectively.

†Whole flaxseeds are not well digested; their alpha-linolenic acid has low bioavailability.[153]

Source: Data from USDA National Nutrient Database for Standard Reference, Release 22, 2009 and manufacturers' information.

Animal studies suggest that LA can actually be synthesized in humans from the fatty acid hexadecadienoate (16:2 n-6), which represents 1–2% of total fatty acids in common edible green vegetables including broccoli and spinach, and ALA can be synthesized from the fatty acid hexadecatrienoate (16:3 n-3), which is present in edible green vegetables at up to 14% of total fatty acids.[51] The endogenous synthesis of these essential fatty acids could play a role in populations consuming vegetarian diets,[52] although no information is available on rates of synthesis in humans.

ARACHIDONIC ACID

Arachidonic acid (AA) can be endogenously produced through the desaturation and elongation of LA, similar to the way that EPA is made from ALA. Rates of conversion of LA to AA are very low; <0.1% of dietary LA is converted to AA.[53] Typical intake of AA by nonvegetarians is limited (approximately 150 mg/d) and mainly comes from meat, eggs, and some fish.[30] Although plant foods do not contain AA and intakes of AA by vegans have been reported as nondetectable,[37] it is not clear that AA tissue or serum content in vegetarians is different from that of nonvegetarians. Some studies show that tissues or cells from vegetarians and vegans contain a lower proportion of AA,[39,45,47,50] whereas others show little or no difference between vegetarians or vegans and nonvegetarians.[39,40,49]

Two intervention studies demonstrate the conflicting nature of this literature; in one, AA levels were reduced significantly when omnivore subjects were placed on a vegan diet for 3 to 5 months after an initial 7- to 10-day fast, but levels returned to their initial values when subjects consumed a lacto vegetarian diet.[54] In the other study, when meat eaters were placed on a vegetarian diet, AA levels increased.[55]

EPA AND DHA

Recently, calls have been made for the IOM to establish specific recommendations for the individual long-chain omega-3 fatty acids DHA and EPA.[56,57] New evidence of DHA and EPA's effects on risk of fatal CHD as well as limited conversion of ALA to DHA and EPA have been proposed as a rationale for establishing Dietary Reference Intakes (DRIs) for these fatty acids.[56]

In 2002, the IOM concluded that only limited data were available to define a DRI for EPA and DHA. EPA and DHA are not currently considered essential nutrients because EPA can be synthesized from ALA, and DHA from EPA (DHA can be retroconverted into EPA)[52,58–60] (Figure 4-1). DHA is believed to be important for brain development and retinal function[61–63] and possibly for reproduction.[64] EPA and DHA reduce the risk of cardiac mortality.[56] Depressed DHA levels have been seen in those with Alzheimer's disease,[65] depression,[66] attention deficit disorder,[67] and schizophrenia.[68] DHA is found in low levels in most cells of the body, in higher levels in sperm and testes, and in very high levels in the brain and retina.[69] Adipose tissue stores of EPA and DHA are very low, suggesting a limited storage of these fatty acids and a need for a regular dietary supply.[69]

Effects of EPA and DHA on CHD

Initial speculation about the cardiovascular benefits of omega-3 fatty acids stemmed from the observation that Eskimos, who consume a diet that is high in omega-3 fatty acids, have a very low rate of CHD despite high total fat intakes.[70] The Greenland Eskimos consume as much as 10 to 11 g of omega-3 fatty acids per day,[71] much more than the 0.8 g/d, and 0.1 to 0.2 g/d consumed by Danish whites[71] and persons in the United States, respectively.[72] Cardioprotective effects of DHA and EPA include decreased risk of arrhythmia,[73] lower plasma triglyceride levels,[74] reduced inflammatory responses,[75] improved endothelial function,[76] reduced heart rate,[77] and reduced platelet aggregation.[78,79] EPA and DHA supplementation has reduced blood pressure in hypertensive individuals.[75] High doses of EPA + DHA (3 to 4 g/d) appear effective in treatment of severe and moderate hypertriglyceridemia.[74] These mechanisms, especially the reduction in cardiac arrhythmias, are likely to account for the reduced risk of sudden cardiac death associated with higher intakes of DHA and EPA.[12,56] Other roles of DHA + EPA in cardiovascular disease such as effects on atherosclerosis progression and a reduction in risk of nonfatal events and stroke are less definitive compared with EPA and DHA's effects on cardiac mortality.[56,80]

Several intervention studies have demonstrated the benefits of omega-3 fatty acids for reducing chronic disease risk.[81–83] For example, in the GISSI Prevenzione trial, patients suffering a previous myocardial infarction who were given 1 g of omega-3 PUFAs (EPA + DHA from fish oil) per day experienced a 45% reduced risk of sudden cardiac death over a 3.5-year period in comparison to the placebo group.[81]

One group estimates that cardiac mortality is reduced by approximately 35% from moderate EPA and DHA consumption in the range of 250 to 500 mg/d.[56] Intakes of approximately 500 mg/d appear to provide the greatest protection according to a recent meta-analysis limited to prospective studies in the United States.[84]

Other Health Effects of EPA and DHA

A number of studies and a recent meta-analysis have found that fish and foods rich in omega-3 fatty acids were associated with a reduced risk of age-related macular degeneration.[85] Some studies suggest that this association is strongest in those consuming lower amounts of LA.[86,87] At this point, results, although promising, do not provide enough evidence to develop recommendations for EPA and DHA based on their potential role in preventing age-related macular degeneration.[85]

Chapter 11 provides information on DHA's role in pregnancy outcome, cognitive development, and visual development.

Interest in DHA's role in reduction of the risk of dementia and Alzheimer's disease arose because DHA is concentrated in many of the most active areas of the brain, and DHA content of the brain decreases with age in animals.[56] Epidemiologic studies have found that higher DHA intakes are associated with a lower risk of Alzheimer's disease,[88] and higher DHA + EPA intakes were associated with a postponement of cognitive decline in elderly men.[89] Higher plasma EPA and DHA levels or EPA levels alone have been associated with a marked reduction in risk of developing dementia and a lower decline in verbal fluency.[65,90,91] One randomized controlled trial found some positive effects of supplemental EPA and DHA in patients with very mild Alzheimer's disease, although overall little effect was seen.[92] Additional trials are being conducted.[56]

Omega-3 fatty acids may play a role in treatment of depressive illness, although study results are inconsistent. For example, a meta-analysis of 12 randomized trials of omega-3 fatty acids in treatment of depression found little evidence of benefit.[93] Another meta-analysis of 10 double-blind, placebo-controlled trials of omega-3 fatty acid in treatment of mood disorders found a significant antidepressive effect.[94] Weighted analysis of omega-3 status in those with mental health problems found no significant differences from controls.[95]

Omega-3 fatty acids, mainly DHA, also appear to play a role in osteoporosis prevention, although there have only been limited studies in this area.[96]

Recommendations for EPA and DHA

The DRI report published in 2002 did not include a recommended dietary allowance for EPA or DHA but did state that up to 10% of the AMDR for ALA can be from EPA and/or DHA (0.06–0.12% of energy).[27] This range was based on median consumption of EPA and DHA in the United States.

Many expert groups and health agencies have issued recommendations for these omega-3 fatty acids or for fish intakes to provide EPA and DHA. Table 4-2 provides examples of these recommendations. Typically, recommendations are near 500 mg/d with higher amounts sometimes recommended for secondary prevention of CHD.[97]

Dietary Intakes of EPA and DHA

The median intake of EPA by adults in the United States ranges from 4 mg/d to 7 mg/d; median DHA intakes are between 66 mg/d and 93 mg/d for men and 52 mg/d to 69 mg/d for women.[27]

Table 4-2 Examples of Recommendations for Omega-3 and Omega-6 Fatty Acid Intakes for Healthy Adults

	ALA	*EPA + DHA*	*Total Omega-3 Fatty Acids*	*Total Omega-6 Fatty Acids*
U.S. Dietary Reference Intakes[27]	1.6 g/d Men 1.1 g/d Women	0.06–0.12% of calories	0.6–1.2% of calories	5–10% of calories
American Heart Association[154]		450–500 mg*		At least 5–10% of calories[30]
American Dietetic Association and Dietitians of Canada[12]	0.6–1.2% of calories	500 mg/d		3–10% of calories
United Kingdom[155]		450–500 mg*		
Australia and New Zealand[156]	1.3 g/d men 0.8 g/d women	610 mg/d men 430 mg/d women		4–10% of calories
The Netherlands[157]		450–500 mg*		
FAO/WHO[158]		450–500 mg*	1–2% of calories	5–8% of calories

*Estimated average daily amount of EPA + DHA from 2 servings of fish, preferably fatty fish, per week.

Table 4-3 DHA and EPA Content of Vegetarian Foods

	EPA (mg)	DHA (mg)
Animal Products		
Egg, 1 large	2	0
Eggs from chickens fed flax,[120] 1 egg		60–100
Eggs from chickens fed microalgae,[120] 1 egg		100–150
Sea Vegetables		
Dulse, dried, 8 g[159]	86.8	
Kelp, dried, 8 g[159]	63.4	
Kelp, raw, ½ cup	0.2	0
Nori, dried, 8 g[159]	198.2	
Nori, raw, 1 sheet	0.2	0
Sea lettuce, dried, 8 g[160]	2.4	7.1
Sea spaghetti, dried, 8 g[159]	42.7	
Wakame, dried, 8 g[159]	79.2	
Wakame, raw, ½ cup	74	0
Foods fortified with microalgae-derived DHA		
DHA-fortified cheese, 1 ounce	0	32
DHA-fortified energy bar, 1	0	50
DHA-fortified juice, 1 cup	0	50
DHA-fortified kefir beverage (dairy), 1 cup	0	32
DHA-fortified milk (dairy), 1 cup	0	32
DHA-fortified canola or olive oil, 1 tbsp	0	25–32
DHA-fortified powdered drink mix, 1 packet	0	100
DHA-fortified soymilk, 1 cup	0	32
DHA-fortified yogurt (dairy), 6 oz		32
Vegan Supplements		
Vegan DHA supplement, 1 capsule or soft gel		200–300
Vegan DHA supplement, liquid, 1 dropper		300
Vegan EPA + DHA supplement, 1 soft gel or capsule	10–50	300–350

Source: Data from USDA National Nutrient Database for Standard Reference, Release 22, 2009 and manufacturers' information except where otherwise identified.

These intakes are based on dietary records and do not include supplements of EPA, DHA, or fish oil. Typically fish oil supplements are higher in EPA, whereas fish provides more DHA.[56] DHA and EPA both appear to be beneficial in terms of reductions of risk; it is not possible at this time to conclude whether the effects are due to primarily to DHA or to EPA or to a specific ratio of these two fatty acids. A ratio of EPA to DHA between 1:2 and 2:1 has been suggested.[56]

Vegetarian DHA and EPA Sources and Intake

Mann et al reported mean daily DHA intakes by moderate meat eaters, lacto-ovo vegetarians, and vegans in Australia to be 70 mg, 10 mg, and 0 mg, respectively, and EPA intakes among these same groups to be 40 mg, 0 mg, and 0 mg.[39] Lacto-ovo vegetarian DHA intake was mainly from eggs. Several other studies including those in the United Kingdom[1,37] and Austria[40] have reported that vegans have very low or no detectable dietary EPA or DHA. DHA intakes of lacto-ovo vegetarians are slightly higher, but EPA intakes are often undetectable.

Vegetarian food sources of DHA and EPA typically contain limited amounts of these fatty acids and include sea vegetables, eggs, and foods fortified with microalgae-derived DHA. (Table 4-3). Sea vegetables mainly provide EPA; there is little information available on their DHA content. Foods fortified with microalgae-derived DHA typically contain 30 to 50 mg of DHA per serving. Microalgae-derived DHA is vegan, although it may be added to nonvegan as well as nonvegetarian foods.

Vegetarian EPA and DHA Status

Most studies have found the proportion of EPA and DHA in blood and/or tissues to be lower in both lacto-ovo vegetarians and vegans compared to nonvegetarians.[1,39,40,45-49] DHA proportions in erythrocytes, plasma, serum, platelet phospholipids, and erythrocyte phosphatidyl ethanolamine are typically ≥50% lower in vegans than in nonvegetarians.[1] DHA proportions in nonvegan vegetarians are also lower than in nonvegetarians although typically not as low as in vegans.[1]

Harris and von Schacky[98] proposed an "omega-3 index" based on the proportion of erythrocyte fatty acids as EPA + DHA. An omega-3 index of ≥8% was designated a cardioprotective target level, and an index of ≤4% was associated with the greatest risk of death from CHD. Two studies suggest that the estimated omega-3 index in vegans is >4%, whereas that of nonvegetarian controls is >4% but not at the cardioprotective target.[46,99]

Limited research suggests that DHA levels are lower in pregnant vegetarian women and in cord blood than in nonvegetarians.[41,48] Reddy et al found lower levels of DHA in breast milk of vegetarian women compared to omnivore women, although levels were higher than in unfortified infant formula.[48]

ENDOGENOUS SYNTHESIS OF LONG-CHAIN PUFA

As Figure 4-1 indicates, EPA and DHA can be endogenously produced from ALA. A key question is whether or not this endogenous conversion is sufficient to meet needs. Nearly 20 studies of ALA conversion to EPA and DHA indicate that, generally, only about 5% of ALA is converted to EPA and <0.5% of ALA is converted to DHA.[53,100] Premenopausal women have been shown to convert more ALA to EPA (2.5-fold more) and DHA (>200-fold more) than similarly aged men.[101] This is believed to be due to estrogen's effect on increasing the activity of the pathway and may help to explain the higher conversion rates seen in pregnancy.[100] During lactation, ALA supplementation does not appear to increase breast milk DHA levels, suggesting that conversion rates are not increased in lactation.[102]

Vegan diets are devoid of DHA, so the DHA found in blood and tissue of long-term vegans must be produced from dietary ALA. Based on the low endogenous synthesis rates of DHA that have been reported in nonvegetarians, vegans might be expected to have clinical symptoms of DHA deficiency; however, this does not seem to occur.[53] Vegans have low but stable plasma levels of DHA[49,50] that do not appear to fall according to the duration of a vegan diet,[49] suggesting there is some basal rate of conversion of ALA to DHA.[1] Additionally, vegans do not seem to markedly increase DHA production in response to ALA supplementation.[103] A lower rate of beta-oxidation of DHA in vegans has been proposed as one possibility to help explain their relative resistance to DHA deficiency.[53] This is certainly an area where additional research is needed.

The synthesis of EPA and DHA is affected by a number of dietary and metabolic factors. A major factor may be either total LA intake or the LA-to-ALA ratio in the diet. This will be discussed in later sections. Inadequate intakes of zinc, iron, and pyridoxine[104] may impair the synthesis of EPA and DHA. In addition, gestational diabetes appears to affect maternal synthesis of omega-3 fatty acids.[41,105]

ENHANCEMENT OF VEGETARIAN DHA AND EPA STATUS

Vegetarians have been shown to have intakes of DHA and EPA that are typically lower than the amounts being recommended for optimal health and to have lower proportions of these fatty acids in blood and tissue than nonvegetarians. A number of possible alternatives could potentially increase vegetarians' blood and tissue concentrations of DHA and EPA. These include indirect supplementation through increased intake of ALA, enhanced endogenous synthesis through a reduction in trans-fat intake along with reduced total LA intake or an altered ratio of LA to ALA, and direct supplementation.

ALA Supplementation

One possible way to increase DHA and EPA synthesis is to provide more of the precursor fatty acid, ALA. It may not be possible, however, to ingest sufficient ALA to achieve blood and tissue levels of DHA + EPA at a cardioprotective target level. In observational studies of both vegetarians and nonvegetarians, intakes of ALA ranging from <1 g/d to >18 g/d result in larger proportions of EPA in plasma and cell lipids but no higher DHA proportions.[69,100,106,107]

Supplementation studies in which vegetarian diets are supplemented short term with ALA show some effect on EPA but not on DHA concentrations. For example, Li et al found that in response to a high-ALA diet in which vegetarian subjects consumed 15.4 g ALA/d for 6 weeks, the proportion of EPA in platelet phospholipids, plasma phospholipids, and plasma triacylglycerols increased while DHA remained unchanged.[43] Specifically, platelet phospholipid EPA increased from 0.2% to 0.5% of total fatty acids, plasma phospholipid EPA increased from 0.4% to 1.4%, and plasma triacylglycerol EPA increased from 0.1% to 0.4%.[43] Sanders and Younger gave vegan subjects 6.5 g/d of ALA from flaxseed oil for 2 weeks and found an increase in plasma EPA but no effect on plasma DHA or platelet EPA or DHA.[108] Fokkema et al gave vegans 2 g of ALA from flaxseed oil for 4 weeks. No significant effect on EPA or DHA levels was seen.[103]

These limited results may be due to a buffering effect of the comparatively high stores of LA in adipose tissue that limit the efficacy of short-term manipulation of the relative amounts of LA and ALA.[1] In addition, due to the larger size of the plasma DHA pool compared to that of EPA, a longer time may be needed to detect changes in DHA levels following ALA supplementation.[107] Sanders concludes that longer-term, randomized controlled studies with a diet reduced in LA are needed in vegetarians.[1] At this point, however, ALA supplementation does not appear to markedly increase DHA and EPA levels.

An additional consideration is that, at an estimated conversion rate of 0.5% for ALA to DHA, even with a daily intake of 1000 mg of ALA, only about 5 mg/d of DHA would be produced, considerably below intakes that are recommended.[53] Even with conversion rates of 10%, a rate higher than has been seen in published studies, a daily intake of ALA of 2000 mg would be needed to produce even 200 mg of DHA.[53]

ALA supplementation, although apparently not effective at increasing DHA levels, may offer other benefits. In the Health Professionals Follow-up Study, in men with little or no EPA or DHA intake, each 1 g/d of ALA intake was associated with a 58% lower risk of nonfatal myocardial infarction and a 47% lower risk of total heart disease and of sudden death. These benefits were not seen in men with higher EPA and DHA intakes.[14] These results may be particularly relevant for those eating vegetarian diets.

Despite some positive findings, randomized controlled trials of ALA in cardiovascular disease[10,81,109] are limited in number and in quality, leaving many questions about ALA's ability to replace DHA + EPA in reducing risk of cardiac death.[110]

In addition, ALA may not duplicate all of the biologic effects of the longer chain omega-3 fatty acids. For example, ALA does not lower triglyceride levels, whereas long-chain omega-3 fatty acids do.[111] Also, fish intake and DHA and EPA intake were found to be associated with a reduced risk of developing macular degeneration,[85] whereas ALA intake was associated with an increased risk.[112] However, this may be because dairy and animal products are often the biggest contributors of ALA to the diet.[113,114] Finally, ALA does not appear as effective as DHA and EPA in terms of anti-inflammatory effects.[115]

Reports of a link between higher intakes or higher blood levels of ALA and prostate cancer[15,16] are concerning and suggest that further research is required before making strong recommendations, especially for those at risk of prostate cancer, to increase ALA intakes.

Altered LA Intake

Dietary modifications have been proposed as a means to increase the rate of conversion of ALA to DHA and EPA. The rate-limiting step in the conversion of ALA to EPA and DHA is the reaction involving Δ6-desaturase (Figure 4-1). The affinity of this desaturase is greater for ALA than for LA, but higher concentrations of LA result in more conversion of LA to AA and a reduced conversion of ALA to EPA and DHA.[100] Proposed dietary modifications center on a reduced dietary ratio of LA to ALA (achieved by decreasing LA intake or increasing ALA intake or both) and a reduced total intake of LA (with less focus on the LA-to-ALA ratio).

Some studies argue that a lower LA intake or a lower LA-to-ALA ratio will enhance synthesis of DHA and EPA from ALA. For example, Ezaki et al found that when elderly Japanese subjects switched from soybean oil to perilla oil (high in ALA), causing the LA-to-ALA ratio to go from 4:1 to 1:1, serum EPA, but not DHA increased after 3 months. Ten months were needed to see a 21% increase in DHA.[116] This study was rather unique because the LA-to-ALA ratio was so low and because of its long duration. Goyens et al[117] decreased the LA-to-ALA ratio of a control diet from 19:1 to 7:1 by either reducing LA while keeping ALA constant or by increasing ALA while keeping LA constant. The rate of conversion of ALA to EPA and DHA increased compared to the control diet when dietary ALA was increased while keeping LA constant but did not change when LA was reduced but ALA was kept constant. These results suggest that the amount of ALA and LA influence ALA conversion to EPA and DHA rather than the ratio of LA to ALA.

Other studies only find positive effects on the conversion of ALA to EPA but not on conversion to DHA with lower intakes of LA. Hussein et al reported increased phospholipid EPA but no change in DHA when the LA-to-ALA ratio went from 27.9:1 to 0.5:1.[118] In addition, Liou et al found that while plasma EPA content was reduced when dietary LA was increased from 3.8% to 10.5% of energy and the ratio of LA-to-ALA went from 4:1 to 10:1, DHA was unaffected.[119]

Although some have downplayed the reduction of dietary LA as a strategy to promote increased EPA and DHA production from ALA,[30] this reduction may offer benefits in those with few or no dietary sources of EPA and DHA,[27] as is typical of both vegetarian and vegan diets. Because of the need for enhanced conversion of ALA to DHA and EPA, vegetarians and vegans may benefit from an LA-to-ALA ratio that is toward the lower end of recommended ranges (5:1 to 10:1 are often suggested as reasonable ranges). Davis and Kris-Etherton[120] have suggested a ratio of 2:1 to 4:1 as optimal for vegetarians and others not consuming preformed EPA and DHA. As shown in Appendix F, the LA-to-ALA ratio in vegetarian diets is frequently higher than most recommendations.

To achieve a lower ratio of LA to ALA, vegetarians can strive for an intake of <1.5% to 2% of calories from ALA and 5.5–8% of calories from LA.[120] Several dietary modifications can help to achieve a lower LA-to-ALA ratio. These include choosing primary cooking oils that are rich in monounsaturated fats and consuming adequate amounts of ALA. Monounsaturated fats by themselves do not affect the LA-to-ALA ratio and, if substituted for oils high in LA, will result in a lower ratio. Foods high in monounsaturated fats include olive oil, canola oil, high-oleic sunflower oil, high oleic-safflower oil, nuts (except walnuts), peanuts, olives, and avocados.[120] Cooking oils that are high in LA, including safflower oil, grapeseed oil, sunflower oil, corn oil, cottonseed oil, and soybean oil (Table 4-1), should not be used as primary cooking oils.

Because of the importance of the question of the efficacy of alteration of LA intakes on EPA and DHA production in those with no dietary EPA or DHA, additional research on vegans and vegetarians is needed before conclusions can be made as to amounts of LA and ALA to recommend for this population.

Dietary Trans-Fatty Acids

Dietary trans-fatty acids (TFA) may interfere with the conversion of ALA to EPA.[120,121] There are few data on the TFA intake of vegetarians. Draper et al reported that the daily intake of TFA by British male and female lacto-ovo vegetarians was 5.4 and 3.4 g, respectively, and for vegan males and females, it was 2.7 and 2.8 g.[42] In comparison, British male and female nonvegetarians reportedly consume 5.5 and 3.9 g of TFA/d, respectively.[42] In a Swedish study involving small numbers of subjects, nonvegetarian, lacto-vegetarian, and vegan diets reportedly contained 2.0%, 1.3%, and 0.5%, respectively, of their calories as TFA (only trans-octadecanoic acids were determined).[122] The level of TFA (18:n-9) in the subcutaneous fat of lacto-ovo vegetarians was reported by Crane et al to be about a third lower than that of nonvegetarians.[123] Finally, lacto-ovo vegetarians in Hong Kong had lower serum trans-fatty acids than nonvegetarians (0.03% compared with 0.5%).[47] Dietary TFA content is expected to decrease due to a reduction in TFA use by the food industry and to greater consumer awareness of health risks of TFA.[124,125]

Direct Supplementation

Some researchers have recommended that vegans use a supplement or fortified foods to supply DHA and EPA because of limited conversion of ALA and because of EPA and DHA's many benefits,[57] although others question the benefit of EPA and DHA supplementation in vegetarians and vegans.[126]

Direct supplementation with DHA-rich microalgae has been suggested as a means to increase blood and tissue DHA and EPA content of vegetarians. Five studies have been reported in which preformed DHA from microalgae was provided to vegetarians. Geppert et al compared the effect of 940 mg of DHA and a placebo for 8 weeks.[127] The proportion of DHA in plasma phospholipids increased from 2.8% to 7.3% and EPA increased from 0.58% to 0.77%.[127] In another report from the same study, erythrocyte lipid DHA proportion increased from 4.4% to 7.9%.[44] Conquer and Holub gave vegetarian subjects 1620 mg of microalgal-derived DHA daily for 6 weeks. Serum phospholipid DHA proportion increased from 2.4% to 8.3% and platelet phospholipid DHA proportion increased from 1.2% to 3.9%. EPA levels also increased.[59] Postmenopausal vegetarian women who received 2.14 g of DHA daily for 6 weeks had higher plasma LDL EPA and DHA.[128] Most of these studies have used amounts of DHA higher than those typically recommended. A single study has reported, in abstract form, use of a lower dose of DHA. In a study of vegans, 200 mg/d of DHA for 3 months increased the proportion of DHA in plasma by 50%.[129] In nonvegetarians, DHA supplementation at doses above approximately 2 g/d produces little additional increase in plasma phospholipid DHA concentration.[69] When DHA is provided in combination with EPA, the DHA saturation dose appears to be 1.2 g/d.[69]

DHA supplementation appears to increase both the DHA and EPA content of blood and tissues. The production of EPA following DHA supplementation appears to be due to retroconversion.[53] EPA concentrations increase by approximately 0.4 g/100 g fatty acid for each 1 g of DHA intake.[69]

Microalgal-derived DHA supplements are available in liquid form and in vegan gelatin capsules. Foods fortified with microalgae-derived DHA include soymilk, energy bars, olive oil, and cow's milk. Table 4-3 provides information on vegetarian sources of DHA and EPA. In addition, microalgal-derived DHA is used to fortify some cow's milk-based and soy-based infant formulas. DHA, whether provided as a supplement (oil in capsules) or in DHA-fortified foods, is bioavailable and well tolerated.[130]

Specific recommendations for amounts of DHA and EPA for vegetarians have not been developed. Guidelines developed for the general public (Table 4-2) may be helpful to vegetarians who opt to use microalgal sources of DHA (or DHA + EPA). Intakes of EPA + DHA up to 1 g/d and of 1.8 g/d of EPA have been used in large studies with no adverse effects.[81–83]

The creation of new plant cultivars that contain fatty acids that are more readily converted to EPA and DHA than ALA is or that contain plant-derived EPA and DHA is being studied,[131–133] suggesting the possibility of new sources of EPA and DHA for vegetarians. Stearidonic acid (SDA, 18:4 n-3) is one such fatty acid. SDA is a metabolic intermediate in the conversion of ALA to EPA. Compared to ALA, SDA was more efficiently converted to EPA, although it did not increase EPA concentrations as much as direct EPA supplementation did.[134,135] Limited research suggests that SDA offers promise as a surrogate for EPA in terms of some physiologic effects.[134]

WOULD VEGETARIANS BENEFIT FROM EATING FISH?

The inefficient conversion of ALA into EPA and DHA, possible differences in biologic effects between ALA and the long-chain omega-3 PUFAs, and the difficulty of ingesting sufficient ALA have led to speculation that the addition of fish to a vegetarian diet might confer health benefits beyond those associated with vegetarian diets alone. The development of microalgae-derived DHA and EPA supplements and fortified foods would seem to eliminate any calls for vegetarians to eat fish or use fish oil. In addition, even if one assumes that fatty fish intake is associated with health benefits in omnivores, this does not imply that vegetarians will have similar benefits because factors common to vegetarian diets may result in similar outcomes even though they do not eat fish. One review of dietary fatty acid requirements states, "For vegans who do not consume any preformed sources of EPA and DHA, additional research is needed before recommendations can be made for these fatty acids, including supplements. It is important to note the absence of reported adverse health effects in this population that consumes no fish."[12]

Numerous observational studies suggest that vegetarians live longer than nonvegetarians and have ≤25% lower death rates from cardiovascular disease.[126,136,137] For example, an analysis of five studies involving >75,000 adults found that mortality from ischemic heart disease was 24% lower in vegetarians than in nonvegetarians.[137] Specifically, compared to regular meat eaters, lacto-ovo vegetarians had a 34% lower risk of death and vegans a 26% lower risk. The number of vegan subjects was quite small, which may have affected results. Subjects who ate fish but not meat had death rates similar to those of vegetarians suggesting that vegetarians do not need to eat fish to reduce risk of death from ischemic heart disease. Fraser et al did not find protective effects of fish consumption against CHD in the Adventist Health Study[138] or in a subset of older vegetarians (≥84 years of age).[139]

Factors in vegetarians that may reduce risk of CHD death include lower rates of overweight and obesity,[140,141] lower blood pressure and lower rates of hypertension,[140] and lower total and LDL cholesterol levels.[142,143]

Protective effects of fatty acids from fish on risk of dementia have also been suggested, although there is not enough evidence to make specific recommendations.[56] Only limited research has been done on the incidence of Alzheimer's disease or dementia in vegetarians. Existing studies find no increased risk of dementia or cognitive impairment in vegetarians or in vegan men.[1,144,145] The Oxford Vegetarian Study found a higher mortality from mental and neurologic disease in vegetarians compared to nonvegetarians, although there were, overall, a small number of deaths from this condition.[146]

In addition, concerns have been raised about the potential environmental and societal impact of the increased fish consumption that is being recommended by some health authorities.[147] Overfishing has led to the extinction of some types of fish and to limited availability of other types.[148] Loss of species has a number of harmful environmental effects.[149,150] Fish farming, although sometimes proposed as a solution, has also been associated with environmental damage.[151] Food security of developing nations is jeopardized by increased exporting of fish.[152] Use of more sustainable vegetarian sources of DHA and EPA, such as microalgae, reduces the environmental and societal impacts of increasing consumption of these long-chain fatty acids.

CONCLUSION

There are many questions about ALA, LA, EPA, and DHA needs for vegetarians that are not resolved. Although we know that ALA and LA are essential fatty acids, we do not know the optimal ratio of these nutrients for vegetarians. Additional research is needed to determine if dietary manipulations such as increased ALA, decreased LA, and/or an altered ratio of LA to ALA can promote EPA and DHA synthesis by vegetarians so that blood and tissue content of these fatty acids are similar to those seen in fish eaters. With the availability of supplemental DHA and EPA derived from microalgae and foods fortified with DHA, there is no need for vegetarians to eat fish or use fish oil to obtain DHA or EPA. Vegetarians can improve their EPA and DHA status by using direct sources of these fatty acids and possibly by increasing dietary ALA and replacing some dietary LA with carbohydrates or monounsaturated fats.

COUNSELING POINTS: MEETING NEEDS FOR KEY FATS

- There are two essential fatty acids: linoleic acid and linolenic acid.
- Linoleic acid is found in whole grains, nuts, seeds, soybeans, and in many vegetable oils. Dietary recommendations for linoleic acid are 12 g/d for adult women and 17 g/d for adult men. Because it is widely available in foods, most people have high intakes of linoleic acid.
- Needs for alpha-linolenic acid can be met by choosing daily servings of ground flaxseed or flaxseed oil, walnuts, hempseed products (such as veggie burgers or cheese made from hemp), canola oil, soybeans, and generous quantities of leafy green vegetables. Dietary recommendations are 1.1 g/d for adult women and 1.6 g/d for adult men. Higher intakes may be beneficial for those with low or no dietary DHA and EPA.
- Due to concerns about an increased risk of prostate cancer in those with higher intakes of alpha-linolenic acid, excessive intakes should be avoided especially by those in risk groups for prostate cancer.

- A lower ratio of linoleic acid to alpha-linolenic acid may be beneficial. Foods high in mono-unsaturated fat such as olive oil, canola oil, high-oleic sunflower oil, high-oleic safflower oil, nuts, peanuts, olives, and avocados should be used judiciously in place of overreliance on oils high in linoleic acid such as safflower oil, grapeseed oil, sunflower oil, corn oil, cotton-seed oil, and soybean oil. Complex carbohydrates can also be used to replace some linoleic acid.

- EPA and DHA are long-chain fats found in fish oils and in limited amounts in some sea vegetables. The body can make some EPA and DHA from other fats, but production is limited. Vegetarians can use nonanimal sources of DHA and EPA by selecting foods fortified with DHA derived from microalgae or by using vegan supplements of DHA or DHA + EPA derived from microalgae. The DHA or DHA + EPA in supplements or fortified foods may offer health advantages to some individuals. Their use should be assessed in view of other risk factors for chronic diseases.

- Microalgae-derived DHA and EPA are vegan sources of DHA and EPA, although they may be added to nonvegan or nonvegetarian foods. Some foods contain added DHA and EPA from fish oil, so label reading is important to determine the source of these fatty acids and to identify nonfish sources for vegetarians.

- Trans-fatty acids may interfere with the synthesis of EPA and DHA. Limit consumption of foods rich in trans-fatty acids such as foods containing partially hydrogenated oils.

Case Study

Dorothy is a 58-year-old woman with a family history of CHD. About 5 years ago she became vegan, with a goal of reducing her risk of heart disease. She eats a generally healthy diet but would like advice on omega-3 fats. After discussing various strategies with Dorothy, she tells you that she wants to modify her diet so that the LA-to-ALA ratio is closer to 4:1 while maximizing her intake of ALA. Her cardiologist has recommended a total fat intake of ≤30% of calories. Dorothy's recommended calorie intake is 2000 calories per day. Develop 2 days of menus for Dorothy that meet her objectives while staying within her fat and calorie limits.

Should Dorothy take supplemental DHA? Why or why not?

REFERENCES

1. Sanders TAB. DHA status of vegetarians. *Prostaglandins Leukot Essent Fatty Acids.* 2009;81(2–3):137–141.
2. Vergroesen AJ. Early signs of polyunsaturated fatty acid deficiency. *Bibl Nutr Dieta.* 1976(23):19–26.
3. Holman RT, Johnson SB. Linolenic acid deficiency in man. *Nutr Rev.* 1982;40:144–147.
4. Mensink RP, Zock PL, Kester AD, Katan MB. Effects of dietary fatty acids and carbohydrates on the ratio of serum total to HDL cholesterol and on serum lipids and apolipoproteins: a meta-analysis of 60 controlled trials. *Am J Clin Nutr.* 2003;77:1146–1155.
5. Grimsgaard S, Bonaa KH, Jacobsen BK, et al. Plasma saturated and linoleic fatty acids are independently associated with blood pressure. *Hypertension.* 1999;34:478–483.
6. Salmeron J, Hu FB, Manson JE, et al. Dietary fat intake and risk of type 2 diabetes in women. *Am J Clin Nutr.* 2001;73:1019–1026.

7. Djousse L, Pankow JS, Eckfeldt JH, et al. Relation between dietary linolenic acid and coronary artery disease in the National Heart, Lung, and Blood Institute Family Heart Study. *Am J Clin Nutr.* 2001;74:612–619.
8. Ascherio A, Rimm EB, Giovannnucci EL, et al. Dietary fat and risk of coronary heart disease in men: cohort follow up study in the United States. *BMJ.* 1996;313:84–90.
9. Campos H, Baylin A, Willett WC. Alpha-linolenic acid and risk of nonfatal acute myocardial infarction. *Circulation.* 2008;118(4):339–345.
10. de Lorgeril M, Salen P, Martin JL, et al. Mediterranean diet, traditional risk factors, and the rate of cardiovascular complications after myocardial infarction: final report of the Lyon Diet Heart Study. *Circulation.* 1999;99(6):779–785.
11. Hu FB, Stampfer MJ, Manson JE, et al. Dietary intake of alpha-linolenic acid and risk of fatal ischemic heart disease among women. *Am J Clin Nutr.* 1999;69(5):890–897.
12. Kris-Etherton PM, Innis S. Position of the American Dietetic Association and Dietitians of Canada: dietary fatty acids. *J Am Diet Assoc.* 2007;107:1599–1611.
13. Albert CM, Oh K, Whang W, et al. Dietary alpha-linolenic acid intake and risk of sudden cardiac death and coronary heart disease. *Circulation.* 2005;112(21):3232–3238.
14. Mozaffarian D, Ascherio A, Hu FB, et al. Interplay between different polyunsaturated fatty acids and risk of coronary heart disease in men. *Circulation.* 2005;111(2):157–164.
15. Simon JA, Chen YH, Bent S. The relation of alpha-linolenic acid to the risk of prostate cancer: a systematic review and meta-analysis. *Am J Clin Nutr.* 2009;89(5):1558S–1564S.
16. Brouwer IA, Katan MB, Zock PL. Dietary alpha-linolenic acid is associated with reduced risk of fatal coronary heart disease, but increased prostate cancer risk: a meta-analysis. *J Nutr.* 2004;134:919–922.
17. Koralek DO, Peters U, Andriole G, et al. A prospective study of dietary alpha-linolenic acid and the risk of prostate cancer (United States). *Cancer Causes Control.* 2006;17(6):783–791.
18. Leitzmann MF, Stampfer MJ, Michaud DS, et al. Dietary intake of n-3 and n-6 fatty acids and the risk of prostate cancer. *Am J Clin Nutr.* 2004;80:204–216.
19. Carayol M, Grosclaude P, Delpierre C. Prospective studies of dietary alpha-linolenic acid intake and prostate cancer risk: a meta-analysis. *Cancer Causes Control.* 2010;21(3):347–355.
20. Kinsella JE, Lokesh B, Broughton S, Whelan J. Dietary polyunsaturated fatty acids and eicosanoids: potential effects on the modulation of inflammatory and immune cells: an overview. *Nutrition.* 1990;6(1):24–44.
21. Kinsella JE, Lokesh B, Stone RA. Dietary n-3 polyunsaturated fatty acids and amelioration of cardiovascular disease: possible mechanisms. *Am J Clin Nutr.* 1990;52(1):1–28.
22. Simopoulos AP. Essential fatty acids in health and chronic disease. *Am J Clin Nutr.* 1999;70(3 suppl):560S–569S.
23. Serhan CN. Lipoxins and aspirin-triggered 15-epi-lipoxins are the first lipid mediators of endogenous anti-inflammation and resolution. *Prostaglandins Leukot Essent Fatty Acids.* 2005;73:141–162.
24. Stanley JC, Elsom RL, Calder PC, et al. UK Food Standards Agency Workshop Report: the effects of dietary n-6:n-3 fatty acid ratio on cardiovascular health. *Br J Nutr.* 2007;98:1305–1310.
25. Node K, Huo Y, Ruan X, et al. Anti-inflammatory properties of cytochrome P450 epoxygenase-derived eicosanoids. *Science.* 1999;285:1276–1279.
26. Leng GC, Smith FB, Fowkes FG, et al. Relationship between plasma essential fatty acids and smoking, serum lipids, blood pressure and haemostatic and rheological factors. *Prostaglandins Leukot Essent Fatty Acids.* 1994;51(2):101–108.
27. Institute of Medicine Food and Nutrition Board. *Dietary Reference Intakes for Energy, Carbohydrate, Fiber, Fat, Fatty Acids, Cholesterol, Protein, and Amino Acids.* Washington, DC: National Academy Press; 2002.
28. Calder PC. Polyunsaturated fatty acids and inflammation. *Prostaglandins Leukot Essent Fatty Acids.* 2006;75:197–202.
29. International Society for the Study of Fatty Acids and Lipids. Recommendations for intake of polyunsaturated fatty acids in healthy adults. 2004. http://www.issfal.org.uk/index.php?option=com_content&task=view&id=23&Itemid=8.
30. Harris WS, Mozaffarian D, Rimm E, et al. Omega-6 fatty acids and risk for cardiovascular disease. A science advisory from the American Heart Association Nutrition Subcommittee of the Council on Nutrition, Physical Activity, and Metabolism; Council on Cardiovascular Nursing; and Council on Epidemiology and Prevention. *Circulation.* 2009;119:902–907.

31. Steinberg D, Parthasarathy S, Carew TE, et al. Beyond cholesterol: modifications of low-density lipoprotein that increase its atherogenicity. *N Engl J Med.* 1989;320:915–924.
32. Galassetti P, Pontello A. Dietary effects on oxidation of low-density lipoprotein and atherogenesis. *Curr Atheroscler Rep.* 2006;8:523–529.
33. Zock PL, Katan MB. Linoleic acid intake and cancer risk: a review and meta-analysis. *Am J Clin Nutr.* 1998;68:142–153.
34. American Soybean Association. Soy Stats 2008. http://www.soystats.com/2008/default.htm.
35. Pan WH, Chin CJ, Sheu CT, Lee MH. Hemostatic factors and blood lipids in young Buddhist vegetarians and omnivores. *Am J Clin Nutr.* 1993;58(3):354–359.
36. Ferrier LK, Caston LJ, Leeson S, et al. alpha-Linolenic acid- and docosahexaenoic acid-enriched eggs from hens fed flaxseed: influence on blood lipids and platelet phospholipids fatty acids in humans. *Am J Clin Nutr.* 1995;62(1):81–86.
37. Roshanai F, Sanders TAB. Assessment of fatty-acid intakes in vegans and omnivores. *Hum Nutr Appl Nutr.* 1984; 38A:345–354.
38. Krajcovicova-Kudlackova M, Blazicek P, Babinska K, et al. Traditional and alternative nutrition—levels of homocysteine and lipid parameters in adults. *Scand J Clin Lab Invest.* 2000;60(8):657–664.
39. Mann M, Pirotta Y, O'Vonnell S, et al. Fatty acid composition of habitual omnivore and vegetarian diets. *Lipids.* 2006;41:637–646.
40. Kornsteiner M, Singer I, Elmadfa I. Very low n-3 long-chain polyunsaturated fatty acid status in Austrian vegetarians and vegans. *Ann Nutr Metab.* 2008;52:37–47.
41. Lakin V, Haggarty P, Abramovich DR, et al. Dietary intake and tissue concentration of fatty acids in omnivore, vegetarian and diabetic pregnancy. *Prostaglandins Leukot Essent Fatty Acids.* 1998;59(3):209–220.
42. Draper A, Lewis J, Malhotra N, Wheeler E. The energy and nutrient intakes of different types of vegetarian: a case for supplements? *Br J Nutr.* 1993;69(1):3–19.
43. Li D, Sinclair A, Wilson A, et al. Effect of dietary alpha-linolenic acid on thrombotic risk factors in vegetarian men. *Am J Clin Nutr.* 1999;69(5):872–882.
44. Geppert J, Kraft V, Demmelmair H, et al. Docosahexaenoic acid supplementation in vegetarians effectively increases omega-3 index: a randomized trial. *Lipids.* 2005;40:807–814.
45. Sanders TA, Roshanai F. Platelet phospholipid fatty acid composition and function in vegans compared with age- and sex-matched omnivore controls. *Eur J Clin Nutr.* 1992;46(11):823–831.
46. Sanders TA, Ellis FR, Dickerson JW. Studies of vegans: the fatty acid composition of plasma choline phosphoglycerides, erythrocytes, adipose tissue, and breast milk, and some indicators of susceptibility to ischemic heart disease in vegans and omnivore controls. *Am J Clin Nutr.* 1978;31(5):805–813.
47. Lee HY, Woo J, Chen ZY, et al. Serum fatty acid, lipid profile and dietary intake of Hong Kong Chinese omnivores and vegetarians. *Eur J Clin Nutr.* 2000;54(10):768–773.
48. Reddy S, Sanders TA, Obeid O. The influence of maternal vegetarian diet on essential fatty acid status of the newborn. *Eur J Clin Nutr.* 1994;48(5):358–368.
49. Rosell MS, Lloyd-Wright Z, Appleby PN, et al. Long-chain n-3 polyunsaturated fatty acids in plasma in British meat-eating, vegetarian, and vegan men. *Am J Clin Nutr.* 2005;82:327–334.
50. Phinney SD, Odin RS, Johnson SB, Holman RT. Reduced arachidonate in serum phospholipids and cholesteryl esters associated with vegetarian diets in humans. *Am J Clin Nutr.* 1990;51(3):385–392.
51. Cunnane SC, Ryan MA, Craig KS, et al. Synthesis of linoleate and alpha-linolenate by chain elongation in the rat. *Lipids.* 1995;30(8):781–783.
52. Cunnane SC. The conditional nature of the dietary need for polyunsaturates: a proposal to reclassify 'essential fatty acids' as 'conditionally- indispensable' or 'conditionally-dispensable' fatty acids. *Br J Nutr.* 2000;84(6):803–812.
53. Plourde M, Cunnane SC. Extremely limited synthesis of long chain polyunsaturates in adults: implications for their dietary essentiality and use as supplements. *Appl Physiol Nutr Metab.* 2007;32:619–634.
54. Haugen MA, Kjeldsen-Kragh J, Bjerve KS, et al. Changes in plasma phospholipid fatty acids and their relationship to disease activity in rheumatoid arthritis patients treated with a vegetarian diet. *Br J Nutr.* 1994;72(4):555–566.
55. Chetty N, Bradlow BA. The effects of a vegetarian diet on platelet function and fatty acids. *Thromb Res.* 1983; 30(6):619–624.

56. Harris WS, Mozaffarian D, Lefevre M. Towards establishing dietary reference intakes for eicosapentaenoic and docosahexaenoic acids. *J Nutr.* 2009;139:804S–819S.
57. Kris-Etherton PM, Grieger JA, Etherton TD. Dietary reference intakes for DHA and EPA. *Prostaglandins Leukot Essent Fatty Acids.* 2009;81(2–3):99–104.
58. Nelson GJ, Schmidt PC, Bartolini GL, Kelley DS, Kyle D. The effect of dietary docosahexaenoic acid on plasma lipoproteins and tissue fatty acid composition in humans. *Lipids.* 1997;32(11):1137–1146.
59. Conquer JA, Holub BJ. Supplementation with an algae source of docosahexaenoic acid increases (n-3) fatty acid status and alters selected risk factors for heart disease in vegetarian subjects. *J Nutr.* 1996;126(12):3032–3039.
60. Conquer JA, Holub BJ. Dietary docosahexaenoic acid as a source of eicosapentaenoic acid in vegetarians and omnivores. *Lipids.* 1997;32(3):341–345.
61. Carlson SE. Docosahexaenoic acid supplementation in pregnancy and lactation. *Am J Clin Nutr.* 2009;89(2):678S–684S.
62. Birch EE, Garfield S, Hoffman DR, et al. A randomized controlled trial of early dietary supply of long-chain polyunsaturated fatty acids and mental development in term infants. *Dev Med Child Neurol.* 2000; 42:174–181.
63. SanGiovanni JP, Berkey CS, Dwyer JT, Colditz GA. Dietary essential fatty acids, long-chain polyunsaturated fatty acids, and visual resolution acuity in healthy full-term infants: a systematic review. *Early Hum Dev.* 2000; 57:165–188.
64. Szajewska H, Horvath A, Koletzko B. Effect of n-3 long-chain polyunsaturated fatty acid supplementation of women with low-risk pregnancies on pregnancy outcomes and growth measures at birth: a meta-analysis of randomized controlled trials. *Am J Clin Nutr.* 2006;83:1337–1344.
65. Schaefer EJ, Bongard V, Beiser AS, et al. Plasma phosphatidylcholine docosahexaenoic acid content and risk of dementia and Alzheimer disease: The Framingham Heart Study. *Arch Neurol.* 2006;63:1545–1550.
66. Tiemeier H, van Tuijl HR, Hofman A, et al. Plasma fatty acid composition and depression are associated in the elderly: the Rotterdam Study. *Am J Clin Nutr.* 2003;78(1):40–46.
67. Antalis CJ, Stevens LJ, Campbell M, et al. Omega-3 fatty acid status in attention-deficit/hyperactivity disorder. *Prostaglandins Leukot Essent Fatty Acids.* 2006;75(4–5):299–308.
68. Joy CB, Mumby-Croft R, Joy LA. Polyunsaturated fatty acid supplementation for schizophrenia. *Cochrane Database Syst Rev.* 2003;(2):CD001257.
69. Arterburn LM, Hall EB, Oken H. Distribution, interconversion, and dose-response of n-3 fatty acids in humans. *Am J Clin Nutr.* 2006;83(suppl):1467S–1476S.
70. Kromann N, Green A. Epidemiological studies in the Upernavik district, Greenland. Incidence of some chronic diseases 1950–1974. *Acta Med Scand.* 1980;208(5):401–406.
71. Bang HO, Dyerberg J, Sinclair HM. The composition of the Eskimo food in north western Greenland. *Am J Clin Nutr.* 1980;33(12):2657–2661.
72. Raper NR, Cronin FJ, Exler J. Omega-3 fatty acid content of the US food supply. *J Am Coll Nutr.* 1992;11(3):304–308.
73. Kang JX, Leaf A. Effects of long-chain polyunsaturated fatty acids on the contraction of neonatal rat cardiac myocytes. *Proc Natl Acad Sci U S A.* 1994;91(21):9886–9890.
74. Jacobson TA. Role of n-3 fatty acids in the treatment of hypertriglyceridemia and cardiovascular disease. *Am J Clin Nutr.* 2008;87(suppl):1981S–1990S.
75. Jung UJ, Torrejon C, Tighe AP, et al. n-3 Fatty acids and cardiovascular disease: mechanisms underlying beneficial effects. *Am J Clin Nutr.* 2008;87(suppl):2003S–2009S.
76. DeCaterina R, Liao JK, Libby P. Fatty acid modulation of endothelial activation. *Am J Clin Nutr.* 2000;71(1 suppl):213S–223S.
77. Dallongeville J, Yarnell J, Ducimetiere P, et al. Fish consumption is associated with lower heart rates. *Circulation.* 2003;108(7):820–825.
78. Adan Y, Shibata K, Sato M, et al. Effects of docosahexaenoic and eicosapentaenoic acid on lipid metabolism, eicosanoid production, platelet aggregation and atherosclerosis in hypercholesterolemic rats. *Biosci Biotechnol Biochem.* 1999;63(1):111–119.
79. Andriamampandry MD, Leray C, Freund M, et al. Antithrombotic effects of (n-3) polyunsaturated fatty acids in rat models of arterial and venous thrombosis. *Thromb Res.* 1999;93(1):9–16.

80. Hooper L, Thompson RL, Harrison RA, et al. Risks and benefits of omega-3 fats for mortality, cardiovascular disease, and cancer: systematic review. *BMJ.* 2006;332:752–760.
81. Dietary supplementation with n-3 polyunsaturated fatty acids and vitamin E after myocardial infarction: results of the GISSI-Prevenzione trial. Gruppo Italiano per lo Studio della Sopravvivenza nell'Infarto miocardico. *Lancet.* 1999;354(9177):447–455.
82. GISSI-HF Investigators. Effect of n-3 polyunsaturated fatty acids in patients with chronic heart failure (the GISSI-HF trial): a randomised, double-blind, placebo-controlled trial. *Lancet.* 2008;372:1223–1230.
83. Yokoyama M, Origasa H, Matsuzaki M, et al. Effects of eicosapentaenoic acid on major coronary events in hypercholesterolaemic patients (JELIS): a randomised open-label, blinded endpoint analysis. *Lancet.* 2007;369:1090–1098.
84. Harris WS, Kris-Etherton PM, Harris KA. Intakes of long-chain omega-3 fatty acid associated with reduced risk for death from coronary heart disease in healthy adults. *Curr Atheroscler Rep.* 2008;10:503–509.
85. Chong EW, Kreis AJ, Wong TY, et al. Dietary omega-3 fatty acid and fish intake in the primary prevention of age-related macular degeneration: a systematic review and meta-analysis. *Arch Ophthalmol.* 2008;126(6):826–833.
86. Seddon JM, George S, Rosner B. Cigarette smoking, fish consumption, omega-3 fatty acid intake, and associations with age-related macular degeneration: The US Twin Study of Age-Related Macular Degeneration. *Arch Ophthalmol.* 2006;124:995–1001.
87. Tan JSL, Wang JJ, Flood V, Mitchell P. Dietary fatty acids and the 10-year incidence of age-related macular degeneration: The Blue Mountains Eye Study. *Arch Ophthalmol.* 2009;127:656–665.
88. Morris MC, Evans DA, Bienias JL, et al. Consumption of fish and n-3 fatty acids and risk of incident Alzheimer disease. *Arch Neurol.* 2003;60(7):940–946.
89. van Gelder BM, Tijhuis M, Kalmijn S, et al. Fish consumption, n-3 fatty acids, and subsequent 5-y cognitive decline in elderly men: the Zutphen Elderly Study. *Am J Clin Nutr.* 2007;85(4):1142–1147.
90. Beydoun MA, Kaufman JS, Satia JA, et al. Plasma n-3 fatty acids and the risk of cognitive decline in older adults: The Atherosclerosis Risk in Communities Study. *Am J Clin Nutr.* 2007;85:1103–1111.
91. Samieri C, Féart C, Letenneur L, et al. Low plasma eicosapentaenoic acid and depressive symptomatology are independent predictors of dementia risk. *Am J Clin Nutr.* 2008;88(3):714–721.
92. Freund-Levi Y, Eriksdotter-Jonhagen M, Cederholm T, et al. Omega-3 fatty acid treatment in 174 patients with mild to moderate Alzheimer disease: OmegAD study: a randomized double-blind trial. *Arch Neurol.* 2006;63:1402–1408.
93. Appleton KM, Hayward RC, Gunnell D, et al. Effects of n-3 long-chain polyunsaturated fatty acids on depressed mood: systematic review of published trials. *Am J Clin Nutr.* 2006;84(6):1308–1316.
94. Lin PY, Su KP. A meta-analytic review of double-blind, placebo-controlled trials of antidepressant efficacy of omega-3 fatty acids. *J Clin Psychiatry.* 2007;68(7):1056–1061.
95. Milte CM, Sinn N, Howe PR. Polyunsaturated fatty acid status in attention deficit hyperactivity disorder, depression, and Alzheimer's disease: towards an omega-3 index for mental health? *Nutr Rev.* 2009;67(10):573–590.
96. Hogstrom M, Nordstrom P, Nordstrom A. n-3 fatty acids are positively associated with peak bone mineral density and bone accrual in healthy men: the NO$_2$ Study. *Am J Clin Nutr.* 2007;85:803–807.
97. Kris-Etherton PM, Harris WS, Appel LJ. Fish consumption, fish oil, omega-3 fatty acids, and cardiovascular disease. *Circulation.* 2002;106:2747–2757.
98. Harris WS, von Schacky C. The Omega-3 Index: a new risk factor for death from coronary heart disease? *Prev Med.* 2004;39(1):212–220.
99. Fokkema MR, Brouwer DA, Hasperhoven MB, et al. Polyunsaturated fatty acid status of Dutch vegans and omnivores. *Prostaglandins Leukot Essent Fatty Acids.* 2000;63(5):279–285.
100. Williams CM, Burdge G. Long-chain n-3 PUFA: plant v. marine sources. *Proc Nutr Soc.* 2006;65:42–50.
101. Burdge GC, Wootton SA. Conversion of alpha-linolenic acid to eicosapentaenoic, docosapentaenoic and docosahexaenoic acids in young women. *Br J Nutr.* 2002;88(4):411–420.
102. Francois CA, Connor SL, Bolewicz LC, et al. Supplementing lactating women with flaxseed oil does not increase docosahexaenoic acid in their milk. *Am J Clin Nutr.* 2003;77:226–233.
103. Fokkema MR, Brouwer DA, Hasperhoven MB, et al. Short-term supplementation of low-dose gamma-linolenic acid (GLA), alpha-linolenic acid (ALA), or GLA plus ALA does not augment LCP omega 3 status of Dutch vegans to an appreciable extent. *Prostaglandins Leukot Essent Fatty Acids.* 2000;63(5):287–292.
104. Cunnane SC. Role of zinc in lipid and fatty acid metabolism and in membranes. *Prog Food Nutr Sci.* 1988;12:151–188.

105. Dijck-Brouwer DA, Hadders-Algra M, Bouwstra H, et al. Impaired maternal glucose homeostasis during pregnancy is associated with low status of long-chain polyunsaturated fatty acids (LCP) and essential fatty acids (EFA) in the fetus. *Prostaglandins Leukot Essent Fatty Acids.* 2005;73(2):85–87.

106. Burdge GC, Calder PC. Conversion of alpha-linolenic acid to longer-chain polyunsaturated fatty acids in human adults. *Reprod Nutr Dev.* 2005;45(5):581–597.

107. Brenna JT, Salem N Jr, Sinclair AJ, Cunnane SC; International Society for the Study of Fatty Acids and Lipids, ISSFAL. alpha-Linolenic acid supplementation and conversion to n-3 long-chain polyunsaturated fatty acids in humans. *Prostaglandins Leukot Essent Fatty Acids.* 2009;80(2–3):85–91.

108. Sanders TA, Younger KM. The effect of dietary supplements of omega-3 polyunsaturated fatty acids on the fatty acid composition of platelets and plasma choline phosphoglycerides. *Br J Nutr.* 1981;45(3):613–616.

109. Natvig H, Borchgrevink CF, Dedichen J, et al. A controlled trial of the effect of linolenic acid on incidence of coronary heart disease. The Norwegian vegetable oil experiment of 1965–66. *Scand J Clin Lab Invest.* 1968;105:S1–S20.

110. Harris WS. Alpha-linolenic acid: a gift from the land? *Circulation.* 2005;111(22):2872–2874.

111. Wendland E, Farmer A, Glasziou P, Neil A. Effect of alpha linolenic acid on cardiovascular risk markers: a systematic review. *Heart.* 2006;92(2):166–169.

112. Cho E, Hung S, Willett WC, et al. Prospective study of dietary fat and the risk of age-related macular degeneration. *Am J Clin Nutr.* 2001;73(2):209–218.

113. Giovannucci E, Rimm EB, Colditz GA, et al. A prospective study of dietary fat and risk of prostate cancer. *J Natl Cancer Inst.* 1993;85(19):1571–1579.

114. Ramon JM, Bou R, Romea S, et al. Dietary fat intake and prostate cancer risk: a case-control study in Spain. *Cancer Causes Control.* 2000;11(8):679–685.

115. Calder PC. n-3 polyunsaturated fatty acids, inflammation, and inflammatory diseases. *Am J Clin Nutr.* 2006;83 (6 suppl):1505S–1519S.

116. Ezaki O, Takahashi M, Shigematsu T, et al. Long-term effects of dietary alpha-linolenic acid from perilla oil on serum fatty acids composition and on the risk factors of coronary heart disease in Japanese elderly subjects. *J Nutr Sci Vitaminol (Tokyo).* 1999;45(6):759–772.

117. Goyens PL, Spilker ME, Zock PL, et al. Conversion of α-linolenic acid in humans is influenced by the absolute amounts of _-linolenic acid and linoleic acid in the diet, and not by the ratio. *Am J Clin Nutr.* 2006;84:44–53.

118. Hussein N, Ah-Sing E, Wilkinson P, et al. Relative rates of long chain conversion of 13C linoleic and alpha-linolenic acid in response to marked changes in their dietary intakes in male adults. *J Lipid Res.* 2005;46:269–280.

119. Liou YA, King DJ, Zibrik D, Innis SM. Decreasing linoleic acid with constant alpha-linolenic acid in dietary fats increases (n-3) eicosapentaenoic acid in plasma phospholipids in healthy men. *J Nutr.* 2007;137(4):945–952.

120. Davis BC, Kris-Etherton PM. Achieving optimal essential fatty acid status in vegetarians: current knowledge and practical implications. Am J Clin Nutr. 2003;78(suppl):640S–646S.

121. Koletzko B. Trans fatty acids may impair biosynthesis of long-chain polyunsaturates and growth in man. *Acta Paediatr.* 1992;81(4):302–306.

122. Akesson B, Johansson BM, Svensson M, Ockerman PA. Content of trans-octadecanoic acid in vegetarian and normal diets in Sweden, analyzed by the duplicate portion technique. *Am J Clin Nutr.* 1981;34(11):2517–2520.

123. Crane MG, Zielinski R, Aloia R. Cis and trans fats in omnivorous, lacto-ovo-vegetarians, and vegans. *Am J Clin Nutr.* 1988;48:920. Abstract P2.

124. Eckel RH, Kris-Etherton P, Lichtenstein AH, et al. Americans' awareness, knowledge, and behaviors regarding fats: 2006–2007. *J Am Diet Assoc.* 2009;109(2):288–296.

125. Teegala SM, Willett WC, Mozaffarian D. Consumption and health effects of trans fatty acids: a review. *J AOAC Int.* 2009;92(5):1250–1257.

126. Mangat I. Do vegetarians have to eat fish for optimal cardiovascular protection? *Am J Clin Nutr.* 2009;89 (suppl):1597S–1601S.

127. Geppert J, Kraft V, Demmelmair H, et al. Microalgal docosahexaenoic acid decreases plasma triacylglycerol in normolipidaemic vegetarians: a randomized trial. *Br J Nutr.* 2006;95:779–786.

128. Wu WH, LU SC, Wang TF, et al. Effects of docosahexaenoic acid supplementation on blood lipids, estrogen metabolism, and in vivo oxidative stress in postmenopausal vegetarian women. *Eur J Clin Nutr.* 2006;60:386–392.

129. Lloyd-Wright Z, Preston R, Gray R, et al. Randomized placebo controlled trial of a daily intake of 200 mg docosahexaenoic acid in vegans. *Proc. Nutr. Soc.* 2003;62:42A.

130. Arterburn LM, Oken HA, Hoffman JP, et al. Bioequivalence of docosahexaenoic acid from different algal oils in capsules and in a DHA-fortified food. *Lipids.* 2007; 42:1011–1024.

131. Graham IA, Larson T, Napier JA. Rational metabolic engineering of transgenic plants for biosynthesis of omega-3 polyunsaturates. *Curr Opin Biotechnol.* 2007;18(2):142–147.

132. Damude HG, Kinney AJ. Enhancing plant seed oils for human nutrition. *Plant Physiol.* 2008;147(3):962–968.

133. Ruiz-López N, Haslam RP, Venegas-Calerón M, et al. The synthesis and accumulation of stearidonic acid in transgenic plants: a novel source of 'heart-healthy' omega-3 fatty acids. *Plant Biotechnol J.* 2009;7(7):704–716.

134. Whelan J. Dietary stearidonic acid is a long chain (n-3) polyunsaturated fatty acid with potential health benefits. *J Nutr.* 2009;139: 5–10.

135. Harris WS. The omega-3 index as a risk factor for coronary heart disease. *Am J Clin Nutr.* 2008;87:S1997–S2002.

136. Fraser GE, Shavlik DJ. Ten years of life: is it a matter of choice? *Arch Intern Med.* 2001;161:1645–1652.

137. Key TJ, Fraser GE, Thorogood M, et al. Mortality in vegetarians and nonvegetarians: detailed findings from a collaborative analysis of 5 prospective studies. *Am J Clin Nutr.* 1999;70(suppl):516S–524S.

138. Fraser GE. Associations between diet and cancer, ischemic heart disease, and all- cause mortality in non-Hispanic white California Seventh-day Adventists. *Am J Clin Nutr.* 1999;70(3 suppl):532S-538S.

139. Fraser GE, Shavlik DJ. Risk factors for all-cause and coronary heart disease mortality in the oldest-old. The Adventist Health Study. *Arch Intern Med.* 1997;157(19):2249–2258.

140. Fraser GE. Vegetarian diets: what do we know of their effects on common chronic diseases? *Am J Clin Nutr.* 2009; 9(suppl):1607S-1612S.

141. Spencer EA, Appleby PN, Davey GK, Key TJ. Diet and body mass index in 38000 EPIC-Oxford meat-eaters, fish-eaters, vegetarians and vegans. *Int J Obesity Res.* 2003;27: 728–734.

142. Appleby PN, Thorogood M, McPherson K, et al. Association between plasma lipid concentrations and dietary, lifestyle, and physical factors in the Oxford Vegetarian Study. *J Hum Nutr Diet.* 1995;8:305–314.

143. Key TJ, Appleby PN, Rosell MS. Health effects of vegetarian and vegan diets. *Proc Nutr Soc.* 2006;65:35–41.

144. Giem P, Beeson WL, Fraser GE, The incidence of dementia and intake of animal products: preliminary findings from the Adventist Health Study. *Neuroepidemiology.* 1993;12:28–36.

145. Fraser GE, Singh PN, Bennett H. Variables associated with cognitive function in elderly Californian Seventh-day Adventists. *Am J Epidemiol.* 1996; 143: 1181–1190.

146. Appleby PN, Key TJ, Thorogood M, et al. Mortality in British vegetarians. *Public Health Nutr.* 2002;5(1):29–36.

147. Jenkins DJ, Sievenpiper JL, Pauly D, et al. Are dietary recommendations for the use of fish oils sustainable? *CMAJ.* 2009;180(6):633–637.

148. Worm B, Barbier EB, Beaumont N, et al. Impacts of biodiversity loss on ocean ecosystem services. *Science.* 2006; 314:787–790.

149. McIntyre PB, Jones LE, Flecker AS, Vanni MJ. Fish extinctions alter nutrient recycling in tropical freshwaters. *Proc Natl Acad Sci U S A.* 2007;104:4461–4466.

150. Taylor BW, Flecker AS, Hall RO. Loss of a harvested fish species disrupts carbon flow in a diverse tropical river. *Science.* 2006;313:833–836.

151. Krkosek M, Ford JS, Morton A, et al. Declining wild salmon populations in relation to parasites from farm salmon. *Science.* 2007;318:1772–1775.

152. Atta-Mills J, Alder J, Rashid Sumaila U. The decline of a regional fishing nation: the case of Ghana and West Africa. *Nat Resource Forum.* 2004;28:13–21.

153. Flax Council of Canada. Flax FAQs. http://www.flaxcouncil.ca/english/index.jsp?p=faq.

154. Lichtenstein AH, Appel LJ, Brands M, et al. American Heart Association Nutrition Committee, Diet and Lifestyle Recommendations Revision 2006: A Scientific Statement from the American Heart Association Nutrition Committee. *Circulation.* 2006;114:82–96.

155. UK Scientific Advisory Committee on Nutrition. Advice on fish consumption: Benefits and risks. April 2004. http://www.sacn.gov.uk/pdfs/fics_sacn_advice_fish.pdf.

156. National Health and Medical Research Council. Nutrient Reference Values for Australia and New Zealand Including Recommended Dietary Intakes. 2006. http://www.nhmrc.gov.au/_files_nhmrc/file/publications/synopses/n35.pdf.

157. Health Council of the Netherlands. Guidelines for a Healthy Diet. 2006. http://www.gezondheidsraad.nl/en/publications/guidelines-healthy-diet-2006.

158. Joint WHO/FAO Expert Consultation on Diet, Nutrition, and the Prevention of Chronic Diseases. Diet, Nutrition and the Prevention of Chronic Diseases: Report of a Joint WHO/FAO expert Consultation. Geneva, Switzerland: WHO; 2002.

159. Sanchez-Machado DI, Lopez-Hernandez J, Paseiro-Losada P, Lopez-Cervantes J. Fatty acids, total lipid, protein and ash contents of processed edible seaweeds. *Food Chem.* 2004;85:439–444.

160. Khotimchenko SV, Vaskovsky VE, Titlyanova TV. Fatty acids of marine algae from the Pacific coast of North California. *Botanica Marina.* 2002; 45:17–22.

CHAPTER 5

Calcium

Developing and maintaining optimal bone health represents the interplay between bone mineralization and resorption, a complex process that is affected by a wide array of factors. Research has demonstrated that even in older persons, lifestyle factors, including dietary measures, not only retard age-related bone loss but actually increase bone mineral density (BMD).[1-3] Thus dietary interventions aimed at the later stages of life should hold promise for reducing fracture rates.

Osteoporosis is a worldwide problem of immense magnitude; in 2000, there were 1.6 million hip fractures worldwide.[4] By one estimate, as many as 40% of all women >50 years of age will experience a fracture in their lifetime.[5] Osteoporosis is the most prevalent metabolic bone disease in the United States and other developed countries.[6] An estimated 10 million people, 8 million of whom are women, have osteoporosis, and 34 million have low bone mass. Bone health is affected by many dietary, lifestyle, and genetic factors, and although calcium is certainly one of the more important ones, adequate calcium alone is not sufficient to ward off fractures.

CALCIUM AND BONES

The adult human body contains between 1000 and 1500 g of calcium, approximately 99% of which is found in bones and teeth. Most of the remaining 1% is found in the soft tissue with smaller amounts in the bloodstream and extravascular fluid.[7] Adequate calcium is critical for optimal bone health; this is particularly true during the years when bones are forming so that peak bone mass is maximized. Although BMD and bone mass are not the only factors determining risk of fracture, they are the predominant ones.[8,9]

Bones are extremely dynamic and are constantly remodeling; as much as 15% of the total bone mass turns over annually,[10] and about 700 mg of calcium exits and enters the bones every day.[11] This active remodeling process gives bone the ability to repair any damage caused by the daily stresses to which it is exposed. Until the end of the third decade or so of life, bone physiology favors bone acquisition and bone mass.[12] Between the ages of 35 and 45 years, peak bone mass is generally maintained, whereas beyond this age resorption dominates, and bone mass gradually decreases. After the age of 45 years, humans lose as much as 0.5% of their total bone mass every year. For many women, this process increases dramatically after menopause, especially at the spine, due to the decrease in circulating estrogen levels. Women lose on average 3% of their bone mass per year for about 5 years just before and after menopause,[13] and over the course of the decade following menopause, cancellous (spongy bone, such as in the spine) bone losses of 20–30%, and cortical (harder bone, such as in the hip) bone losses of 5–10%, are common.[14]

Many large epidemiologic studies including both case-control[15] and prospective studies[16–22] conducted in Western countries fail to show that calcium intake is protective against fracture. In a trial of secondary-fracture prevention, there was no effect on incidence of fractures from calcium supplements, vitamin D supplements, or a combination of the two.[23] Reid et al found a sustained reduction in bone loss and turnover in postmenopausal women taking 1000 mg calcium per day, but effects on fracture risk were unclear.[24] However, the balance of evidence from controlled trials suggests that combined calcium and vitamin D therapy reduces fracture risk.[25–27]

Dairy foods provide two thirds of the calcium in the United States, but there is some disagreement in the literature about the extent to which epidemiologic data support a relationship between dairy consumption and reduced bone fracture risk.[28,29] Heaney has pointed out why randomized controlled trials (RCTs) of calcium supplements and the few trials involving addition of dairy foods to the diet do appear to show protective effects, but case-control and prospective studies often do not. For example, actual calcium content of foods may differ from the amounts listed in databases used to calculate calcium content of the diet, one-day food records are often not representative of dietary intake over time, calcium bioavailability from foods differs markedly, and absorption differs among individuals.[29] It is also important to note that different dairy foods may impact bone health differently because of their widely varying contents of calcium, protein, potassium, and sodium (Table 5-1).

There is much debate over the calcium requirement,[30] but in 1997, the Food and Nutrition Board (FNB) dramatically increased dietary calcium requirements for some groups in comparison to the 1989 recommendations.[31] Many Americans, particularly teenage girls and women, do not

---

Table 5-1 Nutrient Content per 100 g Edible Product for Selected Dairy Foods

Food	Calcium (mg)	Potassium (mg)	Protein (g)	Sodium (mg)	Calcium (mg): Sodium (mg)
Milk, skim	12	156	3.4	42	2.9
Milk, 3.25% fat	113	132	3.1	43	2.6
Yogurt, nonfat	143	177	3.4	59	2.4
Cheddar cheese	721	98	25	621	1.2
American cheese	497	363	19.6	966	0.51
Cottage cheese	61	86	12.3	406	0.15

Source: Data from USDA National Nutrient Database for Standard Reference, Release 22, 2009.

meet the recommended intakes for this nutrient.[32] Average calcium intake for 14- to 50-year-old women is only about 700 mg/d, which is quite a bit lower than the adequate intake value of 1300 mg for girls 13 to 18 years and of 1000 mg for women 19 to 50 years. Data from the 1999–2002 National Health and Nutrition Examination Survey (NHANES) suggests that many ethnic minorities do not meet calcium recommendations.[33]

CALCIUM ABSORPTION

Calcium absorption is affected by both physiologic needs and total calcium intake. Young infants have high calcium needs as a result of new bone growth and can absorb as much as 60% of the calcium in their diet.[34] Fractional calcium absorption declines to about 25% throughout much of the rest of life but then declines further with old age.[35] The total amount of calcium ingested at one time is inversely related to calcium absorption efficiency.[36] For this reason, it is recommended that to use calcium most efficiently, amounts >500 mg should not be taken at one time. However, because the decrease in absorption efficiency with increasing intakes is a gradual one, higher intakes still result in greater absolute calcium absorption.

Calcium absorption varies among individuals and is a critically important determinant of fracture risk. In a study of pre- and perimenopausal women, calcium absorption ranged from 17% to 58%, and women with low fractional calcium absorption were 24% more likely to suffer a hip fracture.[37] Studies have found that differences in calcium absorption account for between 38% and 79% of the variation in calcium balance among women, whereas differences in calcium intake account for only between 2% and 27%.[7] Although there is great variation in calcium absorption among individuals, absorption rates in a given individual are relatively constant over time.[38]

The absorption of calcium is a complicated process. Calcium in food is usually linked to other substances and must be released. It was once thought that because many elderly people do not produce adequate amounts of gastric acid, calcium absorption may be impaired with aging.[39–41] This seems to be relevant only in the case of low-solubility calcium supplements, however, such as calcium carbonate.[42] When calcium is ingested with a meal, lack of gastric acid does not inhibit calcium absorption.[43,44] Vitamin D is important for calcium absorption, although primarily at low calcium intakes. It also acts directly to stimulate calcium uptake by the bones.[45] Perhaps for these reasons, higher intakes of vitamin D have been shown to be related to improved bone health.[21,43,46–48] Older people have lower serum levels of $1,25(OH)_2D3$ and possibly fewer vitamin D receptors; the lower serum vitamin D levels that occur with age reduce calcium absorption, which is associated with lower bone mass.[49]

As is the case for most nutrients, humans have an ability to partially adapt to lower calcium intakes. Although it may take as long as 2 months for absorption rates to increase in response to low calcium intakes,[50] it only takes 1 day for the body to decrease the amount of calcium excreted in the urine.[51] It has been suggested that it may take as long as 2 years for the bones themselves to adjust fully to a lower calcium intake by slowing the rate at which calcium exits and enters the bones,[52] but research suggests that this process may occur within a matter of weeks.[53] However, despite marked increases in calcium absorption efficiency and decreases in urinary calcium excre-

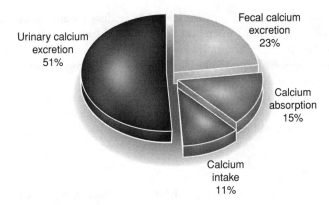

Figure 5-1 Relative impact of factors on the variation in calcium balance among middle-aged women. These data are based on balance/kinetic studies in >500 healthy middle-aged women. *Source*: Data from Heaney RP. Cofactors influencing the calcium requirement—other nutrients. Paper presented at: NIH Consensus Development Conference on Optimal Calcium Intake; June 6–8, 1994; Bethesda, MD.

tion,[54,55] bone calcium content will eventually be compromised in response to chronically low calcium intakes.[54,56,57]

CALCIUM EXCRETION

The kidneys filter about 8000 mg of calcium per day, and although some loss of calcium is normal, about 98% is reabsorbed.[58] With such large amounts of calcium filtered, it is clear that any factor that causes the kidneys to excrete even slightly more calcium can have a detrimental effect on bone health. In fact, research based on data from >500 women shows that urinary calcium loss accounts for >50% of the variation in calcium balance among individuals, whereas calcium intake accounts for only 11% (Figure 5-1).[59] However, although one other study did find a similarly large role for calcium excretion on calcium balance, other studies suggest a smaller role.[7,60] Still, excessive calcium loss is particularly important because, at typical calcium intakes, *net* calcium absorption may be no more than 5–10% (see "Net vs Gross Calcium Absorption," page 124). Consequently, to compensate for a urinary calcium loss of 50 mg, it may be necessary to consume an additional 250 to 500 mg of calcium. Factors that affect urinary calcium excretion include protein, sodium, and potassium.

PROTEIN EFFECTS ON CALCIUM EXCRETION

Protein, Acid-Base Balance, and Calcium Excretion

Protein directly increases glomerular filtration rate, which increases calcium excretion somewhat, but the effect of dietary protein on calcium excretion has been attributed primarily to the sulfur amino acid (SAA) content of protein. The SAAs methionine and cysteine are metabolized to sulfate and hydrogen, resulting in an acid ash, which explains why dietary protein intake is correlated with renal net acid excretion. Because the skeletal system is the largest source of alkali in the body, bone is dissolved in response to production of hydrogen ions, which allows phosphate to be released as a buffering agent.

As discussed later, although the effect of SAAs on calcium excretion has been demonstrated experimentally, recent research has not been supportive of the hypothesis that high protein intake is associated with bone loss and negative calcium balance.

Ecological Findings

The effect of both the amount and type of protein on fracture risk has, for several decades, been the subject of rigorous investigation and debate. The inverse relationship among countries between protein intake and hip fracture incidence is frequently cited in support of a critical role for protein in bone health. For example, in an analysis published in 1992 that included 16 countries, Abelow et al found that animal protein intake was highly positively correlated with hip fracture incidence for women >50 years of age, whereas the intake of calcium was unrelated to incidence.[61] In an analysis that included 33 countries, Frassetto et al observed a similar relationship.[62] Furthermore, although the intake of total protein and animal protein was positively correlated with hip fracture incidence, plant protein intake was inversely related.[62]

These types of studies are often cited as support for the belief, commonly held among some vegetarians, that people who consume low-protein diets have lower calcium requirements. However, because of the many potential confounding variables, limited insight about the relationship of protein and calcium to bone health is provided by such international comparisons. Low animal protein–consuming countries are often populated by blacks and Asians, both of whom may be less likely to suffer from hip fracture for reasons unrelated to dietary intake.[63] Blacks use calcium more efficiently than whites and are less responsive to the effects of parathyroid hormone,[64] and Asians have a shorter hip axis length, which may reduce fracture risk.[65] Ethnic differences in bone strength manifest in childhood and are due to difference in bone structural properties.[66] Asians also suffer fewer falls than whites,[67,68] a potentially important consideration because >90% of all hip fractures occur as a result of trauma.[69]

These observations are consistent with findings that, although Asians do have a lower hip fracture rate than whites,[70,71] their spinal fracture rate and BMD are similar.[72–80]

There are also genetic differences in vitamin D production,[81–83] as well as geographic and even cultural effects on endogenous vitamin D levels that may affect bone health. Also, taller people may be more prone to hip fracture than shorter people.[84,85] Finally, physical activity, the level of which can vary markedly among cultures, has a significant impact on bone health.[86–89]

Despite these caveats, Frasseto et al did find a positive relationship between protein intake and hip fracture risk when their analysis was restricted to the 23 countries of predominantly white population. But in a systematic review of 31 cross-sectional studies, Darling et al found little support for a relationship between protein intake and BMD or bone mineral content within populations.[90] This analysis is similar to the results of a prospective cohort study in which almost 1000 elderly individuals were followed for 5 years. There were positive correlations between baseline protein intake and bone mineral content, perhaps a result of the higher whole body lean mass of the higher protein consumers.[91]

Clinical Data

A number of older studies have found that, under certain experimental conditions, the effect of protein on calcium nutriture can be marked. For example, when subjects were fed 142 g of protein they were in negative calcium balance despite consuming 1400 mg of calcium per day, but were in positive calcium balance when consuming only 500 mg of calcium and 48 g of protein.[92] Similarly, when young men consumed roughly 600 mg of calcium on a low-protein diet they were in positive calcium balance, but when they ate a similar diet with the addition of more protein in the form of meat, the same amount of calcium did not support calcium balance.[93]

Researchers at the University of Connecticut found that increasing a person's daily protein intake by 50 g caused an extra 60 mg of calcium to be excreted.[94] As discussed later, however, positive effects of protein intake on calcium absorption may be part of the explanation for increased calcium excretion.

The effect of SAAs on calcium excretion has some support in earlier research. For example, Breslau et al found that when subjects consumed diets with similar amounts of calcium and total protein (about 75 g), they excreted 150 mg of calcium in their urine per 24 hours when the protein was derived from animal products, but only 103 mg when protein was derived entirely from soy.[95] In a Japanese study involving nearly 800 subjects, urinary calcium excretion was correlated with both protein intake and urinary sulfate excretion.[96]

However, Spencer et al concluded that experiments using isolated proteins such as casein do not accurately reflect dietary conditions because diets high in animal protein are also high in phosphorus; this is not necessarily true of diets based on isolated protein. They found that when whole animal foods were used as primary protein sources, there was no increase in urinary calcium.[97–100] Roughead et al found no increase in urinary calcium loss or effects on calcium retention with a high meat diet (20% energy as protein) compared to a low meat diet (12% energy as protein).[101] And in a meta-analysis of RCTs, Darling et al found no effect of high protein on BMD or bone content.[90]

Phosphorus mitigates the hypercalciuric effect of protein by increasing circulating parathyroid hormone levels, which in turn leads to a decrease in urinary calcium.[102,103] However, phosphorus increases the calcium content of the digestive juice (100 mg of phosphorus increases calcium content by about 6 mg) and therefore increases fecal calcium content to a similar magnitude that it reduces urinary loss. The result is no effect of protein on calcium balance.[98, 103–105]

PROTEIN–CALCIUM INTERACTIONS

Because of the effects of protein on calcium balance, it has been suggested by some that the dietary ratio of calcium (mg) to protein (g) is a better predictor of bone health than total calcium intake alone.[106] However, there is evidence that the total amounts of these two nutrients in the diet as well as the ratio may have an impact on bone health.[107]

Any effect of protein on calcium balance is likely to be most relevant at low calcium intakes. A prospective study in Norway showed that protein increased fracture risk in those with daily calcium intakes below, but not above, 623 mg.[108] In agreement, a prospective study of 40,224 postmenopausal women enrolled in the E3N French Women Study found there was no significant association between protein intake and fracture risk in the whole population, but fracture risk was elevated in those women with high protein and low calcium intakes.[109] And in a cross-sectional study of postmenopausal women, calcium intake was not associated with fracture risk, but high calcium was associated with increased risk when protein intake was low.[110]

In regard to the intervention data, in a controlled feeding study of 27 postmenopausal women, although protein increased urinary calcium losses, it had no effect on calcium balance at either low or high calcium intakes. At lower calcium intake, increased urinary losses were compensated for by increased calcium absorption. At higher calcium intake, protein had no effect on absorption, but the higher calcium intake compensated for urinary losses.[111] Similarly, Dawson-Hughes et al found dietary protein to have favorable effects on bone health in elderly subjects who were meeting calcium needs but not in those with low calcium intakes. They suggested that the positive effects of protein could be optimized and the negative effects minimized by increasing calcium intake and possibly by increasing fruit and vegetable intake to increase the alkali content of the diet.[107] Rapuri et al found that high protein intake was associated with higher BMD only when calcium intake exceeded 408 mg/d.[112]

Importantly, in a meta-analysis that included five RCTs, despite a linear relationship between net acid excretion and urine calcium, there was no relationship between net acid excretion with calcium balance or N-terminal telopeptides, a marker of bone resorption.[113]

A number of studies have found a protective effect of higher protein intakes on overall bone health. Although several prospective studies conducted in the United States and other Western countries have found that high protein (especially animal protein) intake increases fracture risk[114] and the rate of bone loss,[115] other studies have not seen these effects on bone loss[116,117] or have found that higher protein intake is protective against fracture[16] or is associated with higher BMD.[118] An analysis of NHANES III data showed protein intake to be positively correlated with BMD in postmenopausal women, and animal protein consumption and BMD were positively correlated in older men and women.[119] For every 15 g/d increase in animal protein intake, BMD increased by 0.016 g/cm^2 at the hip, 0.012 g/cm^2 at the femoral neck, and 0.015 g/cm^2 at the spine.[120]

Several clinical studies have also found no association between higher protein diets and increased calcium excretion or adverse effects on bone health.[121,122] Protein supplements have been shown to reduce fracture risk in older subjects who consume diets marginal in protein.[123,124]

Protein may positively affect bone health in a number of ways. For example, higher protein diets may increase muscle mass, which would favorably impact bone. Also, protein supplements have been found to increase circulating levels of insulin-like growth factor (IGF)-1, which may stimulate bone formation.[123,125] People consuming plant-based diets have also been found to have lower circulating levels of IGF-1 (which may in theory be protective against cancer).[126] Low serum concentrations of IGF-1 have also been observed in adults following raw foods vegetarian diets.[127] Kerstetter et al found in a series of human studies that feeding low-protein diets (≤0.8 g/kg body weight) significantly decreased fractional calcium absorption (0.19 ± 0.03 vs 0.26 ± 0.03; $P = 0.05$), increased parathyroid hormone levels, and decreased calcium excretion in comparison to feeding higher protein diets.[128–130] However, in a much larger, longer-term study, no association between protein intake and calcium absorption was found.[131,132] But in a study of 13 healthy women (10 young women and 3 postmenopausal), high-protein diets (2.1 g/kg) in comparison with moderate protein diets (1 g/kg) resulted in a significant increase in intestinal calcium absorption that paralleled the increase in urinary calcium excretion. The increase in urinary calcium from a high protein diet was explained, at least acutely, by the increased intestinal absorption and not by bone resorption.[60] It is noteworthy that protein itself is an important structural component of bone, accounting for approximately half of bone volume and a fourth of bone mass, including the skeletal matrix.

Acid-Base Balance and Calcium

Diets high in total protein, and in some cases high in animal protein, appear to have myriad effects on bone health including alterations in the rates of bone resorption, inhibition of vitamin D activation, lower levels of base precursors, and lower levels of potassium. There are competing theories as to the biologic basis for the hypercalciuric effect of protein; in addition to the effects of acid on bone dissolution, in vitro data indicate acidosis stimulates osteoclastic (bone resorption), and inhibits osteoblastic (bone formation), activity.[133] Low pH may also inhibit the activity of 1α-hydroxylase, the enzyme in the kidney responsible for converting vitamin D to its biologically active form, and thus may possibly inhibit calcium absorption.[134] In fact, the consumption of a soy protein diet identical in composition to an animal protein diet, with the exception of protein source, led to higher serum vitamin 1,25 dihydroxyvitamin D levels in young healthy subjects.[95]

Some research indicates that the SAAs account for only part of the hypercalciuric effect of animal foods, such as meat, and that other organic acids in animal foods also play an important role.[135] Frassetto et al concluded that the independent protective effect of plant protein intake on hip fracture risk observed among countries was more likely the result of the higher level of base precursors found in plant-based diets than the lower sulfur amino acid content of plant protein per se.[62] In an analysis of the effects of dietary patterns on bone health in older people, Tucker et al found that high fruit and vegetable consumption was associated with greater BMD.[136] Prynne et al compared bone mineral measurements of the whole body, hip, and spine to dietary intake records in five cohorts (adolescent boys and girls, young women, and older men and women) and concluded that higher fruit and vegetable intakes could have positive effects on bone mineral status in all age groups.[137] Sahni et al suggested a possible protective role for vitamin C for bone health in older men.[138]

In the Northern Ireland Young Hearts Project, 12-year-old girls consuming high amounts of fruit had significantly higher heel bone density[139] and in girls 8 to 13 years, those who consumed fruits and vegetables more than three times per day had lower urinary calcium excretion, larger bone size, and lower parathyroid hormone (PTH) concentrations compared to girls who consumed fruits and vegetables fewer than three times per day.[140] And in a longitudinal study of postmenopausal women, vitamin C, magnesium, and potassium were associated with increased BMD in the femoral neck.[141]

Diets that consist primarily of vegetable foods yield lower rates of endogenous acid production than do mixed diets and result in net base production.[95,142] In contrast to animal foods, vegetables and fruit contain substantial amounts of base (alkaline) precursors, such as organic potassium salts, which yield potassium bicarbonate.[143, 144] Consequently, potassium salts consumed via foods or in the form of supplements reduce urinary calcium excretion.[145]

An excellent example of the effect of potassium on calcium excretion comes from the Dietary Approaches to Stop Hypertension (DASH) study, which was designed to test the effect of diet on blood pressure. In this study, maintaining protein at a constant level, but more than doubling the potassium content of the diet from about 1700 mg/d to about 4000 mg/d by increasing vegetable intake resulted in a decrease in urinary calcium of 47 mg/d.[146,147] Similarly, Kaneko et al found that in young Japanese women, supplementing soy protein with SAAs led to an increase in urinary calcium excretion, whereas no increase was noted when potassium was increased.[148] However, in a review of balance studies, Rafferty and Heaney found that potassium was inversely associated with both urinary calcium excretion and intestinal calcium absorption resulting in no significant net change in calcium balance.[149] Finally, and most importantly, in an analysis of the clinical data, Fenton et al found no support for the acid-ash hypothesis of osteoporosis on calcium balance.[113]

SODIUM AND CALCIUM BALANCE

Sodium and calcium excretion are linked in the proximal renal tubule; that is, they share a common reabsorption pathway.[150] Consequently, high sodium intake results in an increase in urinary sodium and an obligatory increase in urinary calcium.[151] For this reason, high sodium intakes are thought by many to increase risk of osteoporosis,[152,153] and in fact, a study of young girls (8 to 13 years of age) found that urinary sodium excretion was the biggest determinant of urinary calcium excretion.[117]

Sodium intake varies considerably more among populations than does protein intake. In one worldwide survey, sodium intake varied by as much as a factor of 1000 among different geographic regions.[154] In the United States, sodium intake is quite high, about 5 to 10 times more than the estimated biologic requirement of 500 mg/d and the estimated 600 mg provided by the late Paleolithic diet.[155,156]

The effects of sodium on bone health may be quite important as indicated by a prospective study of postmenopausal women that found that urinary sodium excretion was correlated with increased bone loss from the hip.[157] Similarly, a cross-sectional study of 763 Japanese women 50 to 79 years of age found that sodium intake was positively associated with deoxypyridinoline (a marker of bone resorption) excretion ($P < 0.05$).[158] Also, Ginty et al found that increasing sodium intake from 80 to 180 mmol/d (1840 mg to 4140) increased urinary sodium about two-fold in both sodium-sensitive and sodium-non-sensitive individuals, but it increased urinary calcium excretion (by 73%) only in the sodium-sensitive subjects.[159]

However, there was no effect on biochemical markers of bone resorption or formation in either group. This may be because, at least over the 2-week period of this study, subjects in the sodium-sensitive group were able to compensate by increasing calcium absorption.[159]

In general, every gram of sodium ingested increases urinary calcium loss by between 20 and 40 mg.[160,161] Based on findings from a 2-year longitudinal study of bone density in 124 postmenopausal women, it was estimated that when urinary sodium excretion is reduced by 50%

from 3450 mg/d to 1725 mg/d, the effect on bone density is equivalent to an increase in dietary calcium intake of 891 mg.[157] However, in postmenopausal women, the addition of potassium citrate (90 mmol/d) to a high-sodium diet (225 mmol/d) prevented increased excretion of calcium in the urine.[162]

Findings from a randomized crossover trial of 11 postmenopausal women suggest that sodium affects bone health only when calcium intake is high. Low calcium intake (518 mg/d) was associated with negative bone calcium balance with both high (11.2g/d) and low (3.9g/d) salt diets, but when calcium intake was moderately high (1284 mg/d) bone balance was positive with the low salt intake but not with the high salt intake.[163] Finally, in a randomized, parallel-design dietary intervention study involving prehypertensive women 45 to 75 years of age, Nowson et al compared the effects on bone turnover of a low-sodium base-producing DASH-type diet with a high-carbohydrate low-fat diet with a higher acid load (both >800 mg dietary calcium per day). On the former diet, urinary calcium excretion decreased, but bone resorption did not differ between groups.[164]

DIET AND BONE HEALTH: IMPLICATIONS FOR VEGETARIANS

As discussed, evidence in support of the proposed harmful effect of higher SAA-content diets on bone health has weakened in recent years. Interestingly, despite the lower protein intake of vegetarians, it is not even clear that vegetarian diets are lower in SAAs than omnivore diets. The relative SAA (mg/g protein) of beans is lower than that of animal proteins, but the SAA content of grains and many other plant proteins is similar to or higher than animal proteins. Although Krajcovicova-Kudlackova et al found the methionine intake of vegans, lacto-ovo vegetarians, and nonvegetarians was 0.77, 0.92, and 1.46 mg/d, respectively,[165] several studies found that SAA intake is similar between vegetarians and nonvegetarians.[166–168] And, in a study of 42 women (10 vegan, 16 vegetarian, and 16 omnivores) although the differences in urinary pH values between the vegans and omnivores was statistically significant despite very large intraindividual variations, with the urine of the vegans being less acidic than either lacto-ovo vegetarians or omnivores, the differences were not predicted by the essential amino acid content of the diet.[169] Finally, in a cohort study of 1865 peri- and postmenopausal women, higher consumption of foods rich in either meat protein or vegetable protein was associated with decreased risk for wrist fracture.[170]

The extent to which the hypercalciuric effects of sodium are pertinent to differences in calcium requirements between vegetarians and omnivores is not clear because dietary sodium intake data are limited. Also, it is very difficult to quantify sodium intake accurately. Some data suggest that only about 10% of the sodium consumed comes naturally from the food we eat. Fifteen percent comes from salt added during cooking and at the table, and fully 75% comes from salt added during processing and manufacturing.[171–173] Although many agrarian societies, whose diets are primarily vegetarian, consume less sodium than the typical industrialized society,[174,175] the sodium intake of lacto-ovo vegetarians appears to be similar to or only slightly lower than that of omnivores. There are only limited data on vegans, although their sodium intake does appear to be somewhat lower than that of nonvegetarians (Appendix G).

In addition, other dietary factors may affect bone health of vegetarians. Although findings are inconclusive, some research suggests that vitamin K reduces fracture risk and that the effects are independent of bone density.[176] Recent interest has also focused on serum homocysteine (Hcy) concentrations. Inadequate intake of vitamin B_{12}, folate, vitamin B_6, and possibly riboflavin is associated with increased levels of Hcy, and higher levels have been seen in some vegetarian populations (Chapter 7). Both vitamin B_{12}[177] and folate[178] have been associated with increased BMD, and in elderly Japanese, supplements of these two nutrients were effective in reducing hip fractures.[179] Among 5304 subjects in the Rotterdam Study, increased intakes of riboflavin and vitamin B_6 were associated with higher femoral neck BMD.[180] In healthy Slovak women, the higher Hcy levels seen in vegetarian women were associated with bone loss.[181]

BONE HEALTH OF VEGETARIANS

Overall, little evidence suggests that BMD differs significantly between Western omnivores and lacto-ovo vegetarians. Although some early research[182,183] suggested vegetarians had superior bone health, most later research suggests that bone health is similar to or slightly worse than omnivores.[184–190] For example, in a study of Canadian premenopausal women, the BMD of nonvegetarians increased 1.1% over the course of 1 year, whereas lacto-ovo vegetarian BMD was unchanged.[191] And in elderly Chinese living in Hong Kong, Lau et al found that the BMD of lactovegetarians at the femoral neck and Wards' triangle was lower than the BMD of omnivores, although in both groups, calcium intake was very low.[189] In a meta-analysis of three studies,[184,185,186] Anderson found that the BMD of the midradius of postmenopausal U.S. vegetarian women was about 2% lower than in the nonvegetarian controls.[192]

Unfortunately, there is little information about the bone health of vegans. Because their calcium intake is low relative to both lacto-ovo vegetarians and omnivores, vegans certainly absorb more of the calcium they ingest. In fact, one study found that vegetarians are generally more efficient at absorbing calcium than omnivores.[193] It is not known, however, whether this improved absorption compensates fully for a low calcium intake or to what extent the lower protein impacts calcium balance and bone health.

One small study involving only 11 women found that BMD of elderly vegans (age 60 to 90 years) was lower than that of nonvegan vegetarians.[187] The relevance of these findings to lifelong vegans is questionable, though, because subjects were classified as vegans if they had followed this diet for as little as 2 years. In the previously mentioned study of elderly Chinese by Lau et al, there was no difference in BMD between lactovegetarians and vegans, although the BMD of both groups was lower than that of omnivores.[194] But a study of Taiwanese vegetarians, 65% of whom were vegans, found that long-term vegan dietary practice was associated with lower hip BMD and lumbar spine osteomalacia, and with exceeding the BMD threshold associated with fracture risk.[194] It should be noted, however, that calcium intake for all subjects in this study averaged <400 mg/d, so the relevance to Western vegans is unclear. The BMD of semi-vegan rural Chinese who consumed few or no dairy products was somewhat lower than rural Chinese who consumed dairy and who had calcium intakes similar to those of the vegans.[195] No information was provided about the dietary sources of calcium in the vegan diets, however, so that calcium bioavailability of the overall diet is unknown. Also, calcium intakes were only between 300 and 400 mg/d, much less than the calcium intake of vegans in industrialized countries. And although a meta-analysis of nine studies found that vegetarians as a group have a lower BMD than omnivores, with most of the difference due to vegan subjects, the magnitude of the association was clinically insignificant.[196] Finally, in a study of 210 Buddhist nuns, there were no differences in BMD between vegans and omnivores despite the lower median calcium intake of vegans compared to the omnivores (330 ± 205 vs 682 ± 417 mg/d).[197]

A report from EPIC-Oxford, a prospective study of men and women in the United Kingdom, found a 30% higher fracture rate among vegans compared to meat eaters. However, the difference was halved in magnitude by adjustment for energy and calcium intake, and it disappeared altogether when the analysis was restricted to subjects who consumed at least 525 mg/d of calcium.[198]

Clearly, BMD is determined by many lifestyle and dietary factors, and because data on bone health of western vegans are limited, it is difficult to draw conclusions about the relationship of a vegan diet to bone health. For example, vitamin D intake, serum vitamin D, and intact PTH levels in Finnish vegans were shown to be below the normal range,[199] and vitamin D supplementation increased femoral BMD in Finnish vegans but not in lactovegetarians or omnivores.[200] Other research has also found vitamin D status may be compromised in vegans.[201] Interestingly, Anderson has suggested that the lower serum estrogen levels of vegetarians, perhaps resulting from their lower fat or high-fiber intake, is one risk factor for osteoporosis.[192] Other features of vegetarian diets, such as the inclusion of soy products, may be protective (Chapter 9).

MEETING THE CALCIUM ACCEPTED INTAKE ON PLANT-BASED DIETS

Based on current understanding of requirements, vegetarians should strive to meet the calcium recommendations set by the FNB. Dietary recommendations in Western countries tend to be biased toward the inclusion of dairy products in the diet, creating the impression that calcium needs cannot be met by vegan diets. Generally, populations that consume dairy have higher calcium intakes than those who do not.

Estimates are that about two thirds of the world's adult population has difficulty digesting milk.[202,203] In fact, nutritional anthropologists suggest that until 10,000 years ago or so, all human adults were lactose intolerant.[202,203] The ability to digest milk well into adulthood is probably the result of a genetic mutation among northern European populations. In the rest of the world, including Asia, North and South America, Africa, and along the Mediterranean, populations continued to develop normally; that is, they continued to lose their ability to digest milk as they matured. Thus historically, milk has played a limited role in the diet of humans.

To a large extent, however, the prevalence of lactase insufficiency is exaggerated because most lactose-intolerant adults are able to tolerate significant amounts of dairy foods even in populations where lactase insufficiency rates are high.[204-206] In fact, even among lactose maldigesters, lactose is not a major cause of symptoms, such as flatulence and bloating, in response to the ingestion of 1 cup of milk.[207] There is also evidence that the intestinal bacteria adapt to the intake of dairy/lactose, such that symptoms of lactose intolerance lessen over time.[208,209]

Nevertheless, many plant foods are rich sources of calcium. In fact, Eaton and Nelson have estimated that plants provided most of the calcium in our ancestral diets and that we evolved in a calcium-rich environment with average calcium intakes that may have been as high as 3000 mg/d on diets that included no dairy foods.[210] A more recent analysis suggests calcium intake was much lower than this.[211] Interestingly, wild plants are generally much higher in calcium than cultivated ones; nevertheless, commonly consumed vegetables such as broccoli and kale are quite high in calcium.

The absorption efficiency of calcium from a meal is fairly uniform, between 25% and 35%, regardless of the food source of the calcium, except for the high-oxalate foods.[38] Although the calcium in some high-oxalate vegetables—most notably spinach, Swiss chard, beet greens, and rhubarb—is largely unavailable, these foods represent the exception rather than the norm. On average, although only about 20% of the calcium from legumes is absorbed, as much as 50% of the calcium from green leafy vegetables is absorbed[212,213] (Table 5-2). The fractional absorption of calcium from milk and other dairy products is about 30%.[214] Calcium is well absorbed from calcium-fortified apple and orange juice.[215] Calcium absorption from the vast majority of soymilk sold in the United States is similar to that from calcium absorption from cow's milk.[216] Calcium absorption from tofu is also excellent. Finally, Hunt et al found that in premenopausal women, 22% of calcium from a controlled lacto-ovo vegetarian diet was absorbed, which was significantly lower than the 30% absorption of calcium from a nonvegetarian diet.[217]

Calcium is well distributed in the food supply, although many foods contain relatively small amounts of this nutrient. Foods that are fortified with calcium, including some breakfast cereals, orange juice, and some forms of tofu, are also widely available (Table 5-3). Some baked goods

Table 5-2 Availability of Calcium from Cow's Milk and Selected Plant Foods

Food Source[a]	Calcium Content (mg)	Fractional Absorption (%)[b]	Estimated Absorbable Calcium (mg)/Serving
Broccoli	35	52.6	18.4
Brussels sprouts	19	63.8	12.1
Chinese cabbage	79	53.8	42.5
Green cabbage	25	64.9	16.2
Kale	47	58.8	27.6
Milk (1 cup)	300	30.6	91.8
Mustard greens	64	57.8	37.0
Pinto beans	44.7	17.0	7.6
Sesame seeds (1 oz)	37	20.8	7.7
Soymilk fortified with tricalcium phosphate (1 cup)	300	23.7	71.1
Turnip greens	99	51.6	51.1
Tofu, calcium set	258	31.0	80.0

[a]Serving size equals ½ cup unless otherwise indicated.

[b]Absorption rates were adjusted for load (absolute amount of calcium).

Source: Data from Weaver CM, Plawecki KL. Dietary calcium: Adequacy of a vegetarian diet. *Am J Clin Nutr*. 1994;59(suppl):1238–1241; Heaney RP, Dowell SM, Rafferty K, Bierman J. Bioavailability of the calcium in soy imitation milk, with some observations on method. *Am J Clin Nutr*. 2000;71: 1166–1169.

Table 5-3 Calcium Content of Foods

Food	Calcium Content (mg)	Food	Calcium Content (mg)
Legumes, 1 cup cooked		**Nuts and Seeds**, (continued)	
Chickpeas	80	Sesame seeds	140
Great northern beans	120	Sesame tahini	128
Kidney beans	50	**Vegetables**, ½ cup cooked	
Lentils	38	Bok choy	79
Lima beans	32	Broccoli, from fresh	31
Navy beans	126	Broccoli, from frozen	43
Pinto beans	79	Collard greens, from fresh	133
Black beans	102	Kale, from fresh	47
Vegetarian baked beans	86	Kale, from frozen	90
Tofu, 3.5 oz [a]		Mustard greens, from fresh	52
Firm, prepared with nigari	175	Mustard greens, from frozen	76
Firm, prepared with calcium sulfate	683	Butternut squash	23
		Sweet potato	45
Regular, prepared with calcium sulfate	350	Turnip greens, from fresh	98
		Turnip greens, from frozen	125
Soft, prepared with calcium sulfate and nigari	111	**Fruits**	
Other soyfoods		Dried figs, 1 cup	241
Soybeans, 1 cup cooked	175	Orange, medium navel	60
Tempeh, 3.5 oz	111	Raisins, ½ cup	41
TVP, ½ cup rehydrated[b,c]	85	Orange juice, calcium fortified, 1 cup	300
Soymilk, 1 cup unfortified	61	**Other foods**	
Soymilk, 1 cup fortified[c]	250–300	Corn tortilla, 6 inch[c]	50
Soynuts, ¼ cup	60	English muffin, made with calcium propionate	92
Nuts and Seeds, 2 tbsp		Blackstrap molasses, 1 tbsp[c]	
Almonds	24	Fortified almond or rice milk, 1 cup	300
Almond butter	86		
Brazil nuts	15		

[a] Calcium in tofu varies depending on processing. Firmer types and those made with calcium sulfate contain the most calcium.

[b] TVP is a trademark of Archer Daniels Midland Company and is a textured soy protein.

[c] From product package information.

Source: Data from USDA National Nutrient Database for Standard Reference, Release 22, 2009.

contain the preservative calcium propionate, which can contribute to calcium intake as well. Consumption of calcium-rich water has been shown to have an important impact on calcium intake and bone health.[218] Thus calcium needs can be met without consuming dairy foods, but this does require that efforts be made to include specific foods in the diet that are good sources (Exhibit 5-1).

Vegetarians typically consume 50–100% more fiber (Appendix A) and two to three times the amount of phytate as nonvegetarians.[219–221] There is disagreement over the extent to which high-fiber diets may impair calcium absorption. Some investigators have concluded that fiber does not have a significant effect,[222–225] whereas others have concluded it does.[43,53,226,227]

In one study, fiber supplementation markedly decreased calcium absorption and reduced calcium balance in young men, although bone turnover was slowed, suggesting that subjects were adapting to the lower calcium bioavailability.[53] Similarly, although the calcium content of a high-fiber, plant-based rural Mexican diet was higher than that of an urban Mexican diet, both calcium absorption and calcium balance were poorer on the rural diet.[228] Wolf et al found that fractional calcium absorption by pre- and perimenopausal women who consumed low-fat, high-fiber diets was 19% less than those who consumed high-fat low-fiber diets[229] (Figure 5-2).

Total fiber may be less important than the amount of insoluble fiber in the diet, which is more likely to bind calcium. Wolf et al suggested that low-fat, high-fiber diets reduced calcium bio-

---

Exhibit 5-1 Sample Vegan Menu Providing 1000 mg Calcium

Breakfast:	1 cup bran flakes
	½ cup fortified soymilk
	½ sesame seed bagel
	2 tbsp almond butter
	6 oz calcium-fortified orange juice
Lunch:	1 6-inch whole wheat pita
	½ cup hummus spread
	Sliced tomato
	3 dried figs
	1 oatmeal cookie
Dinner:	1 cup baked beans
	1 cup steamed kale
	1 cup brown rice
Snacks:	Soymilk shake with 1 cup fortified soymilk
	½ frozen banana
	½ cup strawberries

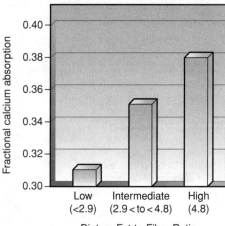

Figure 5-2 Calcium absorption in women ($N = 142$) according to dietary fat to fiber ratios. Ratios based on intake of dietary fat (g) divided by intake of dietary fiber. Trend statistically significant ($P < 0.001$) after adjustment for body mass index, calcium intake, serum vitamin D, parathyroid hormone concentration, and physical activity. *Source.* Data from Eaton SB, Konner MJ, Cordain L. Diet-dependent acid load, Paleolithic nutrition, and evolutionary health promotion. *Am J Clin Nutr*;92(2): 295–297.

availability by increasing intestinal motility, rather than by forming insoluble complexes.[218] Previous work has shown that a faster mouth to cecum transit time reduces calcium absorption[230] and that fat slows, and fiber increases, transit time.[231] However, psyllium, in the form of Metamucil, had essentially no effect on the bioavailability of co-ingested calcium when ingested at typical therapeutic doses.[232] Also, the calcium from kale is extremely well absorbed, although it is a high-fiber food.[233]

In vitro work suggests that it is the phytate, not the fiber, that inhibits calcium absorption.[234] For example, fractional calcium absorption from high-phytate soybeans was about 25% less than from low-phytate soybeans.[235] Components such as oxalate and phytate are already bound to calcium in foods, and so they are unlikely to interfere with calcium absorption from other foods.[236] Only wheat bran, which is very high in phytate, has been shown to decrease calcium absorption from other foods eaten at the same time.[236,237] For a general review on factors affecting calcium bioavailability see Gueguen and Pointillart.[238]

When grain products are leavened with yeast, which hydrolyzes the bond between phytate and calcium, the calcium bioavailability is increased.[237] Germination of beans[218] and fermentation of foods[239] also have been shown to mitigate the effects of phytate on calcium. But even the calcium in unleavened bread products is better absorbed than the calcium from milk, although bread is relatively low in calcium.[237] However, in a study of Nigerian children, dephytinization of maize porridge did not improve calcium absorption.[240]

It is noteworthy that foods naturally high in phytate and fiber tend to have higher mineral contents than refined food, so the total amount of available calcium may be greater in these

---

Net vs Gross (True) Calcium Absorption

There are huge differences in calcium bioavailability among dietary sources of calcium. Fractional calcium absorption from some green leafy vegetables is as high as 0.6, whereas from milk it is approximately 0.3, from many legumes it is 0.2, and from spinach and other oxalate-rich vegetables it is only 0.05. However, these values refer to gross calcium absorption.

Net calcium absorption is the difference between the amount of dietary calcium ingested and the amount excreted in the feces. Calcium is secreted into the intestines during digestion as part of digestive juices. A portion of this calcium is absorbed along with dietary calcium. Daily digestive juice contains approximately 200 mg of calcium, which must be taken into consideration when determining net calcium absorption.[7] For example, if 200 mg of calcium are consumed, and 50% of the total 400 mg of calcium in the gut is absorbed (200 mg from the diet and 200 mg from digestive juices), 200 mg of calcium will be absorbed and 200 mg will be excreted in the feces, making net calcium absorption zero. If 800 mg of calcium is ingested, and 40% of the total 1000 mg in the gut is absorbed (because absorption efficiency decreases with increased intake), then gross calcium absorption is 400 mg. This represents a net calcium absorption of 25% because the difference between calcium consumed (800 mg) and calcium excreted (600 mg) is 200 mg, or 25% of the 800 mg consumed. In addition to the effect of digestive juice calcium content, there is a slight increase in urinary calcium excretion as blood calcium rises in response to newly absorbed calcium.

When taking into consideration the loss of calcium via that in digestive juice, the slight hypercalciuric effect of ingested calcium, and the inverse relationship between fractional calcium absorption and calcium intake, at typical calcium intake levels in the United States, net calcium absorption may be only 5–10%.

---

unprocessed foods despite high phytate and fiber contents. Finally, the oxalate, fiber, and phytate content of a food does not always dictate calcium bioavailability. For example, the calcium in soybeans is well absorbed despite the fact that this food is high in all three of these components.[235] Despite concerns about fiber and phytate, calcium appears to be well absorbed from plant-based diets.

CONCLUSION

A number of dietary factors, including protein, sodium, potassium, phosphorus, fiber, and phytate intake, may affect calcium requirements of vegetarians. However, understanding of the impact of any single dietary factor on bone health is limited, and often data are quite conflicting. For example, research cited in this chapter indicates a protective role for protein in bone health when calcium intake is adequate. Therefore, lower protein and calcium intakes of vegans may adversely affect bone health. At this time, it is prudent for lacto-ovo vegetarians and vegans to meet the acceptable intake for calcium as established by the FNB. Because of the variety of plant foods that are naturally good sources of calcium as well as the growing number of fortified products, it is increasingly easy for vegans to meet calcium requirements provided they are given appropriate information about calcium sources. Although unrefined plant foods are high in fiber and sometimes phytate, both of which may reduce calcium absorption, calcium absorption has been shown to be good from most plant foods. Absorption rates from some vegetables are as much as twice those of calcium from milk. The exceptions are vegetables that are high in oxalates.

COUNSELING POINTS: CALCIUM

- The decreased hip fracture rates seen in countries where calcium intakes are lower may be due to a variety of genetic, lifestyle, and dietary factors and do not reflect calcium needs in other populations.
- Because of conflicting findings regarding the effects of protein on calcium balance and fracture risk, there is currently limited support for a protective effect of lower-protein diets on bone health.
- Pending further evidence, both lacto-ovo vegetarians and vegans should strive to meet the calcium recommendations set by the Institute of Medicine.
- Although dairy foods are the primary sources of calcium in the diets of most Americans, calcium needs can be met by consuming only plant foods
- With the exception of vegetables that are high in oxalates—beet greens, spinach, and chard—the calcium from plant foods is relatively well absorbed.
- Fortified foods—which include fruit juices, cereals, soymilk, and rice milk—can be helpful in meeting calcium needs. For those who do not meet needs, supplements are recommended.
- The following can help to enhance calcium absorption and retention:
  - Consume plenty of fruits and vegetables (high in potassium salts and alkali)
  - Consume adequate protein
  - Reduce sodium intake (decrease processed food intake)
  - If using supplements, spread intake out over the day (increases fractional calcium absorption efficiency)
  - Consume adequate vitamin D (promotes calcium absorption)

Case Study

Kate is a 53-year-old woman referred for nutrition counseling because she is concerned about osteoporosis. She has been a lacto-ovo vegetarian for the past 10 years but would like to adopt a vegan diet.

She currently takes a multivitamin supplement that includes iron and zinc. She is not taking any calcium supplements. Kate would like to plan a diet that includes at least 600 mg of calcium, which she believes is enough to meet the calcium needs of a vegan.

Kate works 40 hours per week in an office. She walks 2 miles every day at lunch and works out in the gym for 45 minutes three mornings per week.

(continued)

Kate's 24-hour recall:

Breakfast
    1 oz bran flakes with ½ cup low-fat milk
    1 banana
    ½ cup orange juice (takes her multivitamin with the orange juice)
    Coffee with cream

Midmorning snack
    ½ bagel with 1 tbsp peanut butter
    Coffee with cream

Lunch
    Sandwich on whole wheat bread with 2 slices Swiss cheese and 1 slice soy "deli meat."
    Apple

Afternoon Snack
    Pretzels

Dinner
    1 cup brown rice
    Stir-fried tofu and vegetables with ½ cup tofu, 1 cup broccoli, ½ cup carrots

To discuss:

    What will you tell Kate about her goals regarding calcium intake?

    What suggestions will you make for replacing the dairy foods in her diet with vegan options?

    What are some ideas for boosting the calcium content of her diet?

    Are there other changes she can make in her diet to promote bone health?

REFERENCES

1. Dawson-Hughes B, Harris SS, Krall EA, Dallal GE. Effect of calcium and vitamin D supplementation on bone density in men and women 65 years of age or older. *N Engl J Med.* 1997;337(10):670–676.
2. Fardellone P, Brazier M, Kamel S, et al. Biochemical effects of calcium supplementation in postmenopausal women: influence of dietary calcium intake. *Am J Clin Nutr.* 1998;67(6):1273–1278.
3. Gregg EW, Cauley JA, Seeley DG, Ensrud KE, Bauer DC. Physical activity and osteoporotic fracture risk in older women. Study of Osteoporotic Fractures Research Group. *Ann Intern Med.* 1998;129(2):81–88.
4. Foundation NO. http://www.nof.org/osteoporosis/diseasefacts.htm.
5. Melton LJ 3rd. Chrischilles EA, Cooper C, Lane AW, Riggs BL. Perspective. How many women have osteoporosis? *J Bone Miner Res.* 1992;7(9):1005–1010.
6. Wasnich RD. Vertebral fracture epidemiology. *Bone.* 1996;18 (3 suppl):179S–183S.
7. Nordin BE. Calcium and osteoporosis. *Nutrition.* 1997;13(7–8):664–686.
8. Heaney RP. Is there a role for bone quality in fragility fractures? *Calcif Tissue Int.* 1993;53 (suppl 1):S3–S6.
9. Faulkner KG. Bone matters: are density increases necessary to reduce fracture risk? *J Bone Miner Res.* 2000;15(2):183–187.
10. Green J. The physiochemical structure of bone: cellular and noncellular elements. *Miner Electrolyte Metab.* 1994;20:7–15.
11. Nilas L. Calcium intake and osteoporosis. *World Rev Nutr Diet.* 1993;73:1–26.

12. Xiaoge D, Eryuan L, Xianping W, et al. Bone mineral density differences at the femoral neck and Ward's triangle: a comparison study on the reference data between Chinese and Caucasian women. *Calcif Tissue Int.* 2000;67(3):195–198.

13. Gallagher JC, Goldgar D, Moy A. Total bone calcium in normal women: effect of age and menopause status. *J Bone Miner Res.* 1987;2(6):491–496.

14. Riggs BL, Khosla S, Melton LJ 3rd. A unitary model for involutional osteoporosis: estrogen deficiency causes both type I and type II osteoporosis in postmenopausal women and contributes to bone loss in aging men [see comments]. *J Bone Miner Res.* 1998;13(5):763–773.

15. Cumming RG, Klineberg RJ. Case-control study of risk factors for hip fractures in the elderly. *Am J Epidemiol.* 1994;139(5):493–503.

16. Munger RG, Cerhan JR, Chiu BC. Prospective study of dietary protein intake and risk of hip fracture in postmenopausal women. *Am J Clin Nutr.* 1999;69(1):147–152.

17. Owusu W, Willett WC, Feskanich D, Ascherio A, Spiegelman D, Colditz GA. Calcium intake and the incidence of forearm and hip fractures among men. *J Nutr.* 1997;127(9):1782–1787.

18. Feskanich D, Willett WC, Stampfer MJ, Colditz GA. Milk, dietary calcium, and bone fractures in women: a 12-year prospective study. *Am J Public Health.* 1997;87(6):992–997.

19. Cumming RG, Cummings SR, Nevitt MC, et al. Calcium intake and fracture risk: results from the study of osteoporotic fractures. *Am J Epidemiol.* 1997;145(10):926–934.

20. Michaelsson K, Melhus H, Bellocco R, Wolk A. Dietary calcium and vitamin D intake in relation to osteoporotic fracture risk. *Bone.* 2003;32(6):694–703.

21. Feskanich D, Willett WC, Colditz GA. Calcium, vitamin D, milk consumption, and hip fractures: a prospective study among postmenopausal women. *Am J Clin Nutr.* 2003;77(2):504–511.

22. Bischoff-Ferrari HA, Dawson-Hughes B, Baron JA, et al. Calcium intake and hip fracture risk in men and women: a meta-analysis of prospective cohort studies and randomized controlled trials. *Am J Clin Nutr.* 2007;86(6):1780–1790.

23. Grant AM, Avenell A, Campbell MK, et al. Oral vitamin D3 and calcium for secondary prevention of low-trauma fractures in elderly people (Randomised Evaluation of Calcium Or vitamin D, RECORD): a randomised placebo-controlled trial. *Lancet.* 2005;365(9471):1621–1628.

24. Reid IR, Mason B, Horne A, et al. Randomized controlled trial of calcium in healthy older women. *Am J Med.* 2006;119(9):777–785.

25. Tang BM, Eslick GD, Nowson C, Smith C, Bensoussan A. Use of calcium or calcium in combination with vitamin D supplementation to prevent fractures and bone loss in people aged 50 years and older: a meta-analysis. *Lancet.* 2007;370(9588):657–666.

26. Bischoff-Ferrari HA, Rees JR, Grau MV, Barry E, Gui J, Baron JA. Effect of calcium supplementation on fracture risk: a double-blind randomized controlled trial. *Am J Clin Nutr.* 2008;87(6):1945–1951.

27. Prince RL, Devine A, Dhaliwal SS, Dick IM. Effects of calcium supplementation on clinical fracture and bone structure: results of a 5-year, double-blind, placebo-controlled trial in elderly women. *Arch Intern Med.* 2006;166(8):869–875.

28. Barger-Lux MJ, Heaney RP. The role of calcium intake in preventing bone fragility, hypertension, and certain cancers. *J Nutr.* 1994;124(8 suppl):1406S-1411S.

29. Heaney RP. Nutrient effects: discrepancy between data from controlled trials and observational studies. *Bone.* 1997;21(6):469–471.

30. Nordin BC. Calcium requirement is a sliding scale. *Am J Clin Nutr.* 2000;71(6):1381–1383.

31. Food and Nutrition Board IoM. *Dietary Reference Intakes for Calcium, Phosphorus, Magnesium, Vitamin D, and Fluoride.* Washington, DC: National Academy Press; 1997.

32. Pennington JA, Schoen SA. Total diet study: estimated dietary intakes of nutritional elements, 1982–1991. *Int J Vitam Nutr Res.* 1996;66:350–362.

33. Ma J, Johns RA, Stafford RS. Americans are not meeting current calcium recommendations. *Am J Clin Nutr.* 2007;85(5):1361–1366.

34. Abrams SA, Wen J, Stuff JE. Absorption of calcium, zinc, and iron from breast milk by five- to seven-month-old infants [published erratum appears in *Pediatr Res.* 1997;41(6):814]. *Pediatr Res.* 1997;41(3):384–390.

35. Heaney RP, Recker RR, Stegman MR, Moy AJ. Calcium absorption in women: relationships to calcium intake, estrogen status, and age. *J Bone Miner Res.* 1989;4(4):469–475.
36. Heaney RP, Saville PD, Recker RR. Calcium absorption as a function of calcium intake. *J Lab Clin Med.* 1975; 85:881–890.
37. Ensrud KE, Duong T, Cauley JA, et al. Low fractional calcium absorption increases the risk for hip fracture in women with low calcium intake. Study of Osteoporotic Fractures Research Group. *Ann Intern Med.* 2000;132(5): 345–353.
38. Heaney RP, Weaver CM, Fitzsimmons ML, Recker RR. Calcium absorptive consistency. *J Bone Miner Res.* 1990; 5(11):1139–1142.
39. Recker RR. Calcium absorption and achlorhydria. *N Engl J Med.* 1985;313(2):70–73.
40. Heaney RP, Gallagher JC, Johnston CC, Neer R, Parfitt AM, Whedon GD. Calcium nutrition and bone health in the elderly. *Am J Clin Nutr.* 1982;36(5 suppl):986–1013.
41. Parfitt AM, Gallagher JC, Heaney RP, Johnston CC, Neer R, Whedon GD. Vitamin D and bone health in the elderly. *Am J Clin Nutr.* 1982;36(5 suppl):1014–1031.
42. Heaney RP, Recker RR, Weaver CM. Absorbability of calcium sources: the limited role of solubility. *Calcif Tissue Int.* 1990;46(5):300–304.
43. Knox TA, Kassarjian Z, Dawson-Hughes B, et al. Calcium absorption in elderly subjects on high- and low-fiber diets: effect of gastric acidity. *Am J Clin Nutr.* 1991;53(6):1480–1486.
44. Weaver CM. Age related calcium requirements due to changes in absorption and utilization. *J Nutr.* 1994;124(8 suppl):1418S–1425S.
45. Anderson JJB. Nutritional biochemistry of calcium and phosphorus. *J Nutr Biochem.* 1991;2:300–307.
46. Heaney RP. Lessons for nutritional science from vitamin D [editorial; comment]. *Am J Clin Nutr.* 1999;69(5):825–826.
47. Morris HA, Morrison GW, Burr M, Thomas DW, Nordin BE. Vitamin D and femoral neck fractures in elderly South Australian women. *Med J Aust.* 1984;140(9):519–521.
48. Riggs BL, Jowsey J, Kelly PJ, Hoffman DL, Arnaud CD. Effects of oral therapy with calcium and vitamin D in primary osteoporosis. *J Clin Endocrinol Metab.* 1976;42(6):1139–1144.
49. Agnusdei D, Civitelli R, Camporeale A, et al. Age-related decline of bone mass and intestinal calcium absorption in normal males. *Calcif Tissue Int.* 1998;63(3):197–201.
50. Leitch I, Aitken FC. The estimation of calcium requirement: a re-examination. *Nutr Abstr Rev.* 1959;29:393–411.
51. Adams ND, Gray RW, Lemann J Jr. The effects of oral CaCO3 loading and dietary calcium deprivation on plasma 1,25-dihydroxyvitamin D concentrations in healthy adults. *J Clin Endocrinol Metab.* 1979;48(6):1008–1016.
52. Kanis JA, Passmore R. Calcium supplementation of the diet—II [see comments]. *BMJ.* 1989;298(6668):205–208.
53. O'Brien KO, Allen LH, Quatromoni P, et al. High fiber diets slow bone turnover in young men but have no effect on efficiency of intestinal calcium absorption. *J Nutr.* 1993;123(12):2122–2128.
54. O'Brien KO, Abrams SA, Liang LK, Ellis KJ, Gagel RF. Increased efficiency of calcium absorption during short periods of inadequate calcium intake in girls [see comments]. *Am J Clin Nutr.* 1996;63(4):579–583.
55. Lee WT, Leung SS, Xu YC, et al. Effects of double-blind controlled calcium supplementation on calcium absorption in Chinese children measured with stable isotopes (42Ca and 44Ca). *Br J Nutr.* 1995;73(2):311–321.
56. Bonner F. Adaptation and nutritional needs. *Am J Clin Nutr.* 1997;65:1570.
57. O'Brien K. Reply to WTK Lee. *Am J Clin Nutr.* 1995;64:827–828.
58. Bleich HL, Moore MJ, Lemann J Jr, Adams ND, Gray RW. Urinary calcium excretion in human beings. *N Engl J Med.* 1979;301(10):535–541.
59. Heaney RP. Cofactors influencing the calcium requirement—other nutrients. Paper presented at the NIH Consensus Development Conference on Optimal Calcium Intake; June 6–8, 1994; Bethesda, MD.
60. Kerstetter JE, O'Brien KO, Caseria DM, Wall DE, Insogna KL. The impact of dietary protein on calcium absorption and kinetic measures of bone turnover in women. *J Clin Endocrinol Metab.* 2005;90(1):26–31.
61. Abelow BJ, Holford TR, Insogna KL. Cross-cultural association between dietary animal protein and hip fracture: a hypothesis. *Calcif Tissue Int.* 1992;50(1):14–18.
62. Frassetto LA, Todd KM, Morris RC Jr, Sebastian A. Worldwide incidence of hip fracture in elderly women: relation to consumption of animal and vegetable foods. *J Gerontol A Biol Sci Med Sci.* 2000;55(10):M585–592.

63. Heaney RP. Calcium, dairy products and osteoporosis. *J Am Coll Nutr.* 2000;19(2 suppl):83S–99S.

64. Aloia JF, Mikhail M, Pagan CD, Arunachalam A, Yeh JK, Flaster E. Biochemical and hormonal variables in black and white women matched for age and weight [see comments]. *J Lab Clin Med.* 1998;132(5):383–389.

65. Faulkner KG, Cummings SR, Black D, Palermo L, Gluer CC, Genant HK. Simple measurement of femoral geometry predicts hip fracture: the study of osteoporotic fractures. *J Bone Miner Res.* 1993;8(10):1211–1217.

66. Wetzsteon RJ, Hughes JM, Kaufman BC, et al. Ethnic differences in bone geometry and strength are apparent in childhood. *Bone.* 2009;44(5):970–975.

67. Aoyagi K, Ross PD, Davis JW, Wasnich RD, Hayashi T, Takemoto T. Falls among community-dwelling elderly in Japan. *J Bone Miner Res.* 1998;13(9):1468–1474.

68. Davis JW, Ross PD, Nevitt MC, Wasnich RD. Incidence rates of falls among Japanese men and women living in Hawaii. *J Clin Epidemiol.* 1997;50(5):589–594.

69. Lauritzen JB. Hip fractures: incidence, risk factors, energy absorption, and prevention. *Bone.* 1996;18(1 suppl):65S–75S.

70. Ho SC, Bacon WE, Harris T, Looker A, Maggi S. Hip fracture rates in Hong Kong and the United States, 1988 through 1989. *Am J Public Health.* 1993;83(5):694–697.

71. Ross PD, Norimatsu H, Davis JW, et al. A comparison of hip fracture incidence among native Japanese, Japanese Americans, and American Caucasians. *Am J Epidemiol.* 1991;133(8):801–809.

72. Ross PD, He Y, Yates AJ, et al. Body size accounts for most differences in bone density between Asian and Caucasian women. The EPIC (Early Postmenopausal Interventional Cohort) Study Group. *Calcif Tissue Int.* 1996; 59(5):339–343.

73. Russell-Aulet M, Wang J, Thornton JC, Colt EW, Pierson RN Jr. Bone mineral density and mass in a cross-sectional study of white and Asian women. *J Bone Miner Res.* 1993;8(5):575–582.

74. Ross PD, Huang C. Hip fracture incidence among Caucasians in Hawaii is similar to Japanese. A population-based study. *Aging (Milano).* 2000;12(5):356–359.

75. Ross PD, Fujiwara S, Huang C, et al. Vertebral fracture prevalence in women in Hiroshima compared to Caucasians or Japanese in the US. *Int J Epidemiol.* 1995;24(6):1171–1177.

76. Lau EM, Chan HH, Woo J, et al. Normal ranges for vertebral height ratios and prevalence of vertebral fracture in Hong Kong Chinese: a comparison with American Caucasians. *J Bone Miner Res.* 1996;11(9):1364–1368.

77. Dennison E, Yoshimura N, Hashimoto T, Cooper C. Bone loss in Great Britain and Japan: a comparative longitudinal study. *Bone.* 1998;23(4):379–382.

78. Tsai K, Twu S, Chieng P, Yang R, Lee T. Prevalence of vertebral fractures in Chinese men and women in urban Taiwanese communities. *Calcif Tissue Int.* 1996;59(4):249–253.

79. Kin K, Lee JH, Kushida K, et al. Bone density and body composition on the Pacific rim: a comparison between Japan-born and U.S.-born Japanese-American women. *J Bone Miner Res.* 1993;8(7):861–869.

80. Tsai K, Huang K, Chieng P, Su C. Bone mineral density of normal Chinese women in Taiwan. *Calcif Tissue Inter.* 1991;48:161–166.

81. Anderson JJ, Pollitzer WS. Ethnic and genetic differences in susceptibility to osteoporotic fractures. *Adv Nutr Res.* 1994;9:129–149.

82. Pollitzer WS, Anderson JJ. Ethnic and genetic differences in bone mass: a review with a hereditary vs environmental perspective [published erratum appears in *Am J Clin Nutr.* 1990;52(1):181]. *Am J Clin Nutr.* 1989;50(6):1244–1259.

83. Morrison NA, Qi JC, Tokita A, et al. Prediction of bone density from vitamin D receptor alleles [see comments] [published erratum appears in *Nature.* 1997; 387(6628):106]. *Nature.* 1994;367(6460):284–287.

84. Hemenway D, Azrael DR, Rimm EB, Feskanich D, Willett WC. Risk factors for hip fracture in US men aged 40 through 75 years. *Am J Public Health.* 1994;84(11):1843–1845.

85. Reid IR, Chin K, Evans MC, Jones JG. Relation between increase in length of hip axis in older women between 1950s and 1990s and increase in age specific rates of hip fracture [see comments]. *BMJ.* 1994;309(6953):508–509.

86. Anderson JJB, Metz JA. Contributions of dietary calcium and physical activity to primary prevention of osteoporosis in females. *J Am Coll Nutr.* 1993;12:378–383.

87. Chalmers J, Ho KC. Geographic variations in senile osteoporosis. The association with physical activity. *J Bone Joint Surg [Br].* 1970;52:667–675.

88. Wallace BA, Cumming RG. Systematic review of randomized trials of the effect of exercise on bone mass in pre- and postmenopausal women. *Calcif Tissue Int.* 2000;67(1):10–18.

89. Tudor-Locke C, McColl RS. Factors related to variation in premenopausal bone mineral status: a health promotion approach. *Osteoporos Int.* 2000;11(1):1–24.

90. Darling AL, Millward DJ, Torgerson DJ, Hewitt CE, Lanham-New SA. Dietary protein and bone health: a systematic review and meta-analysis. *Am J Clin Nutr.* 2009;90(6):1674–1692.

91. Meng X, Zhu K, Devine A, Kerr DA, Binns CW, Prince RL. A 5-year cohort study of the effects of high protein intake on lean mass and BMC in elderly postmenopausal women. *J Bone Miner Res.* 2009;24(11):1827–1834.

92. Linkswiler HM, Zemel MB, Hegsted M, Schuette S. Protein-induced hypercalciuria. *Fed Proc.* 1981;40(9):2429–2433.

93. Schuette SA, Linkswiler HM. Effects on Ca and P metabolism in humans by adding meat, meat plus milk, or purified proteins plus Ca and P to a low protein diet. *J Nutr.* 1982;112(2):338–349.

94. Kerstetter JE, Allen LH. Dietary protein increases urinary calcium. *J Nutr.* 1990;120(1):134–136.

95. Breslau NA, Brinkley L, Hill KD, Pak CY. Relationship of animal protein-rich diet to kidney stone formation and calcium metabolism. *J Clin Endocrinol Metab.* 1988;66(1):140–146.

96. Itoh R, Nishiyama N, Suyama Y. Dietary protein intake and urinary excretion of calcium: a cross-sectional study in a healthy Japanese population [see comments]. *Am J Clin Nutr.* 1998;67(3):438–444.

97. Spencer H, Kramer L, Osis D. Do protein and phosphorus cause calcium loss? *J Nutr.* 1988;118(6):657–660.

98. Spencer H, Kramer L, Osis D, Norris C. Effect of phosphorus on the absorption of calcium and on the calcium balance in man. *J Nutr.* 1978;108(3):447–457.

99. Spencer H, Kramer L, DeBartolo M, Norris C, Osis D. Further studies of the effect of a high protein diet as meat on calcium metabolism. *Am J Clin Nutr.* 1983;37(6):924–929.

100. Spencer H, Kramer L. Does dietary protein increase urinary calcium? [letter; comment]. *J Nutr.* 1991;121(1):151–152.

101. Roughead ZK, Johnson LK, Lykken GI, Hunt JR. Controlled high meat diets do not affect calcium retention or indices of bone status in healthy postmenopausal women. *J Nutr.* 2003;133(4):1020–1026.

102. Heaney RP, Recker RR. Effects of nitrogen, phosphorus, and caffeine on calcium balance in women. *J Lab Clin Med.* 1982;99(1):46–55.

103. Heaney RP, Recker RR. Determinants of endogenous fecal calcium in healthy women. *J Bone Miner Res.* 1994; 9(10):1621–1627.

104. Heaney RP. Protein intake and the calcium economy. *J Am Diet Assoc.* 1993;93(11):1259–1260.

105. Spencer H, Kramer L, Rubio N, Osis D. The effect of phosphorus on endogenous fecal calcium excretion in man. *Am J Clin Nutr.* 1986;43(5):844–851.

106. Recker RR, Davies KM, Hinders SM, Heaney RP, Stegman MR, Kimmel DB. Bone gain in young adult women [see comments]. *JAMA.* 1992;268(17):2403–2408.

107. Dawson-Hughes B, Harris SS. Calcium intake influences the association of protein intake with rates of bone loss in elderly men and women. *Am J Clin Nutr.* 2002;75(4):773–779.

108. Meyer HE, Pedersen JI, Loken EB, Tverdal A. Dietary factors and the incidence of hip fracture in middle-aged Norwegians. A prospective study. *Am J Epidemiol.* 1997;145(2):117–123.

109. Dargent-Molina P, Sabia S, Touvier M, et al. Proteins, dietary acid load, and calcium and risk of postmenopausal fractures in the E3N French women prospective study. *J Bone Miner Res.* 2008;23(12):1915–1922.

110. Zhong Y, Okoro CA, Balluz LS. Association of total calcium and dietary protein intakes with fracture risk in postmenopausal women: the 1999–2002 National Health and Nutrition Examination Survey (NHANES). *Nutrition* 2009;25(6):647–654.

111. Hunt JR, Johnson LK, Fariba Roughead ZK. Dietary protein and calcium interact to influence calcium retention: a controlled feeding study. *Am J Clin Nutr.* 2009;89(5):1357–1365.

112. Rapuri PB, Gallagher JC, Haynatzka V. Protein intake: effects on bone mineral density and the rate of bone loss in elderly women. *Am J Clin Nutr.* 2003;77(6):1517–1525.

113. Fenton TR, Lyon AW, Eliasziw M, Tough SC, Hanley DA. Meta-analysis of the effect of the acid-ash hypothesis of osteoporosis on calcium balance. *J Bone Miner Res.* 2009;24(11):1835–1840.

114. Feskanich D, Willett WC, Stampfer MJ, Colditz GA. Protein consumption and bone fractures in women. *Am J Epidemiol.* 1996;143(5):472–479.

115. Sellmeyer DE, Stone KL, Sebastian A, Cummings SR. A high ratio of dietary animal to vegetable protein increases the rate of bone loss and the risk of fracture in postmenopausal women. *Am J Clin Nutr.* 2001;73(1):118–122.

116. Hannan MT, Tucker KL, Dawson-Hughes B, Cupples LA, Felson DT, Kiel DP. Effect of dietary protein on bone loss in elderly men and women: the Framingham Osteoporosis Study. *J Bone Miner Res.* 2000;15(12):2504–2512.

117. Matkovic V, Ilich JZ, Andon MB, et al. Urinary calcium, sodium, and bone mass of young females [see comments]. *Am J Clin Nutr.* 1995;62(2):417–425.

118. Devine A, Dick IM, Islam AF, Dhaliwal SS, Prince RL. Protein consumption is an important predictor of lower limb bone mass in elderly women. *Am J Clin Nutr.* 2005;81(6):1423–1428.

119. Kerstetter JE, Looker AC, Insogna KL. Low dietary protein and low bone density. *Calcif Tissue Int.* 2000;66(4):313.

120. Promislow JH, Goodman-Gruen D, Slymen DJ, Barrett-Connor E. Protein consumption and bone mineral density in the elderly: the Rancho Bernardo Study. *Am J Epidemiol.* 2002;155(7):636–644.

121. Hunt JR, Gallagher SK, Johnson LK, Lykken GI. High- versus low-meat diets: effects on zinc absorption, iron status, and calcium, copper, iron, magnesium, manganese, nitrogen, phosphorus, and zinc balance in postmenopausal women. *Am J Clin Nutr.* 1995;62(3):621–632.

122. Pannemans DL, Schaafsma G, Westerterp KR. Calcium excretion, apparent calcium absorption and calcium balance in young and elderly subjects: influence of protein intake. *Br J Nutr.* 1997;77(5):721–729.

123. Schurch MA, Rizzoli R, Slosman D, Vadas L, Vergnaud P, Bonjour JP. Protein supplements increase serum insulin-like growth factor-I levels and attenuate proximal femur bone loss in patients with recent hip fracture. A randomized, double-blind, placebo-controlled trial. *Ann Intern Med.* 1998;128(10):801–809.

124. Delmi M, Rapin CH, Bengoa JM, Delmas PD, Vasey H, Bonjour JP. Dietary supplementation in elderly patients with fractured neck of the femur. *Lancet.* 1990;335(8696):1013–1016.

125. Khalil DA, Lucas EA, Juma S, Smith BJ, Payton ME, Arjmandi BH. Soy protein supplementation increases serum insulin-like growth factor-I in young and old men but does not affect markers of bone metabolism. *J Nutr.* 2002;132(9):2605–2608.

126. Allen NE, Appleby PN, Davey GK, Kaaks R, Rinaldi S, Key TJ. The associations of diet with serum insulin-like growth factor 1 and its main binding proteins in 292 women meat-eaters, vegetarians, and vegans. *Cancer Epidemiol Biomarkers Prev.* 2002;11(11):1441–1448.

127. Fontana L, Shew JL, Holloszy JO, Villareal DT. Low bone mass in subjects on a long-term raw vegetarian diet. *Arch Intern Med.* 2005;165(6):684–689.

128. Kerstetter JE, Caseria DM, Mitnick ME, et al. Increased circulating concentrations of parathyroid hormone in healthy, young women consuming a protein-restricted diet. *Am J Clin Nutr.* 1997;66(5):1188–1196.

129. Kerstetter JE, O'Brien KO, Insogna KL. Dietary protein affects intestinal calcium absorption. *Am J Clin Nutr.* 1998;68(4):859–865.

130. Kerstetter JE, Svastisalee CM, Caseria DM, Mitnick ME, Insogna KL. A threshold for low-protein-diet-induced elevations in parathyroid hormone. *Am J Clin Nutr.* 2000;72(1):168–173.

131. Heaney RP. Dietary protein and phosphorus do not affect calcium absorption. *Am J Clin Nutr.* 2000;72(3):758–761.

132. Barr SI, McCarron DA, Heaney RP, et al. Effects of increased consumption of fluid milk on energy and nutrient intake, body weight, and cardiovascular risk factors in healthy older adults. *J Am Diet Assoc.* 2000;100(7):810–817.

133. Krieger NS, Sessler NE, Bushinsky DA. Acidosis inhibits osteoblastic and stimulates osteoclastic activity in vitro. *Am J Physiol.* 1992;262(3 Pt 2):F442–F448.

134. Giovannucci E. Dietary influences of 1,25(OH)2 vitamin D in relation to prostate cancer: a hypothesis [see comments]. *Cancer Causes Control.* 1998;9(6):567–582.

135. Zemel MB, Schuette SA, Hegsted M, Linkswiler HM. Role of the sulfur-containing amino acids in protein-induced hypercalciuria in men. *J Nutr.* 1981;111(3):545–552.

136. Tucker KL, Chen H, Hannan MT, et al. Bone mineral density and dietary patterns in older adults: the Framingham Osteoporosis Study. *Am J Clin Nutr.* 2002;76(1):245–252.

137. Prynne CJ, Mishra GD, O'Connell MA, et al. Fruit and vegetable intakes and bone mineral status: a cross sectional study in 5 age and sex cohorts. *Am J Clin Nutr.* 2006;83(6):1420–1428.

138. Sahni S, Hannan MT, Gagnon D, et al. High vitamin C intake is associated with lower 4-year bone loss in elderly men. *J Nutr.* 2008;138(10):1931–1938.

139. McGartland CP, Robson PJ, Murray LJ, et al. Fruit and vegetable consumption and bone mineral density: the Northern Ireland Young Hearts Project. *Am J Clin Nutr.* 2004;80(4):1019–1023.

140. Tylavsky FA, Holliday K, Danish R, Womack C, Norwood J, Carbone L. Fruit and vegetable intakes are an independent predictor of bone size in early pubertal children. *Am J Clin Nutr.* 2004;79(2):311–317.

141. Macdonald HM, New SA, Golden MH, Campbell MK, Reid DM. Nutritional associations with bone loss during the menopausal transition: evidence of a beneficial effect of calcium, alcohol, and fruit and vegetable nutrients and of a detrimental effect of fatty acids. *Am J Clin Nutr.* 2004;79(1):155–165.

142. Blatherwick NR. The specific role of foods in relation to the composition of urine. *Arch Intern Med.* 1914;14:409–450.

143. Remer T, Manz F. Potential renal acid load of foods and its influence on urine pH. *J Am Diet Assoc.* 1995;95(7):791–797.

144. Halperin ML. Metabolism and acid-base physiology. *Artif Organs.* 1982;6(4):357–362.

145. Green TJ, Whiting SJ. Potassium bicarbonate reduces high protein-induced hypercalciuria in adult men. *Nutr Rev.* 1994;14:991–1002.

146. Appel LJ, Moore TJ, Obarzanek E, et al. A clinical trial of the effects of dietary patterns on blood pressure. DASH Collaborative Research Group. *N Engl J Med.* 1997;336(16):1117–1124.

147. Barzel US. Dietary patterns and blood pressure. *N Engl J Med.* 1997;337(9):637; discussion 638.

148. Kaneko K, Masaki U, Aikyo M, et al. Urinary calcium and calcium balance in young women affected by high protein diet of soy protein isolate and adding sulfur-containing amino acids and/or potassium. *J Nutr Sci Vitaminol (Tokyo)* 1990;36(2):105–116.

149. Rafferty K, Heaney RP. Nutrient effects on the calcium economy: emphasizing the potassium controversy. *J Nutr.* 2008;138(1):166S–171S.

150. Shortt C, Flynn A. Sodium-calcium inter-relationships with specific reference to osteoporosis. *Nutr Res Rev.* 1990;3:101–115.

151. Kurtz TW, Al-Bander HA, Morris RC Jr. "Salt-sensitive" essential hypertension in men. Is the sodium ion alone important? *N Engl J Med.* 1987;317(17):1043–1048.

152. MacGregor GA, Cappuccio FP. The kidney and essential hypertension: a link to osteoporosis? *J Hypertens.* 1993;11(8):781–785.

153. Cirillo M, Ciacci C, Laurenzi M, Mellone M, Mazzacca G, De Santo NG. Salt intake, urinary sodium, and hypercalciuria. *Miner Electrolyte Metab.* 1997;23(3–6):265–268.

154. Intersalt Cooperative Research Group. Intersalt: an international study of electrolyte excretion and blood pressure. Results for a 24 hour urinary sodium and potassium excretion. *BMJ.* 1988;297:319–328.

155. Kaplan NM. The dietary guideline for sodium: should we shake it up? No. *Am J Clin Nutr.* 2000;71(5):1020–1026.

156. US Department of Agriculture. Nationwide Food Consumption Survey. Individuals in 48 States, Year 1977–78 (report 1–2). Hyattsville, MD: Consumer Nutrition Division, Human Nutrition Information Service; 1984.

157. Devine A, Criddle RA, Dick IM, Kerr DA, Prince RL. A longitudinal study of the effect of sodium and calcium intakes on regional bone density in postmenopausal women [see comments]. *Am J Clin Nutr.* 1995;62(4):740–745.

158. Itoh R, Suyama Y, Oguma Y, Yokota F. Dietary sodium, an independent determinant for urinary deoxypyridinoline in elderly women. A cross-sectional study on the effect of dietary factors on deoxypyridinoline excretion in 24-h urine specimens from 763 free-living healthy Japanese. *Eur J Clin Nutr.* 1999;53(11):886–890.

159. Ginty F, Flynn A, Cashman KD. The effect of dietary sodium intake on biochemical markers of bone metabolism in young women. *Br J Nutr.* 1998;79(4):343–350.

160. McBean LD, Forgac T, Finn SC. Osteoporosis: visions for care and prevention—a conference report. *J Am Diet Assoc.* 1994;94:668–671.

161. Nordin BEC, Polley KJ. Metabolic consequences of the menopause. A cross-sectional, longtitudinal, and intervention study on 557 normal postmenopausal women. *Calcif Tissue Int.* 1987;41:S1–S59.

162. Sellmeyer DE, Schloetter M, Sebastian A. Potassium citrate prevents increased urine calcium excretion and bone resorption induced by a high sodium chloride diet. *J Clin Endocrinol Metab.* 2002;87(5):2008–2012.

163. Teucher B, Dainty JR, Spinks CA, et al. Sodium and bone health: impact of moderately high and low salt intakes on calcium metabolism in postmenopausal women. *J Bone Miner Res.* 2008;23(9):1477–1485.

164. Nowson CA, Patchett A, Wattanapenpaiboon N. The effects of a low-sodium base-producing diet including red meat compared with a high-carbohydrate, low-fat diet on bone turnover markers in women aged 45–75 years. *Br J Nutr.* 2009;102(8):1161–1170.

165. Krajcovicova-Kudlackova M, Blazicek P, Babinska K, et al. Traditional and alternative nutrition—levels of homocysteine and lipid parameters in adults. *Scand J Clin Lab Invest.* 2000;60(8):657–664.

166. Kunkel ME, Beauchene RE. Protein intake and urinary excretion of protein-derived metabolites in aging female vegetarians and nonvegetarians. *J Am Coll Nutr.* 1991;10(4):308–314.

167. Hardinge MG, Crooks H, Stare FJ. Nutritional studies of vegetarians. *J Am Diet Assoc.* 1966;48(1):25–28.

168. Register UD, Sonnenberg LM. The vegetarian diet. Scientific and practical considerations. *J Am Diet Assoc.* 1973;62(3):253–261.

169. Ausman LM, Oliver LM, Goldin BR, Woods MN, Gorbach SL, Dwyer JT. Estimated net acid excretion inversely correlates with urine pH in vegans, lacto-ovo vegetarians, and omnivores. *J Ren Nutr.* 2008;18(5):456–465.

170. Thorpe DL, Knutsen SF, Beeson WL, Rajaram S, Fraser GE. Effects of meat consumption and vegetarian diet on risk of wrist fracture over 25 years in a cohort of peri- and postmenopausal women. *Public Health Nutr.* 2008;11(6):564–572.

171. Sanchez-Castillo CP, Warrender S, Whitehead TP, James WP. An assessment of the sources of dietary salt in a British population. *Clin Sci.* 1987;72(1):95–102.

172. Sanchez-Castillo CP, Branch WJ, James WP. A test of the validity of the lithium-marker technique for monitoring dietary sources of salt in man. *Clin Sci.* 1987;72(1):87–94.

173. Mattes RD, Donnelly D. Relative contributions of dietary sodium sources. *J Am Coll Nutr.* 1991;10(4):383–393.

174. Page LB. Nutritional determinants of hypertension. *Curr Concepts Nutr.* 1981;10:113–126.

175. McCarron DA, Henry HJ, Morris CD. Human nutrition and blood pressure regulation, an integrated approach. *Hypertension.* 1982;4 (suppl 3):2–13.

176. Iwamoto J, Sato Y, Takeda T, Matsumoto H. High-dose vitamin K supplementation reduces fracture incidence in postmenopausal women: a review of the literature. *Nutr Res.* 2009;29(4):221–228.

177. Morris MS, Jacques PF, Selhub J. Relation between homocysteine and B-vitamin status indicators and bone mineral density in older Americans. *Bone.* 2005;37(2):234–242.

178. Cagnacci A, Baldassari F, Rivolta G, Arangino S, Volpe A. Relation of homocysteine, folate, and vitamin B12 to bone mineral density of postmenopausal women. *Bone.* 2003;33(6):956–959.

179. Sato Y, Honda Y, Iwamoto J, Kanoko T, Satoh K. Effect of folate and mecobalamin on hip fractures in patients with stroke: a randomized controlled trial. *JAMA.* 2005;293(9):1082–1088.

180. Yazdanpanah N, Zillikens MC, Rivadeneira F, et al. Effect of dietary B vitamins on BMD and risk of fracture in elderly men and women: the Rotterdam study. *Bone.* 2007;41(6):987–994.

181. Krivosikova Z, Krajcovicova-Kudlackova M, Spustova V, et al. The association between high plasma homocysteine levels and lower bone mineral density in Slovak women: the impact of vegetarian diet. *Eur J Nutr.* 2010;49(3):147–153.

182. Ellis FR, Holesh S, Ellis JW. Incidence of osteoporosis in vegetarians and omnivores. *Am J Clin Nutr.* 1972;25(6):555–558.

183. Sanchez TV, Mickelson O, Marsh AG, Garn SM, Mayor GH. Bone mineral density in elderly vegetarian and omnivorous females. In: Mazeness RB, ed. *Proceedings of the 4th International Conference on Bone Mineral Measurements.* Bethesda, MD: National Institute of Arthritis, Metabolism, and Digestive Diseases; 1980:94–98.

184. Tylavsky FA, Anderson JJ. Dietary factors in bone health of elderly lactoovovegetarian and omnivorous women. *Am J Clin Nutr.* 1988;48(3 suppl):842–849.

185. Tesar R, Notelovitz M, Shim E, Kauwell G, Brown J. Axial and peripheral bone density and nutrient intakes of postmenopausal vegetarian and omnivorous women. *Am J Clin Nutr.* 1992;56(4):699–704.

186. Reed JA, Anderson JJ, Tylavsky FA, Gallagher PN Jr. Comparative changes in radial-bone density of elderly female lacto-ovo vegetarians and omnivores [published erratum appears in *Am J Clin Nutr.* 1994;60(6):981]. *Am J Clin Nutr* 1994;59(5 suppl):1197S–1202S.

187. Marsh AG, Sanchez TV, Michelsen O, Chaffee FL, Fagal SM. Vegetarian lifestyle and bone mineral density. *Am J Clin Nutr.* 1988;48(3 suppl):837–841.

188. Hunt IF, Murphy NJ, Henderson C, et al. Bone mineral content in postmenopausal women: comparison of omnivores and vegetarians. *Am J Clin Nutr.* 1989;50(3):517–523.

189. Lau EM, Kwok T, Woo J, Ho SC. Bone mineral density in Chinese elderly female vegetarians, vegans, lacto-vegetarians and omnivores. *Eur J Clin Nutr.* 1998;52(1):60–64.
190. Ellis FR, Holesh S, Sanders TAB. Osteoporosis in British vegetarians and omnivores. *Am J Clin Nutr.* 1974;27:769–770.
191. Barr SI, Prior JC, Janelle KC, Lentle BC. Spinal bone mineral density in premenopausal vegetarian and nonvegetarian women: cross-sectional and prospective comparisons. *J Am Diet Assoc.* 1998;98(7):760–765.
192. Anderson JJ. Plant-based diets and bone health: nutritional implications. *Am J Clin Nutr.* 1999;70(3 suppl):539S–542S.
193. Nnakwe N, Kies C. Calcium and phosphorus utilization by omnivorous and lacto-ovo- vegetarians fed laboratory controlled lacto-ovo-vegetarian diets. *Nutr Rep Int.* 1985;31:1009–1014.
194. Chiu JF, Lan SJ, Yang CY, et al. Long-term vegetarian diet and bone mineral density in postmenopausal Taiwanese women. *Calcif Tissue Int.* 1997;60(3):245–249.
195. Hu JF, Zhao XH, Jia JB, Parpia B, Campbell TC. Dietary calcium and bone density among middle-aged and elderly women in China. *Am J Clin Nutr.* 1993;58(2):219–227.
196. Ho-Pham LT, Nguyen ND, Nguyen TV. Effect of vegetarian diets on bone mineral density: a Bayesian meta-analysis. *Am J Clin Nutr.* 2009;90(4):943–950.
197. Ho-Pham LT, Nguyen PL, Le TT, et al. Veganism, bone mineral density, and body composition: a study in Buddhist nuns. *Osteoporos Int.* 2009;20(12):2087–2093.
198. Appleby P, Roddam A, Allen N, Key T. Comparative fracture risk in vegetarians and nonvegetarians in EPIC-Oxford. *Eur J Clin Nutr.* 2007;61(12):1400–1406.
199. Outila TA, Karkkainen MU, Seppanen RH, Lamberg-Allardt CJ. Dietary intake of vitamin D in premenopausal, healthy vegans was insufficient to maintain concentrations of serum 25-hydroxyvitamin D and intact parathyroid hormone within normal ranges during the winter in Finland. *J Am Diet Assoc.* 2000;100(4):434–441.
200. Outila TA, Lamberg-Allardt CJ. Ergocalciferol supplementation may positively affect lumbar spine bone mineral density of vegans [letter]. *J Am Diet Assoc.* 2000;100(6):629.
201. Lamberg-Allardt C, Karkkainen M, Seppanen R, Bistrom H. Low serum 25- hydroxyvitamin D concentrations and secondary hyperparathyroidism in middle-aged white strict vegetarians. *Am J Clin Nutr.* 1993;58(5):684–689.
202. Montgomery RK, Buller HA, Rings EH, Grand RJ. Lactose intolerance and the genetic regulation of intestinal lactase- phlorizin hydrolase. *Faseb J.* 1991;5(13):2824–2832.
203. Simoons FJ. The geographic hypothesis and lactose malabsorption. *Dig Dis Sci.* 1989;23:963–980.
204. Johnson AO, Semenya JG, Buchowski MS, Enwonwu CO, Scrimshaw NS. Adaptation of lactose maldigesters to continued milk intakes. *Am J Clin Nutr.* 1993;58(6):879–881.
205. Suarez FL, Savaiano D, Arbisi P, Levitt MD. Tolerance to the daily ingestion of two cups of milk by individuals claiming lactose intolerance. *Am J Clin Nutr.* 1997;65(5):1502–1506.
206. Suarez FL, Adshead J, Furne JK, Levitt MD. Lactose maldigestion is not an impediment to the intake of 1500 mg calcium daily as dairy products [see comments]. *Am J Clin Nutr.* 1998;68(5):1118–1122.
207. Savaiano DA, Boushey CJ, McCabe GP. Lactose intolerance symptoms assessed by meta-analysis: a grain of truth that leads to exaggeration. *J Nutr.* 2006;136(4):1107–1113.
208. Hertzler SR, Savaiano DA. Colonic adaptation to daily lactose feeding in lactose maldigesters reduces lactose intolerance. *Am J Clin Nutr.* 1996;64(2):232–236.
209. Pribila BA, Hertzler SR, Martin BR, Weaver CM, Savaiano DA. Improved lactose digestion and intolerance among African-American adolescent girls fed a dairy-rich diet. *J Am Diet Assoc.* 2000;100(5):524–528; quiz 9–30.
210. Eaton SB, Nelson DA. Calcium in evolutionary perspective. *Am J Clin Nutr.* 1991;54(1 suppl):281S–287S.
211. Eaton SB, Konner MJ, Cordain L. Diet-dependent acid load, Paleolithic nutrition, and evolutionary health promotion. *Am J Clin Nutr.* 2010;91(2):295–297.
212. Weaver CM, Proulx WR, Heaney R. Choices for achieving adequate dietary calcium with a vegetarian diet. *Am J Clin Nutr.* 1999;70(3 suppl):543S–548S.
213. Weaver CM, Plawecki KL. Dietary calcium: adequacy of a vegetarian diet. *Am J Clin Nutr.* 1994;59(5 suppl):1238S–1241S.
214. Nickel KP, Martin BR, Smith DL, Smith JB, Miller GD, Weaver CM. Calcium bioavailability from bovine milk and dairy products in premenopausal women using intrinsic and extrinsic labeling techniques. *J Nutr.* 1996;126(5):1406–1411.

215. Andon MB, Peacock M, Kanerva RL, DeCastro JA. Calcium absorption from apple and orange juice fortified with calcium citrate malate (CCM). *J Am Coll Nutr.* 1996;15:313–316.

216. Zhao Y, Martin BR, Weaver CM. Calcium bioavailability of calcium carbonate fortified soymilk is equivalent to cow's milk in young women. *J Nutr.* 2005;135(10):2379–2382.

217. Hunt JR, Matthys LA, Johnson LK. Zinc absorption, mineral balance, and blood lipids in women consuming controlled lactoovovegetarian and omnivorous diets for 8 wk. *Am J Clin Nutr.* 1998;67(3):421–430.

218. Ghanem KZ, Hussein L. Calcium bioavailability of selected Egyptian foods with emphasis on the impact of fermentation and germination. *Int J Food Sci Nutr.* 1999;50(5):351–356.

219. Brune M, Rossander L, Hallberg L. Iron absorption: no intestinal adaptation to a high-phytate diet. *Am J Clin Nutr.* 1989;49(3):542–545.

220. Ellis R, Morris ER, Hill AD, Smith JC Jr. Phytate:zinc molar ratio, mineral, and fiber content of three hospital diets. *J Am Diet Assoc.* 1982;81(1):26–29.

221. Ellis R, Kelsay JL, Reynolds RD, Morris ER, Moser PB, Frazier CW. Phytate:zinc and phytate X calcium:zinc millimolar ratios in self- selected diets of Americans, Asian Indians, and Nepalese. *J Am Diet Assoc.* 1987;87(8):1043–1047.

222. van Dokkum W. The relative significance of dietary fibre for human health. *Front Gastrointest Res.* 1988;14:135–145.

223. Rattan J, Levin N, Graff E, Weizer N, Gilat T. A high-fiber diet does not cause mineral and nutrient deficiencies. *J Clin Gastroenterol.* 1981;3:389–393.

224. Spencer H, Norris C, Derler J, Osis D. Effect of oat bran muffins on calcium absorption and calcium, phosphorus, magnesium and zinc balance in men. *J Nutr.* 1991;121(12):1976–1983.

225. Shah M, Chandalia M, Adams-Huet B, et al. Effect of a high-fiber diet compared with a moderate-fiber diet on calcium and other mineral balances in subjects with type 2 diabetes. *Diabetes Care.* 2009;32(6):990–995.

226. Sandstead HH. Fiber, phytates, and mineral nutrition. *Nutr Rev.* 1992;50(1):30–31.

227. Moynahan EJ. Nutritional hazards of high-fibre diet [letter]. *Lancet.* 1977;1(8012):654–655.

228. Rosado JL, Lopez P, Morales M, Munoz E, Allen LH. Bioavailability of energy, nitrogen, fat, zinc, iron and calcium from rural and urban Mexican diets. *Br J Nutr.* 1992;68(1):45–58.

229. Wolf RL, Cauley JA, Baker CE, et al. Factors associated with calcium absorption efficiency in pre- and perimenopausal women. *Am J Clin Nutr.* 2000;72(2):466–471.

230. Barger-Lux MJ, Heaney RP, Lanspa SJ, Healy JC, DeLuca HF. An investigation of sources of variation in calcium absorption efficiency [published erratum appears in *J Clin Endocrinol Metab.* 1995;80(7):2068]. *J Clin Endocrinol Metab.* 1995;80(2):406–411.

231. Heaney RP, Weaver CM, Barger-Lux MJ. Food factors influencing calcium availability. *Challenges Mod Med.* 1995;7:229–241.

232. Heaney RP, Weaver CM. Effect of psyllium on absorption of co-ingested calcium. *J Am Geriatr Soc.* 1995;43(3):261–263.

233. Heaney RP, Weaver CM. Calcium absorption from kale. *Am J Clin Nutr.* 1990;51(4):656–657.

234. Kennefick S, Cashman KD. Inhibitory effect of wheat fibre extract on calcium absorption in Caco-2 cells: evidence for a role of associated phytate rather than fibre per se. *Eur J Nutr.* 2000;39(1):12–17.

235. Heaney RP, Weaver CM, Fitzsimmons ML. Soybean phytate content: effect on calcium absorption. *Am J Clin Nutr.* 1991;53(3):745–747.

236. Heaney RP. Optimal calcium intake [letter; comment]. *JAMA.* 1995;274(13):1012–1013.

237. Weaver CM, Heaney RP, Martin BR, Fitzsimmons ML. Human calcium absorption from whole-wheat products. *J Nutr.* 1991;121(11):1769–1775.

238. Gueguen L, Pointillart A. The bioavailability of dietary calcium. *J Am Coll Nutr.* 2000;19(2 suppl):119S–136S.

239. Levrat-Verny MA, Coudray C, Bellanger J, et al. Wholewheat flour ensures higher mineral absorption and bioavailability than white wheat flour in rats. *Br J Nutr.* 1999;82(1):17–21.

240. Thacher TD, Obadofin MO, O'Brien KO, Abrams SA. The effect of vitamin D2 and vitamin D3 on intestinal calcium absorption in Nigerian children with rickets. *J Clin Endocrinol Metab.* 2009;94(9):3314–3321.

CHAPTER 6

Minerals

Plant-based diets can provide adequate amounts of all minerals. Three minerals, however, have been the focus of much attention regarding their levels and/or bioavailability in vegetarian diets. These are calcium (discussed in Chapter 5), iron, and zinc.

PHYTATE AND MINERAL BIOAVAILABILITY

One of the most important inhibitors of mineral absorption in vegetarian diets is phytic acid. Phytate (inositol hexaphosphate, IP_6) is a phosphorus-containing organic compound found in plant foods including whole grains legumes, seeds, nuts, and to a lesser extent in vegetables (see Table 6-1). It is an excellent chelator of metal ions, particularly iron and zinc. Humans are not able to hydrolyze phytate so that minerals bound to phytate are very poorly absorbed.

Refining whole grains can remove much of the phytate but also much of the minerals. Other food-processing techniques, such as soaking, malting, and fermenting, and high-temperature thermal processing, result in phytate hydrolysis.[1,2] This leads to the production of lower phosphorylated forms of phytate (IP_1, IP_2, IP_3, IP_4, and IP_5). IP_3, IP_4, and IP_5 are still able to bind iron, but IP_1 and IP_2 cannot; only IP_5 binds zinc.[3,4] Because of the hydrolysis of phytate that occurs during fermentation and the baking process, mineral bioavailability from leavened breads is much higher than from unleavened breads.[5–8] Sourdough fermentation, occurring over a period of several days, almost completely degrades the phytate in the wheat flour and increases iron bioavailability.[9]

Although phytic acid interferes with the absorption of some minerals, particularly iron and zinc, there may be some advantage to consuming phosphorus in the form of phytic acid because it is a potent antioxidant[10–13] and may favorably influence signal transduction, thereby regulating cell growth.[14] Even the hydrolysis products of phytate are potent antioxidants.[15] For these reasons it is hypothesized that phytate reduces risk of several chronic diseases including various forms of cancer.[16]

Data are limited, but the average phytate intake of Western omnivores eating diets low in phytate-rich plant foods ranges between about 200 and 350 mg/d with higher intakes (500 to 800 mg/d) in those eating more whole grains and legumes.[17] Vegetarian diets have been reported to contain ≥1000 mg/d.[17] Dietary choices affect the phytate intake of vegetarians. Although

Table 6-1 Phytate Phosphorus Content (mg/100 g product unless indicated)[a] of Selected Plant Foods

Food	Phytate	Food	Phytate
Legumes		**Vegetables**	
Black	262	Corn	24
Red	271	Mushrooms	13
White	269	Yellow onion	16
Mung	188	Brussels sprouts	11
Brown	185	Broccoli	10
Lentils	132	**Fruits and berries**	
Chickpeas	140	Kiwi	10
Nuts and seeds		Blueberry	6
Walnut	303	Strawberry	4
Sunflower	576	Orange	2
Sweet almond	296	Currants, black	78
Sesame	576	Currants, red	55
Cereals and cereal products			
Wheat bran	680–1189	Oat bran	399–628
Crisp bread		Rice flour	27
Rye, thin	72–86	Long grain rice	53–64
Rye, fiber	114–193	Parboiled rice	71
Rice cakes	113	Wild, Brown rice	181–215
Millet		Oats, rolled	282
Sorghum	217	Spaghetti	
Red	279	Buitoni	6
White	389	Barilla	71
Wheat germ	467	Corn flakes	12
Soybeans and soy products			
Tofu (mg/100 g EP)	469	Soybeans (μmol/g dry wt)	12.5
Tofu (mmol/kg dry wt)	23.26	Soy isolate (mmol/kg dry wt)	23.26
Fried soy burgers (mmol/kg dry wt)	9.28	Soy isolate (μg/g dry wt)	7440
Tofu (μg/g dry wt)	5850	Tempeh (μg/g dry wt)	3950
Soy flour, defatted (μg/g dry wt)	5900	Hulls (μg/g dry wt)	340

[a]1 mg phytate phosphorus equals 3.5 mg phytic acid, which equals 5.56 μmol phytic acid.
Sources: Hallberg L, Hulthen L. Prediction of dietary iron absorption: an algorithm for calculating absorption and bioavailability of dietary iron. *Am J Clin Nutr* 2000; 71:1147–1160; Turnland JR, Weaver CM, Kim SK, et al. Molybdenum absorption and utilization in humans from soy and kale intrinsically labelled with stable isotopes of molybdenum. *Am J Clin Nutr* 1999;69:1217–1223; Harland BF, Morris ER. Phytate: a good or bad food component? *Nutr Res* 1995; 15:733–754; Phillippy BG, Johnston MR, Tao S-H, Fox MRS. Inositol phosphates in processed foods. *J Food Sci* 1988; 53:496–499.

Table 6-2 A Comparison of Mineral Recommendations for Premenopausal Vegetarian Women

Mineral	RDA[18]	WHO[23]
Iron (mg/d)	33[a]	29.4[b]
Zinc (mg/d)	8[c]	4.9[d]
Selenium (μg/d)	55	26
Magnesium (mg/d)	310/320[e]	220
Iodine	150 μg/d	2 μg/kg per day

[a]Based on bioavailability of 10%. For bioavailability of 5%, RDA increases to 66 mg/d.
[b]Based on bioavailability of 10%. For bioavailability of 5%, recommendation increases to 58.8 mg/d.
[c]Vegetarians with a high phytate diet may need as much as 12 mg/d.
[d]Based on moderate bioavailability. For low bioavailability, recommendation increases to 9.8 mg/d. Moderate bioavailability is defined as lacto-ovo, ovo-vegetarian, or vegan diets not based primarily on unrefined cereal grains or high-extraction-rate flours. Phytate-to-zinc molar ratio of total diet within the range 5 to 15, or not exceeding 10 if >50% of the energy intake is accounted for by unfermented, unrefined cereal grains and flours and the diet is fortified with inorganic calcium salts (>1g Ca^{2+}/d). Low bioavailability is defined as a phytate-to-zinc molar ratio of total diet >15; high-phytate, soy-protein products constitute the primary protein source; diets in which, singly or collectively, approximately 50% of the energy intake is accounted for by the following high-phytate foods: high-extraction-rate (≥90%) wheat, rice, maize, grains and flours, oatmeal, and millet; chapatti flours and *tanok*; and sorghum, cowpeas, pigeon peas, grams, kidney beans, black-eyed beans, and groundnut flours.[23]
[e]The first amount is for 19- to 30-year-olds, the second for age 31 to 50 years.

vegan diets would be expected to be higher in phytate because of larger intakes of beans, grains, nuts, and seeds; no recent studies have examined the phytate intakes of vegans. Because of the effects of phytate (as well as other factors) on mineral absorption, the Food and Nutrition Board (FNB) established a specific iron recommended dietary allowance (RDA) for vegetarians and noted that zinc needs of vegetarians may be 50% higher than nonvegetarians.[18] Consequently, this chapter focuses most on these two minerals with briefer discussions of the rest of the minerals.

Table 6-2 compares U.S. Dietary Reference Intakes and World Health Organization (WHO) recommendations for a number of minerals.

IRON

Iron deficiency is considered the most common nutritional deficiency worldwide. WHO estimates that approximately 25% of the global population, >1.6 billion people, has anemia, mainly due to iron deficiency.[19] In developing countries, the likelihood of having iron deficiency is greatly enhanced because of iron losses resulting from parasitic infections and repeated pregnancies. In the United States, impaired iron status has been estimated to occur in ≤3% of men age ≥16 years and ≤9% of women ≥50 years but to occur in 12% of women 12 to 49 years of age.[20] Higher rates of iron deficiency are seen in black and Mexican American women.[20] Iron intake is most likely to be inadequate during four periods of life: 6 months to 4 years, adolescence, during the female reproductive period, and during pregnancy.

Approximately 40% of the iron in meat products is heme iron, whereas 60% of the iron in meat and all the iron in plant foods is nonheme iron. Because heme iron is better absorbed than nonheme iron, vegetarians, whose diet consists solely of iron in the nonheme form, typically absorb less iron than nonvegetarians.

Biologic Iron Requirements

The primary function of iron is to transport oxygen. On average, total body iron in men and women is about 3.8 g and 2.3 g, respectively,[21] and approximately three fourths of this iron is contained in hemoglobin (65%) and myoglobin (10%). Although a small amount of iron is used by enzymes, the remaining 25% of total body iron is considered storage iron. In most adults, each 1 μg/L of serum ferritin indicates the presence of about 8 to 10 mg of storage iron.[22] In children and small adults, 1 μg/L of serum ferritin indicates iron stores of about 120 μg/kg body weight.[22] Serum ferritin concentrations <12 μg/L indicate that iron stores are depleted.[19] Although the absence of iron stores may not lead to any immediate adverse effect, low ferritin levels indicate an increased risk of inadequate iron supply to various sites. The average nonvegetarian male in the United States has about 1000 to 1400 mg of stored iron[21] or enough to supply iron needs for about 3 years. Nonvegetarian females on average have only about 360 to 400 mg[18] or enough to supply needs for about 6 months. Men lose about 1.0 mg of iron per day, whereas premenopausal women lose about 1.5 mg/d. Although menstrual losses generally average 0.5 mg of iron per day, averaged over the entire 28-day menstrual cycle, about 5% of the female population loses three times this much.[23]

In men and postmenopausal women, iron loss comes primarily from small amounts of intestinal blood loss or sloughing off of intestinal cells. Some iron is also lost via the urine and skin. Because humans have a limited ability to excrete iron, body levels are controlled primarily through changes in absorption.

Iron-Deficiency Anemia

When iron needs are not adequately met, iron stores begin to decrease. Once stores are depleted, serum iron levels decrease, and hemoglobin production is depressed. Eventually, hemoglobin production decreases to a point where iron-deficiency anemia, characterized as microcytic hypochromic anemia, appears. Another indication of low iron levels is an increase in total iron binding capacity. Iron is transported in the blood by transferrin; normally, about a third of the available iron binding sites on transferrin are filled. When iron levels decrease, the number of available iron binding sites on transferrin increases.

Iron-deficiency anemia results in functional impairment due to inadequate oxygen delivery and abnormal enzyme function. Impairments include reduced physical endurance and decreased work performance, altered immune response, improper temperature regulation, developmental delay, and decreased cognitive function.[18,24,25] Tests to diagnose iron-deficiency anemia include hemoglobin concentration, mean cell volume, hematocrit, transferrin saturation, and erythrocyte protoporphyrin concentration.[18]

Dietary Iron Intake in the United States

Although iron is one of the earth's most abundant elements and widely distributed in food (Table 6-3), it is relatively insoluble and consequently poorly absorbed. Since 1909, the availability of iron in the U.S. food supply has increased by about 25%, mainly due to the enrichment of flour and other grain products beginning in the 1940s.[26] This was no doubt a contributing factor to the decline in the prevalence of anemia that was observed in the 1970s and 1980s in infants and children[27] and in adult women.[28] Iron fortification of foods like breakfast cereals and the increased use of iron supplements and oral contraceptives may have also contributed to these lower rates.[28]

The median iron intake by men in the United States is 16 to 18 mg.[18] However, the median intake of pre- and postmenopausal women is 12 mg,[18] which indicates that iron intakes of premenopausal women are often inadequate. Grains (including fortified ready-to-eat cereals) provide almost 50% of the iron in the diet of adults in the United States; beef provides about 9%, poultry about 3%, legumes about 3%, and fruits and vegetables about 5%, with smaller amounts derived from eggs and other foods like fish and coffee.[29]

Approximately 23% of women[30] and 16% of men[18] in the United States use supplements containing iron. Among nonpregnant, nonlactating women who consume iron-containing supplements, the mean iron intake from supplements is close to 30 mg/d.[30] Among older adults, the median iron intake from supplements appears to be close to 7 mg/d for men and 4 mg/d for women.[31]

Iron Bioavailability

A number of factors impact iron absorption. Although the primary one is iron status,[32] depending on the composition of a meal, iron absorption can vary 20-fold.[33] Nonheme iron is much more sensitive than heme iron to factors affecting absorption. Nonheme iron absorption has been shown to be 10 times higher (2.0–22.5%), but heme iron absorption is only four times higher (10–40%) in iron-deficient compared with iron-replete individuals.[32,34] The total amount of iron ingested at any one time also strongly influences the amount of iron absorbed. For example, when the nonheme iron content of a meal increased fourfold from 1.5 mg to 6.0 mg, absorption decreased threefold from 18% to 6%; consequently, there was little difference in the actual amount of iron absorbed.[35] In contrast, 20% of the heme iron was absorbed regardless of whether 1.5 or 6.0 mg of iron was ingested.[35]

Inhibitors of Iron Absorption

By far, phytate appears to be the most important inhibitor of iron absorption for most populations. Under experimental conditions, phytate can inhibit iron absorption by as much as 90%,[36-38] and there is no intestinal adaptation to these inhibitory effects.[36] In an analysis of 49 strains of maize, iron absorption from the maize was directly correlated with phytate content.[39] Generally, as the phytate and fiber content of a food or diet increases, so does the iron content. Consequently, consuming foods high in these components will have less of an effect on iron status than one might expect. In one study, for example, when subjects were switched from a diet containing a low-fiber white bread to one containing whole wheat bread, daily iron intake increased from

Table 6-3 Iron Content of Foods

Food	Iron Content (mg)	Food	Iron Content (mg)
Breads, cereals, grains		**Fruits**	
Bread, white, 1 slice	0.9	Apricots, dried, ¼ cup	0.9
Bread, whole wheat, 1 slice	0.9	Prunes, ¼ cup	1.2
Bran flakes, 1 cup	10.5	Prune juice, 6 oz	2.3
Kashi Go Lean cereal, 1 cup	1.8	Raisins, ¼ cup	0.8
Product 19, 1 cup	18.0	**Legumes,** ½ cup cooked	
Total, ¾ cup	18.0	Black beans	1.8
Cream of Wheat, ½ cup, cooked	5.8	Black-eyed peas	2.2
Oatmeal, instant, 1 packet	8.2	Garbanzo beans	2.4
Barley, pearled, ½ cup, cooked	1.0	Kidney beans	2.0
Pasta, enriched, ½ cup, cooked	0.9	Lentils	3.3
Rice, brown, ½ cup, cooked	0.4	Lima beans	2.2
Wheat germ, 2 tbsp	1.4	Navy beans	2.3
Vegetables, ½ cup cooked unless otherwise indicated		Pinto beans	2.2
		Split peas	1.3
Asparagus	0.8	Vegetarian baked beans	1.7
Beet greens	1.4	**Soyfoods**	
Bok choy	0.9	Soybeans, ½ cup, cooked	4.4
Broccoli rabe	1.0	Soymilk, 1 cup	1.1 to 1.8[a]
Brussels sprouts	0.9	Tempeh, ½ cup	1.3
Collard greens	1.1	Tofu, firm, ½ cup	6.6
Peas	1.2	Textured vegetable protein, ¼ cup, dry	1.4
Pumpkin	1.7		
Spinach	3.2	Veggie "meats," fortified, 1 oz	0.8 to 2.1[a]
Sun-dried tomatoes	2.4	**Nuts and seeds,** 2 tbsp	
Swiss chard	2.0	Cashews	1.0
Tomato juice, 1 cup	1.0	Pumpkin seeds	2.5
Tomato sauce	0.9	Sunflower seeds	1.2
Sea Vegetables, 8 g dry weight		Tahini	2.7
Dulse, dry	6.4	**Other foods**	
Kombu, dry	22.1	Blackstrap molasses, 1 tbsp	3.6
Nori, dry	3.7	Dark chocolate, 1 oz	3.9
Wakame, dry	3.3	Energy bars, fortified, 1 bar	1.4 to 4.5[a]

[a] Indicates a range of iron found in different soymilks, fortified veggie "meats," and energy bars.
Source: Data from USDA National Nutrient Database for Standard Reference, Release 22, 2009 and manufacturers' information. Values for sea vegetables from MacArtain P, Gill CIR, Brooks M, et al. Nutritional value of edible seaweeds. *Nutr Rev.* 2007;65:535–543.

8.3 to 12.2 mg, but iron status was unaffected. The higher iron intake compensated for poorer bioavailability.[40]

Other inhibitors of iron absorption include tannic acids (see Hallberg and Hulthen[41] for tannin content of foods) in tea that can reduce nonheme iron absorption by as much as half.[42] Some herb teas also inhibit iron absorption.[43] Many Indian spices, such as turmeric, coriander, chilies, and tamarind, also contain tannins.[44] Coffee can also inhibit iron absorption, and adding milk to coffee exacerbates this effect.[45]

Calcium inhibits the absorption of both heme and nonheme iron. Inhibition is not seen when a meal contains <40 mg of calcium.[46] No further inhibition of absorption is seen when the meal's calcium content is >300 mg.[46] These results indicate that, when possible, high calcium foods and supplements should not be consumed at the same time as high iron foods, especially for those with high iron requirements.

Enhancers of Iron Absorption

In single-meal studies, vitamin C can largely counteract the effects of phytate.[33,47] For example, researchers found that nonheme iron absorption from a vegetarian meal high in phytate increased 2.5-fold just by the addition of about a half cup of cauliflower, which is rich in vitamin C.[47] Vitamin C, which is abundant in vegetarian diets, enhances absorption of nonheme iron by reducing dietary ferric iron to ferrous iron, which forms a soluble iron–ascorbic acid complex in the stomach. To enhance absorption, the vitamin C source and iron must be consumed at about the same time.[48] Five fluid ounces of orange juice containing 75 mg of vitamin C can enhance iron absorption from a meal by as much as a factor of 4.[49]

In addition to vitamin C, fruits and vegetables contain small amounts of other organic acids that can also enhance iron absorption, and the effect of citric acid (which is found in citrus fruits) is additive to the effect of ascorbic acid.[50,51] Because vitamin C and organic acids enhance iron absorption by releasing nonheme iron bound to inhibitors of iron absorption, the effect of vitamin C is most pronounced in meals containing high levels of inhibitors such as phytic acid and tannins.[18]

Research suggests that the effects on iron absorption are much less pronounced when vitamin C is consumed as part of the daily diet[52] compared to effects of vitamin C on iron absorption from a single meal.[53] Hunt et al found, for example, that vitamin C supplementation of 1500 mg/d had little effect on iron status over a 5-week period in premenopausal women with low iron stores.[53] This lack of effect may have been at least partially due to the relative insensitivity of iron stores as a marker of iron status over the short term. But Cook and Monsen did find that iron absorption was increased only 35% over a 5-day period when the vitamin C content of diets varied from 51 mg to 247 mg,[52] and yet this same range of intake in single-meal studies was associated with a 100% increase in iron absorption.[54] Nevertheless, epidemiologic studies do show a relationship between vitamin C intake and iron stores.[55]

Other factors may increase iron absorption. Factors in meat enhance the absorption of both nonheme and heme iron.[56] Finally, some research suggests that vitamin A and β-carotene can improve nonheme iron absorption from plant foods such as rice, wheat, and corn.[57] Vitamin A and β-carotene may form a complex with iron, keeping it soluble in the intestinal lumen and thereby preventing the inhibitory effect of phytates and polyphenols on iron absorption. Not all studies support an enhancing effect of vitamin A; this may only occur in those with poor vitamin A status.[58]

As mentioned previously, most studies have looked at how factors affect the absorption of iron from a single meal. These effects appear to be less important when iron absorption from the overall diet is considered because mixed diets contain an assortment of both iron inhibitors and iron enhancers.[53,59,60] Exhibit 6-1 summarizes inhibitors and enhancers of iron absorption.

A number of algorithms for estimating iron absorption from whole diets have been developed based on enhancers and inhibitors of iron absorption.[41,61–64] Although these may prove useful in some cases, they have limitations including the inclusion of animal products, which makes their use with vegetarians questionable. Several equations appear to underestimate iron absorption[65] and may require information about food content of factors such as inositol phosphate forms, hemicelluloses, and tannins that are not found in standard nutrient databases.[64]

Vegetarian Iron Requirements

Concern over the iron status of vegetarians is based not on the iron content of vegetarian diets but rather on the poor bioavailability of iron from plant foods. Vegetarian and plant-based diets generally contain as much or more iron than animal-based diets (Appendix H). Vegan diets are generally higher in iron than lacto-ovo vegetarian diets because dairy foods contain relatively little iron.

Because of the differences in bioavailability between vegetarian and nonvegetarian diets, the FNB has established a separate iron RDA for vegetarians of 14 mg for men and postmenopausal women and 33 mg for premenopausal women not using oral contraceptives.[18] (The RDA for iron is 8 mg for adult men and postmenopausal women and 18 mg for premenopausal women.[18]) These values assume the bioavailability of iron from a vegetarian diet is approximately 10% compared to 18% for nonvegetarian diets. This assumption is based on limited data using a diet that was very high in inhibitors of iron absorption and limited in enhancers,[59] however, and this may not reflect the way most Western vegetarians eat. However, the FNB also indicated that iron bioavailability on some types of vegetarian diets might be as low as 5%, which would double the

Exhibit 6-1 Summary of Inhibitors and Enhancers of Iron Absorption in Vegetarian Diets

Inhibiting Factors

Phytates (whole grains, legumes including soy, nuts, seeds, vegetables)

Tea, coffee, cocoa

Some spices

Calcium from foods and supplements

Enhancing Factors

Vitamin C (ascorbic acid)

Other organic acids including citric acid

Fermented foods including sauerkraut, soy sauce, and sourdough bread

RDA to 66 mg for premenopausal vegetarian women. Support for very low iron bioavailability in some vegetarian diets comes from the research of Hunt et al, who found that nonheme iron absorption from a controlled lacto-ovo vegetarian diet high in vitamin C was only 1.1%, and even bioavailability from the nonvegetarian diet in this study was only 3.8%.[66]

The RDA values for vegetarians in other age groups can be estimated by multiplying the iron RDA for nonvegetarians by a factor of 1.8 (the difference between the adult RDA and adult vegetarian RDA). However, the iron RDA for infants from birth to 6 months is based on the iron content of breast milk, and the RDA for infants age 7 to 12 months is based on a bioavailability of 10% rather than the 18% bioavailability that is used for other age groups. Thus no adjustment needs to be made for infants on vegetarian diets.

Concerns about the lower bioavailability of iron in vegetarian diets are also expressed by the Joint Food and Agriculture Organization (FAO)/WHO Expert Consultation on Human Vitamin and Mineral Requirements, which concluded that iron bioavailability ranged from 5% to 15% depending on the relative amount of enhancers and inhibitors of iron absorption in the diet.[23] The FAO recommendations for iron intake for premenopausal women consuming a diet with 10% iron bioavailability was 29.4 mg,[23] lower than the 33 mg set by the FNB for premenopausal vegetarian women. FAO recommendations for men and postmenopausal women were similar to those of the FNB (13.7 and 11.3 mg, respectively). Recommended iron intakes for those whose diets had 5% iron bioavailability were 58.8 mg for premenopausal women, 27.4 mg for men, and 22.6 mg for postmenopausal women.[23]

Committees responsible for establishing recommendations for iron intake for the United States, the United Kingdom, and Australia all suggest that iron intake be increased and that enhancers of iron absorption, such as vitamin C, be increased in vegetarian diets.[18,67,68]

Vegetarian Iron Intake

Most studies, but not all,[69-71] show that vegetarians consume more iron than nonvegetarians. Vegans tend to consume more iron than lacto-ovo vegetarians because, as noted earlier, dairy products contain relatively little iron.[72,73] Plant-based diets tend to be high in iron. For example, the diets of rural Chinese and Mexicans, which are almost completely vegan, were found to contain on average 34 mg[74] and >17 mg[75] of iron per day, respectively. Dutch researchers designed typical vegan, lacto vegetarian, and nonvegetarian diets and found them to contain 20.4, 17.4, and 13.6 mg of iron per day, respectively.[76] These figures agree with a nationwide survey of the Dutch population, which found that vegetarians consumed as much or more iron than the general nonvegetarian population.[77]

Similarly, typical 2600-calorie vegetarian diets constructed by investigators from the Veterans Administration Hospital in Hines, Illinois, contained 19.2, 15.0, and 16.3 mg of iron for vegan, lacto, and lacto-ovo vegetarian diets, respectively,[78] and Indian researchers designed typical Indian vegetarian diets and found them to contain >38 mg of iron.[79] This value is consistent with data showing that in India, where approximately 30% of the population is vegetarian, adult iron intake is very high, between 23 and 35 mg/d.[80] Finally, in an analysis of three hospital diets, iron content was 13.4, 14.3, and 24.4 mg/d for a nonvegetarian, lacto-ovo vegetarian, and soy-based vegetarian diet, respectively.[81]

Although the data are limited on iron intake among vegetarian children, in a study involving 23 British vegan preschool children, the average iron intake was 10 mg/d (which is the U.S. RDA for nonvegetarians), and their diet was nearly twice as iron dense as diets of preschool omnivores.[82] A more recent study of British preschoolers found similar iron intakes in lacto-ovo vegetarians and omnivores and mean iron intakes in both groups that were below the RDA.[83] Lacto-ovo vegetarian preschool children had higher mean iron intakes than their nonvegetarian peers.[84] Total iron intakes of vegetarian teens from Britain were not significantly different from those of omnivores.[85] Swedish vegan teens had similar (males) and higher (females) iron intakes than nonvegetarians.[86]

Although well-planned vegetarian diets can be quite high in iron, vegetarians, especially premenopausal women (not on oral contraceptives), may not meet the higher recommendations for iron without the use of iron-fortified foods or iron supplements. Exhibit 6-2 shows a sample menu providing 33 mg of iron.

Exhibit 6-2 Sample Vegetarian Menu Providing Approximately 33 mg of Iron

Meal/Snack	Food	Iron (mg)
Breakfast	1 package instant oatmeal	8.2
	with 1 tbsp blackstrap molasses	3.6
	1 cup soymilk	1.8
	½ cup strawberries (vitamin C source)	0.3
	1 slice whole wheat toast with margarine or jam	0.9
Lunch	1 cup lentil soup	5.0
	6-inch whole wheat pita bread	2.0
	Tossed salad with ½ avocado	0.6
	Chocolate chip cookie	0.4
	½ cup orange juice (vitamin C source)	
Snack	1 cup tomato juice (vitamin C source)	1.0
	1 slice whole wheat bread	0.9
	1 tbsp tahini	1.4
Dinner	1 cup barbecued firm tofu (BBQ sauce: vitamin C source)	4.0
	1 cup brown rice	0.8
	1 cup steamed collard greens	2.2
	Tossed salad with 1 tbsp pumpkin seeds	0.5
	½ cup mixed fruit (vitamin C source)	
Total		33.6

Source: Data from USDA National Nutrient Database for Standard Reference, release 22, 2009 and manufacturers' information.

Vegetarian Iron Status

Incidence of iron deficiency anemia among vegetarians is similar to that of nonvegetarians (Appendix H). Older men consuming a lacto-ovo vegetarian diet for 12 weeks did not experience any adverse effects on iron status.[87]

Typically, the iron stores of vegetarians are within the normal range, although they are frequently substantially lower than those of omnivores (Appendix H).[69,70,82,88–90] Male vegetarians often have iron stores that are closer to levels of premenopausal omnivorous women than to those of male omnivores[70,73,88,91] (Figure 6-1). Furthermore, several studies indicate that more vegetarians are likely to have iron stores considered to be deficient or only marginally adequate in comparison to nonvegetarians.[69, 88, 89, 91–94]

In Australia, vegetarian women consumed only 10.7 mg of iron per day, and yet their average serum ferritin level was 25.0 μg/L, although this was about half the level seen in the omnivore controls, despite similar iron intakes.[69] Although 18% of the vegetarians did have serum ferritin levels <12 μg/L, so did 12% of omnivores, and the difference between the two groups was not statistically significant.[69] In a group of women in New Zealand, serum ferritin levels were 50.4 μg/L among vegetarians and 59.6 μg/L among omnivore controls; the iron intake of these two groups was 14.7 and 12.8 mg, respectively. Serum hemoglobin levels were also similar between

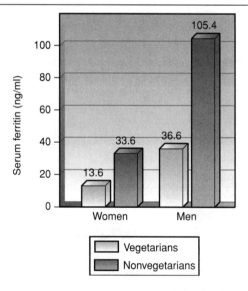

Figure 6-1 Iron stores in vegetarians and omnivores. Values are for 36 females and 14 male vegetarians and for equal numbers of nonvegetarians. Of the 36 female vegetarians, 31 were lacto-ovo vegetarians and 5 were vegans. Differences between the vegetarians and nonvegetarians were statistically significant for both men and women (*P* < 0.01; Mann-Whitney *U* test). The mean age of the female and male vegetarians was 26 and 28 years, respectively. The omnivorous controls were aged within 1 year of the vegetarians. *Source:* Alexander D, Ball MJ, Mann J. Nutrient intake and haematological status of vegetarians and age-sex matched omnivores. *Eur J Clin Nutr* 1994; 48:538–546.

the two groups, and 2 of 12 vegetarian women and 1 of 12 omnivore women had levels below the lower reference range.[70] Other studies have also found similar dietary iron intakes and serum ferritin levels between vegetarians and nonvegetarians.[95] Haddad et al found that vegan premenopausal females had serum ferritin levels that were similar to the nonvegetarians and a similar percentage of each group had serum ferritin levels ≤12 μg/L. Average serum ferritin levels were 27 μg/L and 22 μg/L for vegans and nonvegetarians, respectively, and the percentage of subjects with ferritin levels <12 μg/L was 27% and 20% for vegans and nonvegetarians, respectively. However, dietary iron intake (26.4 mg vs 15.0 mg; $P < 0.001$) and total iron intake including supplements (43.4 vs 20.9 mg) was higher among vegan females in comparison to nonvegetarians, which suggests iron bioavailability was poor because iron stores did not differ between these two groups.[73] A study of German vegan women found low ferritin levels despite generally adequate iron intakes, suggesting that iron bioavailability was low in their diets whose major iron sources were vegetables, fruits, and cereals.[96]

Data in children are limited. Among those consuming a restricted macrobiotic diet, about 15% had poor iron status even though iron intake was adequate.[97,98] Significantly more British vegetarian preschoolers (age 1.5 to 3 years) had serum ferritin levels that were <12 μg/L than omnivores, although there was no significant difference in incidence of low hemoglobin levels.[83] British vegetarian girls age 11 to 18 years, particularly those age 15 to 18 years, were more likely to have lower hemoglobin, serum ferritin, and transferrin saturation than nonvegetarians.[85] In contrast, vegetarian children 6 to 12 years of age had iron-related blood values that were not significantly different from those of similarly aged nonvegetarian children.[99] Swedish adolescent vegans also had iron-related blood values that were not significantly different from nonvegetarians.[86]

There may be some advantage to the lower-normal serum ferritin levels commonly seen in vegetarians. One study of lacto-ovo vegetarians found a positive correlation between serum ferritin and insulin resistance.[90] In addition, when body iron stores of male nonvegetarians were reduced to a level similar to that of lacto-ovo vegetarians, a marked reduction in insulin resistance was seen.[90]

Adaptation

Given the fact that iron intakes of many vegetarians, but especially premenopausal females, are typically lower than recommendations, it could be expected that among premenopausal women in particular, serum ferritin levels would be low. However, many studies suggest there is little difference, if any, in parameters of iron status such as hemoglobin, hematocrit, total iron binding capacity, and serum iron levels between vegetarians and nonvegetarians (Appendix H).[36,70,73,89,91,92,100–104]

Collectively, the data suggest that iron bioavailability is lower on a vegetarian diet, but that the iron status of premenopausal women as not as poor as one would expect considering that their iron intake is typically far below recommendations for vegetarians. There are several explanations for this discrepancy. One is that subjects may have followed a vegetarian diet for a relatively short period of time. The second is that vegetarians may adapt to low intakes. Hunt and Roughead found that in response to the 70% lower nonheme iron bioavailability from vegetarian diets, subjects excreted far less fecal ferritin compared to omnivores (1.0 vs 6.6 μg/d; $P < 0.01$).[66] Furthermore, Hunt and

Roughead found that in men, nonheme iron absorption differed nearly fivefold between low-iron-bioavailability and high-iron-bioavailability diets initially, but after 10 weeks the difference in absorption was only twofold.[105] There appears to be both an ability to conserve iron losses and to increase iron absorption in response to the consumption of diets with poor iron bioavailability. This may suggest that iron needs are not as high for vegetarians as the RDAs indicate. Nevertheless, pending further evidence, vegetarians should strive to meet the recommendations set by the FNB.

Athletes

According to the FNB, there are several mechanisms by which iron needs of athletes may be increased. These include a shorter biologic half-life for iron[106] and increased rate of red blood cell turnover and fragility.[107] These effects result in greater whole body iron losses among athletes,[108] and for this reason the FNB concluded that the EAR for iron will conservatively be 30% higher for those who engage in regular intense exercise but could be as much as 70% higher for certain subpopulations of athletes.[18] Much of the research on iron needs of athletes has been conducted in runners, and iron losses seen in this group are not necessarily representative of those in other athletes. However, if intense exercise, especially running, increases iron needs, vegetarian premenopausal women who engage in such activity must be particularly mindful of consuming, at the very least, the vegetarian RDA, monitoring iron status, and supplementing as necessary.[109]

ZINC

Animal products, and meat in particular, provide more than half of the zinc in the typical American diet with a fourth of zinc intake coming from beef.[29] Ready-to-eat cereal was the second-ranking source of zinc.[29] Vegetarian zinc intake is similar to or somewhat lower than nonvegetarian intake (Appendix I). The FNB does not specify a RDA for zinc for vegetarians. However, because the absorption of zinc from plants is somewhat lower than from animal products, the FNB recommends a zinc intake 50% higher than the RDA for vegetarians whose diet contains generous amounts of grains and legumes so that their phytate-to-zinc molar ratio is >15:1.[18]

Zinc Deficiency

In humans, outright zinc deficiency was first observed in Middle Eastern men and was associated with a condition called hypogonadism (small and underdeveloped testicles), which leads to dwarfism.[110] Turkish investigators have observed zinc deficiency in growth-stunted children who indulge in geophagia, the practice of eating clay,[111] which inhibits zinc absorption. In the 1980s, Chinese investigators have reported that as many as 30% of Chinese children were stunted from zinc deficiency.[112]

In addition to geophagia, other predisposing factors contribute to zinc deficiency. For instance, zinc deficiency in school-age boys in some Middle East countries was associated with blood loss from parasitic infestations, geophagia, and excessive loss of zinc related to excessive perspiration.[110,113] Boys from the same population without these predisposing factors were not overtly zinc deficient.[114]

For North Americans, marginal zinc deficiency is more likely to occur than overt deficiency. Marginal or mild zinc deficiency has been observed in several studies of children and has been associated in many cases with poor appetite, suboptimal growth, and impaired taste acuity.[115,116] In one U.S. survey, about 3% of the children between the ages of 3 and 8 years had low serum zinc levels.[117] The dietary zinc intake of low-income children in the United States is particularly low.[118] Both children and pregnant women, because of increased needs, appear to be vulnerable to zinc deficiency.

When zinc-deficient diets are fed in research studies, zinc losses from the intestines and skin as well as urinary zinc are reduced and zinc absorption is increased so that serum zinc levels and activities of zinc-containing enzymes can be maintained for several months.[23,119]

Zinc is thought to be a cofactor for more than 300 enzymes and is also involved in nonenzymatic reactions.[23] Zinc is needed for genetic expression. Adequate zinc is needed for optimal cell growth, which explains why, in patients with low zinc levels, zinc supplements increase the rate of wound healing, a process involving rapid cell division.[120] Zinc also plays a role in protein synthesis and blood formation. In addition, zinc is involved in the immune system;[121] zinc supplements have improved immune function in elderly adults with low plasma zinc levels.[122]

Dietary Requirements for Zinc

Zinc absorption increases in individuals with poor zinc status, and zinc losses can be reduced by as much as 80% in response to low zinc intakes.[119] Consequently, it takes little zinc to maintain a low zinc status and much more to maintain a high zinc status. The attainment of zinc balance, however, does not necessarily imply that normal zinc concentrations are maintained in all body tissues and fluids.[123] It is not known to what extent a marginal zinc status hinders optimal health.

The adult RDAs for zinc are 11 mg and 8 mg for men and women, respectively,[18] and they are higher than those of the FAO/WHO.[23] In calculating the adult RDA, average fractional absorption of zinc was estimated to be 0.41 for men and 0.48 for women. However, according to the FNB, some vegetarians may need to consume 50% more zinc than nonvegetarians because of the poorer bioavailability of zinc from vegetarian diets.[18] The FAO/WHO bases zinc recommendations on estimated bioavailability as shown in Table 6-2.

Regulation of Zinc Absorption

In the classic research first identifying human zinc deficiency in the Middle East, dietary zinc intake was adequate, but bioavailability was not. Because none of the zinc in foods is present as the free ion, digestion greatly impacts zinc bioavailability. Upon digestion, zinc is able to bind to exogenous and endogenous constituents in the intestinal lumen that can affect absorption. A considerable amount of zinc in the intestines is from endogenous sources such as pancreatic secretions. Regulation of zinc metabolism is achieved mainly by changes in absorption and secretion of endogenous zinc in response to dietary zinc intakes.[18] Zinc losses may range from <1 mg/d in response to a diet low in zinc to >5 mg/d with a zinc-rich diet, a difference that reflects the regulatory role that the intestinal tract serves in zinc homeostasis. In one study of young Chinese women, those consuming a diet low in zinc reduced fecal zinc losses to such an extent that they were able to maintain zinc balance when consuming just 5 mg/d of zinc.[124] Dietary factors that affect zinc absorption can impact both the absorption of dietary zinc and the reabsorption of endogenous zinc.[125]

Zinc Bioavailability

Zinc bioavailability of vegetarian diets is lower than that of nonvegetarian diets.[75,126,127] Zinc absorption from foods varies dramatically depending on the type of meal consumed; studies have shown that zinc absorption can vary fourfold, from as little as 8.2% to as high as 38.2%.[128,129] In these studies, the two most important factors affecting zinc absorption were animal protein and total zinc content, the former increasing relative absorption and the latter decreasing it.[128–131]

Phytate is a potent inhibitor of zinc absorption. For example, zinc absorption from whole grain cereal meals with a high phytate content is only 5%.[8] When phytate levels are reduced by fermentation to about a third the initial level, however, absorption increases fourfold.[8] Although phytate is likely to be a problem only when consumed in large amounts, as noted at the onset, the phytate content of plant-based diets can be quite high. Some reports have suggested there is an intestinal adaptation to the inhibitory effects of phytate, but others have found this not to be the case.[36,132,133] In a controlled experiment in which premenopausal women were fed lacto-ovo vegetarian and omnivore diets for 8 weeks in random order, Hunt et al found that zinc absorption on the vegetarian diet was 26% versus 33% for the omnivore diet. There was no apparent adaptation or compensatory response to the lower zinc absorption among vegetarians, and somewhat surprisingly (because plasma zinc is a relatively insensitive indicator of zinc status), there was a significant 5% reduction in plasma zinc concentrations.[134]

A phytate-to-zinc ratio above the range of 6 to 10 (on a molar basis) leads to a decline in zinc absorption; above a ratio of 15, zinc absorption is <15%.[23] Several studies have concluded that, based on the phytate-to-zinc ratios seen in vegetarian diets, zinc bioavailability would be compromised on at least some vegetarian diets.[81,135–137]

The bioavailability of zinc in vegetarian diets can be improved by reducing the phytate content. Refining grains reduces their phytate content but also reduces zinc content so the effects of refining on zinc availability, overall, are limited.[23] Phytases, present in most phytate-containing foods, can be activated through germination (sprouting) of cereals and legumes. Microbial or fungal phytases can be added to phytate-containing foods.[23] Low-phytate cereals and legumes can be produced through plant breeding.[39] Leavening of bread, soaking, and fermentation have also been shown to reduce the effects of phytate.[138–140] Fermentation of cornmeal, soybeans, cowpeas, and lima beans can remove ≥90% of phytate.[141]

Boiling root vegetables can reduce their phytate content somewhat.[141] Soaking followed by disposal of the soaking water is effective for reducing the phytate content of unrefined cereal and legume flours but not whole grains or seeds.[142,143] Organic acids (citric, lactic, acetic, etc.) naturally found in foods or produced during fermentation can also improve zinc absorption but probably to a lesser extent than for iron absorption.[7,144] Foods containing these organic acids include yogurt, sauerkraut, and fermented soy sauce.

Fiber may also bind zinc,[145] but the effect is probably minor because no adverse effects of fiber on zinc absorption have been seen.[146] Also, whole grain products are higher in zinc than refined ones, so that the absolute amount of zinc absorbed is often not compromised. For example, although relative zinc absorption was higher from refined white bread, total zinc absorbed was higher from whole wheat bread because of the higher zinc content.[128] Similarly, when subjects in one study were switched from a diet containing a low-fiber white bread to one containing whole wheat bread, daily zinc intake increased from 9.0 to 12.7 mg, but zinc status was unaffected, indicating that the higher zinc intake compensated for the poorer bioavailability.[40]

The role of calcium on the absorption of zinc is an area of active research. When calcium is added to low-phytate meals, zinc absorption does not appear to be affected.[147] However, calcium may potentiate the inhibitory effects of phytate on zinc absorption,[130] so it has been proposed that the amount of phytate and calcium relative to zinc is the key factor in determining zinc absorption.[132] This idea is contradicted by a recent study that found no effect of calcium (at levels as high as 1700 mg/d) contributing to phytate's inhibition of zinc absorption at phytate-to-zinc molar ratios as high as 15.6.[147] Milk or yogurt added to a high-phytate plant-based diet appear to increase zinc bioavailability.[148]

Iron supplements, but not dietary iron, also appear to impair zinc absorption,[149–151] although this has not been seen in all studies.[152] Most studies have shown an effect with iron supplements of ≥30 mg/d; however, one study[153] reported lower plasma zinc concentrations following use of a multivitamin/mineral supplement with only 18 mg of iron. In some cases the combination of 15 mg of supplemental zinc used with iron supplements has led to improved zinc status.[154] If iron supplements are used, there may be some advantage to taking them between meals to limit their effect on zinc absorption.[155]

Generally speaking, higher levels of dietary protein have a positive effect on zinc bioavailability.[7] Casein in milk has an inhibitory effect on zinc absorption, whereas soy protein does not appear to interfere with zinc absorption beyond the interference due to its phytate content.[7]

Vegetarian Zinc Intake and Status

In healthy individuals, plasma, urinary, and hair zinc can be used to assess zinc status.[156] Plasma, red blood cell, hair, and urine zinc are decreased in severe zinc deficiency; other conditions such as stress and pregnancy can affect these levels. On a population basis, reduced plasma zinc levels, low zinc intakes, and prevalence of stunting in children <5 years of age indicate a problem with zinc adequacy.[23,157]

Median zinc intakes for adult men and women in the United States are 13 mg/d and 9 mg/d, respectively.[18] Canadian Seventh-day Adventist lacto-ovo vegetarian women with an average age of 50 years had a zinc intake of approximately 9 mg/d, which is slightly above the RDA. Similar intake values were found in two studies from the United Kingdom.[158,159] Several other studies have found vegetarian zinc intake to be similar to or even slightly higher than nonvegetarians, but others have reported low intakes among vegetarians[70] (Appendix I). Especially noteworthy is a study showing that among African American male and female lacto-ovo vegetarians, zinc intake was only 8.7 mg/d, versus 11.4 and 10.6 mg/d, respectively, for male and female nonvegetarians.[72] In a cross-sectional study of zinc status of Australian vegetarians, Ball and Auckland found that the zinc intake of male omnivores, lacto-ovo vegetarians, and vegans was 12.8, 11.4, and 10.9 mg/d, respectively, but the intake of omnivorous and vegetarian women was only 8.3 and 6.8 mg/d.[160] However, serum zinc concentrations did not differ between the vegetarian and nonvegetarian females, and they were actually higher in lacto-ovo vegetarian men than nonvegetarian men.

In studies of vegan[82] and vegetarian[83] preschool children, the zinc density of the diet (milligrams of zinc per 1000 kcal) was identical to the average zinc density of the diet of nonvegetarian preschoolers. Zinc intake among Canadian children age 4 to 7 years was reported to be 8.5 mg/d,[161] and among female Canadian lacto-ovo vegetarians age 14 to 20 years, it was found to be 7 mg/d.[162] The RDA for 4- to 8-year-olds is 5 mg/d; for 14- to 18-year-old women it is 9 mg/d.[18]

Studies of pregnant women have found no difference in zinc status between vegetarians and nonvegetarians.[126,163,164] Levels of zinc in hair, saliva, and serum are in the normal range for vegetarians, although they are lower than in nonvegetarians.[165–167] Also, in some studies, greater numbers of vegetarians in comparison to nonvegetarians had very low blood zinc levels.[101,167]

The fact that zinc intake among vegetarians appears to be relatively similar to the intake of nonvegetarians but their zinc status is somewhat poorer is most likely due to reduced zinc absorption. Although overt zinc deficiency is typically not seen among vegetarians, because of the difficulty of determining zinc status and the uncertainty over the effects of a marginally lower zinc

Exhibit 6-3 Sample Vegetarian Menu Providing More Than 20 mg of Zinc

Meal/Snack	Food	Zinc (mg)
Breakfast	1½ cups quick oatmeal	3.5
	2 tbsp wheat germ	2.7
	1 tbsp maple syrup	0.8
	½ cup strawberries	0.1
	1 whole wheat English muffin	1.1
	1 cup orange juice	0.2
Lunch	2 slices whole wheat bread	0.6
	2 ounces zinc-fortified veggie deli slices	4.6
	1 wedge watermelon	0.3
	1 cup soymilk	0.6
	¼ cup peanuts	2.2
Snack	½ cup hummus	2.2
	5 wheat crackers	0.2
	½ cup carrot and celery sticks	0.1
Dinner	¾ cup curried chickpeas	1.8
	1½ cups quinoa	3.0
	¾ cup peas	0.7
	Pineapple chunks	0.1
Total		**24.8**

Source: Data from USDA National Nutrient Database for Standard Reference, Release 22, 2009.

status on overall health, it is appropriate for vegetarians to strive for intakes that meet the RDA. Vegetarians consuming high phytate diets based on grains and legumes should strive for an intake of 50% above the RDA.

With appropriate food selections, vegetarian menus can provide as much as 20 mg of zinc.[75,76,168] Exhibit 6-3 shows a sample menu providing 20 mg of zinc. Table 6-4 illustrates food sources of zinc. Experimental diets designed to represent the typical intake of vegetarians found zinc levels to be about 10 mg in one case[78] and 17 mg in a second.[79] A typical Indian vegetarian diet designed by researchers contained >20 mg of zinc.[79] Vegetarian-designed hospital diets were found to contain 9.7 mg of zinc for lacto-ovo vegetarian diets and 15.0 mg for a vegan-type diet in comparison to 12.2 mg for the nonvegetarian diet.[81] Intervention trials have designed vegan diets containing 18 mg/d[169] and 3.4 mg/1000 kcal[170] of zinc from food alone.

SELENIUM

Selenium is a cofactor for the enzyme glutathione peroxidase, which is present in red blood cells and other tissues and helps prevent oxidative damage by neutralizing lipid hydroperoxides and hydrogen peroxides. It works closely in conjunction with vitamin E. Selenium also regulates thyroid hormone action. Useful markers of selenium status include plasma, erythrocyte, and whole-blood selenium; plasma selenoprotein P; and plasma, platelet, and whole-blood glutathione peroxidase activity.[171]

The selenium content of foods varies widely. Although Table 6-5 provides information about the selenium content of foods from the nutrient database of the U.S. Department of Agriculture (USDA), these values can under- or overestimate the actual selenium content of a specific food item.[172] Large variations in selenium content have been reported in similar food items produced by different manufacturers.[172] In plants and foods made from plants, the selenium content largely depends on the amount of selenium in the soil. In China, for example, in an area where human selenosis (excess selenium) occurs, the selenium concentration of corn, rice, and soybeans is 1000 times higher than the selenium concentration of those crops grown in an area of China where selenium deficiency is common.[173] Variation in the selenium concentration of animal products is not nearly as great because animals can conserve selenium when intakes are low and excrete more selenium when intakes are high.

Selenium intake varies considerably among countries. In the United States, median selenium intake is 106.7 μg/d for men and 78.5 μg/d for women.[174] A Canadian study found average intakes to range from 113 to 220 μg/d.[175] Median intakes in Japan are 177.5 μg/d in men and 139.8 μg/d in women.[176] These values compare favorably to the adult RDA of 55 μg.[18]

In many parts of the world, selenium status is often affected more by the selenium content of soil in a given region than by dietary pattern. However, in the United States the effect of soil selenium content is reduced due to efficient food distribution. Studies of North American vegetarians suggest there is little difference in selenium status between vegetarians and nonvegetarians.[177,178] Although animal products are the most important sources of selenium in many Northern European countries, this tends to be the case only when dietary selenium content is otherwise low, generally as a result of low soil selenium.[179] This explains the low selenium intake of Swedish subjects placed on a lacto-ovo vegetarian diet[180] and the reports showing Swedish vegetarian diets, particularly vegan diets, to be low in selenium.[86,181,182]

Table 6-4 Zinc Content of Foods

Food	Zinc Content (mg)	Food	Zinc Content (mg)
Breads, cereals, grains		Lentils	1.3
Bran flakes, 1 cup	2.0	Navy beans	0.9
Granola, ¼ cup	1.3	Pinto beans	0.8
Grape-Nuts, ½ cup	3.2	Split peas	1.0
Oatmeal, instant, 1 packet	1.0	**Soyfoods**	
Product 19, 1 cup	15	Soybeans, ½ cup, cooked	1.0
Total, ¾ cup	15	Tempeh, ½ cup, cooked	1.0
Barley, pearled, ½ cup, cooked	0.6	Tofu, firm, ½ cup	1.1
Millet, ½ cup, cooked	0.8	Veggie "meats," fortified, 1 oz	1.4–1.8[a]
Quinoa, ½ cup, cooked	1.0	**Nuts and seeds,** 2 tbsp	
Rice, brown, ½ cup, cooked	0.6	Almond butter	1.0
Wheat germ, 2 tbsp	2.7	Brazil nuts	0.7
Vegetables ½ cup cooked, unless otherwise indicated		Cashews	0.9
		Peanut butter	0.9
Asparagus	0.5	Peanuts	1.1
Avocado, ½	0.6	Pumpkin/squash seeds	1.1
Broccoli	0.4	Sunflower seeds	0.9
Corn	0.5	Tahini	1.4
Mushrooms	0.7	**Animal products**	
Peas	0.5	Milk, 1 cup	0.9
Spinach	0.7	Cheese	
Legumes, ½ cup cooked		Cheddar, 1 oz	0.9
Adzuki beans	2.0	Swiss, 1 oz	1.2
Black-eyed peas	1.1	Yogurt, 1 cup	2.0
Chickpeas	1.2	**Other foods**	
Hyacinth beans	2.8	Chocolate, dark, 1 oz	1.0
Kidney beans	0.9	Energy bar, 1 bar	3.0–5.2[a]
Lima beans	0.9		

[a] Indicates a range of zinc found in different fortified veggie "meats" and energy bars.
Source: Data from USDA National Nutrient Database for Standard Reference, Release 22, 2009 and manufacturers' information.

Table 6-5 Selenium Content of Foods

Food	Selenium Content (μg)	Food	Selenium Content (μg)
Breads, cereals, grains		**Legumes and soyfoods, ½ cup, cooked**	
Bread, whole wheat, 1 slice	7.2	Chickpeas	3
English muffin, 1	12.8	Lima beans	4.2
Bran flakes, 1 cup	4.1	Pinto beans	5.3
Grape-Nuts, ½ cup	5.3	Soybeans	6.3
Oatmeal, ½ cup, cooked	6.3	Tofu, firm	12.5
Barley, pearled, ½ cup, cooked	6.8	**Nuts and seeds**	
Pasta, whole wheat, ½ cup, cooked	18.1	Brazil nuts, 2 tbsp	319
Rice, brown, ½ cup, cooked	9.6	**Animal products**	
		Egg, 1 large	15.4
		Yogurt, 1 cup	12

Source: Data from USDA National Nutrient Database for Standard Reference, Release 22, 2009.

These observations agree with two studies conducted in Slovakia that found parameters of selenium status (plasma levels of selenium and glutathione, and glutathione peroxidase activity) were lower in vegetarians than nonvegetarians.[183,184] The selenium content of soil in Slovakia is low relative to many other countries.

Experimental vegan diets in the United States were reported to contain 50 μg/1000 kcal of selenium[170] and 140 μg/d.[169] In experimental diets designed to represent typical omnivore, lacto-ovo vegetarian, and vegan diets consumed in the United States, selenium content was 92.7, 84.8, and 85.9 mg/d, respectively, all surpassing the RDA.[185] These results are similar to those reported for Canadian vegetarians.[186] Cereals, which provided more than a third of the selenium intake of both vegetarians and nonvegetarians in the Canadian study, are much higher in selenium when grown in Canada than cereals grown in many northern European countries. Interestingly, one study found that, although daily selenium intake did not differ between lactating lacto-ovo vegetarians and nonvegetarians (101 vs 106 μg), breast milk selenium concentration and glutathione peroxidase activity were significantly greater in vegetarians.[177] This may give added protection against oxidative damage to the infants of vegetarian mothers.

In a study in India that involved subjects occupationally exposed to selenium, hair selenium content was lower (1.55 μg/g selenium vs 1.15 μg/g; $P < 0.05$) in vegetarians than vegetarians, suggesting vegetarian selenium intake from dietary sources may have been lower.[187] However, the value of hair selenium as an indicator of selenium status in free-living populations is unclear.[188] Other studies in the United States and New Zealand indicate that vegetarian intake is similar to omnivores (Appendix I). In low-selenium areas, however, all individuals, including vegetarians, need to identify good sources of selenium.

COPPER

Copper has been used therapeutically since at least 400 BC when Hippocrates prescribed copper compounds for pulmonary disorders and other diseases.[189] The adult copper RDA for both men and women is 900 μg, with an upper tolerable limit set at 10 mg (10,000 μg).[18] Median intakes in the United States are 1.2 mg/d for men and 1.0 mg/d for women.[174] Outright copper deficiency is rare, and it generally occurs only in unusual circumstances such as patients on copper-deficient formula diets or total parenteral nutrition solutions.[18] There are a number of important copper-containing proteins and enzymes, some of which are essential for the proper utilization of iron.

The efficiency of copper absorption is better at lower intakes (e.g., 75% absorption at an intake of only 400 μg but only 12% absorption at an intake of 7.5 mg).[190,191] Generally, diet

Table 6-6 Copper Content of Foods

Food	Copper Content (mg)	Food	Copper Content (mg)
Breads, cereals, grains		**Legumes,** ½ cup, cooked	
Bread, whole wheat, 1 slice	0.04	Chickpeas	0.29
Bran flakes, 1 cup	0.25	Lentils	0.25
Millet, ½ cup, cooked	0.14	Split peas	0.18
Pasta, whole wheat, ½ cup, cooked	0.12	**Soyfoods,** ½ cup, cooked	
Quinoa, ½ cup, cooked	0.18	Soybeans	0.35
Vegetables, ½ cup, cooked, unless otherwise indicated		Tempeh	0.46
		Tofu, firm	0.27
Avocado, ½	0.19	**Nuts and seeds,** 2 tbsp	
Mushrooms	0.39	Almond butter	0.29
Potato	0.15	Almonds	0.20
Spinach	0.16	Brazil nuts	0.29
Sweet potato	0.16	Cashews	0.33
Tomato juice, 1 cup	0.15	Peanuts	0.22
Turnip greens	0.18	Pumpkin/squash seeds	0.19
Sea vegetables, 8 g dry weight		Sunflower seeds	0.30
Dulse, dry	0.2	Tahini	0.48
Kombu, dry	0.14	**Other foods**	
Nori, dry	0.07	Chocolate, dark, 1 ounce	0.53
Wakame, dry	0.16		

Source: Data from USDA National Nutrient Database for Standard Reference, Release 22, 2009 and manufacturers' information. Values for sea vegetables from MacArtain P, Gill CIR, Brooks M, et al. Nutritional value of edible seaweeds. *Nutr Rev.* 2007;65:535–543.

composition has little effect on copper bioavailability because the main determinant of absorption is copper intake and need.

Zinc well in excess of dietary levels can inhibit copper absorption but when zinc to copper ratios of 2:1, 5:1, and 15:1 were fed to humans, there was little effect on copper absorption.[192] Phytate does not appear to affect copper absorption nearly as much as it does zinc and iron.[193] Turnlund et al found no effect of either cellulose or phytate on absorption in young men,[194] a finding supported by other studies.[195]

Some concerns have been raised about the bioavailability of copper on vegetarian diets. Several factors pertinent to vegetarian diets may positively affect copper absorption and/or requirements, however. Some reports suggest that high protein may decrease copper requirements, whereas high zinc may slightly increase them; thus for vegans, who consume relatively low amounts of zinc and protein, these factors might negate one another.[196,197] Although data are limited, lacto-ovo vegetarians consume somewhat more copper, and vegans considerably more, than omnivores (Appendix I). Thus one would surmise that the higher intake should override any possible concerns about absorption. However, some research indicates that vegetarians have lower serum copper levels[198] and that, when switching from an omnivore diet to a vegetarian one, serum copper levels decrease.[180] Hunt et al found that copper absorption, measured by the copper balance method, from a controlled lacto-ovo vegetarian diet was slightly lower (18% vs 24%) than from an omnivore diet and that plasma copper concentrations were significantly lower.[134] In a study using stable isotopes of copper, Hunt et al found that copper absorption from a controlled lacto-ovo vegetarian diet was 33% compared to 42% from a nonvegetarian diet.[216] However, because the vegetarian diet contained around 50% more copper than the nonvegetarian diet, total copper absorption was actually greater from the vegetarian diet. In this study, there was no effect of diet on plasma copper or ceruloplasmin levels.[199] Table 6-6 lists vegetarian sources of copper.

MAGNESIUM

Magnesium may have a role in more diverse functions than any other single nutrient; >300 enzymes are thought to require magnesium for activation.[200] Magnesium plays a major role in bone and mineral homeostasis, and about half the body content of magnesium (body content is about 25 g) is found in bone.[201] The male and female adult RDA for magnesium is 420 and 310 mg, respectively.[201] Whole grains are extremely rich in magnesium. A slice of whole wheat bread, for example, contains 12 mg, but a slice of white bread contains only half as much. During refinement, >80% of the magnesium is lost by removal of the germ and outer layer of cereal grains.[202] The magnesium content of vegetarian type foods is generally higher than that of nonvegetarian-type foods.[203]

In one survey of nearly 600 men and women, approximately half of the participants consumed less than two thirds of the RDA for magnesium.[204] Median intakes in the United States are 283 mg/d for men and 211 mg/d for women.[174] Magnesium deficiency may result from alcoholism, malabsorption, renal disease, and some medications.[201]

Some research has suggested that an inadequate magnesium intake is associated with diabetes, hypertension, and atherosclerosis.[205,206] Supplemental magnesium has also been shown to decrease blood pressure,[207] although not all studies support this.[208] Some evidence also suggests that supplemental magnesium can improve bone health.[209]

Vegetarian diets are generally much higher in magnesium than nonvegetarian diets (Appendix I). When subjects were placed on a vegetarian diet, magnesium intake increased 34% in one study.[210] Similarly, experimentally designed vegan diets were shown to contain more magnesium than lacto and lacto-ovo vegetarian diets.[78] One study found that pregnant lacto-ovo vegetarians had higher mean magnesium intakes than nonvegetarians.[211] In macrobiotic and nonmacrobiotic vegetarian children, magnesium intake was markedly higher than the RDA,[97] and in vegetarian macrobiotic adult women serum magnesium levels were about 10% higher.[212] Several studies have examined the effects of vegetarian diets on magnesium status but with somewhat conflicting results. In one, although magnesium content was higher on the vegetarian diet, urinary magnesium excretion was not affected.[213] In two other studies, one found that a vegetarian diet was associated with higher plasma magnesium levels,[180] whereas the other found slightly lower levels.[134] Elderly Taiwanese vegans and lacto-ovo vegetarians had serum magnesium levels that were similar to nonvegetarians, although dietary magnesium intake was significantly lower in vegans than in nonvegetarians.[214] The lower magnesium intakes in this study may have been due to the vegetarians' use of processed soy products in preference to whole grains and legumes.

Approximately 50% of dietary magnesium is absorbed from a typical diet, but high fiber intake decreases absorption. Men consuming 355 mg of magnesium were in positive magnesium balance on a low-fiber diet (9 g/d) but in negative balance on a high-fiber diet.[215] Similar effects have been observed in women.[216] Although phytate and fiber, which are high in vegetarian diets, may reduce magnesium absorption,[215,217,218] absorption is still adequate,[219] and the reduced absorption may be compensated for by higher magnesium content of unrefined products. In general, the higher magnesium content of many vegetarian diets should compensate for any lower absorption. Table 6-7 lists vegetarian sources of magnesium.

PHOSPHORUS

Approximately 85% of the total amount of phosphorus in the body (about 700 g) is in the bone in a 1:2 ratio with calcium. Although phosphorus has a critical role in bone development and maintenance, it has other functions as well. For example, the body stores and releases energy by breaking and making phosphate bonds via adenosine triphosphate (ATP). The adult phosphorus RDA is 700 mg/d.[201] On a mixed diet, net absorption of phosphorus ranges from 55% to 70% in adults but is higher in children. Absorption rates are typically lower in vegetarian diets because most of the phosphorus in these diets is derived from phytate, which is not absorbed as well as inorganic phosphorous. In controlled vegetarian diets, phosphorus absorption was 54% compared to 65% absorption from controlled omnivore diets containing similar amounts of phosphorus but containing markedly less phytate than the vegetarian diets.[134] Phosphorus absorption is also reduced by the ingestion of aluminum-containing antacids and by pharmacologic doses of calcium carbonate but not by typical calcium intakes. Absorption efficiency does not decrease with higher intakes, in contrast to other minerals.

Estimates are that nonvegetarian men and women consume approximately 1350 mg and 1000 mg of phosphorus per day, respectively.[174] The phosphorus intake of vegetarians (Appendix G) is similar to or higher than that of omnivores and, despite potentially lower rates of absorption, is

Table 6-7 Magnesium Content of Foods

Food	Magnesium Content (mg)	Food	Magnesium Content (mg)
Breads, cereals, grains		Orange juice, 1 cup	27
Bread, whole wheat, 1 slice	12	**Legumes,** ½ cup, cooked	
Bran flakes, 1 cup	83	Black-eyed peas	46
Oatmeal, ½ cup, cooked	32	Kidney beans	37
Millet, ½ cup, cooked	38	Lima beans	40
Pasta, whole wheat, ½ cup, cooked	21	Navy beans	48
Quinoa, ½ cup cooked	57	Pinto beans	43
Rice, brown, ½ cup, cooked	42	Split peas	35
Wheat germ, 2 tbsp	53	**Soyfoods,** ½ cup, cooked	
Vegetables, ½ cup, cooked, unless otherwise indicated		Soybeans	74
		Tempeh	67
Avocado, ½	29	Tofu, firm	47
Beet greens	49	**Nuts and seeds,** 2 tbsp	
Beets	20	Almond butter	97
Okra	29	Almonds	49
Peas	18	Brazil nuts	63
Pumpkin	28	Cashews	44
Spinach	78	Peanuts	31
Sweet potato	27	Peanut butter	51
Swiss chard	75	Pumpkin/squash seeds	81
Butternut squash	30	Sunflower seeds	21
Sea vegetables, 8 g dry weight		**Other foods**	
Dulse, dry	49	Chocolate, dark, 1 ounce	68
Kombu, dry	196	Energy bar, 1 bar	100
Nori, dry	76	**Animal products**	
Wakame, dry	66	Milk, 1 cup	24
Fruits		Yogurt, 1 cup	39
Banana, 1 medium	32		

Source: Data from USDA National Nutrient Database for Standard Reference, Release 22, 2009 and manufacturer's information. Values for sea vegetables from MacArtain P, Gill CIR, Brooks M, et al. Nutritional value of edible seaweeds. *Nutr Rev.* 2007;65:535–543.

frequently considerably above recommendations. This relatively high intake of phosphorus by vegetarians makes it unlikely that phosphorus deficiency will occur.

MANGANESE

Manganese is involved in bone formation and in metabolism of carbohydrate, cholesterol, and amino acids. It activates a number of metalloenzymes. Manganese deficiency has never been observed in noninstitutionalized human populations because of the abundant supply of manganese in edible plant materials compared with the relatively low requirement.[220]

The adequate intake (AI) for manganese for adults is 2.3 mg for men and 1.8 mg for women, respectively.[18] The tolerable upper level of intake is set at 11 mg/d.[18] Median daily intake in the United States for men and women was reported in one study to be 2.3 mg for men and 1.8 mg for women.[18] Only a small percentage of dietary manganese is actually absorbed; in some studies <5%.[221] Absorption of manganese from manganese chloride was 8.9% but was only 5.2% from lettuce, 3.81% from spinach, 2.16% from wheat, and 1.71% from sunflower seeds.[222] Phytate has some effect on manganese absorption that is not countered by the addition of ascorbic acid.[223]

In a study of college-age men consuming a vegetarian diet, manganese absorption was quite good.[224] Similarly, Hunt et al found that in experimentally designed diets, the manganese content of the vegetarian diet was about twice (5.9 mg vs 2.5 mg) that of the nonvegetarian diet, and manganese absorption was 11% and 4% from the vegetarian and nonvegetarian diets, respectively.[134]

Whole grains and cereal products are the richest dietary sources of manganese, but nuts, seeds, soyfoods, legumes, and fruits and vegetables also are good sources (Table 6-8). Dairy products, meat, fish, and poultry are all low in manganese. Based on the Total Diet Study, grain products contributed 37% of dietary manganese; tea, 20%; and vegetables, 18%, to the adult male diet.[225] Although data are limited, manganese intake in vegetarians is as much as 50–100% higher than that in nonvegetarians (Appendix I).[161,186,226] Indian diets high in foods of plant origin provide a daily average intake of >8 mg, suggesting that vegetarian diets typically provide adequate amounts of manganese.[227]

IODINE

In many parts of the world, iodine deficiency, characterized by goiter and cretinism, is a major problem. Approximately 2 billion people worldwide have an inadequate iodine intake; in 47 countries iodine deficiency is considered a public health problem.[228] Iodine deficiency at critical stages of development in fetal life and early childhood remains the world's single most important and preventable cause of brain damage.[228] Even mild iodine deficiency in childhood can prevent children from attaining their full intellectual potential.[229]

Iodine is an integral part of the thyroid hormones, thyroxine and triiodothyronine. The adult iodine RDA is 150 µg.[18] The median intake of iodine in the United States is approximately 240 to 300 µg/d for men and 190 to 210 µg/d for women.[18] Although median urinary iodine levels in the United States declined from the 1960s to the late 1980s,[230] these levels appear to have stabilized[231] and to be within a reasonable range.

Table 6-8 Manganese Content of Foods

Food	Manganese Content (mg)	Food	Manganese Content (mg)
Breads, cereals, grains		**Legumes,** ½ cup, cooked	
Bran flakes, 1 cup	1.39	Black-eyed peas	0.41
Oatmeal, ½ cup, cooked	0.68	Chickpeas	0.84
Shredded wheat, ½ cup	2.0	Lentils	0.49
Pasta, whole wheat, ½ cup, cooked	0.96	Lima beans	0.48
Quinoa, ½ cup, cooked	0.58	**Soyfoods,** ½ cup, cooked	
Rice, brown, ½ cup, cooked	0.88	Soybeans	0.71
Wheat germ, 2 tbsp	3.20	Tempeh	1.08
Vegetables, ½ cup, cooked		Tofu, firm	0.79
Beet greens	0.37	**Nuts and seeds,** 2 tbsp	
Collard greens	0.56	Almond butter	0.75
Peas	0.22	Peanut butter	0.58
Spinach	0.84	Pumpkin/squash seeds	0.66
Sweet potato	0.50	Sunflower seeds	0.35
Turnip greens	0.24	**Other foods**	
Fruits		Chocolate, dark, 1 oz	0.58
Banana, 1 medium	0.32	Energy bar, 1 bar	0.5 to 0.7
Pineapple, ½ cup	0.76	Tea, brewed, 8 oz	0.52
Strawberries, ½ cup, sliced	0.32		

Source: Data from USDA National Nutrient Database for Standard Reference, Release 22, 2009 and manufacturers' information.

In the United States, the incidence of endemic goiter fell sharply after the introduction of iodized salt in 1924.[232] Universal salt iodization is recommended worldwide to ensure sufficient intake of iodine by all individuals.[233] Many populations are at risk of iodine deficiency because they live in an iodine-deficient environment where iodine has been removed from soil by glaciation, high rainfall, or flood. This situation occurs most often in mountainous areas, such as the Himalayan region, the Andean region, and the vast mountain ranges of China. Low-lying areas subject to flooding, however, as in the Ganges Valley in India and Bangladesh, are also severely iodine deficient.

In coastal areas, seafood, water, and iodine-containing mist from the ocean are important sources. Farther inland, the iodine content of plants is variable, depending on the geochemical environment and on fertilizing and food processing practices. Food composition tables may over- or underestimate iodine intake due to lack of data for some foods and incorrect values for others.[234] Variable sources of dietary iodine include iodates that are sometimes still used as dough conditioners in commercial bread production, although their use has declined; dairy products whose iodine content is affected by iodine-containing disinfectants used on cows' teats and milking equipment; and iodized salt use in food processing.[235,236]

Iodized salt is an excellent source of iodine. In the United States, iodized salt contains 46 mg I/kg.[237] One-quarter teaspoon of commercially available iodized salt provides 45% of the daily value or about 68 µg. Iodized salt is used by about half of the U.S. population.[18] Food processors are not required to use iodized salt. Virtually none of the salt used by the pre-prepared or the fast-food industry is iodized.[237] Kosher salt and salty seasonings such as tamari and soy sauce are not iodized. Commercial sea salt contains variable amounts of iodine; at least one brand is iodized.

The iodine content of sea vegetables varies widely; some may contain substantial amounts of iodine, potentially leading to toxicity with regular and generous consumption.[238] Hypothyroidism in newborn and nursing infants in Japan has been linked to their mothers' consumption of seaweed containing from 2300 to 3200 µg iodine per day.[239]

Some data suggest vegetarians who do not use iodized salt may be at increased risk of developing iodine deficiency.[240] No studies have been conducted of vegetarians in the United States. In a study of British vegetarians, iodine intake (not including iodized salt) was found to be 70% and 40% below recommendations in males and female vegans, respectively ($N = 38$) even when supplements were included, but it was more than adequate for lacto-ovo vegetarians ($N = 52$) and fish-eating lacto-ovo vegetarians ($N = 37$).[159] These findings are in agreement with those of another study involving Finnish vegans. Average iodine intake of vegan subjects was 29 µg of iodine per day compared to 222 µg for the omnivores in this study. However, thyroid function based on hormone levels was still normal, and the vegans consumed a rather restricted diet that included only uncooked food and no salt.[241] In a small study of six lacto vegetarians in Sweden, a low-iodine area, iodine intake was 82 µg/d and 58 µg/d, respectively, for males and females.[194] None of the vegetarians in this study exhibited clinical signs of iodine deficiency as assessed by thyroid hormone levels.[181] Data from a study of Swedish vegans showed intake per 1000 calories was only 39 µg compared to 156 µg for an omnivore diet.[182] Although British vegans consumed an average of 751 µg of iodine per day, more than five times the British recommendation, 24% of the 39 subjects did not consume the lower reference nutrient intake established by the Department of Health in the United Kingdom.[242]

Remer et al looked at both intake and iodine excretion in healthy German subjects on experimentally designed vegetarian and nonvegetarian diets.[240] These diets did not include fish or iodized salt. Iodine intake was 15.6 µg/d on the vegetarian diet compared to 35.2 µg/d on the omnivore diet. Vegetarian iodine excretion was also about 50% lower than in the omnivores. Vegetarians and vegans in Slovakia also had markedly lower urine iodine levels than nonvegetarians.[243] Finally, Key et al measured serum thyroid hormone levels in 48 adult vegans and 53 omnivores. They found that thyroid stimulating hormone (TSH) levels, although within the normal range, were significantly higher (29%) in vegans than in omnivores, which is suggestive of a low iodine intake.[244] Furthermore, three of the five vegan subjects with the highest TSH values used kelp tablets or powder. This may be because of the variability of iodine content of kelp leading to discrepancies between the labeled and actual content of iodine in kelp-based supplements.[245]

Prior to absorption, dietary iodine is converted to the iodide ion, which is almost completely absorbed.[18] Foods that may be eaten by vegetarians including soy products, cruciferous vegetables, and sweet potatoes contain naturally occurring goitrogens (Chapter 9). These goitrogens are not problematic in healthy people except in those with a deficient iodine intake.[18,246] Therefore, vegetarians, particularly vegans, should use either iodized salt or make sure they are consuming other reliable sources of iodine.

SODIUM

Sodium is the primary regulator of extracellular fluid volume but has several other important functions. It is involved in the regulation of acid-base balance and the membrane potential of cells. On average, higher sodium intakes are linked to higher blood pressure.[247] Reducing sodium intake to below the current recommendations reduces blood pressure to a greater extent than reducing it to the recommended levels, and the hypotensive effects of sodium restriction occur in subjects who are already consuming blood-pressure-lowering diets.[248,249]

The average intake of sodium by adults in the United States is >3500 mg/d.[250] *Dietary Guidelines for Americans, 2005,* from the U.S. Department of Health and Human Services and USDA, recommend that adults in the United States consume no more than 2300 mg of sodium per day with a lower intake of 1500 mg/d recommended for specific groups (i.e., all persons with hypertension, all middle-aged and older adults, and all blacks).[247] Close to 70% of adults in the United States are in one or more groups who should aim for the lower intake of sodium.[251]

Although many agrarian societies with primarily vegetarian diets consume less sodium than Westerners, the sodium intake of vegetarians in industrialized countries is similar to that of omnivores (Appendix G). A study in the United States found that the sodium intake of African American vegans was about 30% lower than of lacto-ovo vegetarians.[72]

Because unprocessed foods are naturally low in sodium, sodium intake is not determined so much by the intake of different food groups but by the amount of processed foods. Estimates are that in Western countries, only about 10% of sodium intake comes naturally from food, about 15% from salt added during cooking and at the table, and fully 75% from salt added during processing and manufacturing.[247] Consumers eating lower sodium foods typically do not add table salt to compensate for the lower sodium content.[247] To reduce sodium intake substantially, a reduction in processed food consumption is required.

The sodium content of convenience foods commonly marketed to vegetarians such as veggie burgers and dogs and prepared entrees varies widely (Table 6-9). Dietitians can help consumers select lower sodium products, reduce the sodium contribution from other foods if convenience foods are key dietary components, and identify recipes for home preparation of foods like burgers so that the sodium content can be reduced. Strategies such as draining the canning brine and rinsing canned beans and vegetables can reduce their sodium content.[252]

CHLORIDE

Chloride plays a critical role in maintaining fluid and electrolyte balance, and it is a key component of gastric juice. Because the intake of chloride from food as well as its loss from the body

Table 6-9 Sodium Content of Some Common Vegetarian Processed Foods

Food	Sodium Content (mg)
Frozen entree, 1 serving	550–780
Seitan, commercially prepared, 1 oz	130–160
Vegetarian chili, canned, 1 cup	460–680
Vegetarian cup of soup, 1 package	310–680
Vegetarian refried beans, canned, ½ cup	390–530
Vegetarian soup, canned, 1 cup	340–890
Veggie bacon, 1 slice	140
Veggie burger, 1 burger	280–400
Veggie deli slices, 1 oz	160–270
Veggie dog, 1	300–560
Veggie sausage, 1 oz	155–230

Source: Manufacturers' information. Values indicate ranges in commonly available foods.

under normal conditions parallel those of sodium, the requirements specified for all age and sex groups (with the exception of infants) are similar to those for sodium. Dietary chloride comes almost exclusively from sodium chloride (ordinary salt). Chloride intake is similar between vegetarians and nonvegetarians, as determined from the limited direct dietary intake data and the similarity in sodium intake between these two groups.

POTASSIUM

Potassium is the principal intracellular cation; its concentration in cells is 30 times higher than that in blood. Potassium in the blood plays an important role in controlling skeletal muscle contractions and nerve impulses and in maintaining normal blood pressure.

Potassium is widely distributed in foods (Table 6-10). Fruits and vegetables are especially rich in this mineral as are dried beans and peas. Vegetarians tend to consume somewhat more potassium than nonvegetarians (Appendix G); potassium intakes of vegans are similar to those of lacto-ovo vegetarians.[253,254] Potassium intake has been linked with increased bone calcium retention, reduced risk of cardiovascular disease, and lower blood pressure.[247,255] The daily median adult intake in the United States is about 2800 mg/d for men and 2100 mg/d for women.[174] The recommended intake of potassium for adolescents and adults is 4700 mg/d, considerably higher than current median intakes.[255]

FLUORIDE

The decline in dental caries in industrialized countries during the past 40 years is primarily attributed to the widespread use of fluoride. Through extensive epidemiologic studies of communities with naturally fluoridated water in the United States in the 1930s, the protective properties

Table 6-10 Potassium Content of Foods

Food	Potassium Content (mg)	Food	Potassium Content (mg)
Breads, cereals, grains		Nori, dry	212
Bran flakes, 1 cup	240	**Fruits**	
Vegetables, ½ cup, cooked, unless otherwise indicated		Banana, 1 medium	422
		Orange juice, 1 cup	443
Avocado, ½	487	**Legumes,** ½ cup, cooked	
Asparagus	202	Black-eyed peas	239
Beet greens	654	Chickpeas	239
Beets	259	Kidney beans	358
Broccoli	229	Lentils	365
Parsnips	286	Lima beans	478
Plantain	465	Navy beans	354
Potato	296	Pinto beans	373
Pumpkin	252	Soybeans	443
Spinach	419	Split peas	355
Acorn squash	322	**Nuts and seeds**	
Sweet potato	475	Almond butter, 2 tbsp	243
Swiss chard	480	Peanut butter, 2 tbsp	238
Stewed tomatoes	264	**Animal products**	
Tomato juice, 1 cup	556	Milk, 1 cup	322
Sea vegetables, 8 g dry weight		Yogurt, 1 cup	537
Dulse, dry	585		
Kombu, dry	976		

Source: Data from USDA National Nutrient Database for Standard Reference, Release 22, 2009. Values for sea vegetables from MacArtain P, Gill CIR, Brooks M, et al. Nutritional value of edible seaweeds. *Nutr Rev.* 2007;65:535–543.

of fluoride in the prevention of dental caries were fully recognized. Although fluoride is best known for its prevention of tooth decay,[201] some evidence suggests that fluoride may promote bone health.[256]

For adults, the AI is 4 mg/d for men and 3 mg/d for females.[201] Fluoridated drinking water is an important source of this mineral and accounts for much of the difference in fluoride intake among different areas of the United States.[201] Brewed tea is a good source of fluoride as are other foods prepared with fluoridated water.[201]

Fluoride toxicity, referred to as skeletal fluorosis, adversely affects bone health and possibly muscle and nerve function. This condition occurs only after years of intake of 20 to 80 mg/d, however, which is greatly in excess of U.S. intake. Mottling of teeth in children has been observed at 2 to 8 mg fluoride/kg body weight. No published reports on the fluoride intake of vegetarians were identified, but because fluoridated water directly and indirectly accounts for most of the fluoride intake in the United States, there is not likely to be any difference between vegetarians and nonvegetarians.

CHROMIUM

Chromium is generally accepted as an essential nutrient that potentiates insulin action and thus influences overall metabolism, although the precise biologic manner in which this effect occurs is poorly understood. Anderson concluded that supplemental chromium has beneficial effects without any documented side effects on people with varying degrees of glucose intolerance.[257] Chromium supplementation does not appear to have a significant effect on lipid or glucose metabolism in people without diabetes.[258] For adults, the AI is 35 μg/d for men and 25 μg/d for women.[18] Athletes may have higher needs for chromium than sedentary individuals due to losses in sweat.[259] Chromium intake in the United States appears to be close to the AI.[260] Several dietary factors may increase chromium absorption including vitamin C and oxalate.[18]

Chromium is widely distributed in the food chain, but most foods have small amounts. Dairy products, fruits, and vegetables contain low amounts of chromium, whereas whole grain products, including ready-to-eat bran cereals, processed meats, and spices, are the best sources. Considerable amounts of chromium are lost when grains are refined.[261] Conversely, substantial amounts can be added to the food supply during processing and preparation because chromium can be leached from stainless steel containers, particularly when acidic juices are heated in them.[262] Some beers also contain significant amounts of chromium, although brands vary quite a bit in their content.[263]

Although chromium absorption is thought to be relatively low, in a study of Indian vegetarian or largely vegetarian diets, chromium intake was generally between 100 and 200 μg/d, and absorption was quite good.[219] The chromium intake of Western vegetarians has not been assessed.

MOLYBDENUM

Molybdenum functions as a constituent of several enzymes, including aldehyde oxidase, xanthine oxidase, and sulfite oxidase. Molybdenum may play an important role in the detoxification of foreign compounds. The RDA for adult men and women is 45 μg/d.[18] The average intake in the United States is 109 μg/d in men and 76 μg/d in women.[264] Vegetarian intake is likely to be adequate because the foods that are staples of many vegetarian diets including legumes, grain products, nuts, seeds, and vegetables are good sources of molybdenum.[265] Although molybdenum in soybeans was not absorbed as well as molybdenum in kale, it does not appear that the presence of soy in a meal interferes with molybdenum absorption from other sources.[266]

COUNSELING POINTS: IRON AND ZINC

- Whole grains and legumes contain phytates, which can reduce absorption of minerals, especially iron and zinc. However, because these foods are also good sources of iron and zinc, and because a number of factors can reduce the effects of phytates in vegetarian diets, whole grains and legumes should be included in vegetarian diets.

- Refined grains are lower in phytate but they are also lower in iron and zinc. Choose whole grains often to increase iron and zinc intake.
- Some dietary factors affect the activity of phytate and the absorption of minerals. Absorption of iron and zinc are better from leavened grain products like bread than from unleavened products like crackers.
- Fermentation increases absorption of some minerals so that absorption is improved from sourdough bread and from soy foods like tempeh and miso.
- Soaking grains and beans so that they germinate can improve mineral absorption.
- Organic acids that occur naturally in fruits and vegetables increase absorption of zinc and iron.
- Vitamin C improves iron absorption when these two nutrients are included in the same meal. It is important for vegetarians to include a source of vitamin C at every meal. Vegetarians with marginal iron status whose diet already contains generous amounts of vitamin C may need to use an iron supplement to improve iron status.[96]
- Calcium inhibits iron absorption, and a high calcium and phytate intake may reduce zinc absorption. It is important to take calcium supplements between meals so they don't interfere with mineral absorption.
- Although vegetarian diets are often higher in iron than omnivore diets, many vegetarians, especially premenopausal women, may not meet the RDA, which is much higher for vegetarians than for nonvegetarians. Choose a diet that includes a wide range of iron-rich foods to make sure recommendations are met.
- Although overt zinc deficiency is rare, vegetarians often have zinc intakes that are lower than those of omnivores and their needs may be 50% higher. Choose a diet that includes zinc-rich foods.

COUNSELING POINTS: IODINE

- Iodine is needed for normal thyroid function.
- Certain foods, like soy foods and vegetables in the cabbage family, contain compounds that can interfere with thyroid function, but their effects are important only if iodine intake is too low.
- Vegetarians, particularly vegans, should use iodized salt or other foods that are good sources of iodine or take a supplement containing iodine.

Case Studies

Susan is a 25-year-old avid runner and is training for her first marathon. She has experienced some difficulty with hills and, after a physical examination and lab work, has been diagnosed with iron-deficiency anemia. Susan is a lacto-ovo vegetarian. She is 5′2″ tall and weighs 105 pounds (body mass index: 19.2). Her weight is stable. Due to a family history of osteoporosis, she takes a 500-mg calcium supplement twice daily—at breakfast and dinner. She does not use other supplements.

(continued)

A typical day's intake is:

⅓ cup bran cereal with a banana and ½ cup low-fat milk, 2 biscuits, and 2 cups of tea for breakfast.

1½ cups of vanilla yogurt, 8 saltines, a medium apple, 2 tablespoons of peanut butter, and a glass of iced tea for lunch.

1½ cups of macaroni and cheese, 1 cup of tossed salad with dressing, ½ cup of baby carrots, and ½ cup of ice cream for dinner.

16 oz of Gatorade and an energy bar for snacks.

What are some possible explanations for Susan's iron-deficiency anemia?

What is Susan's current iron intake (approximately)? Is it adequate?

What suggestions will you make to Susan with regard to dietary changes? Should she take an iron supplement? If so, what level of supplementary iron do you suggest?

Alan is a middle-aged man who has recently been divorced. He lives alone and says that he is not a particularly good cook. He has recently learned that he has high blood pressure and wants to try to reduce his blood pressure without medication. His doctor has agreed to a 6-month trial of diet. Alan became vegan about 10 years ago when his daughter persuaded the entire family to try a vegan diet. He is about 20 pounds overweight and has recently joined a gym, hoping that more exercise will help him lose weight. His doctor suggests that he reduce his sodium intake, and Alan has heard that increasing potassium might be good as well.

A typical day might include:

Breakfast:
   2 toaster waffles with 1 tablespoon maple syrup and 1 tablespoon margarine
   1 cup grape juice
   5 veggie sausage links

Lunch:
   Sandwich with ½ package (about 2.5 oz) veggie deli slices, mustard, and lettuce
   1 instant soup cup
   1 medium banana
   1 cup enriched soymilk

Dinner:
   Vegan frozen entree
   1 cup unsweetened applesauce
   Vegan frozen dessert

Snacks:
   Tortilla chips and salsa, salted nuts, pear

What suggestions can you give Alan to help him reduce his sodium intake and increase his potassium intake? Keep his limited cooking skills in mind when you develop suggestions.

REFERENCES

1. Sandberg AS, Andersson H. Effect of dietary phytase on the digestion of phytate in the stomach and small intestine of humans. *J Nutr.* 1988;118:469–473.
2. Sandberg AS. Bioavailability of minerals in legumes. *Br J Nutr.* 2002;88(suppl 3):S281–S285.

3. Sandberg AS, Brune M, Carlsson NG, et al. Inositol phosphates with different numbers of phosphate groups influence iron absorption in humans. *Am J Clin Nutr.* 1999;70:240–246.

4. Lonnerdal B, Sandberg AS, Sandström B, Kunz C. Inhibitory effects of phytic acid and other inositol phosphates on zinc and calcium absorption in suckling rats. *J Nutr.* 1989;119:211–214.

5. Larsson M, Rossander-Hulthen L, Sandstrom B, Sandberg AS. Improved zinc and iron absorption from breakfast meals containing malted oats with reduced phytate content. *Br J Nutr.* 1996;76:677–688.

6. Brune M, Rossander-Hulthen L, Hallberg L, et al. Iron absorption from bread in humans: inhibiting effects of cereal fiber, phytate and inositol phosphates with different numbers of phosphate groups. *J Nutr.* 1992;122:442–449.

7. Lonnerdal B. Dietary factors influencing zinc absorption. *J Nutr.* 2000;130:1378S–1383S.

8. Navert B, Sandstrom B, Cederblad A. Reduction of the phytate content of bran by leavening in bread and its effect on zinc absorption in man. *Br J Nutr.* 1985;53:47–53.

9. Dallman PR. Biochemical basis for the manifestations of iron deficiency. *Annu Rev Nutr.* 1986;6:13–40.

10. Shamsuddin AM. Metabolism and cellular functions of IP6: a review. *Anticancer Res.* 1999; 19:3733–3736.

11. Owen RW, Spiegelhalder B, Bartsch H. Phytate, reactive oxygen species and colorectal cancer. *Eur J Cancer Prev.* 1998;7(suppl 2):S41–S54.

12. Zhou JR, Erdman JW. Phytic acid in health and disease. *Crit Rev Food Sci Nutr.* 1995;35:495–508.

13. Graf E, Eaton JW. Antioxidant functions of phytic acid. *Free Radic Biol Med.* 1990;8:61–69.

14. Weber G, Shen F, Yang H, et al. Regulation of signal transduction activity in normal and cancer cells. *Anticancer Res.* 1999;19:3703–3709.

15. Miyamoto S, Kuwata G, Imai M, et al. Protective effect of phytic acid hydrolysis products on iron-induced lipid peroxidation of liposomal membranes. *Lipids.* 2000;35:1411–1413.

16. Vucenik I, Shamsuddin AM. Protection against cancer by dietary IP6 and inositol. *Nutr Cancer.* 2006;55:109–125.

17. Schlemmer U, Frolich W, Prieto RM, et al. Phytate in foods and significance for humans: food sources, intake, processing, bioavailability, protective role and analysis. *Mol Nutr Food Res.* 2009,53,S330–S375.

18. Institute of Medicine, Food and Nutrition Board. *Dietary Reference Intakes for Vitamin A, Vitamin K, Arsenic, Boron, Chromium, Copper, Iodine, Iron, Manganese, Molybdenum, Nickel, Silicon, Vanadium, and Zinc.* Washington, DC: National Academy Press; 2001.

19. WHO Global Database on Anaemia. *Worldwide Prevalence of Anaemia 1993–2005.* Geneva, Switzerland: World Health Organization; 2008.

20. Centers for Disease Control and Preventions. Iron Deficiency—United States, 1999–2000. *MMWR.* 2002;51:897–899.

21. Centers for Disease Control and Prevention. Recommendations to prevent and control iron deficiency in the United States. *MMWR.* 1998;47 (No. RR-3):1–28.

22. Finch CA, Bellotti V, Stray S, et al. Plasma ferritin determination as a diagnostic tool. *West J Med.* 1986;145(5):657–663.

23. Joint FAO/WHO Expert Consultation on Human Vitamin and Mineral Requirements. *Vitamin and Mineral Requirements in Human Nutrition.* 2nd ed. Geneva, Switzerland: World Health Organization and Food and Agriculture Organization of the United Nations; 2004.

24. Beard JL. Iron biology in immune function, muscle metabolism, and neuronal functioning. *J Nutr.* 2001;131:568S–580S.

25. Murray-Kolb LE, Beard JL. Iron treatment normalizes cognitive functioning in young women. *Am J Clin Nutr.* 2007;85:778–787.

26. Committee on Diet and Health FNB, Commission on Life Sciences, National Research Council. *Diet and Health, Implications for Reducing Chronic Disease Risk.* Washington, DC: National Academy Press; 1989.

27. Yip R, Walsh KM, Goldfarb MG, Binkin NJ. Declining prevalence of anemia in childhood in a middle-class setting: a pediatric success story? *Pediatrics.* 1987;80:330–334.

28. Dallman PR, Yip R, Johnson C. Prevalence and causes of anemia in the United States, 1976 to 1980. *Am J Clin Nutr.* 1984;39:437–445.

29. Cotton PA, Subar AF, Friday JE, Cook A. Dietary sources of nutrients among US adults, 1994 to 1996. *J Am Diet Assoc.* 2004;104:921–930.

30. Cogswell ME, Kettel-Khan L, Ramakrishnan U. Iron supplement use among women in the United States: science, policy, and practice. *J Nutr.* 2003;133:1974S–1977S.

31. Ervin RB, Kennedy-Stephenson J. Mineral intakes of elderly adult supplement and non- supplement users in the Third National Health and Nutrition Examination Survey. *J Nutr.* 2002;132:3422–3427.

32. Cook JD. Adaptation in iron metabolism. *Am J Clin Nutr.* 1990;51:301–308.

33. Hallberg L, Rossander L. Absorption of iron from Western-type lunch and dinner meals. *Am J Clin Nutr.* 1982; 35:502–509.

34. Hallberg L, Hulthen L, Gramatkovski E. Iron absorption from the whole diet in men: how effective is the regulation of iron absorption? *Am J Clin Nutr.* 1997;66:347–356.

35. Bezwoda WR, Bothwell TH, Charlton RW, et al. The relative dietary importance of haem and non-haem iron. *S Afr Med J.* 1983;64:552–556.

36. Brune M, Rossander L, Hallberg L. Iron absorption: no intestinal adaptation to a high-phytate diet. *Am J Clin Nutr.* 1989;49:542–545.

37. Hurrell RF, Juillerat MA, Reddy MB, et al. Soy protein, phytate, and iron absorption in humans. *Am J Clin Nutr.* 1992;56:573–578.

38. Hallberg L, Rossander L, Skanberg AB. Phytates and the inhibitory effect of bran on iron absorption in man. *Am J Clin Nutr.* 1987;45:988–996.

39. Mendoza C, Viteri FE, Lonnerdal B, et al. Effect of genetically modified, low-phytic acid maize on absorption of iron from tortillas. *Am J Clin Nutr.* 1998;68:1123–1127.

40. Van Dokkum W, Wesstra A, Schippers FA. Physiological effects of fibre-rich types of bread. 1. The effect of dietary fibre from bread on the mineral balance of young men. *Br J Nutr.* 1982;47:451–460.

41. Hallberg L, Hulthen L. Prediction of dietary iron absorption: an algorithm for calculating absorption and bioavailability of dietary iron. *Am J Clin Nutr.* 2000;71:1147–1160.

42. Rossander L, Hallberg L, Bjorn-Rasmussen E. Absorption of iron from breakfast meals. *Am J Clin Nutr.* 1979;32: 2484–2489.

43. Hurrell RF, Reddy M, Cook JD. Inhibition of non-haem iron absorption in man by polyphenolic-containing beverages. *Br J Nutr.* 1999;81:289–295.

44. Narasinga R, Prabhavathi T. Tannin content of foods commonly consumed in India and its influence on ionizable iron. *J Sci Food Agric.* 1982;33:89–96.

45. Morck TA, Lynch SR, Cook JD. Inhibition of food iron absorption by coffee. *Am J Clin Nutr.* 1983;37:416–420.

46. Hallberg L. Does calcium interfere with iron absorption? *Am J Clin Nutr.* 1998;68(1):3–4.

47. Siegenberg D, Baynes RD, Bothwell TH, et al. Ascorbic acid prevents the dose-dependent inhibitory effects of polyphenols and phytates on nonheme-iron absorption. *Am J Clin Nutr.* 1991;53:537–541.

48. Cook JD. Absorption of food iron. *Fed Proc.* 1977;36:2028–2032.

49. Monsen ER, Balintfy JL. Calculating dietary iron bioavailability: refinement and computerization. *J Am Diet Assoc.* 1982;80:307–311.

50. Gillooly M, Bothwell TH, Torrance JD, et al. The effects of organic acids, phytates and polyphenols on the absorption of iron from vegetables. *Br J Nutr.* 1983;49:331–342.

51. Ballot D, Baynes RD, Bothwell TH, et al. The effects of fruit juices and fruits on the absorption of iron from a rice meal. *Br J Nutr.* 1987;57:331–343.

52. Cook JD, Reddy MB. Effect of ascorbic acid intake on nonheme-iron absorption from a complete diet. *Am J Clin Nutr.* 2001;73:93–98.

53. Hunt JR, Gallagher SK, Johnson LK. Effect of ascorbic acid on apparent iron absorption by women with low iron stores. *Am J Clin Nutr.* 1994;59:1381–1385.

54. Cook JD, Monsen ER. Vitamin C, the common cold, and iron absorption. *Am J Clin Nutr.* 1977;30:235–241.

55. Fleming DJ, Jacques PF, Dallal GE, et al. Dietary determinants of iron stores in a free-living elderly population: The Framingham Heart Study. *Am J Clin Nutr.* 1998;67:722–733.

56. Hallberg L Bjørn-Rasmussen E, Howard L, et al. Dietary heme iron absorption. A discussion of possible mechanisms for the absorption-promoting effect of meat and for the regulation of iron absorption. *Scan J Gastroenterol.* 1979;14:769–779.

57. Garcia-Casal MN, Layrisse M, Solano L, et al. Vitamin A and beta-carotene can improve nonheme iron absorption from rice, wheat and corn by humans. *J Nutr.* 1998;128:646–650.

58. Walczyk T, Davidson L, Rossander-Hulthen L, et al. No enhancing effect of vitamin A on iron absorption in humans. *Am J Clin Nutr.* 2003;77:144–149.

59. Cook JD, Dassenko SA, Lynch SR. Assessment of the role of nonheme-iron availability in iron balance. *Am J Clin Nutr.* 1991;54:717–722.
60. Cook JD, Watson SS, Simpson KM, et al. The effect of high ascorbic acid supplementation on body iron stores. *Blood* 1984;64:721–726.
61. Reddy MB, Hurrell RF, Cook JD. Estimation of nonheme-iron bioavailability from meal composition. *Am J Clin Nutr.* 2000;71:937–943.
62. Du S, Zhai F, Wang Y, Popkin BM. Current methods for estimating dietary iron bioavailability do not work in China. *J Nutr.* 2000;130:193–198.
63. Rickard AP, Chatfield MD, Conway RE, et al. An algorithm to assess intestinal iron availability for use in dietary surveys. *Br J Nutr.* 2009;102:1672–1685.
64. Chiplonkar SA, Agte VV. Statistical model for predicting non-heme iron bioavailability from vegetarian meals. *Int J Food Sci Nutr.* 2006;57:434–450.
65. Beard JL, Murray-Kolb LE, Haas JD, et al. Iron absorption prediction equations lack agreement and underestimate iron absorption. *J Nutr.* 2007;137:1741–1746.
66. Hunt JR, Roughead ZK. Nonheme-iron absorption, fecal ferritin excretion, and blood indexes of iron status in women consuming controlled lactoovovegetarian diets for 8 wk. *Am J Clin Nutr.* 1999;69:944–952.
67. Panel on Dietary Reference Values of the Committee on Medical Aspects of Food Policy—Department of Health. Dietary reference values for food energy and nutrients for the United Kingdom. Report of the Panel on Dietary Reference Values of the Committee on Medical Aspects of Food Policy. *Rep Health Soc Subj.* 1991;41:1–210.
68. National Health and Medical Research Council of Australia (NHMRC). *Nutrient Reference Values for Australia and New Zealand Including Recommended Dietary Intakes.* 2006.
69. Ball MJ, Bartlett MA. Dietary intake and iron status of Australian vegetarian women. *Am J Clin Nutr.* 1999;70:353–358.
70. Harman SK, Parnell WR. The nutritional health of New Zealand vegetarian and non-vegetarian Seventh-day Adventists: selected vitamin, mineral and lipid levels. *N Z Med J.* 1998;111:91–94.
71. Huang Y-C, Lin W-J, Cheng C-H, Su K-H. Nutrient intakes and iron status of healthy young vegetarians and non-vegetarians. *Nutr Res.* 1999;19:663–674.
72. Toohey ML, Harris MA, DeWitt W, et al. Cardiovascular disease risk factors are lower in African-American vegans compared to lacto-ovo-vegetarians. *J Am Coll Nutr.* 1998;17:425–434.
73. Haddad EH, Berk LS, Kettering JD, et al. Dietary intake and biochemical, hematologic, and immune status of vegans compared with nonvegetarians. *Am J Clin Nutr.* 1999;70:586S–593S.
74. Campbell TC, Junshi C. Diet and chronic degenerative diseases: perspectives from China. *Am J Clin Nutr.* 1994;59:1153S–1161S.
75. Rosado JL, Lopez P, Morales M, et al. Bioavailability of energy, nitrogen, fat, zinc, iron and calcium from rural and urban Mexican diets. *Br J Nutr.* 1992;68:45–58.
76. Van Dokkum W, Wesstra JA, Schippers FA. Effect of lactovegetarian, vegan and mixed diets on mineral utilization. Paper presented at: 5th International Symposium on Trace Elements in Man and Animals; 1986; Ziest, The Netherlands.
77. Van Dokkum W. Significance of iron bioavailability for iron recommendations. *Biol Trace Elem Res.* 1992;35:1–11.
78. Kramer LB, Osis D, Coffey J, Spencer H. Mineral and trace element content of vegetarian diets. *J Am Coll Nutr.* 1984;3:3–11.
79. Couzy F, Kastenmayer P, Mansourian R, et al. Zinc absorption in healthy elderly humans and the effect of diet. *Am J Clin Nutr.* 1993;58:690–694.
80. Hambraeus L. Animal- and plant-food-based diets and iron status: benefits and costs. *Proc Nutr Soc.* 1999;58:235–242.
81. Ellis R, Morris ER, Hill AD, Smith JC Jr. Phytate:zinc molar ratio, mineral, and fiber content of three hospital diets. *J Am Diet Assoc.* 1982;81:26–29.
82. Sanders TA, Purves R. An anthropometric and dietary assessment of the nutritional status of vegan preschool children. *J Hum Nutr.* 1981;35:349–357.
83. Thane CW, Bates CL. Dietary intakes and nutrient status of vegetarian preschool children from a British national survey. *J Hum Nutr Diet.* 2000;13:149–162.
84. Yen CE, Yen CH, Huang MC, et al. Dietary intake and nutritional status of vegetarian and omnivorous preschool children and their parents in Taiwan. *Nutr Res.* 2008;28:430–436.

85. Thane CW, Bates CJ, Prentice A. Risk factors for low iron intake and poor iron status in a national sample of British young people aged 4–18 years. *Public Health Nutr.* 2003;6:485–496.

86. Larsson CL, Johansson GK. Dietary intake and nutritional status of young vegans and omnivores in Sweden. *Am J Clin Nutr.* 2002;76:100–106.

87. Wells AM, Haub MD, Fluckey J, et al. Comparisons of vegetarian and beef-containing diets on hematological indexes and iron stores during a period of resistive training in older men. *J Am Diet Assoc.* 2003;103(5):594–601.

88. Alexander D, Ball MJ, Mann J. Nutrient intake and haematological status of vegetarians and age-sex matched omnivores. *Eur J Clin Nutr.* 1994;48:538–546.

89. Worthington-Roberts BS, Breskin MW, Monsen ER. Iron status of premenopausal women in a university community and its relationship to habitual dietary sources of protein. *Am J Clin Nutr.* 1988;47:275–279.

90. Hua NW, Stoohs RA, Facchini FS. Low iron status and enhanced insulin sensitivity in lacto- ovo vegetarians. *Br J Nutr.* 2001;86:515–519.

91. Shaw NS, Chin CJ, Pan WH. A vegetarian diet rich in soybean products compromises iron status in young students. *J Nutr.* 1995;125:212–219.

92. Reddy S, Sanders TA. Haematological studies on pre-menopausal Indian and Caucasian vegetarians compared with Caucasian omnivores. *Br J Nutr.* 1990;64:331–338.

93. Brants HA, Lowik MR, Westenbrink S, et al. Adequacy of a vegetarian diet at old age (Dutch Nutrition Surveillance System). *J Am Coll Nutr.* 1990;9:292–302.

94. Helman AD, Darnton-Hill I. Vitamin and iron status in new vegetarians. *Am J Clin Nutr.* 1987;45:785–789.

95. Lacong A. Nutritional status and dietary intake of a selected sample of young adult vegetarians. *Can Med Assoc J.* 1986;47:101–108.

96. Waldmann A, Koschizkea JW, Leitzmannb C, et al. Dietary iron intake and iron status of German female vegans: Results of the German Vegan Study. *Ann Nutr Metab.* 2004;48:103–108.

97. Dagnelie PC, van Staveren WA, Vergote FJ, et al. Increased risk of vitamin B12 and iron deficiency in infants on macrobiotic diets. *Am J Clin Nutr.* 1989;50:818–824.

98. Dwyer JT, Dietz WH Jr, Andrews EM, Suskind RM. Nutritional status of vegetarian children. *Am J Clin Nutr.* 1982;35:204–216.

99. Kim YC. *The Effect of a Vegetarian Diet on the Iron and Zinc Status of School-Age Children.* Amherst: University of Massachusetts Press; 1988.

100. Donovan UM, Gibson RS. Iron and zinc status of young women aged 14 to 19 years consuming vegetarian and omnivorous diets. *J Am Coll Nutr.* 1995;14:463–472.

101. Latta D, Liebman M. Iron and zinc status of nonvegetarian males. *Nutr Rep Int.* 1984;30:141–149.

102. Tungtrongchitr R, Pongpaew P, Prayurahong B, et al. Vitamin B12, folic acid and haematological status of 132 Thai vegetarians. *Int J Vitam Nutr Res.* 1993;63:201–207.

103. Anderson BM, Gibson RS, Sabry JH. The iron and zinc status of long-term vegetarian women. *Am J Clin Nutr.* 1981;34:1042–1048.

104. Armstrong BK, Davis RE, Nicol DJ, et al. Hematological, vitamin B12, and folate studies on Seventh-day Adventist vegetarians. *Am J Clin Nutr.* 1974;27:712–718.

105. Hunt JR, Roughead ZK. Adaptation of iron absorption in men consuming diets with high or low iron bioavailability. *Am J Clin Nutr.* 2000;71(1):94–102.

106. Ehn L, Carlmark B, Hoglund S. Iron status in athletes involved in intense physical activity. *Med Sci Sports Exerc.* 1980;12:61–64.

107. Lampe JW, Slavin JL, Apple FS. Iron status of active women and the effect of running a marathon on bowel function and gastrointestinal blood loss. *Int J Sports Med.* 1991; 12:173–179.

108. Weaver CM, Rajaram S. Exercise and iron status. *J Nutr.* 1992;122:782–787.

109. Rodriguez NR, DiMarco NM, Langley S, et al. Position of the American Dietetic Association, Dietitians of Canada, and the American College of Sports Medicine: Nutrition and athletic performance. *J Am Diet Assoc.* 2009;109:509–527.

110. Prasad AS, Miale AJ, Sanstead HH, Schulert AR. Zinc metabolism in patients with syndrome of iron deficiency anemia, hepatosplenomegaly, dwarfism, and hypogonadism. *Lab Clin Med.* 1961;61:537–549.

111. Arcasoy A, Cavdar AO, Babacan E. Decreased iron and zinc absorption in Turkish children with iron deficiency and geophagia. *Acta Haematol.* 1978;60:76–84.

112. Chen XC, Yin TA, He JS, et al. Low levels of zinc in hair and blood, pica, anorexia, and poor growth in Chinese preschool children. *Am J Clin Nutr.* 1985;42:694–700.

113. Prasad AS, Schulert AR, Sandstead HH. Zinc and iron deficiencies in male subjects with dwarfism but without ancylostomiasis, schistosomiasis, or severe anemia. *Am J Clin Nutr.* 1963;12:437–444.

114. Ronaghy HA, Reinhold JG, Mahloudji M, et al. Zinc supplementation of malnourished schoolboys in Iran: increased growth and other effects. *Am J Clin Nutr.* 1974;27:112–121.

115. Gibson RS, Vanderkooy PD, MacDonald AC, et al. A growth-limiting, mild zinc-deficiency syndrome in some southern Ontario boys with low height percentiles. *Am J Clin Nutr.* 1989;49:1266–1273.

116. Vanderkooy PD, Gibson RS. Food consumption patterns of Canadian preschool children in relation to zinc and growth status. *Am J Clin Nutr.* 1987;45:609–616.

117. Pilch SM, Senti FR. Analysis of zinc data from the second National Health and Nutrition Examination Survey (NHANES II). *J Nutr.* 1985;115:1393–1397.

118. Hambidge KM, Walravens PA, Brown RM, et al. Zinc nutrition of preschool children in the Denver Head Start program. *Am J Clin Nutr.* 1976;29:734–738.

119. Johnson PE, Hunt CD, Milne DB, Mullen LK. Homeostatic control of zinc metabolism in men: zinc excretion and balance in men fed diets low in zinc. *Am J Clin Nutr.* 1993; 57:557–565.

120. Scholl D, Langkamp-Henken B. Nutrient recommendations for wound healing. *J Intraven Nurs.* 2001;24(2):124–132.

121. Failla ML. Trace elements and host defense: recent advances and continuing challenges. *J Nutr.* 2003;133:1443S–1447S.

122. Prasad AS. Clinical, immunological, anti-inflammatory and antioxidant roles of zinc. *Exp Gerontol.* 2008;43(5):370–377.

123. King JC. Assessment of techniques for determining human zinc requirements. *J Am Diet Assoc.* 1986;86:1523–1528.

124. Sian L, Mingyan X, Miller LV, et al. Zinc absorption and intestinal losses of endogenous zinc in young Chinese women with marginal zinc intakes. *Am J Clin Nutr.* 1996;63:348–353.

125. Cousins RJ. Theoretical and practical aspects of zinc uptake and absorption. *Adv Exp Med Biol.* 1989;249:3–12.

126. Campbell-Brown M, Ward RJ, Haines AP, et al. Zinc and copper in Asian pregnancies—is there evidence for a nutritional deficiency? *Br J Obstet Gynaecol.* 1985;92:875–885.

127. Pecoud A, Donzel P, Schelling JL. Effect of foodstuffs on the absorption of zinc sulfate. *Clin Pharmacol Ther.* 1975;17:469–474.

128. Sandstrom B, Arvidsson B, Cederblad A, Bjorn-Rasmussen E. Zinc absorption from composite meals. I. The significance of wheat extraction rate, zinc, calcium, and protein content in meals based on bread. *Am J Clin Nutr.* 1980;33:739–745.

129. Sandstrom B, Cederblad A. Zinc absorption from composite meals. II. Influence of the main protein source. *Am J Clin Nutr.* 1980;33:1778–1783.

130. Sandstrom B, Almgren A, Kivisto B, Cederblad A. Effect of protein level and protein source on zinc absorption in humans. *J Nutr.* 1989;119:48–53.

131. Zheng JJ, Mason JB, Rosenberg IH, Wood RJ. Measurement of zinc bioavailability from beef and a ready-to-eat high- fiber breakfast cereal in humans: application of a whole-gut lavage technique. *Am J Clin Nutr.* 1993;58:902–907.

132. Ellis R, Kelsay JL, Reynolds RD, et al. Phytate:zinc and phytate X calcium:zinc millimolar ratios in self- selected diets of Americans, Asian Indians, and Nepalese. *J Am Diet Assoc.* 1987;87:1043–1047.

133. Reinhold JG, Nasr K, Lahimgarzadeh A, Hedayati H. Effects of purified phytate and phytate-rich bread upon metabolism of zinc, calcium, phosphorus, and nitrogen in man. *Lancet* 1973;1:283–288.

134. Hunt JR, Matthys LA, Johnson LK. Zinc absorption, mineral balance, and blood lipids in women consuming controlled lactoovovegetarian and omnivorous diets for 8 wk. *Am J Clin Nutr.* 1998;67:421–430.

135. Harland BF, Peterson M. Nutritional status of lacto-ovo vegetarian Trappist monks. *J Am Diet Assoc.* 1978;72:259–264.

136. Oberleas D, Harland BF. Phytate content of foods: effect on dietary zinc bioavailability. *J Am Diet Assoc.* 1981; 79:433–436.

137. Bindra GS, Gibson RS. Iron status of predominantly lacto-ovo vegetarian East Indian immigrants to Canada: a model approach. *Am J Clin Nutr.* 1986;44:643–652.
138. Reinhold JG, Parsa A, Karimian N, et al. Availability of zinc in leavened and unleavened wholemeal wheaten breads as measured by solubility and uptake by rat intestine in vitro. *J Nutr.* 1974;104:976–982.
139. Gibson RS, Yeudall F, Drost N, et al. Dietary interventions to prevent zinc deficiency. *Am J Clin Nutr.* 1998; 68(suppl):484S–487S.
140. Gibson RS, Perlas L, Hotz C. Improving the bioavailability of nutrients in plant foods at the household level. *Proc Nutr Soc.* 2006;65:160–168.
141. Hotz C, Gibson RS. Traditional food-processing and preparation practices to enhance the bioavailability of micro-nutrients in plant-based diets. *J Nutr.* 2007;137:1097–1100.
142. Perlas L, Gibson RS. Use of soaking to enhance the bioavailability of iron and zinc from rice-based complementary foods used in the Philippines. *J Sci Food Agric.* 2002;82:1115–1121.
143. Hotz C, Gibson RS. Assessment of home-based processing methods to reduce phytate content and phytate/zinc molar ratios of white maize (Zea mays). *J Agric Food Chem.* 2001;49:692–698.
144. Pabon M, Lonnerdal B. Effect of citrate on zinc bioavailability from milk, milk fractions and infant formula. *Nutr Res.* 1992;13:103–111.
145. Wisker E, Nagel R, Tanudjaja TK, Feldheim W. Calcium, magnesium, zinc, and iron balances in young women: effects of a low-phytate barley-fiber concentrate. *Am J Clin Nutr.* 1991;54:553–559.
146. Behall KM, Scholfield DJ, Lee K, et al. Mineral balance in adult men: effect of four refined fibers. *Am J Clin Nutr.* 1987;46:307–314.
147. Hunt JR, Beiseigel JM. Dietary calcium does not exacerbate phytate inhibition of zinc absorption by women from conventional diets. *Am J Clin Nutr.* 2009;89:839–843.
148. Rosado JL, Diaz M, Gonzalez K, et al. The addition of milk or yogurt to a plant-based diet increases zinc bioavail-ability but does not affect iron bioavailability in women. *J Nutr.* 2005;135:465–468.
149. O'Brien KO, Zavaleta N, Caulfield LE, et al. Prenatal iron supplements impair zinc absorption in pregnant Peru-vian women. *J Nutr.* 2000;130:2251–2255.
150. Chung CS, Nagey DA, Veillon C, et al. A single 60-mg iron dose decreases zinc absorption in lactating women. *J Nutr.* 2002;132:1903–1905.
151. Solomons NW. Competitive interaction of iron and zinc in the diet: consequences for human nutrition. *J Nutr.* 1986;116:927–935.
152. Donangelo CM, Woodhouse LR, King SR, et al. Supplemental zinc lowers measures of iron status in young women with low iron reserves. *J Nutr.* 2002;132:1860–1864.
153. Dawson EB, Albers J, McGanity WJ. Serum zinc changes due to iron supplementation in teen-age pregnancy. *Am J Clin Nutr.* 1989;50:848–852.
154. Caulfield LE, Zavaleta N, Gigueroa A. Adding zinc to prenatal iron and folate supplements improves maternal and neonatal zinc status in a Peruvian population. *Am J Clin Nutr.* 1999;69:1257–1263.
155. Ruz M, Codeceo J, Rebolledo A, et al. Effects of iron supplementation on zinc absorption in Chilean women [abstract]. *Ann Nutr Metab.* 2001;45(suppl):363.
156. Lowe NM, Fekete K, Decsi T. Methods of assessment of zinc status in humans: a systematic review. *Am J Clin Nutr.* 2009;89(suppl):2040S–2051S.
157. Gibson RS, Hess SY, Hotz C, et al. Indicators of zinc status at the population level: a review of the evidence. *Br J Nutr.* 2008;99 (suppl):S14–S23.
158. Davies GJ, Crowder M, Dickerson JW. Dietary fibre intakes of individuals with different eating patterns. *Hum Nutr Appl Nutr.* 1985;39:139–148.
159. Draper A, Lewis J, Malhotra N, Wheeler E. The energy and nutrient intakes of different types of vegetarian: a case for supplements? *Br J Nutr.* 1993;69:3–19.
160. Ball MJ, Ackland ML. Zinc intake and status in Australian vegetarians. *Br J Nutr.* 2000;83:27–33.
161. Gibson RS. Content and bioavailability of trace elements in vegetarian diets. *Am J Clin Nutr.* 1994;59: 1223S–1232S.
162. Houghton LA, Green TJ, Donovan UM, et al. Association between dietary fiber intake and the folate status of a group of female adolescents. *Am J Clin Nutr.* 1997;66:1414–1421.

163. King JC, Stein T, Doyle M. Effect of vegetarianism on the zinc status of pregnant women. *Am J Clin Nutr.* 1981; 34:1049–1055.

164. Abu-Assal MJ. The zinc status of pregnant vegetarian women. *Nutr Rep Int.* 1984;29:485–494.

165. Morris ER, Ellis R, Hill AD. Apparent zinc and iron balance of adult men consuming three levels of phytate. [abstract]. *Fed Proc.* 1986;45:819.

166. Freeland-Graves JH, Bodzy PW, Eppright MA. Zinc status of vegetarians. *J Am Diet Assoc.* 1980;77:655–661.

167. Srikumar TS, Ockerman PA, Akesson B. Trace element status in vegetarians from southern India. *Nutr. Res.* 1992;12:187–198.

168. Agte V, Chiplonkar S, Joshi N, Paknikar K. Apparent absorption of copper and zinc from composite vegetarian diets in young Indian men. *Ann Nutr Metab.* 1994;38:13–19.

169. Dewell A, Weidner G, Sumner MD, et al. A very-low-fat vegan diet increases intake of protective dietary factors and decreases intake of pathogenic dietary factors. *J Am Diet Assoc.* 2008;108:347–356.

170. Turner-McGrievy GM, Barnard ND, Scialli AR, et al. Effects of a low-fat vegan diet and a Step II diet on macro- and micronutrient intakes in overweight postmenopausal women. *Nutrition.* 2004;20:738–746.

171. Ashton K, Hooper L, Harvey LJ, et al. Methods of assessment of selenium status in humans: a systematic review. *Am J Clin Nutr.* 2009;89(suppl):2025S–2039S.

172. Finley JW. Selenium accumulation in plant foods. *Nutr Rev.* 2005;63:196–202.

173. Yang GQ, Wang SZ, Zhou RH, Sun SZ. Endemic selenium intoxication of humans in China. *Am J Clin Nutr.* 1983;37:872–881.

174. Ervin RB, Wang CY, Wright JD, Kennedy-Stephenson J. Dietary intake of selected minerals for the United States population: 1999–2000. *Adv Data.* 2004;341:1–5.

175. Thompson JN, Erdody P, Smith DC. Selenium content of food consumed by Canadians. *J Nutr.* 1975;105:274–277.

176. Yoneyama S, Miura K, Itai K, et al. Dietary intake and urinary excretion of selenium in the Japanese adult population: the INTERMAP Study Japan. *Eur J Clin Nutr.* 2008;62(10):1187–1193.

177. Debski B, Finley DA, Picciano MF, et al. Selenium content and glutathione peroxidase activity of milk from vegetarian and nonvegetarian women. *J Nutr.* 1989;119:215–220.

178. Shultz TD, Leklem JE. Selenium status of vegetarians, nonvegetarians, and hormone-dependent cancer subjects. *Am J Clin Nutr.* 1983;37:114–118.

179. Gissel-Nielsen G, Gupta UC, Lamand M, Westermarck T. Selenium in soils and plants and its importance in livestock and human nutrition. *Adv Agron.* 1984;37:397–464.

180. Srikumar TS, Johansson GK, Ockerman PA, et al. Trace element status in healthy subjects switching from a mixed to a lactovegetarian diet for 12 mo. *Am J Clin Nutr.* 1992; 55:885–890.

181. Abdulla M, Aly KO, Andersson I, et al. Nutrient intake and health status of lactovegetarians: chemical analyses of diets using the duplicate portion sampling technique. *Am J Clin Nutr.* 1984;40:325–338.

182. Abdulla M, Andersson I, Asp NG, et al. Nutrient intake and health status of vegans. Chemical analyses of diets using the duplicate portion sampling technique. *Am J Clin Nutr.* 1981;34:2464–2477.

183. Nagyova A, Ginter E, Kovacikova Z. Low glutathione levels and decreased glutathione peroxidase activity in the blood of vegetarians. *Int J Vitam Nutr Res.* 1995;65:221.

184. Kadrabova J, Madaric A, Kovacikova Z, Ginter E. Selenium status, plasma zinc, copper, and magnesium in vegetarians. *Biol Trace Elem Res.* 1995;50:13–24.

185. Ganapathy SN, Dhandra R. Selenium content of omnivorous and vegetarian diets. *J Nutr Diet.* 1980;17:53–59.

186. Gibson RS, Anderson BM, Sabry JH. The trace metal status of a group of post-menopausal vegetarians. *J Am Diet Assoc.* 1983;82:246–250.

187. Srivastava AK, Gupta BN, Bihari V, et al. Hair selenium as a monitoring tool for occupational exposures in relation to clinical profile. *J Toxicol Environ Health.* 1997;51:437–445.

188. Salbe AD, Levander OA. Effect of various dietary factors on the deposition of selenium in the hair and nails of rats. *J Nutr.* 1990;120:200–206.

189. Mason KE. A conspectus of research on copper metabolism and requirements of man. *J Nutr.* 1979;109:1979–2066.

190. Turnlund JR, Keyes WR, Anderson HL, Acord LL. Copper absorption and retention in young men at three levels of dietary copper by use of the stable isotope 65Cu. *Am J Clin Nutr.* 1989;49:870–878.

191. Turnlund JR, Keyes WR, Peiffer GL, Scott KC. Copper absorption, excretion, and retention by young men consuming low dietary copper determined by using the stable isotope 65Cu. *Am J Clin Nutr.* 1998;67:1219–1225.

192. August D, Janghorbani M, Young VR. Determination of zinc and copper absorption at three dietary Zn-Cu ratios by using stable isotope methods in young adult and elderly subjects. *Am J Clin Nutr.* 1989;50:1457–1463.

193. Wapnir RA. Copper absorption and bioavailability. *Am J Clin Nutr.* 1998;67(5 suppl):1054S–1060S.

194. Turnlund JR, King JC, Gong B, et al. A stable isotope study of copper absorption in young men: effect of phytate and alpha-cellulose. *Am J Clin Nutr.* 1985;42:18–23.

195. Lyon DB. Studies on the solubility of Ca, Mg, Zn, and Cu in cereal products. *Am J Clin Nutr.* 1984;39:190–195.

196. Sandstead HH. Copper bioavailability and requirements. *Am J Clin Nutr.* 1982;35:809–814.

197. Greger JL, Snedeker SM. Effect of dietary protein and phosphorus levels on the utilization of zinc, copper and manganese by adult males. *J Nutr.* 1980;110:2243–2253.

198. Judd PA, Long A, Butcher M, et al. Vegetarians and vegans may be most at risk from low selenium intakes. *BMJ.* 1997;314:1834.

199. Hunt JR, Vanderpool RA. Apparent copper absorption from a vegetarian diet. *Am J Clin Nutr.* 2001;74:803–807.

200. Garfinkel L, Garfinkel D. Magnesium regulation of the glycolytic pathway and the enzymes involved. *Magnesium.* 1985;4:60–72.

201. Institute of Medicine, Food and Nutrition Board. *Dietary Reference Intakes for Calcium, Phosphorus, Magnesium, Vitamin D, and Fluoride.* Washington, DC: National Academy Press; 1997.

202. Marier JR. Magnesium content of the food supply in the modern-day world. *Magnesium.* 1986;5:1–8.

203. McNeill DA, Ali PS, Song YS. Mineral analyses of vegetarian, health, and conventional foods: magnesium, zinc, copper, and manganese content. *J Am Diet Assoc.* 1985;85:569–572.

204. Hallfrisch J, Muller DC. Does diet provide adequate amounts of calcium, iron, magnesium, and zinc in a well-educated adult population? *Exp Gerontol.* 1993;28:473–483.

205. Sontia B, Touyz RM. Role of magnesium in hypertension. *Arch Biochem Biophys.* 2007;458(1):33–39.

206. Barbagallo M, Dominguez LJ, Resnick LM. Magnesium metabolism in hypertension and type 2 diabetes mellitus. *Am J Ther.* 2007;14(4):375–385.

207. Witteman JC, Grobbee DE, Derkx FH, et al. Reduction of blood pressure with oral magnesium supplementation in women with mild to moderate hypertension. *Am J Clin Nutr.* 1994;60:129–135.

208. Yamamoto ME, Applegate WB, Klag MJ, et al. Lack of blood pressure effect with calcium and magnesium supplementation in adults with high-normal blood pressure. *Ann Epidemiol.* 1995;5:96–107.

209. Rude RK, Gruber HE. Magnesium deficiency and osteoporosis: animal and human observations. *J Nutr Biochem.* 2004;15(12):710–716.

210. Rouse IL, Beilin LJ, Armstrong BK, Vandongen R. Vegetarian diet, blood pressure and cardiovascular risk. *Aust N Z J Med.* 1984;14:439–443.

211. Koebnick C, Leitzmann R, Garcia AL, et al. Long-term effect of a plant-based diet on magnesium status during pregnancy. *Eur J Clin Nutr.* 2005;59:219–225.

212. Specker BL, Tsang RC, Ho M, Miller D. Effect of vegetarian diet on serum 1,25- dihydroxyvitamin D concentrations during lactation. *Obstet Gynecol.* 1987;70:870–874.

213. Siener R, Hesse A. Influence of a mixed and a vegetarian diet on urinary magnesium excretion and concentration. *Br J Nutr.* 1995;73:783–790.

214. Wang JL, Shaw NS, Yeh HY, Kao MD. Magnesium status and association with diabetes in the Taiwanese elderly. *Asia Pac J Clin Nutr.* 2005;14:263–269.

215. Kelsay JL, Behall KM, Prather ES. Effect of fiber from fruits and vegetables on metabolic responses of human subjects, II. Calcium, magnesium, iron, and silicon balances. *Am J Clin Nutr.* 1979;32:1876–1880.

216. Wisker E, Nagel R, Tanudjaja TK, Feldheim W. Calcium, magnesium, zinc, and iron balances in young women: effects of a low-phytate barley-fiber concentrate. *Am J Clin Nutr.* 1991;54:553–559.

217. Reinhold JG, Faradji B, Abadi P, Ismail-Beigi F. Decreased absorption of calcium, magnesium, zinc and phosphorus by humans due to increased fiber and phosphorus consumption as wheat bread. *J Nutr.* 1976;106:493–503.

218. Schwartz R, Spencer H, Welsh JJ. Magnesium absorption in human subjects from leafy vegetables, intrinsically labeled with stable 26Mg. *Am J Clin Nutr.* 1984;39:571–576.

219. Rao CN, Rao BS. Absorption and retention of magnesium and some trace elements by man from typical Indian diets. *Nutr Metab.* 1980;24:244–254.

220. Underwood EJ. The incidence of trace element deficiency diseases. *Philos Trans R Soc Lond B Biol Sci.* 1981;294:3–8.

221. Finley JW, Johnson PE, Johnson LK. Sex affects manganese absorption and retention by humans from a diet adequate in manganese. *Am J Clin Nutr.* 1994;60:949–955.

222. Johnson PE, Lykken GI, Korynta ED. Absorption and biological half-life in humans of intrinsic and extrinsic 54Mn tracers from foods of plant origin. *J Nutr.* 1991;121:711–717.

223. Davidsson L, Almgren A, Juillerat MA, Hurrell RF. Manganese absorption in humans: the effect of phytic acid and ascorbic acid in soy formula. *Am J Clin Nutr.* 1995;62:984–987.

224. Lang VM, North BB, Morse LM. Manganese metabolism in college men consuming vegetarian diets. *J Nutr.* 1965: 132–138.

225. Pennington JA, Young BE. Total diet study nutritional elements, 1982–1989. *J Am Diet Assoc.* 1991;91:179–183.

226. Kelsay JL, Frazier CW, Prather ES, et al. Impact of variation in carbohydrate intake on mineral utilization by vegetarians. *Am J Clin Nutr.* 1988;48:875–879.

227. Bindra GS, Gibson RS. Mineral intakes of predominantly lacto-ovo vegetarian east Indian adults. *Biol Trace Elem Res.* 1986;10:223–234.

228. deBenoist B, McLean E, Andersson M, et al. Iodine deficiency in 2007: global progress since 2003. *Food Nutr Bull.* 2008;3:195–202.

229. Gordon RC, Rose MC, Skeaff SA, et al. Iodine supplementation improves cognition in mildly iodine-deficient children. *Am J Clin Nutr.* 2009;90:1264–1271.

230. Hollowell J, Staehling NW, Hannon WH, et al. Iodine nutrition in the United States. Trends and public health implications: iodine excretion data from National Health and Nutrition Examination Surveys I and III (1971–1974 and 1988–1994). *J Clin Endocrinol Metab.* 1998;83:3401–3408.

231. Fields C, Dourson M, Borak J. Iodine-deficient vegetarians: a hypothetical perchlorate-susceptible population? *Regul Toxicol Pharmacol.* 2005;42:37–46.

232. Brush BE, Altland JK. Goiter prevention with iodized salt. Results of a thirty-year study. *J Clin Endocrinol Metab.* 1952;12:1380–1388.

233. WHO, UNICEF, ICCIDD. *Assessment of Iodine Deficiency Disorders and Monitoring Their Elimination.* 3rd ed. Geneva, Switzerland: WHO Press; 2007.

234. Lightowler HJ, Davies GJ. Assessment of iodine intake in vegans: weighted dietary record vs duplicate portion technique. *Eur J Clin Nutr.* 2002;56:765–770.

235. Dunn JT. What's happening to our iodine? *J Clin Endocrinol Metab.* 1998;83:3398–3400.

236. Pearce EN, Pino S, He X, et al. Sources of dietary iodine: bread, cows' milk, and infant formula in the Boston area. *J Clin Endocrinol Metab.* 2004;89:3421–3424.

237. Dasgupta PK, Liu Y, Dyke JV. Iodine nutrition: iodine content of iodized salt in the United States. *Environ Sci Technol.* 2008;42:1315–1323.

238. Teas J, Pino S, Critchley A, et al. Variability of iodine content in common commercially available seaweeds. *Thyroid.* 2004;14:836–841.

239. Nishiyama S, Mikeda T, Okada T, et al. Transient hypothyroidism or persistent hyperthyrotropinemia in neonates born to mothers with excessive iodine intake. *Thyroid.* 2004;14:1077–1083.

240. Remer T, Neubert A, Manz F. Increased risk of iodine deficiency with vegetarian nutrition. *Br J Nutr.* 1999;81:45–49.

241. Rauma AL, Tormala ML, Nenonen M, Hanninen O. Iodine status in vegans consuming a living food diet. *Nutr Res.* 1994;14:1789–1795.

242. Lightowler HJ, Davis GJ. The effect of self-selected dietary supplements on micronutrient intakes in vegans. *Proc Nutr Soc.* 1998;58:35A.

243. Krajcovicova M, Buckova K, Klimes I, Sebokova E. Iodine deficiency in vegetarians and vegans. *Ann Nutr Metab.* 2003;47:183–185.

244. Key TJA, Thorogood M, Keenant J, Long A. Raised thyroid stimulating hormone associated with kelp intake in British vegan men. *J Human Nutr Diet.* 1992;5:323–326.

245. Leung AM, Pearce EN, Braverman LE. Iodine content of prenatal multivitamins in the United States [letter]. *N Engl J Med.* 2009;360:939–940.

246. Messina M, Redmond G. Effects of soy protein and soybean isoflavones on thyroid function in healthy adults and hypothyroid patients: a review of the relevant literature. *Thyroid.* 2006;16:249–258.

247. U.S. Department of Health and Human Services and U.S. Department of Agriculture. *Dietary Guidelines for Americans, 2005.* 6th ed. Washington, DC: U.S. Government Printing Office; 2005.

248. Sacks FM, Svetkey LP, Vollmer WM, et al. Effects on blood pressure of reduced dietary sodium and the Dietary Approaches to Stop Hypertension (DASH) diet. *N Engl J Med.* 2001;344:3–10.

249. Mohan S, Campbell NR. Salt and high blood pressure. *Clin Sci (Lond).* 2009;117(1):1–11.

250. U.S. Department of Agriculture, Agricultural Research Service. 2008. Nutrient intakes from food: mean amounts consumed per individual, by race/ethnicity and age, one day, 2005–2006. www.ars.usda.gov/ba/bhnrc/fsrg.

251. Centers for Disease Control and Prevention (CDC). Application of lower sodium intake recommendations to adults—United States, 1999–2006. *MMWR Morb Mortal Wkly Rep.* 2009;58(11):281–283.

252. Vermeulen RT, Sedor FA, Kimm SY. Effect of water rinsing on sodium content of selected foods. *J Am Diet Assoc.* 1983;82(4):394–396.

253. Davey GK, Spencer EA, Appleby PN, et al. EPIC—Oxford: lifestyle characteristics and nutrient intakes in a cohort of 33,883 meat-eaters and 31,546 non meat-eaters in the UK. *Public Health Nutr.* 2003;6:259–268.

254. Appleby PN, Davey GK, Key TJ. Hypertension and blood pressure among meat eaters, fish eaters, vegetarians and vegans in EPIC-Oxford. *Public Health Nutr.* 2002;5:645–654.

255. Food and Nutrition Board, Institute of Medicine. *Dietary Reference Intakes for Water, Potassium, Sodium, Chloride, and Sulfate.* Washington, DC: National Academies Press; 2005.

256. Vestergaard P, Jorgensen NR, Schwarz P, Mosekilde L. Effects of treatment with fluoride on bone mineral density and fracture risk—a meta-analysis. *Osteoporos Int.* 2008;19(3):257–268.

257. Anderson RA. Chromium, glucose intolerance and diabetes. *J Am Coll Nutr.* 1998;17:548–555.

258. Balk EM, Tatsioni A, Lichtenstein AH, et al. Effect of chromium supplementation on glucose metabolism and lipids. A systematic review of randomized controlled trials. *Diab Care.* 2007;30:2154–2163.

259. Kobla HV, Volpe SL. Chromium, exercise, and body composition. *Crit Rev Food Sci Nutr.* 2000;40:291–308.

260. Anderson RA, Bryden NA, Polansky MM. Dietary intake of calcium, chromium, copper, iron, magnesium, manganese, and zinc: duplicate plate values corrected using derived nutrient intake. *J Am Diet Assoc.* 1993;93:462–464.

261. Schroeder HA. Losses of vitamins and trace minerals resulting from processing and preservation of foods. *Am J Clin Nutr.* 1971;24:562–573.

262. Offenbacher EG, Pi-Sunyer FX. Temperature and pH effects on the release of chromium from stainless steel into water and fruit juices. *J Agric Food Chem.* 1983;31:89–92.

263. Anderson RA, Bryden NA. Concentration, insulin potentiation, and absorption of chromium in beer. *J Agric Food Chem.* 1983;31:308–311.

264. Pennington JA, Jones JW. Molybdenum, nickel, cobalt, vanadium, and strontium in total diets. *J Am Diet Assoc.* 1987;87:1644–1650.

265. Choi M-K, Kang M-H, Kim M-H. The analysis of copper, selenium, and molybdenum contents in frequently consumed foods and an estimation of their daily intake in Korean adults. *Biol Trace Elem Res.* 2009;128:104–117.

266. Turnland JR, Weaver CM, Kim SK, et al. Molybdenum absorption and utilization in humans from soy and kale intrinsically labelled with stable isotopes of molybdenum. *Am J Clin Nutr.* 1999;69:1217–1223.

267. Harland BF, Morris ER. Phytate: a good or bad food component? *Nutr Res.* 1995;15:733–754.

268. Phillippy BG, Johnston MR, Tao S-H, Fox MRS. Inositol phosphates in processed foods. *J Food Sci.* 1988;53:496–499.

269. Thompson DB, Erdman JWJ. Phytic acid determination in soybeans. *J Food Sci.* 1982; 47:513–517.

CHAPTER 7

Vitamins

VITAMIN B$_{12}$ (COBALAMIN)

All the vitamin B$_{12}$ in nature is produced by microorganisms, bacteria, fungi, and algae; plants and animals cannot synthesize vitamin B$_{12}$. Animal foods are sources of this vitamin because animals ingest vitamin B$_{12}$-containing microorganisms or because they absorb some of the vitamin B$_{12}$ produced by their intestinal bacteria. Plant foods may contain some vitamin B$_{12}$ if they are contaminated with vitamin B$_{12}$-producing bacteria, but in most instances vitamin B$_{12}$ content is negligible. In the United States and other developed countries, it is likely that most or all of this B$_{12}$ is removed when the food is cleaned.

The current recommended dietary allowance (RDA) for vitamin B$_{12}$ is 2.4 μg for adults, but some research suggests that optimal intakes may be as high as 4 to 7 μg.[1] Concerns over the vitamin B$_{12}$ status of vegetarians have precipitated much discussion within the professional and vegetarian communities. Because plant foods do not naturally contain vitamin B$_{12}$, unsupplemented vegan diets are theoretically completely lacking in this nutrient. Symptomatic vitamin B$_{12}$ deficiency is rare within vegan populations that use supplements or fortified foods regularly.

Terminology

It is worthwhile to discuss some terminology related to the structure of vitamin B$_{12}$ because some foods contain vitamin B$_{12}$ analogs. Not only do these analogs not possess any biologic activity, but they can actually impair the utilization of vitamin B$_{12}$ by blocking its absorption and may even accelerate nerve damage in vitamin B$_{12}$-deficiency states. In many "vitamin B$_{12}$-rich foods," between 5% and 30% of the vitamin B$_{12}$ is analog.[2] In some foods, the B$_{12}$ is nearly all analog.[2]

The core structure of vitamin B$_{12}$ is a macrocyclic ring designated as corrin, which comprises four reduced pyrrole rings linked together. Compounds containing this ring are designated as corrinoids. Cobalt is at the center of the corrin structure. All molecules containing the corrin ring with attached cobalt are considered cobalamins. A number of chemical constituents may be attached to the cobalt. In active vitamin B$_{12}$ either a methyl group or 5′-deoxyadenosyl is attached to form either methylcobalamin or 5′-deoxyadenosyl cobalamin. These are the only two active forms of vitamin B_{12}.

Most commercially available vitamin B_{12} supplements contain cyanocobalamin, which has a cyanide molecule attached to cobalt that stabilizes the vitamin. This form is converted to metabolically active vitamin B_{12} in the body by removal of the cyanide. There is a rare genetic disorder, however, in which infants are unable to remove the cyanide and thus are unable to use this type of vitamin B_{12} preparation.[3] Supplements containing non-cyanocobalamin forms of vitamin B_{12} are available.

Virtually all the vitamin B_{12} within human cells is bound to the only two vitamin B_{12}-dependent enzymes. Methylmalonyl coenzyme A mutase uses vitamin B_{12} for the metabolism of certain amino acids and odd-chain fatty acids. Methionine synthase requires vitamin B_{12} to convert homocysteine (Hcy) to methionine.

Vitamin B_{12} Digestion and Absorption

Vitamin B_{12} digestion begins in the stomach, where gastric secretions and proteases split vitamin B_{12} from the peptides to which it is attached in foods. Vitamin B_{12} is then free to bind to R factor, which is present in many bodily fluids. Pancreatic secretions then partially degrade the R factor, and vitamin B_{12} becomes bound by intrinsic factor (IF), which is secreted by the gastric parietal cells. IF binds to specific receptors on the ileal brush border (the lower small intestine) and facilitates absorption of vitamin B_{12}. Vitamin B_{12} is one of the few nutrients absorbed primarily from the lower half of the small bowel. The formation of the vitamin B_{12}-IF complex protects vitamin B_{12} against bacterial degradation and against the hydrolytic action of pepsin and chymotrypsin.

Atrophy of the gastric mucosa and gradual loss of gastric acid, which is common with aging, can reduce absorption of food-bound cobalamin but not crystalline vitamin B_{12} found in fortified foods and supplements. As many as 30–40% of the elderly may have compromised absorption of food-bound vitamin B_{12}.[4] Based on 1999–2002 National Health and Nutrition Examination Survey data, prevalence of vitamin B_{12} deficiency as assessed by serum B_{12} concentrations was ≤3% for ages 20 to 39 years, about 4% for ages 40 to 59 years, and about 6% for age 70 years.[5] In the Sacramento Area Latino Study on Aging, a study of 1600 California Hispanics ≥60 years of age, 6% had plasma vitamin B_{12} in the range of deficiency and 16% had marginal levels.[6] Evidence suggests that some of the cognitive decline seen in aging could be associated with inadequate or marginal vitamin B_{12} status,[7] although not all research supports this relationship.[8] Vitamin B_{12} deficiency has also been seen in older vegetarians.[9,53]

Vitamin B_{12} is transported in the plasma bound to the protein transcobalamin and eventually is transferred to R proteins. In contrast to the situation with other B vitamins, considerable amounts of vitamin B_{12} relative to need are stored. Approximately 60% of the total body vitamin B_{12} is stored in the liver, and about 30% is stored in the muscles.

Small amounts of vitamin B_{12} are excreted in the urine, but the primary mode of excretion is in the bile and, ultimately, the feces. Only about 0.1–0.2% of total body reserves (2 to 5 μg) is excreted into the bile each day, however, regardless of the amount stored. About 65–75% of the vitamin B_{12} excreted into the bile is actually reabsorbed as a result of an extremely efficient enterohepatic circulation. This helps explain why the RDA for vitamin B_{12} is so low and why deficiency symptoms may not develop for many years in people who consume no vitamin B$_{12}$ but develop very quickly in people who cannot reabsorb this vitamin. Interestingly, vitamin B$_{12}$ analogs seem to be preferentially excreted, whereas cobalamins are largely reabsorbed.[10]

Vitamin B$_{12}$ Deficiency

Vitamin B$_{12}$ deficiency causes red blood cells to increase in size because cell division is inhibited but the cell itself continues to grow. This same type of megaloblastic anemia is also seen in folate deficiency. Vitamin B$_{12}$ deficiency is also associated with demyelinization of peripheral nerves, the spinal cord, the cranial nerves, and the brain, resulting in nerve damage and neuropsychiatric abnormalities. Symptoms include decreased sensation, difficulty in walking, loss of control of bowel and bladder, optic atrophy, memory loss, dementia, depression, general weakness, and psychosis.[11] In infants, symptoms resulting from a vitamin B$_{12}$ deficiency include failure to thrive, movement disorders, and developmental delay and regression. Nerve damage due to B$_{12}$ deficiency can be irreversible. The developmental delays resulting from vitamin B$_{12}$ deficiency in infancy can persist for many years.[12]

Although neuropsychiatric symptoms are clearly associated with vitamin B$_{12}$ deficiency, the biologic explanation for why this is so is unclear. It has been proposed that perhaps a deficiency of a third enzyme that requires vitamin B$_{12}$, or a combined deficiency of the two known vitamin B$_{12}$-requiring enzymes along with some other genetic or environmental factor, is responsible. Other possibilities include impaired methionine production leading to altered myelin synthesis and an accumulation of unusual fatty acids due to the enzyme deficiency that can lead to abnormal nerve function.[13]

As noted, vitamin B$_{12}$ deficiency can take many years to develop, at least with regard to neurologic symptoms. However, signs of vitamin B$_{12}$ deficiency have been detected in adults within 2 years of beginning a vegan diet, suggesting it is important for vegans to use reliable sources of vitamin B$_{12}$ regularly regardless of the duration of their vegan diet.[14-16]

High levels of folate can mask B$_{12}$ deficiency to some degree because normal red blood cells continue to be produced even in the presence of B$_{12}$ deficiency. In this case, anemia, an early and reversible symptom of B$_{12}$ deficiency, is not apparent, so that the B$_{12}$ deficiency may not be detected until the more serious and irreversible nerve damage is observed. This may be of some concern for vegans because their intake of vitamin B$_{12}$ may be low and their intake of folate is generally quite high. The recent fortification of enriched flour with folate has also raised concern about the possibility that high folate intakes may mask B$_{12}$ deficiency[17-19] and have led to recommendations by some public health experts for vitamin B$_{12}$ fortification of flour.[20]

Vitamin B$_{12}$, along with folate, riboflavin, and vitamin B$_6$, is involved in Hcy metabolism. Low intakes of these vitamins have been linked to an increase in blood levels of Hcy, which may raise risk for heart disease,[21] dementia,[8,22] and possibly osteoporosis. (See "B Vitamins and Homocysteine" later in this chapter.) Blood Hcy levels >10 μmol/L are believed to raise heart disease risk.[23]

The extent of animal product consumption has been related to homocysteine levels with low levels seen in meat eaters, intermediate levels in lacto-ovo or lacto vegetarians, and higher levels in vegans.[24-32] Among vegetarians, a lower prevalence of elevated homocysteine levels was seen in those who used supplements containing vitamin B$_{12}$ and vitamin B6.[30] Not unexpectedly, studies have found a negative correlation between homocysteine levels and serum B$_{12}$ levels in vegetarians.[25,30,31] Although epidemiologic studies have found a lower death rate from heart disease among vegetarian men compared to omnivore men, it is possible that risk would be even lower with higher B$_{12}$ intakes. To this point, in a study of Taiwanese postmenopausal women, carotid atherosclerosis was similar between vegetarians and nonvegetarians, despite lower vegetarian low-density lipoprotein (LDL) levels.[9] The investigators suggested that the vegetarians' higher homocysteine levels may have been part of the explanation for the lack of a protective effect on cardiovascular health.

Vitamin B status may also be a factor in bone health. In a study of adolescents who had been raised on a macrobiotic diet up to the age of 6 years, followed by a lacto-ovo vegetarian diet, impaired vitamin B$_{12}$ status was associated with lower bone mineral density (BMD).[33]

Assessing Vitamin B$_{12}$ Status

Disagreements over the vitamin B$_{12}$ status of lacto-ovo vegetarians and vegans exist in part because there is no gold standard for assessing status. A number of hematologic indexes that are not specific to vitamin B$_{12}$ deficiency are sometimes used. Nearly 2 decades ago, Herbert identified four stages of vitamin B$_{12}$ depletion.[34] Stage I is identified by low-serum holotranscobalamin II (the protein that transports vitamin B$_{12}$ in serum) levels. In stage II, holohaptocorrin is also decreased.[35] In both stage I and stage II, plasma and cell stores of vitamin B$_{12}$ are becoming depleted. In stage III, plasma homocysteine and/or methylmalonic acid (MMA) levels are elevated. In stage IV, clinical signs of a vitamin B$_{12}$ deficiency are present.

Blood levels of vitamin B$_{12}$ can be measured using microbiologic or radiodilution methods. In some of these assays, both active vitamin B$_{12}$ and analog levels are included in the measure, so that levels of active vitamin B$_{12}$ can be overestimated.[36] In fact, as much as 30% of the vitamin B$_{12}$ in serum may be analog.[2] This same problem exists when the B$_{12}$ content of foods is determined. Thus measurement of total serum vitamin B$_{12}$ does not rule out a functional cobalamin deficiency.[26,34] In addition, the lowest acceptable value of serum vitamin B$_{12}$ was determined using some individuals who could have appeared to be healthy but who actually had marginal vitamin B$_{12}$ status.[35] Herrmann and Geisel have proposed a higher reference level for vitamin B of >360 pmol/L (>267 pg/ml) to improve the ability to predict marginal vitamin B$_{12}$ status.[35]

Other tests of vitamin B$_{12}$ status include measurement of serum holotranscobalamin II, urinary or serum MMA, total homocysteine levels, and the deoxyuridine suppression test. A combination of these tests appears to be useful in diagnosing and staging vitamin B$_{12}$ deficiency because each test has advantages and disadvantages.[26,34,37,38] Using both serum holotranscobalamin II and total vitamin B$_{12}$ has been found to give a better assessment of B$_{12}$ status than either test alone.[39]

Vegetarians and Vitamin B$_{12}$ Status

Approximately 95% of the known cases of vitamin B$_{12}$ deficiency occur in individuals who are not able to absorb this vitamin because of the lack of IF or because of a reduction in gastric acid

B Vitamins and Homocysteine

Four of the B vitamins, vitamins B$_{12}$ and B$_6$, riboflavin, and folate, are involved in metabolism of the amino acid homocysteine (Hcy), and deficiencies of each of these vitamins have been associated with elevated blood Hcy levels. Hcy levels also increase with age and may be a consequence of renal decline.[40] The significance of elevated Hcy levels remains controversial. Some research has linked higher levels to increased risk of cardiovascular disease,[41] but recent trials have failed to show a benefit of Hcy-lowering therapies.[42–44] For example, in the Nurses' Health Study, a supplement containing folic acid, vitamin B$_6$, and vitamin B$_{12}$ lowered Hcy levels in women at high risk for heart disease but had no effect on total cardiovascular events.[45]

Elevated Hcy may also be a risk factor in cognitive decline associated with aging, although, again, the evidence for a protective effect of Hcy-lowering therapy using B vitamins is uncertain.[46] More recently, it has been suggested that high levels of Hcy increase fracture risk. Cross-sectional data have shown that superior vitamin B$_{12}$[47] and folate[48] status is associated with increased bone mineral density (BMD). Further, in a randomized cross-over study in Japanese stroke patients, vitamin B$_{12}$ and folate supplements were effective in reducing hip fractures.[49] And among 5304 subjects in the Rotterdam Study, increased intakes of riboflavin and vitamin B$_6$ were associated with higher femoral neck BMD.[50] Finally, in a study of healthy Slovak women, higher levels of Hcy among vegetarians were associated with less bone loss.[51] These types of observations have led to the suggestions that either Hcy or the B vitamins directly affect bone cells.[52]

Health effects of elevated Hcy may be of particular concern to vegetarian populations because a number of studies have found elevated Hcy in groups of both lacto-ovo vegetarians and vegans. For example, in the German Vegan Study, Hcy levels were higher among strict vegans than moderate vegans, who consumed up to 5% of total energy from eggs or dairy foods.[53]

or in the gastric enzymes required to cleave vitamin B$_{12}$ from the proteins in food. Reported cases of symptomatic vitamin B$_{12}$ deficiency due to inadequate intake are rare, although they do exist.

There are several possible explanations for the scarcity of published observations of overt symptoms of vitamin B$_{12}$ deficiency among vegans, a population that consumes no natural sources of this vitamin. First, there have been relatively few studies of long-term vegans who do not use supplements or fortified foods. For example, Sanders et al studied 34 vegans and found no signs of vitamin B$_{12}$ deficiency, but most of the subjects had followed their vegan diet for <5 years.[54] Second, food and drinking water contaminated with vitamin B$_{12}$-producing bacteria may contribute significant B$_{12}$, particularly in developing countries. It is likely, however, that all Western vegans consuming unsupplemented diets will eventually develop vitamin B$_{12}$ deficiency, although it may take decades for this to occur.

Although overt symptoms of deficiency are infrequently observed, plasma levels of vitamin B$_{12}$ tend to be much lower in both vegans[16,32,54–57] and lacto-ovo vegetarians[14,26,31,32,57–63] than in the general population (Figure 7-1). Ellis and Montegriffo[56] studied 26 vegans, 7 of whom did not take vitamin B$_{12}$ supplements, and they found no blood abnormalities related to vitamin B$_{12}$ deficiency. Serum vitamin B$_{12}$ levels were low, however, and three subjects had vitamin B$_{12}$ levels indicative of deficiency (30, 50, and 60 pg/ml). Interestingly, four vegans who had been on this diet for 13 years and longer without supplements had normal vitamin B$_{12}$ levels. A study of Thai vegetarians, however, illustrates the effect of duration of vegetarian diet on serum vitamin B$_{12}$ levels (Figure 7-2).[64]

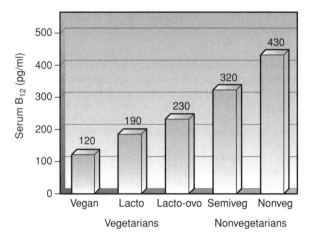

Figure 7-1 Serum vitamin B_{12} levels in five dietary groups (values are in picograms per milliliter). Subjects were recruited from the American Natural Hygiene Society and included a mixture of men and women with an approximate age range of 30 to 60 years. These vegetarians were atypical in that their dietary intake included few grains and legumes and mostly raw fruits, vegetables, nuts, and seeds. Values for men and women were averaged for each group and included 13 vegans, 28 lacto vegetarians, 15 lacto-ovo vegetarians, 10 semi-vegetarians, and 4 omnivores. Vegetarians had been vegetarians for, on average, between 10 and 17 years. None of the 70 subjects reported taking vitamin B_{12} supplements. Serum vitamin B_{12} levels were determined using a radioassay. Normal levels for this assay are between 200 and 900 pg/ml. Values among the five dietary groups were statistically significant at the 1% level (F ratio = 12.1). Subjects with values <100 pg/ml were considered deficient in vitamin B_{12}. *Source:* Data from Allen LH. How common is vitamin B-12 deficiency? *Am J Clin Nutr* 2009:89(2):693S–696S.

In agreement with Ellis and Montegriffo,[56] an Israeli study also found that despite having low blood levels of vitamin B_{12}, vegans had no hematologic abnormalities; however, they complained of weakness, fatigue, and poor mental concentration, symptoms often associated with neurologic disturbances stemming from a lack of vitamin B_{12}. Upon administration of B_{12}, their blood levels increased and, most important, their symptoms improved.[55]

In another study of Thai vegetarians, vitamin B_{12} blood level values were a tenth those of the omnivores, although all the vegans appeared healthy, and none displayed any symptoms of vitamin B_{12} deficiency anemia.[65] This was also the case in an Indian study, where it was found that, although lacto vegetarians had low vitamin B_{12} blood levels (121 versus 366 pg/ml for omnivores), none of the vegetarians had any apparent signs or symptoms of vitamin B_{12} deficiency.[66] Similarly, studies of macrobiotics reveal low levels of vitamin B_{12} in this population.[15,67]

Among vegans who do not use vitamin B_{12} supplements, blood levels of this vitamin tend to be lower the longer the diet is followed.[68–70] Crane et al investigated vitamin B_{12} levels in individuals who had been vegans for between 12 and 340 months and who reported not consuming vitamin B_{12} supplements or fortified foods for at least 1 year prior to the study (Figure 7-3). Of the 78 vegans, 60% had vitamin B_{12} levels <200 pg/ml (normal values are considered to be >200) and 46% had levels <160 pg/ml. In comparison, the mean serum vitamin B_{12} level of vegans ($N = 12$) who used soymilk fortified with B_{12} was 389 pg/ml. Four vegans in the unsup-

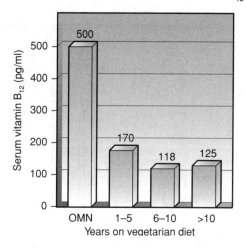

Figure 7-2 Effects of duration of vegetarian diet on serum vitamin B$_{12}$ levels. All subjects were female lacto vegetarians. Vegetarian subjects were grouped according to duration of consuming a vegetarian diet: 1 to 5 years
($N = 22$), 6 to 10 years ($N = 29$), and >10 years ($N = 17$); values were compared to a group of female omnivores (ON) controls ($N = 22$). Differences between the omnivores and the vegetarians were statistically significant ($P < 0.05$ using the Kruskal-Wallis analysis of variance and multiple comparison. *Source:* Data from
Herrmann W, Schorr H, Obeid R, Geisel J. Vitamin B-12 status, particularly holotranscobalamin II and methylmalonic acid concentrations, and hyperhomocysteinemia in vegetarians. *Am J Clin Nutr* 2003;78(1):131–136.

plemented group had a mean corpuscular volume >100 (normal values, 79–100 fl), an indication of abnormal red cell blood synthesis.[70]

Somewhat surprisingly, a study of Australian Seventh-day Adventist ministers who did not use
supplements showed no difference in serum B$_{12}$ levels between the vegans and lacto-ovo vegetarians.[61] However, 53% of the vegetarians (vegans and lacto-ovo vegetarians combined) had levels
below the reference range for the method used (171 pmol/Lor 127 pg/ml), and 73% had levels below
the lower limit of normal (221 pmol/L or 164 pg/ml). In a study of 63 longtime Norwegian
lacto-ovo vegetarians, Solberg et al found no difference in plasma levels of vitamin B$_{12}$ between
the vegetarians and nonvegetarian controls.[71] Van Dusseldorp et al[68] found that among Dutch
adolescents who had consumed a macrobiotic diet early in life, a substantial number still had
impaired cobalamin function despite consumption of moderate amounts of animal products.
Majchrzak et al assessed plasma B$_{12}$ levels in 42 vegans, 36 lacto-ovo vegetarians, and 40 omnivores in Austria. Mean vitamin B$_{12}$ concentrations were within the normal range for all three
groups but were lower in the vegan group than in the omnivores.[72]

Vitamin B$_{12}$ is believed to be the main determinant of homocysteine levels when folate nutrition
is adequate.[73] In the German Vegan Study, elevated Hcy levels were found in both strict vegans and
moderate vegans (defined as those who consumed a maximum of 5% of calories from eggs and
dairy). Furthermore, prevalence of elevated Hcy increased with longer time on a vegan diet. However, cobalamin intake was higher among the strict vegans due to greater use of fortified foods.[74]

Elevated Hcy levels have also been found in Turkish lacto-ovo vegetarian and semi-vegetarian
women,[75] in Taiwanese lacto-ovo vegetarian adults,[76,9] and in rural and urban men in India.[77] As
noted earlier, plasma Hcy concentrations are typically elevated before signs of overt B$_{12}$ deficiency

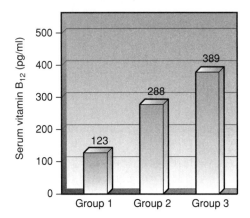

Figure 7-3 Effect of vegan diet on serum vitamin B_{12} levels. Subjects were primarily residents of the Weimer Institute in California and had consumed a vegan diet for 12 to 340 months, avoiding not only eggs and milk but also added free fats and sugars. After analysis of the data, subjects were divided into groups. Individuals in groups 1 and 2 were placed in their respective groups according to whether their serum B_{12} levels were below the value considered to be normal, 200 pg/mL (group 1) or above 200 pg/mL (group 2). Groups 1 (25 males and 22 females) and 2 (16 males and 15 females) consisted of individuals who did not use vitamin B_{12}-fortified foods or B_{12} supplements for 1 year prior to the study, whereas individuals in group 3 (6 males and 6 females) used vitamin B_{12}-fortified soymilk. In another study by these authors, when subjects consuming a lacto-ovo vegetarian diet adopted a strict vegan diet, serum vitamin B_{12} levels decreased from a mean of 417 to 268 pg/ml after 2 months and remained at about that level (276 pg/ml) for the 5 months of the study. *Source:* Data from Dhonukshe-Rutten RA, van Dusseldorp M, Schneede J, de Groot LC, van Staveren WA. Low bone mineral density and bone mineral content are associated with low cobalamin status in adolescents. *Eur J Nutr* 2005;44(6):341–347.

manifest. Huang et al found that subjects with hyperhomocysteinemia had inadequate vitamin B intake but were not necessarily in the deficient stage of B_{12}.[31]

Although a number of studies show lower serum B_{12} levels among lacto-ovo vegetarians compared to omnivores, clinical findings of deficiency do not appear to be common in this group. But in a population consuming a raw foods diet, which also included small amounts of meat and fish, only 21% had adequate B_{12} status and 50% had elevated Hcy.[78] Other indicators of vitamin B_{12} status have also been shown to be abnormal in lacto-ovo vegetarians, suggesting it is important for all vegetarians and perhaps semi-vegetarians, to use reliable sources of vitamin B_{12}.[26,28,32] In addition, some impairment of function can occur without a marked reduction in serum vitamin B_{12} levels. For example, Fata et al found that subtle immunologic impairment may occur with only slight B_{12} deficiency in older subjects.[79] And Louwman et al found that subtle deficiency in the absence of hematologic signs could lead to impaired cognitive performance in adolescents.[12]

Nonanimal Sources of Vitamin B_{12}: Fact or Fantasy?

As noted previously, the standard assay for determining B_{12} content does not distinguish between biologically active forms of vitamin B_{12} and analogs.[2] This has caused considerable confusion about the presence of vitamin B_{12} in plant foods. Foods that have been reported to contain vitamin B_{12} include fermented foods (such as tempeh), sea vegetables, algae and Spirulina, various greens, grains, and legumes.[80–85] Even rainwater has been reported to be a source of vitamin B$_{12}$.[86] (Exhibit 7-1).

In an analysis of 40 plant foods, however, van den Berg et al found that most did not contain vitamin B$_{12}$.[84] Using an assay specific for active vitamin B$_{12}$, the investigators determined that none of the fermented soy products tested, which included tempeh, shoyu, tamari, rice miso, and barley miso, and none of the fermented nonsoy products, such as amesake rice and umeboshi plums, contained any active vitamin B$_{12}$. Neither did tofu.[82] Tiny amounts (0.02 to 0.50 mg/100 g) were found in barley malt syrup, sourdough bread, parsley, and shiitake mushrooms. Only the algae nori (*Porphyra tenera*) and Spirulina contained appreciable amounts. Herbert et al,[87] Herbert and Drivas,[88] and Watanabe et al,[89,90] however, reported that the vitamin B$_{12}$ in Spirulina is mostly analog, and Dagnelie et al[91] reported that the consumption of nori, spirulina, kombu, whole-meal sourdough bread, and barley malt syrup did not improve mean corpuscular volume or mean corpuscular hemoglobin mass despite an increase in vitamin B$_{12}$ plasma volume. This suggests that the vitamin B$_{12}$ in these products is also mostly analog. It has been reported, however, that the consumption of sea vegetables (arame, wakame, and kombu) by a lactating woman led to an improvement in the vitamin B$_{12}$ status of her breastfed infant.[67] The consumption of nori and chlorella sea vegetables was also associated with higher serum B$_{12}$ levels in subjects adhering to a raw foods vegan diet, although serum levels of B$_{12}$ were low among all of the subjects. These studies suggest that sea vegetables may in fact provide some active vitamin B$_{12}$, although the levels in these foods, when consumed in reasonable amounts, is not sufficient to meet vitamin B$_{12}$ needs.[92] More recently, active vitamin B$_{12}$ has been isolated from purple laver[93] and button mushrooms,[94,95] but the biologic significance of these sources has not yet been determined.

The presence of analogs is a particularly important issue because, as noted earlier, some reports have found that high levels of cobalamin analogs are associated with neurologic abnormalities in cases of cobalamin deficiency.[96] Research from Japan suggests that, although raw nori contains true B$_{12}$, dried nori, which is the type most available to Western vegetarians, contains primarily inactive analog.[97] This may explain some of the conflicting findings already noted.

Exhibit 7-1 Foods Reported in the Popular Literature to Be Good Sources of Vitamin B$_{12}$ But Shown by Analysis to Contain Either No Vitamin B$_{12}$ or Only Analog

Alfalfa	Rainwater	Soybeans
Algae	Sea vegetables	Spinach
Amaranth	Shiitake mushrooms	Spirulina
Barley malt syrup	arame*	Tamari
Comfrey	wasake*	Tempeh
Legumes	kombu*	Tofu
Miso	Shoyu	Turnip greens
Peanuts	Sourdough bread	Umeboshi plums

*Recent studies indicate that some sea vegetables may contain some active vitamin B$_{12}$.

As briefly mentioned, some plant foods may be contaminated with vitamin B_{12}-producing bacteria, whose value was demonstrated many years ago. Iranian vegans maintain normal B_{12} status by consuming vegetables that were grown in night soil (human manure) and are not thoroughly washed before being eaten.[98] This demonstrates not only the potential contribution of bacterial contamination but also the fact the human feces contains active vitamin B_{12}, a point discussed later.

Legumes, such as soybeans, possess root nodules that can be inhabited by bacteria. These bacteria may produce small amounts of both active B_{12} and analog. U.S. Department of Agriculture data indicate, however, that soybeans and other legumes contain no vitamin B_{12}. These foods should not be considered a reliable source of this vitamin. Research conducted by Mozafar and Oertli suggests that plants grown in soil treated with manure may take up small amounts of vitamin B_{12}. However, it is not clear whether the B_{12} is active or analog, and the amounts are too small to be of dietary significance.[99]

Endogenous Production of Vitamin B_{12}

Bacteria in the digestive tract of humans produce considerable amounts of active vitamin B_{12}, but the extent to which this is available for absorption is unclear. Most of this B_{12} is produced too far down in the colon to be absorbed,[100] and most of it ends up in the feces.[2] Smaller amounts of vitamin B_{12} may be produced in the small intestine, and there is evidence that some of this could be absorbed.[101,102]

Intestinal synthesis of B_{12} has been proposed as one explanation for why vitamin B_{12} deficiency is uncommon among the largely vegetarian population of India.[103] Vegetarian diets may modify the types of bacteria in the gut; Indian vegetarians reportedly have a larger growth of microflora than nonvegetarians.[103] The extent to which bacteria in the small intestines contribute to vitamin B_{12} status is still poorly understood, however. Indian immigrants to the United Kingdom experience a higher incidence of vitamin B_{12} deficiency, which theoretically could be due to changes in the microecology of the gut but is more likely due to improved hygiene and a reduced intake of food and water contaminated with vitamin B_{12}-producing bacteria.[104]

In Egyptian children with elevated Hcy, yogurt containing probiotics was effective in increasing B_{12}-producing bacteria in the gut.[105] In an earlier study, however, abnormally high urine MMA levels were not normalized following use of probiotics for 3 months.[16]

Finally, the oral cavity does produce vitamin B_{12}, although only in small amounts, and studies demonstrating this did not distinguish between active B_{12} and analog.[106] In any event, the quantity of vitamin B_{12} produced is not sufficient to meet daily requirements, although it might contribute to intake.

Vitamin B_{12} Deficiency in Breastfed Infants of Vegan Women

There have been many reports of vitamin B_{12} deficiency in breastfed infants of vegan or near-vegan mothers,[13,67,107–123] although many of these are findings from macrobiotic populations, in which infant feeding practices differ markedly from those in the general vegan population. The fetus obtains its initial store of B_{12} via the placenta. Under normal conditions, full-term infants have enough stored vitamin B_{12} to last for approximately 3 months on a diet that does not contain vitamin B_{12}.[124] Newborn vitamin B_{12} stores are normally about 14.7 to 18.4 nmol. In contrast, neonates of deficient mothers can have stores as low as 1.5 to 3.7 nmol.[125] At birth, however, these infants have much higher serum vitamin B_{12} levels than their mothers, [126,127] and in most instances they show no signs of B_{12} deficiency.

Serum vitamin B_{12} levels of normal infants decrease progressively and reach a nadir at 6 months.[114,127] This decrease is probably accentuated in breastfed infants of vitamin B_{12}-deficient mothers because the vitamin B_{12} content of the milk reflects maternal serum levels and because these infants will have smaller storage levels. Lactation also can decrease vitamin B_{12} stores in mothers. In repeated pregnancies, especially when the mother's diet is inadequate in vitamin B_{12}, infants may be at risk for vitamin B_{12} deficiency.[128] Interestingly, in numerous reports of nutritional vitamin B_{12} deficiency in infants, the mothers had no clinical manifestation or hematologic abnormality.[110,115,129–131] Some studies have shown improvement when deficient infants are given vitamin B_{12}, but questions remain about the long-term neurologic consequences of nutritional vitamin B_{12} deficiency during infancy.[112,131]

One study involving infants with poor vitamin B_{12} status found that infant MMA levels were not related to the length of time the mother had been practicing a vegetarian diet, even though women who had been vegetarian the longest had the lowest serum levels of vitamin B_{12}.[67] This suggests, as was proposed some time ago, that it is only newly absorbed vitamin B_{12} that is transported readily across the placenta or is present in human milk.[132] In contrast, one study found that vitamin B_{12} concentration in breast milk decreased with increasing time on a vegetarian diet, suggesting that vitamin B_{12} stores may in fact contribute to vitamin B_{12} levels in human milk.[114] When maternal serum vitamin B_{12} levels are low, breast milk vitamin B_{12} levels will also be low, resulting in inadequate vitamin intake in infants.[114,133,134]

Counseling Vegetarian Clients

The biologic need for vitamin B_{12} is about ≤ 1.0 μg/d; in fact, as little as 0.1 μg/d may be enough to satisfy the requirements of most people.[10] Although the RDA for this nutrient was lowered from 3.0 to 2.0 μg in the 1989 version of the RDAs, it was raised in the most recent version of these recommendations to 2.4 μg/d for adults.

A strict vegan diet is theoretically devoid of this nutrient. In the European Prospective Investigation into Cancer (EPIC)-Oxford study, vitamin B_{12} intakes increased progressively with animal product intake, averaging 0.4 μg for vegans, 2.6 μg for lacto-ovo vegetarians, 5.0 μg for those who ate fish, and 7.2 μg for omnivores.[135] Although some foods may be contaminated with this nutrient, these foods are not reliable sources. Therefore, all vegans need a regular, reliable source of B_{12} in their diet, either in fortified foods or as a vitamin supplement.

Supplements and fortified foods have been shown to be effective in maintaining vitamin B_{12} status in nonvegetarians. In the Framingham Offspring Study omnivores who used supplements were less likely to have low plasma B_{12} levels (<85 pmol/L or 137 pg/ml) than those who did not.[136] Subjects who consumed fortified cereal more than four times per week were also less likely to have low levels. Increased dairy consumption also reduced the likelihood of low plasma B_{12} levels. However, there was no difference in plasma B_{12} levels between those in the lowest and highest tertile of meat intake. The researchers suggested that the use of supplements, fortified cereals, and dairy foods protected against low plasma vitamin B_{12}, which implies that vegetarians can easily plan diets to achieve adequate intakes.

Vitamin B_{12} intakes of lacto-ovo vegetarians are often close to recommended intake levels (Appendixes J, M, and Q). However, depending on food choices, lacto and lacto-ovo vegetarians can have diets that are quite low in vitamin B_{12}. Thus individual assessment is important in counseling vegetarians on vitamin B_{12}.

Furthermore, there is a great deal of misinformation in the popular vegetarian literature about foods that are purported to contain vitamin B_{12} but actually contain only analog.

Many foods that are acceptable to vegans are excellent sources of vitamin B_{12} (Table 7-1). Nutritional yeast is one of the best. Only nutritional yeast that has been grown on a vitamin B_{12}-rich medium is a good source of this vitamin, however. Red Star brand nutritional yeast T6635 (called Vegetarian Support Formula) is one that is reliably high in vitamin B_{12} (Table 7-2). A tablespoon provides 4 μg of vitamin B_{12}. Daily consumption of vitamin B_{12}-fortified nutritional yeast for 3 months led to normalization of urine MMA levels in five of eight vegans eating mostly raw foods.[16]

A number of commercial soymilks and some brands of tofu are fortified with vitamin B_{12}. Some meat analogs are also good sources of vitamin B_{12}. Finally, many commercial breakfast cereals are rich in vitamin B_{12}, although fortification varies among brands and in the same brand over time.

Although vitamin B_{12} is an important issue in vegan nutrition, it is an easily resolved one. Regular (two to three servings daily) use of fortified foods provides adequate B_{12} for vegans.[137] Dietitians should also be able to provide suggestions for brand names of B_{12} supplements that are vegan.

Some B_{12} supplements provide as much as 500 μg per dose. At these high levels of intake, however, vitamin B_{12} absorption efficiency decreases markedly. Therefore, clients should be counseled to

Table 7-1 Vitamin B_{12} Content of Foods

Food	Vitamin B_{12} Content (μg)
Kellogg's corn flakes	2.65
Cheerios	1.74
Veggie "meat" analogs, fortified	1.0–3.0 (varies by brand)
Soymilk, fortified, 1 cup	1.2–2.9 (varies by brand)
Milk, 2%, 1 cup	1.29
Cheddar cheese, 1 oz	0.24
Egg, 1 large	0.56
Protein bar (fortified)	1.0–2.0 (varies by brand)
Nutritional yeast, Vegetarian Support Formula, 1 tbsp	4.0
Marmite yeast extract, 1 tsp	0.9

Source: Data from USDA National Nutrient Database for Standard Reference, Release 22, 2009 and manufacturers' information.

Table 7-2 B-Vitamin Content of 2 Heaping tbsp (Large Flake) or 1.5 Heaping tbsp (Mini Flake) Vegetarian Support Formula Nutritional Yeast (Red Star Brand)

Thiamin	9.6 mg
Riboflavin	9.6 mg
Niacin	56 mg
Vitamin B$_6$	9.6 mg
Folic acid	240 μg
Vitamin B$_{12}$	8 μg
Pantothenic acid	1.0 mg
Biotin	20.8 μg

Source: Manufacturers' information.

take supplements daily (5 to 10 μg) or weekly (2000 μg) even though it may appear that one vitamin pill will provide enough B$_{12}$ for several weeks.[137] Most importantly, research indicates that for B$_{12}$ to be well absorbed, B$_{12}$ pills need to be chewed before swallowing or allowed to dissolve under the tongue. This allows for the vitamin to combine with the R factor. In patients with absorption problems, holding tablets providing 2000 μg of B$_{12}$ under the tongue for 30 minutes daily for 7 to 12 days resulted in increases in serum B$_{12}$ from 127.9 ($\pm$42.6) to 515.7 ($\pm$235) pg/ml.[138] Vitamin B$_{12}$ administered intranasally was also shown to increase B$_{12}$ concentrations in patients with B$_{12}$ deficiency.[139]

Summary

Although unwashed produce, bacterial production in the gut, and enterohepatic circulation may all help protect against deficiency in vegans, none is sufficiently reliable to promote adequate vitamin B$_{12}$ status. It is likely that all Western vegans whose diets are unsupplemented will eventually develop vitamin B$_{12}$ deficiency.

Also, although vitamin B$_{12}$-related anemia is rare in vegans, studies consistently show that vegans have low serum levels of vitamin B$_{12}$ and that many have levels considered inadequate and/or marginally deficient. Furthermore, serum levels of vitamin B$_{12}$ have been shown to underestimate the prevalence of deficiency.[140] This appears to be the case even in individuals without anemia who are apparently healthy. There are two concerns related to these findings. One is that individuals with such low levels will be ill equipped to adapt sufficiently during times when vitamin B$_{12}$ needs are increased (e.g., during aging or in the presence of infection).

Much more important, however, anemia is not by any means the only clinical consequence of low vitamin B$_{12}$. Vitamin B$_{12}$ deficiency even in the absence of anemia may have deleterious effects on the nervous system.[141, 142] It is possible that subtle neurologic damage could be occurring even though anemia is not evident. This possibility is increased in vegans because they consume more folate than nonvegetarians. Folate delays or prevents vitamin B$_{12}$-related anemia and thus could prevent early detection of B$_{12}$ deficiency.

Arguments have been made that the lack of vitamin B_{12} in the vegan diet implies that this is not a natural or recommended way of eating. Actually, the evidence suggests that humans evolved to function on a minute intake of vitamin B_{12}. It seems reasonable to speculate that the original diet of humans contained only the smallest amounts of B_{12} because the body conserves it so carefully. It is likely that, until recently, vitamin B_{12} needs could be met entirely through regular consumption of foods contaminated with bacteria or contaminated drinking water. It is only as the food supply has become more hygienic and the risks associated with contaminated food have become better appreciated that additional sources of this vitamin have become necessary.

Counseling Points for Vitamin B_{12}

- The only food sources of vitamin B_{12} are animal products and fortified foods. Fermented soyfoods like tempeh and miso do not contain vitamin B_{12}.
- Vitamin B_{12} deficiency can cause anemia and neurologic symptoms. The neurologic symptoms are sometimes irreversible. B_{12} deficiency can also raise risk for heart disease.
- Although vitamin B_{12} deficiency is not common among vegetarians, it is a serious issue.
- Subtle neurologic symptoms associated with B_{12} deficiency can sometimes occur even when blood levels are in the low-normal range and anemia absent.
- All vegans should have a reliable source of vitamin B_{12} in their diet. Good vegan sources of this include fortified cereals, some fortified meat analogs, some fortified milks, Red Star brand T6635 nutritional yeast (Vegetarian Support Formula), or a vitamin supplement.
- When supplements are the main source of vitamin B_{12}, requirements can be met by a daily supplement providing 5 to 10 μg or a weekly supplement of 2000 μg. Chewing vitamin B_{12} tablets or allowing them to dissolve under the tongue improves absorption.
- Foods such as sea vegetables, algae, and spirulina may contain vitamin B_{12} analogs. These are B_{12}-like compounds that have no vitamin activity in the body. Because they can also interfere with absorption of active vitamin B_{12}, depending on these foods for B_{12} can actually increase the risk of deficiency.
- Production of vitamin B_{12} in the body is either too small—as in the case of that produced by saliva—or produced too far down in the colon to be of nutritional significance.
- Blood levels of vitamin B_{12} tend to be low in vegans who do not use fortified foods or supplements. Vitamin B_{12} status should be assessed in these individuals.
- Vitamin B_{12} from the mother's stores may not be available to the fetus or breast-feeding babies. Therefore, pregnant vegans should use vitamin B_{12} supplements. When babies are being breastfed, either the infant or the vegan mother should receive B_{12} supplements.

THIAMIN (VITAMIN B_1)

Thiamin, as thiamin pyrophosphate, is a coenzyme required for the metabolism of carbohydrates, and therefore requirements for this vitamin are tied to caloric intake. Recent research suggests that thiamin also has non-coenzyme functions in the body and that it plays a structural role in nervous tissue.[143] The RDA is 1.2 and 1.1 mg for men and women, respectively.[144]

Thiamin is widely distributed in foods (Table 7-3), but most foods contain only low concentrations of this vitamin. Yeasts (e.g., dried brewer's yeast and baker's yeast) are particularly good

Table 7-3 Thiamin Content of Foods

Food	Thiamin Content (mg)	Food	Thiamin Content (mg)
Breads, cereals, grains		**Sea vegetables** *(continued)*	
English muffin, 1 whole	0.14	Nori	0.078
White bread, 1 slice	0.10	Wakame	0.4
Whole wheat bread, 1 slice	0.10	**Fruit**	
Bran flakes, 1 cup	0.50	Figs, 10	0.07
Cheerios, 1 cup	0.54	Orange, 1 medium	0.09
Cream of Wheat, ½ cup	0.17	Orange juice, 1 cup	0.20
Grits, enriched, ½ cup	0.1	Pineapple, 1 cup chunks	0.13
Oatmeal, instant, 1 pkt	0.29	Watermelon, 1 cup cubes	0.05
Oatmeal, regular, ¾ cup, cooked	0.13	**Legumes,** ½ cup, cooked	
Barley, whole, ½ cup, cooked	0.59	Kidney beans	0.14
Pasta, enriched, ½ cup, cooked	0.31	Lentils	0.17
Pasta, whole wheat, ½ cup, cooked	0.07	Navy beans	0.21
Quinoa, ½ cup cooked	1.0	Pinto beans	0.16
Rice, brown, ½ cup, cooked	0.09	Split peas	0.19
Rice, white, enriched, ½ cup, cooked	0.13	**Soyfoods**	
Wheat germ, 2 tbsp	0.23	Soybeans, ½ cup, cooked	0.13
Vegetables, ½ cup, cooked		Soymilk, 1 cup	0.15
Peas	0.21	**Nuts/seeds**	
Potatoes	0.08	Peanuts, ¼ cup	0.234
Winter squash	0.12	Tahini, 2 tbsp	0.37
Sea vegetables (8 g dry portion)		**Other**	
Dulce	0.02	Marmite yeast extract, 1 tbsp	0.35
Kombu	0.011	Nutritional yeast, 1 tbsp	4.8

Source: Data from USDA National Nutrient Database for Standard Reference, Release 22, 2009 and manufacturers' information. Values for sea vegetables from MacArtain P, Gill CIR, Brooks M, et al. Nutritional value of edible seaweeds. *Nutr Rev.* 2007;65:535–543.

sources, but enriched, fortified, and whole grain products represent the most important dietary sources of thiamin in most diets. In omnivore diets, about 43% of the thiamin comes from grains and about 16% from meat, fish, and poultry.[145]

Interestingly, there are a number of heat-stable thiamin antagonists in food, such as polyphenols (caffeic acid, chlorogenic acid, and tannic acid) and flavonoids (quercitin and rutin), that can inhibit thiamin absorption. Also, some foods, such as raw fish, tea, betel nuts, blueberries, and red cabbage, contain thiaminases, which are enzymes that can inactivate thiamin by altering its structure.[146,167] Excessive reliance on these foods could contribute to thiamin deficiency.[147]

The average daily thiamin intake of adult men and women in the United States is reported to be nearly 2.0 mg and 1.5 mg, respectively.

The intake of thiamin has increased fairly substantially (by about 25%) since the early part of the 20th century, despite a decrease in grain consumption, because of enrichment of refined flours and cereals. With few exceptions, studies indicate that vegetarians consume adequate thiamin and that their thiamin status is good (Appendix J).[148,149]

RIBOFLAVIN

Riboflavin, commonly called vitamin B_2, is a yellow fluorescent compound that is widely distributed among the plant and animal kingdoms. Data from the 1995 Continuing Survey of Food Intakes by Individuals (CSFII) show that milk is the greatest contributor of riboflavin to the diet followed by bread and fortified cereals.[144]

Riboflavin forms part of the coenzymes flavin mononucleotide and flavin adenine dinucleotide (FAD), both of which are required by many enzymes involved primarily in oxidation and reduction reactions. Riboflavin status is assessed by measuring urinary levels or measuring the activity of glutathione reductase, a FAD-requiring enzyme. Overt deficiency of riboflavin is uncommon in Western countries.

The adult RDA for riboflavin is 1.1 mg for women and 1.3 mg for men.[144] Most Americans meet or exceed these requirements.[150–152] Early clinical studies, in which dietary riboflavin intake was well below the RDA, reported that signs of deficiency rarely if ever resulted.[153,154] The RDA value allows for greater reserves of riboflavin and greater variability among individuals, however, and even without clinical signs of deficiency, riboflavin status can still be subnormal and may result in impaired function.[155,156] Inadequate riboflavin has been associated with elevated homocysteine levels. For example, in Portuguese subjects age 60 to 94 years, riboflavin supplementation (10 mg/d) was effective in lowering plasma homocysteine in subjects with low riboflavin status.[157] Other researchers have found that riboflavin may be effective in lowering plasma homocysteine only in a subset of the population with deficient levels of an enzyme involved in homocysteine metabolism.[158]

Lacto-ovo vegetarians generally have little difficulty meeting the RDA for riboflavin (Appendix J). However, relatively few studies have examined the riboflavin intake of vegans. Limited data suggest intake of this group is similar to or only slightly lower than that of lacto-ovo vegetarians and omnivores (Appendix J). In a study of Austrian omnivores, lacto-ovo vegetarians, and vegans, vegan subjects had lower mean urinary riboflavin levels than omnivores or lacto-ovo vegetarians; furthermore, 38% of the vegans showed inadequate riboflavin status based on urinary riboflavin excretion. However, when measured per millimole of creatinine, riboflavin status was adequate in all groups. Clinical signs of riboflavin deficiency have not been observed in vegan subjects.[149,159–161]

Riboflavin is stable to heat but not to sunlight (irradiation); exposure of milk to sunlight can result in the destruction of more than half the riboflavin content within just 1 day, so that most milk is now sold in opaque containers. Also, substantial amounts of riboflavin can be lost via the water used to boil vegetables.

About half the riboflavin in whole grain rice and more than a third of that of whole wheat is lost when these grains are milled. However, when refined grains are enriched, the riboflavin content can be twice that of the whole grain. Enriched white rice does not contain riboflavin because the yellow tinge it provides is considered undesirable. Parboiled (converted) rice contains most of the riboflavin of the parent grain.

Although whole grains are a relatively poor source of riboflavin, generous use of these foods can make a substantial contribution to intake. Vegetables such as broccoli, many leafy green vegetables, and sea vegetables are reasonably good sources of riboflavin, whereas legumes provide moderate amounts (0.1 mg per cup) with the exception of soybeans, which are an excellent source of riboflavin, providing about 0.48 mg per cup.

Nutritional yeast that is grown on a riboflavin-rich medium contains more than twice the RDA for riboflavin in 1 tbsp. Many ready-to-eat cereals and many brands of soymilk are fortified with this nutrient, so that a meal of fortified cereal with fortified soymilk can provide between 33% and 150% of the RDA for riboflavin, depending on the brands used (Table 7-4).

NIACIN

Niacin functions as part of the coenzymes nicotinamide adenine dinucleotide and nicotinamide adenine dinucleotide phosphate, which are used in many metabolic reactions, including the metabolism of glucose and fatty acids, and in tissue respiration. Niacin has been used in therapeutic doses in treatments to raise high-density lipoprotein cholesterol levels.[162] Pellagra is the deficiency disease most closely associated with niacin; its symptoms include dermatitis, diarrhea, and dementia. Pellagra often occurs in individuals suffering from a deficiency of several B vitamins. Today, pellagra is largely absent from industrialized countries but still occurs in India, China, and parts of Africa.

Niacin is somewhat different from the other vitamins in that a substantial part of the daily requirement is met by consumption of the amino acid tryptophan. Sixty milligrams of tryptophan yields 1 mg of niacin, which is significant considering that omnivore adults consume approximately 50 to 100 g of protein per day and approximately 1% of that is tryptophan (Animal products are somewhat higher and plant products somewhat lower). Conversion is decreased by inadequate iron, riboflavin, or vitamin B_6 status.

The RDA is expressed as niacin equivalents (NEs); for adult men and women the RDA is 16 and 14 mg NE, respectively.[143] One NE is equal to 1 mg of niacin or 60 mg of tryptophan. In the United States, median niacin intake for women is 17 to 20 mg.[144] In the Boston Nutritional Status Survey of the Elderly, median intake for people >60 years was 21 mg/d for men and 17 mg/d for women.[144] These values consider only preformed niacin.

Niacin in grains is poorly absorbed because it is present in covalently bound complexes with small peptides and carbohydrates.[163] Diets based on corn, in particular, can be problematic because the niacin in corn is largely unavailable for absorption and because corn is low in tryptophan. A common practice in Latin American cultures, however, where corn products are frequently consumed, is to soak corn used for preparation of corn tortillas in lime-treated water, which makes the niacin available for absorption and also greatly increases the calcium content.[164] Also, synthetic niacin added to refined grains is well absorbed. Beans also contain niacin in the

Table 7-4 Riboflavin Content of Foods

Food	Riboflavin Content (mg)	Food	Riboflavin Content (mg)
Breads, cereals, grains		**Sea vegetables** *(continued)*	
Bran flakes, ¾ cup	0.42	Kombu	0.01
Cheerios, 1 cup	0.45	Nori	0.27
Corn flakes, 1 cup	0.74	Wakame	0.94
Barley, whole, ½ cup	0.26	**Fruit**	
Pasta, enriched, ½ cup	0.15	Banana, 1 medium	0.09
Pasta, whole wheat, ½ cup	0.03	**Legumes,** ½ cup cooked	
Quinoa, ½ cup	0.1	Kidney beans	0.05
White bread, 1 slice	0.9	Soybeans	0.24
Whole wheat bread	0.06	Split peas	0.06
Vegetables		**Soyfoods**	
Asparagus	0.06	Soymilk, 1 cup	0.5 (varies by brand)
Beet greens	0.2	Veggie "meats"	0.17 (varies by brand)
Collard greens	0.10	**Animal products**	
Mushrooms	0.23	Egg, 1 large	0.26
Peas	0.08	Milk, 1 cup	0.45
Spinach	0.21	Yogurt, 1 cup	0.57
Sweet potatoes	0.08	**Miscellaneous**	
Sea vegetables (8 g dry portion)		Nutritional yeast, Vegetarian Support Formula, 1 tbsp	4.8
Dulse	0.08		
		Marmite yeast extract	0.42

Source: Data from USDA National Nutrient Database for Standard Reference, Release 22, 2009 and manufacturers' information. Values for sea vegetables from MacArtain P, Gill CIR, Brooks M, et al. Nutritional value of edible seaweeds. *Nutr Rev.* 2007;65:535–543.

free form, which is well absorbed. Both vegan and lacto-ovo vegetarian niacin intake is adequate (Table 7-5 and Appendix J).

VITAMIN B₆

Vitamin B_6 is composed of three compounds—pyridoxol, pyridoxal, and pyridoxamine—all of which are converted to pyridoxal phosphate and pyridoxamine, the active forms of the vitamin. Vitamin B_6 functions as a coenzyme for >60 enzymes, most of which are involved in amino

Table 7-5 Niacin Content of Foods

Food	Niacin Content (mg)	Food	Niacin Content (mg)
Breads, cereals, grains		**Vegetables** (continued)	
Bran flakes, fortified, ¾ cup	5.0	Mushrooms	3.5
Cheerios, 1 cup	5.35	Peas	1.2
Corn flakes, 1 cup	6.8	Potatoes	1.1
Rice Krispies, 1¼ cups	65.0	**Sea Vegetables** (8 g dry portion)	
Shredded wheat, 1 cup mini wheats	2.7	Dulse	0.8
		Kombu	4.9
Bread, white, 1 slice	1.1	Nori	0.7
Bread, whole wheat, 1 slice	1.3	Wakame	7.2
Corn tortillas (enriched), 1	1.5	**Nuts/seeds**	
Barley, whole, ½ cup, cooked	4.2	Peanuts, ¼ cup	4.4
		Peanut butter, 2 tbsp	4.3
Bulgur, ½ cup, cooked	0.9	Tahini, 2 tbsp	1.6
Pasta, white enriched	1.9	**Soyfoods**	
Pasta, whole wheat, ½ cup, cooked	0.5	Edamame (green immature soybeans), ½ cup	1.1
Quinoa, ½ cup	0.38	Tempeh, ½ cup	2.2
Rice, brown, ½ cup, cooked	1.5	**Miscellaneous**	
Rice, white, enriched, ½ cup, cooked	1.17	Marmite yeast extract	9.6
Vegetables, ½ cup cooked unless otherwise indicated		Nutritional yeast, Vegetarian Support Formula, 1 tbsp	28
Avocado, ½ raw	1.8		
Corn	1.2		

Source: Data from USDA National Nutrient Database for Standard Reference, Release 22, 2009 and manufacturers' information. Values for sea vegetables from MacArtain P, Gill CIR, Brooks M, et al. Nutritional value of edible seaweeds. *Nutr Rev.* 2007;65:535–543.

acid metabolism. Vitamin B$_6$ may also have some antioxidant properties, and supplements have been shown to improve glucose tolerance in diabetics.[165]

The adult RDA is 1.3 mg for both men and women age 19 to 50 years, 1.7 mg for men ≥51 years, and 1.5 mg for women ≥51 years. Data from the 1995 CSFII indicate that the greatest contribution to vitamin B$_6$ intake among U.S. adults comes from fortified cereals, mixed foods whose main ingredient is meat, fish, or poultry; white potatoes and other starchy vegetables; and noncitrus fruits.[144] In the EPIC-Europe study, meat was the most important contributor to the intake of B vitamins including vitamin B_6.[166] Fortified cereals, organ meats, and fortified soy-based meat substitutes are especially rich sources of vitamin B_6.

Vitamin B_6 participates in the conversion of homocysteine to cystathionine. Low serum levels of vitamin B_6 have been associated with increased levels of homocysteine,[167,168] and perhaps for this reason, vitamin B_6 supplementation has been associated with protection against myocardial infarction.[169] Inadequate vitamin B_6 may be a risk factor for heart disease and stroke independent of homocysteine status, however.[170] Vitamin B_6 has also been studied in relation to cognitive function, although it does not appear to have an effect on cognitive decline.[8]

Some animal work has suggested that low-quality proteins increase vitamin B_6 requirements, but other studies indicate that B_6 from plant foods may meet needs more efficiently than vitamin B_6 from meat. One study found that, in men, vitamin B_6 status correlated inversely with both total protein intake and animal protein intake but not with the intake of plant protein.[171] Consistent with this finding, a 1982 study reported that female subjects depleted of vitamin B_6 required 25% more vitamin B_6 to return B_6 status to normal when protein from animal foods was consumed in comparison with plant proteins (2.0 mg vs 1.5 mg of vitamin B_6).[172] More recent research from this same group of investigators indicated, however, that the amount of vitamin B_6 required to replete vitamin B_6-depleted women was the same whether they were fed a high-animal protein or a high-plant protein diet.[173] In contrast, Huang et al found that vegetarians had slightly lower plasma pyridoxal phosphate concentrations than nonvegetarians despite similar intakes of vitamin B_6.[31]

The high fiber content of plant foods may be a factor in vitamin B_6 bioavailability because this vitamin was shown to be more poorly absorbed from whole wheat bread than from white bread, although blood levels of vitamin B_6 were not affected.[174] In one study, the addition of bran to diets did reduce the absorption of vitamin B_6 but only by 17%.[175] However, a prospective study of 283 adult women found there was no relationship between fiber intake and absorption of vitamin B_6.[176] Furthermore, although 16% of subjects in the German Vegan Study had insufficient vitamin B_6 blood concentrations despite high intakes, neither fiber nor protein intakes were associated with this finding, and the authors suggested that vitamin B_6 status of vegans may be influenced by unknown factors.[177] Any adverse effect of fiber may be offset by the fact that fiber-rich foods tend also to be rich in vitamin B_6, and in most populations a high fiber intake does not seem to interfere with B_6 status.[178,179]

Some concerns have been expressed about the effects of processing on vitamin B_6 bioavailability. This vitamin can form complexes with amino acids during food processing, cooking, and digestion, which can reduce utilization. Vitamin B_6 is stable under acidic conditions but not neutral or alkaline ones, particularly when exposed to heat or light. Of the several forms of the vitamin, however, the kind most often found in plant foods (pyridoxine) is more stable than the forms found in animal foods.

Studies have generally shown that both the intake of vitamin B_6[135,178,180–182] and the vitamin B_6 status[57,178,180] of vegetarians is adequate and similar to nonvegetarians (Appendix J). However, one study did find that the vitamin B_6 intake of elderly vegetarians (65 to 97 years of age) was below recommended levels.[178,193]

Vitamin B_6 is well distributed among different groups of plant foods (Table 7-6). Good sources include many ready-to-eat cereals, potatoes, bananas, figs, chickpeas, soybeans, and brewer's yeast.

Table 7-6 Vitamin B$_6$ Content of Foods

Food	Vitamin B$_6$ Content (mg)	Food	Vitamin B$_6$ Content (mg)
Bread, cereals, grains		**Fruits**	
Bran flakes, 1 cup	0.5	Banana, 1 medium	0.43
Cheerios, 1 cup	0.50	Elderberries, ½ cup	0.17
Corn flakes, 1 cup	0.96	Figs, 10	0.09
Shredded Wheat, 1 cup mini wheats	0.2	Orange juice, 1 cup	0.2
Oatmeal, instant, 1 pkt	0.43	Raisins, ½ cup	0.07
Quinoa, ½ cup	0.11	Watermelon, 1 cup cubes	0.07
Rice, brown, ½ cup, cooked	0.14	**Legumes,** ½ cup cooked	
Vegetables, ½ cup cooked unless otherwise indicated		Chickpeas	0.11
Asparagus	0.04	Kidney beans	0.11
Avocado, ½ raw	0.26	Lentils	0.17
Peas	0.09	Lima beans	0.15
Plantain	0.18	Navy beans	0.12
Potatoes	0.23	Pinto beans	0.19
Spinach	0.22	**Soyfoods**	
Sweet potatoes	0.27	Soybeans, ½ cup	0.20
Tomato juice, 1 cup	0.27	Soymilk, plain, 1 cup	0.24
Winter squash	0.12–0.20	Soynuts, ¼ cup	0.1
Sea vegetables (8 g dry portion)		Tempeh, ½ cup	0.18
Dulse	0.002	**Nuts/seeds**	
Kombu	0.5	Sunflower seeds, 2 tbsp	0.1
Nori	0.1	**Animal products**	
Wakame	0.26	Egg, 1 large	0.0

Source: Data from USDA National Nutrient Database for Standard Reference, Release 22, 2009 and manufacturers' information. Values for sea vegetables from MacArtain P, Gill CIR, Brooks M, et al. Nutritional value of edible seaweeds. *Nutr Rev.* 2007;65:535–543.

FOLATE

Folate functions in the body as a coenzyme that participates in the transfer of single carbon fragments. This function is particularly important in the metabolism of amino acids and in the synthesis of nucleic acids. In prolonged deficiency, the impaired DNA synthesis results in macrocytic anemia. Folate and vitamin B$_{12}$ function together in the synthesis of DNA. As discussed previously, large amounts of folate replace the need for vitamin B$_{12}$ in the synthesis of nucleic acids and thereby prevent vitamin B_{12}-deficiency anemia. Nevertheless, folate cannot substitute for vitamin B_{12} in its role in the nervous system. The role of folate in preventing neural tube defects in the developing embryo is well established and was the impetus for mandatory fortification of refined flour products with folic acid. Folate is also important for maintaining normal levels of homocysteine.

Evidence from both controlled metabolic and epidemiologic studies indicate that plasma homocysteine and blood folate levels are inversely related. In agreement, many studies show that plasma homocysteine is elevated in folate deficient individuals,[11,183,184] although the relationship of folate to cardiovascular disease risk remains unclear.[44,185] In addition, inadequate folate status has been linked to an increased risk for colon cancer.[186–188] Adult lacto-ovo vegetarians and vegans typically consume 25–50% more folate than omnivores (Appendix J).

Folate is widely distributed in foods (Table 7-7). Much of the folate in foods, however, may be destroyed during household preparation, food processing, and storage because folate is destroyed by heat and oxygen exposure. Eating folate-rich fruits and vegetables raw can minimize folate losses.

Folate intake and requirements are expressed as dietary folate equivalents (DFE) to adjust for the nearly 50% lower bioavailability of food folate compared to synthetic folic acid. One DFE equals 1 µg of food folate or 0.5 µg synthetic folic acid taken on an empty stomach or 0.6 µg synthetic folic acid taken with food. The current RDA for adults is 400 µg DFE.

In the past, average daily intakes for men and women in the United States were reported to be between 200 and 250 µg/d. However, since January 1998, all enriched grains (bread, pasta, breakfast cereals, and flour) have been fortified with 1.4 mg folic acid per kilogram grain. Based on National Health and Nutrition Examination Survey (NHANES) data post-fortification, intake of folate averages 450 to 670 DFE/d.[152]

Adequate iron and vitamin C status is necessary for proper folate absorption. Some research suggests there is a positive relationship between fiber intake and folate status.[189] Synthesis of folate by intestinal bacteria may influence folate status.[190]

In general, folate intakes and folate status of vegetarians are equal to or superior to those of nonvegetarians (Appendix J). Among Austrian vegetarians, vegans had superior folate status and were less likely to exhibit folate deficiency.[70] And in a case-control study in Slovakia, serum folate levels were significantly higher in vegetarians compared to nonvegetarians. There were no cases of folate deficiency in the vegetarians compared to 8% among the nonvegetarians.[191]

BIOTIN

Although biotin is an essential nutrient, there are minimal data on which to base intake recommendations. The adequate intake (AI) for adults is 30 µg. Biotin can be synthesized in the large intestine, although the amount that is absorbed is uncertain.[192] Biotin serves as a coenzyme for enzymes involved in the synthesis of glucose and fatty acids and the metabolism of amino acids. Symptoms of biotin deficiency, which occurs only rarely in humans, include anorexia, nausea, vomiting, glossitis, and mental depression. One way of producing biotin deficiency is by ingesting avidin, which is a biotin-binding protein found only in raw egg white.[193]

There is relatively little information about biotin with respect to dietary intake in either vegetarians or nonvegetarians. One study of Seventh-day Adventists found that vegetarians had higher

Table 7-7 Folate Content of Foods

Food	Folate Content (µg)	Food	Folate Content (µg)
Breads, cereals, grains		**Fruits** *(continued)*	
Bran flakes, ¾ cup	100	Grapefruit, ½ pink or red	15
Corn flakes, 1 cup	222	Orange juice, 1 cup	47
Oatmeal, instant, 1 pkt	140	Orange, 1 medium	48
Pasta, enriched, ½ cup	137	Strawberries, ½ cup sliced	20
Rice Krispies, 1¼ cups	104	**Legumes,** ½ cup, cooked	
Rice, white enriched, ½ cup	77	Black beans	128
Wheat germ, 2 tbsp	20	Black-eyed peas	105
Vegetables, ½ cup, cooked unless otherwise indicated		Kidney beans	115
		Lentils	179
Asparagus	134	Lima beans	78
Avocado, ½ raw	81	Pinto beans	147
Beets	68	Soybeans, mature	46
Broccoli	84	Soybeans, immature green (edamame)	100
Brussels sprouts	47	Split peas	64
Cauliflower	27	Tempeh	20
Collard greens	88	**Nuts/seeds**	
Mustard greens	51	Peanuts, ¼ cup	88
Parsnips	45	Peanut butter, 2 tbsp	24
Spinach	131	Sunflower seeds, 2 tbsp	40
Sweet potatoes	10	Tahini, 2 tbsp	29
Turnip greens	85	**Animal products**	
Tomato juice, 1 cup	49	Yogurt, 1 cup	29
Fruits		**Miscellaneous**	
Banana, 1 medium	24	Marmite yeast extract	160
Cantaloupe, 1 cup chunks	34		

Source: Data from USDA National Nutrient Database for Standard Reference, Release 22, 2009 and manufacturers' information.

plasma levels of biotin than nonvegetarians and that vegans had higher levels than lacto-ovo vegetarians.[194] Good sources of this vitamin include egg yolk, soy flour, and cereals, but there is as much as a 10-fold variation in the amount of biotin found in different cereals. Fruit and meat are poor sources. Brewer's yeast is rich in biotin (Table 7-8).

Table 7-8 Biotin Content of Foods

Food	Biotin Content (μg)	Food	Biotin Content (μg)
Breads, Cereal, Grains		**Legumes** (½ cup, cooked)	
Oat bran, ½ cup, cooked	7.0	Black-eyed peas	10.7
Oatmeal, instant, one packet	7.0	Lentils	13.0
Barley, pearled, ½ cup, cooked	3.0	Textured vegetable protein	17.5
Vegetables (½ cup, cooked)		**Nuts/Seeds** (2 tbsp)	
Corn	4.9	Almonds	23.0
Mushrooms	7.6	Peanut butter	12.8
Spinach	7.2	**Animal Products**	
		Egg, 1 medium	11.0

Source: Data from *Bowes & Church's Food Value of Portions Commonly Used*. 16th ed., by J. Pennington, Lippincott-Raven, 1994.

PANTOTHENIC ACID

Pantothenic acid is widely distributed in nature and is abundant in many foods. Some synthesis by intestinal bacteria may also occur. Pantothenic acid plays a role as a coenzyme in the release of energy from carbohydrates, in the synthesis of glucose, and in the synthesis and degradation of fatty acids; it has many other functions as well. The AI for adults is 5 mg. Not surprising, because pantothenic acid is so widely distributed in food, deficiencies in free-living populations have not been reliably documented. The average U.S. intake has been reported to be around 6 mg/d, which appears to be quite adequate,[195,196] although there are very little recent data on pantothenic acid intake. Because plant foods are rich in this vitamin, vegetarians should have no problem meeting requirements for pantothenic acid. In one study, however, lacto vegetarians consumed only about 4 mg of pantothenic acid per day, slightly less than the suggested intake. Conversely, vegans consumed >5 mg/d, slightly more than the omnivores in the study.[149]

VITAMIN C (ASCORBIC ACID)

Dietary deficiency of vitamin C leads to scurvy, a serious disorder that is characterized by weakening of collagen. Vitamin C has many diverse functions in the body, some of which are only partly understood. It is used as a cosubstrate for the formation of collagen, but it also appears to be involved in reactions affecting the immune system. Although the value of vitamin C against the common cold is still under debate, research suggests that it may reduce the duration of episodes and the severity of the symptoms.[197–199] Because of its role as an antioxidant, vitamin C may help to reduce risk for cardiovascular disease and certain types of cancer.[200]

Vegetables and fruits, such as green peppers, broccoli, tomatoes, and oranges, contain high concentrations of vitamin C (Table 7-9). Grains, meat (except for organ meats and meats pro-

Table 7-9 Vitamin C Content of Food

Food	Vitamin C Content (mg)	Food	Vitamin C Content (mg)
Fruits		**Vegetables,** *(continued)*	
Banana, 1 medium	10	Broccoli	58
Blackberries, ½ cup	15	Brussels sprouts	48
Blueberries, ½ cup	7	Butternut squash	15
Cantaloupe, 1 cup chunks	59	Cabbage	28
Elderberries, ½ cup	26	Cauliflower	27
Grapefruit, ½ medium	39	Collards	17
Grapefruit juice, 6 oz	67	Edamame (immature green soybeans)	15
Guava, 1 medium	125		
Honeydew melon, 1 cup chunks	30	Hubbard squash	10
Kiwi, 1 medium	64	Kale	26
Mango, 1 medium	57	Kohlrabi	45
Orange, 1 medium	83	Mustard greens	18
Orange juice, 1 cup	84	Okra	13
Papaya, 1 medium	188	Parsnips	10
Persimmon, 1 medium	16	Pepper (sweet bell)	60
Pineapple, 1 cup chunks	79	Potatoes	10
Raspberries, ½ cup	16	Rutabaga	23
Strawberries, ½ cup sliced	49	Spinach	9
Tangerine, 1 medium	26	Sweet potato	21
Watermelon, 1 cup chunks	12	Swiss chard	16
		Tomato, 1 medium	23
Vegetables, ½ cup, cooked unless otherwise indicated		Tomato juice, 1 cup	44
Acorn squash	8	Turnips	9
Asparagus	3.5	Turnip greens	20
Beet greens	18		

Source: Data from USDA National Nutrient Database for Standard Reference, Release 22, 2009.

cessed with sodium ascorbate), fish, poultry, and dairy products, however, contain essentially none. Average intakes among American adults range from 70 to 100 mg.[152] Most studies show vitamin C intake among vegetarians to be higher than among omnivores, and vegan intake to be higher than that of lacto-ovo vegetarians (Appendix J). In older vegetarian women in Slovakia, oxidative damage of DNA was lower than in nonvegetarians, and vegetarians also had higher plasma values of both β-carotene and vitamin C, suggesting that these nutrients could reduce age-related oxidative damage.[201] Among Hong Kong vegetarians, plasma vitamin C levels appeared to correlate well with other markers of disease risk and served as a useful indicator of overall health status.[202]

VITAMIN D

Although vitamin D is classified as a fat-soluble vitamin, it is not an essential nutrient. With sufficient exposure to sunlight, endogenous synthesis can adequately meet biologic requirements for vitamin D. There are many circumstances under which people do not make adequate vitamin D, however, in which case a dietary source becomes necessary. Most dietary sources of vitamin D are fortified foods because this vitamin has a very limited distribution in nature. It is found primarily in fish oils and the flesh of fatty fish and in eggs from hens that have been fed vitamin D. Cholecalciferol (D_3) is the form of vitamin D found in animal foods. Naturally occurring ergocalciferol does not generally make a significant contribution to vitamin D intake, although one study found it to be well absorbed from some types of wild mushrooms.[203]

In children, inadequate vitamin D leads to rickets, characterized by bowed legs, knock-knees, curvatures of the upper and/or lower arms, swollen joints, and/or enlarged heads. Rickets is associated with urbanization and industrialization and was the scourge of the cities in northern Europe and the United States until the early part of the 20th century. In fact, around the turn of the 19th century, estimates were that nearly 80% of the children in London had rickets, and for that reason rickets became known as the English disease. Rickets was also common in other European countries at this time. For example, in the Netherlands autopsies of young children revealed that 80–90% had residual evidence of rickets. Rickets was rare or nonexistent in southern Europe, however.

In adults, vitamin D deficiency leads to undermineralization of the bone matrix osteoid, which can result in excessive bone loss and osteomalacia. The symptoms of osteomalacia are typically more generalized than those of rickets and include muscular weakness and bone tenderness. Mild vitamin D insufficiency may result in osteoporosis due to decreased calcium absorption.[204,205] Vitamin D deficiency has also been associated with muscle weakness and may lead to falls in elderly people.[206] In a meta-analysis of five randomized clinical trials involving 1237 participants, vitamin D therapy reduced risk of falling in older people by >20%.[207]

Cod liver oil was long used as an effective medicine to prevent rickets. It was not until the early part of the 20th century, however, that the antirachitic factor vitamin D was actually discovered. Soon thereafter, it was shown that skin is fully capable of making vitamin D upon exposure to ultraviolet light. As early as 1822, the importance of exposure to the outdoors and sunlight for the prevention and cure of rickets had been recognized by at least some of the clinical community.

The primary function associated with vitamin D is calcium regulation or homeostasis. Vitamin D stimulates the absorption of phosphorus and calcium (particularly at low levels of calcium intake), decreases urinary calcium excretion, and causes bone demineralization, thereby releasing calcium into the bloodstream. This last action is done in conjunction with parathyroid hormone. All three actions of vitamin D work to increase blood calcium levels.

It appears that physiologic effects of vitamin D are manifest in a wide range of tissues and organs, including the immune system, the skin, and the pancreas. Vitamin D may have roles in reducing risk for cardiovascular disease,[208] diabetes,[209] colon cancer,[210] multiple sclerosis,[211] and dementia.[212]

Vitamin D Requirements

In 1969, on the basis of observed vitamin D deficiency in seven patients, several of whom were vegetarians and consumed no natural sources of vitamin D, the daily requirement for vitamin D was estimated to be 2.5 μg.[213] The current AI for adults is 5.0 μg (200 IU) for ages 19 to 50 years, 10 μg (400 IU) for ages 51 to 70 years, and 15 μg (600 IU) for those >70 years.[214] Endogenous synthesis decreases with aging, making dietary sources more important for older people. This is reflected in the higher recommendations for this group.

Several studies have raised questions about the adequacy of current recommendations. Some experts have suggested that children and adults who do not have adequate sun exposure should consume between 800 and 1000 IU vitamin D daily.[215] For example, a study of veiled Muslim women found that sunlight deprivation resulted in vitamin D deficiency even when the diet was relatively high in vitamin D. The authors concluded that dietary needs could be as high as 25 μg/d in sunlight-deprived individuals.[216] In addition, close to a third of African American women who consumed 5 μg of vitamin D daily from supplements had low serum 25(OH)D concentrations.[217]

There are few data on vitamin D intakes in the United States. According to NHANES II data, the median intake from food for young women was 2.9 μg/d.[218] In general, children have higher vitamin D intakes than adults and males consume more than females.[219]

Based on studies of vitamin D synthesis in infants, it is estimated that adults can synthesize adequate vitamin D by exposing hands and face to sunlight for 10 to 15 minutes, two to three times per week during the summer months.[220,221] Brief exposure to sunlight is thought to be the same as ingesting 5 μg of vitamin D.[222] Because so many factors affect vitamin D synthesis, however, it is unwise to depend entirely on endogenous synthesis to meet vitamin D requirements unless sun exposure is routine. Also, the elderly and dark-skinned people require longer sun exposure to meet vitamin D needs. The significance of poor synthesis in blacks is unclear, however, because low 25(OH)D serum levels in this group do not correlate with lower bone mass or fracture risk.[223]

Unless vitamin D is regularly included in the diet, sufficient stores must be achieved during summertime sun exposure to last through the winter months. In fact, variation in circulating vitamin D levels is usually attributed to seasonal changes. In most people, even in the winter, the concentration of vitamin D in the serum is not determined by current vitamin D intake but rather by the amount of exposure to solar radiation the previous summer.[224] Vitamin D levels tend to be lowest in the winter months. In one study of lacto vegetarians, for example, serum values of 25(OH)D$_3$ in January, March, May, and August were 10.1, 11.9, 18.0, and 27.9 μg/L, respectively (Figure 7-4).[225]

Factors Affecting Vitamin D Synthesis

Both season and latitude affect vitamin D synthesis. This was clearly illustrated by a study conducted in Boston, Massachusetts that used foreskin taken from circumcised infants to monitor vitamin

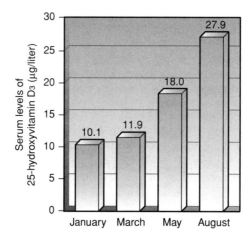

Figure 7-4 Effects of season on vitamin D levels in Finnish lacto vegetarians. Serum vitamin D (25(OH) D) values are for 17 lacto vegetarians who were not taking supplements. Values for May and August were significantly different ($P < 0.05$) from January and March. *Source:* Data from Baker SJ, Jacob E, Rajan KT, Swaminathan SP. Vitamin B12 deficiency in pregnancy and the puerperium. *Br Med J* 1962;16:1658–1661.

D synthesis. When exposed to sunlight (cloudless days) for 3 hours per month, skin was able to synthesize vitamin D during the months of April through October but was unable to do so during the winter months of November and February.[226] Synthesis also took place during the months of November through March in Los Angeles and Puerto Rico but not in Edmonton, Canada, demonstrating the importance of latitude.

Vitamin D synthesis is poorer in dark skin.[227] Six times the amount of simulated solar irradiation was shown to be required in individuals with dark skin to raise serum levels of vitamin D_3 to the same extent as in light-skinned individuals.[227] In one study, >40% of African American women had hypovitaminosis D compared to <5% of white women.[217] Air pollution and sunscreen also block ultraviolet light and inhibit vitamin D synthesis. In fact, it has been shown that topical application of a sunscreen with a sun protection factor of 8 can completely block the photosynthesis of vitamin D in the skin.[228–230] In addition, experts debate the merit of sun exposure for vitamin D synthesis because of increased risk of skin cancer with exposure to ultraviolet rays. Some recommend the consistent use of sunscreen and the regular use of vitamin D supplements.[231,232]

Vegetarians and Vitamin D

Vitamin D deficiency is rare in the general population. For example, of 100,000 pediatric admissions in the 266 teaching hospitals in the United States between 1956 and 1960, only 0.4% of cases were reported as being due to rickets. These results are consistent with two other large U.S. surveys involving thousands of subjects, where it was found that between 0.1% and 0.2% of the children had signs of rickets. Similarly, in Oslo, Norway, no cases of rickets were reported in the pediatric departments between 1967 and 1974.[233] However, rickets has been seen in breastfed

African American infants[234–236] and some white infants in northern climates.[237] In addition, one review of the literature found that marginal vitamin D status is common among U.S. children.[238]

Vitamin D deficiency has been reported in vegetarians, particularly Asian vegetarians.[239–241] Lower circulating levels of vitamin D have also been seen in Asian vegetarians.[242–244] In some studies, though, dietary intake of vitamin D was actually higher than in omnivore populations, suggesting that problems with vitamin D nutriture were a result of inadequate sun exposure rather than a low level of vitamin D intake. The darker skin of Asians reduces their ability to synthesize vitamin D in comparison with light-skinned people. Consistent with this hypothesis, Henderson et al found that the prevalence of rickets in Asians residing in England rose from south to north and that the incidence of rickets was inversely associated with daylight outdoor exposure.[245] However, Awumey et al found that vitamin D metabolism is altered in Asian Indians, placing them at greater risk for vitamin D deficiency.[246] In the Adventist Health Study, white but not black vegetarians had lower vitamin D intakes than nonvegetarians, but there was no association between serum levels of 25(OH)D and vegetarian status in either black or white cohorts.[247]

Findings indicate that exposure to sunlight is the dominant factor affecting risk of rickets and that in an environment where exposure is limited, dietary factors play a pivotal role. In Finland, where dietary fortification of foods is low, vitamin D intake of vegans was insufficient to maintain serum vitamin D within normal ranges in the winter months. Vegans also had lower BMD than omnivores, possibly as a result of vitamin D deficiency.[248] Dietary fiber may decrease vitamin D absorption[249] or increase its excretion.[250] This may be especially relevant for vegetarians when sun exposure is poor and vitamin D dietary intake is marginal, given their higher intake of fiber. A vegetarian diet high in fiber and phytate was associated with decreased vitamin D and calcium absorption in Asian children in Britain.[251]

Vitamin D deficiency has also been reported in U.S. macrobiotic children. Vitamin D, calcium, and phosphorus intakes in macrobiotic preschoolers were marginal and were much less than those of other vegetarians.[252] Instances of rickets have also been reported in macrobiotics in other countries, such as England[253] and the Netherlands.[254] In the Dutch study, between 25% and 50% of the infants examined showed signs of rickets. In addition to the low levels of vitamin D, low availability of calcium was an independent risk factor for rickets.[255] Over a 6-year period, several cases of rickets in vegetarians, thought to be due to low vitamin D intake, were identified in Norway.[233] The lower sunlight exposure in Norway may predispose to rickets. Vitamin D intake has been found to be lower in both vegans and lacto-ovo vegetarians than in omnivores (Appendix K), although in several studies serum levels of vitamin D were similar among the groups.[56,225]

Vitamin D Fortification/Supplementation and Hypervitaminosis D

Because vitamin D is poorly supplied in foods, endogenous vitamin D synthesis may have met most or all of the vitamin D needs throughout history. Modern humans, however, have less sun exposure as a result of urbanization, smog, greater population density at northern latitudes, and less time spent outdoors. Thus a regular source of vitamin D in the diet is good insurance for all people. Except under ideal circumstances, endogenous synthesis by itself should not be viewed as

Table 7-10 Vitamin D Content of Foods

Food	Vitamin D Content (μg)
Corn flakes, 1 cup	1.0
Cheerios, 1 cup	1.0
Fortified soymilk, almond or rice milk, 1 cup	2.5–3.0 μg (varies by brand)
Milk, 2% fat, fortified,1 cup	2.9
Egg, 1 large	0.6
Margarine, fortified, 1 tsp	0.5

Source: Data from USDA National Nutrient Database for Standard Reference, Release 22, 2009 and manufacturers' information.

an adequate means of meeting vitamin D needs. Because there are few natural food sources of vitamin D, fortified foods (Table 7-10) are nearly always relied on to provide dietary vitamin D.

Fortification with vitamin D needs to be monitored because vitamin D is potentially toxic, especially in young children. The effects of excessive vitamin D intake include hypercalcemia and hypercalciuria, which lead to the deposition of calcium in soft tissues and irreversible renal and cardiovascular damage. Elevated vitamin D levels have also been associated with bone resorption.[256] Consumption of as little as 45 μg of vitamin D_3 per day in young children has been associated with signs of hypervitaminosis D.[257] Because of this, dietary supplements should be used with caution, especially where children may already be consuming vitamin D–fortified cow's milk. The tolerable upper limit for vitamin D is 50 μg.[214]

In the United States, milk has been fortified with vitamin D since the 1930s; according to federal regulations, it should contain 400 IU (10 μg) of vitamin D per quart.[258] Fortification was also common in Great Britain, but as a result of toxicity problems this practice has been halted.[259,260] Variation in actual amounts of vitamin D in milk has been of some concern. Three surveys have found that up to 70% of milk sampled throughout North America did not contain the allowed levels of vitamin D per quart, and 62% of milk samples had <8 μg/quart and 14% of skim milk samples had no detectable vitamin D.[261–263] In the United States, hypervitaminosis D in eight individuals was linked to consumption of milk, which in some cases contained vitamin D at concentrations 500 times higher than regulations permit.[264] Because vitamin D is added to large volumes of milk at one time, there is some concern that it is not thoroughly mixed. As a result, vitamin D content of individual samples of milk can vary significantly. Prolonged exposure to sun will not result in vitamin D toxicity because the vitamin D is converted into two biologically inert and harmless isomers.[265]

Vitamin D_3 versus Vitamin D_2

Although fortified milk is traditionally viewed as the most important dietary source of vitamin D, many other foods are also fortified with this vitamin. Many commercial cereals are good sources, although the fortificant in most brands of cereal is vitamin D_3 derived from lanolin from sheep's wool that is not suitable for vegans. Both soymilk and rice milk are often fortified with vitamin D_2, derived from the ultraviolet irradiation of ergosterol obtained from yeast. The type of supplementary vitamin D used may be of some relevance, however, because it is not clear that the two types are bioequivalent. Armas et al found that vitamin D_2 potency was less than a third that of D_3 in healthy adult males given pharmacologic doses.[266] Although the two forms were absorbed comparably, and produced similar increases in serum 25(OH)D, levels declined more rapidly in the men treated with D_2 after 3 days. Similar findings have been reported by other investigators.[267,268] And in a study of 95 hip fracture patients with vitamin D insufficiency, Glendenning et al found that 1000 IU/d of vitamin D_3 was more effective than an equal amount of vitamin D_2 in raising levels of 25(OH)D, although effects on parathyroid hormone lowering were similar.[269] However, in a randomized clinical trial that included 68 healthy adults, Holick et al found that 1000 IU of vitamin D_2 per day was as effective as the same amount of vitamin D_3 in maintaining plasma 25(OH)D levels.[270] And in 489 elderly women (ages 65 to 77 years), both vitamin D_2 and D_3 supplements (based on self-reported intakes) contributed equally to circulating 25(OH)D levels.[271] Vitamin D_2 was also equally effective in treating infants and toddlers with low vitamin D status.[272] Finally, Thacher et al found vitamin D_2 to be bioequivalent to D_3 in children with rickets.[273] Currently, most evidence suggests that vitamin D_2, when provided in nonpharmacologic doses, is effective in raising 25(OH)D levels.

VITAMIN A

Night blindness, as well as several other eye ailments, were treated by the ancient Egyptians with the topical application of juice squeezed from cooked liver or by prescribing liver in the diet, illustrating an early use of vitamin A long before the actual vitamin was identified.[274]

Vitamin A refers to a group of compounds—retinol, retinaldehyde, and retinoic acid—that are essential for vision, growth, cellular differentiation and proliferation, reproduction, and the integrity of the immune system. Although rare in the United States, vitamin A deficiency is a major nutritional problem in some parts of the world, causing a number of the more than 500,000 new cases of active corneal lesions that occur annually in children.[275] Vitamin A deficiency is found most commonly in children <5 years of age. In addition to eye disorders, synthetic vitamin A-related compounds (retinoids) are being studied for their anticancer effects.

Preformed vitamin A is found only in animal products. Vitamin A can be synthesized from the provitamin carotenoids, however, which are widely distributed in many fruits and vegetables (Table 7-11). There are as many as 600 carotenoids in nature, and about 50 of these can be converted into vitamin A, including α- and β-carotene and β-cryptoxanthin. The best known and most active is β-carotene.[276] The carotenoids are yellow-orange pigments, but the color of fruits and vegetables is a poor indicator of carotenoid content because chlorophyll often overshadows the carotenoid color, as in the case of spinach and other leafy green vegetables. The RDA for vitamin A is expressed as micrograms of retinol. Men and women need 900 and 700 μg of retinol per day, respectively.

The provitamin A content of fruits and vegetables is expressed as retinol activity equivalents (RAE). The Food and Nutrition Board (FNB) has determined that relative absorption of

Table 7-11 Vitamin A Content of Foods

Food	Vitamin A Content (μg RAE)	Food	Vitamin A Content (μg RAE)
Vegetables, ½ cup cooked unless otherwise indicated		**Vegetables** (continued)	
		Sweet potatoes	1291
Beet greens	276	Swiss chard	268
Broccoli	60	Tomato, 1 medium	76
Bok choy	180	Tomato juice, 1 cup	56
Butternut squash	572	**Fruits**	
Carrots, 1 medium, raw	509	Apricots, 3 raw	101
Carrots	665	Cantaloupe, 1 cup chunks	270
Chicory greens, 1 cup raw	166	Mango, 1 medium	80
Collards	148	Nectarine, 1 medium	50
Dandelion greens	356	Papaya, 1 medium	167
Hubbard squash	382	**Animal Products**	
Kale	2443	Milk, 2%, 1 cup	134
Mustard greens	221	Milk, whole, 1 cup	112
Pumpkin, canned	953	Cheese, cheddar, 1 oz	75
Spinach	472		

Source: Data from USDA National Nutrient Database for Standard Reference, Release 22, 2009.

β-carotene from a mixed vegetable diet, compared to that from purified β-carotene in oil, is half what was previously believed. Therefore, 12 μg of β-carotene from food yields 1 μg retinol. Some food composition tables are based on the earlier assumption that 6 μg β-carotene produced 1 μg retinol. Vitamin A activity for α-carotene and β-cryptoxanthin is approximately half that of β-carotene. Therefore, the following conversions are used for provitamin A carotenoids.

- 2 μg supplemental β-carotene provides 1 μg retinol
- 12 μg dietary β-carotene provides 1 μg retinol
- 24 μg α-carotene or β-cryptoxanthin provides 1 μg retinol

Although carotenoids are highly bioavailable from supplements, their bioavailability from foods varies widely. Absorption for β-carotene from vegetables ranges from 18% to 26% for carrots[277] to 5% for spinach.[278] One study found that, although a β-carotene-enriched wafer when fed to women markedly improved serum retinol levels, a similar amount of β-carotene when fed in the form of green leafy vegetables had no effect.[279] Similarly, although van net Hof et al[280] found that consumption of spinach did not affect plasma levels of β-carotene, when the spinach matrix was disrupted through liquification, β-carotene absorption was enhanced.[278,280]

Because carotenoids are fat soluble, absorption may be compromised by very low-fat diets. Research suggests that cooking enhances absorption of some carotenoids such as lycopene.[281] In one recent study, serum levels of lycopene were low in subjects following a raw foods diet.[282] However, cooking for prolonged periods at high temperatures can reduce the bioavailability of some carotenoids.

In the United States, provitamin A carotenoids contribute 26 and 34% of vitamin A consumed by men and women, respectively, using the new RAE. In lacto-ovo vegetarians, this ratio increases, and in vegans, all the vitamin A comes from carotenoids. However, because vitamin A content of fruits and vegetables is only half what has been shown in food composition tables, vegan intake is half what has been reported in earlier studies, and some vegans and lacto-ovo vegetarians may not meet the vitamin A RDA. However, it should be relatively easy for vegetarians to meet vitamin A needs if foods rich in the provitamin A carotenoids are chosen frequently.

Not surprisingly, carotenoid intake[283,284] and serum carotenoid levels are about twice as high in vegetarians as in nonvegetarians.[56,180,285,286] Many of the carotenoids, such as β-carotene and lycopene, are excellent antioxidants. In contrast, retinol has no antioxidant activity.[276,287] Carotenoids may reduce cancer risk and heart disease[288–290] and help prevent the development of cataracts[291,292] and macular degeneration.[293,294] There also appear to be potentially important synergistic effects between β-carotene and vitamin E.[295] Finally, even in vitamin A-sufficient animals, carotenoids, both with and without provitamin A activity, enhance the immune system.[296] Consequently, there seems to be considerable advantage to meeting vitamin A needs via the carotenoids.

Although vitamin A is toxic in large amounts, the carotenoids are not. The tolerable upper intake level for vitamin A is 3000 μg. A benign condition called carotenodermia characterized by a jaundice-like yellowing of the skin and high plasma carotenoid concentrations can occur when large amounts of carotene-rich foods are ingested.[297] This condition, however, which is harmless, is most likely to occur only when juices made from carotenoid-rich foods or dietary supplements are consumed.

VITAMIN E

Vitamin E was not recognized formally by the National Research Council as an essential nutrient until 1968. Vitamin E deficiency occurs rarely and has been seen in premature, very low-birthweight infants fed formulas high in polyunsaturated fatty acids and low in vitamin E, in individuals who do not absorb fat normally, and in those with defects in the gene for α-tocopherol transfer protein. In adults, it may take 5 to 10 years of malabsorption for deficiency symptoms, which are primarily neurologic, to appear.

The two main forms of vitamin E found in foods are tocopherol and tocotrienols. Within each main group are four members, each with differing amounts of vitamin E activity. The main forms of vitamin E are α-tocopherol, β-tocopherol, γ-tocopherol, and δ-tocopherol. However, only α-tocopherol contributes toward meeting the vitamin E requirements, and therefore, in a departure from previous reports that based vitamin E recommendations on α-tocopherol equivalents, new recommendations for vitamin E by the FNB are based only on the α-tocopherol form of the vitamin.[298] The RDA for vitamin E for those ≥14 years of age is 15 mg of α-tocopherol.[298]

A number of different forms of α-tocopherol are found in chemically synthesized vitamins, most of which do not occur naturally in foods. The chemically synthesized form has 50% the vitamin activity of natural α-tocopherol.

The primary and best understood function of vitamin E is as an antioxidant. Vitamin E is found in cellular membranes in association with polyunsaturated fatty acids (PUFAs). Vitamin E traps free radicals, thereby preventing the oxidation of PUFAs, which are susceptible to oxidation. Increased amounts of free radicals are associated with many diseases, most notably heart disease and cancer but also cataracts and arthritis; they may even hasten the aging process.[299] One symptom of a lack of vitamin E is the hemolysis of erythrocytes. The membranes of red blood cells become more fragile without the protection of vitamin E.

Two studies involving >87,000 female and about 40,000 male health professionals found that people who consumed the largest amounts of vitamin E had about a 33% reduced risk of coronary heart disease.[300,301] However, in the more recent Physicians' Health II study, a randomized placebo-controlled trial of 14,641 men, vitamin E supplementation of 400 IU/d in combination with 500 mg vitamin C per day did not reduce risk for cardiovascular events.[302] A study of >34,000 postmenopausal women found a reduction in heart disease risk only with vitamin E from foods, not from supplements.[303] Vitamin E has also been investigated in relationship to prostate cancer risk, but the results have been disappointing. Vitamin E supplementation had no effect on cancer risk in the Physicians' Health Study[304] or in the Selenium and Vitamin E Cancer Prevention Trial.[305] Among subjects with vascular disease or diabetes, vitamin E supplementation had no effect on cancer risk or cardiovascular events.[306]

Because vitamin E protects PUFAs from oxidation, the biologic requirements for vitamin E are based on the relative amount of dietary PUFA consumed, although the relationship between vitamin E and PUFA intake is complex. However, increased vitamin E is needed when PUFA intake is high. It is thought that 0.4 mg of RRR-α-tocopherol is needed for every gram of PUFA consumed.[307] In extreme situations, the need for α-tocopherol may vary by as much as a factor of 4 depending on the type of diet consumed. Not surprisingly, vegetarians tend to consume more polyunsaturated fat than saturated fat. Vegetarians' absolute intake of PUFA in many studies is similar to omnivores due to their overall lower fat intake (Appendix A). In other studies, however, PUFA intake is as much as 50% higher than in nonvegetarians.

Based on CSFII data, the median dietary intake of vitamin E is 7.5 mg for men and 5.4 mg for women.[298] Most studies show that vegetarians consume about 50–100% more vitamin E than omnivores (Appendix K). Therefore, although vegetarians may need more vitamin E because of their higher PUFA intake, in most instances, the vitamin E to PUFA dietary intake ratio is higher among vegetarians than nonvegetarians, providing greater protection against the potentially harmful effects of free radicals.

Foods high in PUFA are also high in vitamin E. Thus vegetable oils are rich sources, but many oils, such as soybean oil, corn oil, and rapeseed oil, have excessive amounts of PUFAs relative to their vitamin E content.[308] On the basis of ratios of vitamin E to PUFA, olive oil and sunflower oil are good sources of vitamin E, whereas soybean oil, corn oil, and rapeseed oil are not. Some vegetables are also rich in vitamin E. Half an avocado contains 1.3 mg of vita-

Table 7-12 Vitamin E Content of Foods

Food	Vitamin E Content (mg ATE)	Food	Vitamin E Content (mg ATE)
Breads, cereals, grains		**Legumes**	
Wheat germ, 2 tbsp	2.5	Soybeans, ½ cup	0.3
Quinoa, ½ cup	0.58	**Nuts/seeds**	
Vegetables, ½ cup cooked unless otherwise indicated		Almond butter, 2 tbsp	8.3
		Almonds, ¼ cup	7.8
Avocado, ½ raw	2	Hazelnuts, ¼ cup	4.32
Kohlrabi	0.43	Peanuts, ¼ cup	3
Mustard greens	0.85	Peanut butter, 2 tbsp	2.9
Parsnips	0.8	**Vegetable oils,** 1 tsp	
Pumpkin, canned	1.3	Canola oil	0.79
Kelp	0.9	Corn oil	0.64
Spinach	1.9	Olive oil	0.65
Swiss chard	1.6	Peanut oil	0.71
Stewed tomatoes	1.1	Safflower oil	1.53
Turnip greens	1.35	Soybean oil	0.37
Fruits, 1 medium		Sunflower oil	1.85
Apple	0.33	Wheat germ oil	6.72
Mango	2.3	Mayonnaise	0.3–1.3 (varies by brand)
Pear	0.28	Margarine, 1 tsp	2–3 (varies by brand)
Pomegranate	1.7		
Miscellaneous			
Almond Breeze brand almond milk, 1 cup	10.0		

Source: Data from USDA National Nutrient Database for Standard Reference, Release 22, 2009 and manufacturers' information.

min E, and ½ cup of turnip greens, mustard greens, pumpkin, or Swiss chard contains >1 mg (Table 7-12).

Because of their higher vitamin E intake and lower serum cholesterol levels, most studies, but not all, indicate that vegetarians have higher serum ratios of vitamin E to cholesterol,[309–312] suggesting that their LDL cholesterol will be more resistant to oxidation.[225,286,309–311,312] Vitamin C levels are also higher in vegetarians, and vitamin C, vitamin E, and perhaps β-carotene may work together to inhibit oxidation. Although all the fat-soluble vitamins can cause toxic effects when consumed in excessive amounts, vitamin E is relatively nontoxic even when consumed at levels >50 times the RDA.[314,254]

VITAMIN K

Compounds with vitamin K activity are essential for the formation of prothrombin and at least five other proteins involved in the regulation of blood clotting. Vitamin K deficiency results in defective coagulation. Vitamin K is also required for the synthesis of other proteins found in plasma, bone, and kidney. There are two different forms of vitamin K. Phylloquinone (vitamin K_1), is the only form found in plants and is the primary dietary source of vitamin K. Menaquinone (vitamin K_2), is made by bacteria and makes only a minor contribution to vitamin K intake. Its absorption appears to be limited.[315] Animal foods contain both types of vitamin K.

Although stores of vitamin K are relatively small, vitamin K deficiency in adults is rare for at least three reasons. First, vitamin K is widely distributed in plants and animals, although many foods contain only small amounts. Second, the body tends to conserve this vitamin. Third, human colon bacteria synthesize significant quantities of vitamin K, although the extent to which bacterial synthesis contributes to vitamin K nutriture is unclear. Some reports suggest that it plays a key role,[316] whereas others suggest only a minor role, if any.[317]

For these reasons, only adults treated chronically with broad-spectrum antibiotics (which reduce bacterial synthesis of vitamin K) or people who suffer from malabsorption are at risk of acute vitamin K deficiency. Many older hospitalized patients have low blood levels of vitamin K, however, and respond to vitamin K administration.[318] These findings in the elderly may be particularly important because new insight into the biologic functions of vitamin K suggest that it may have an important role in bone health. For example, research has shown that elderly women with hip fractures have much lower serum levels of vitamin K than elderly women without hip fracture[319] and that men and pre- and postmenopausal women who consumed more vitamin K had a lower risk for hip fracture.[320,321] Low dietary vitamin K intakes have been associated with reduced BMD in women.[322] Vitamin K supplements were also associated with improved bone metabolism in female elite athletes.[323] Lower circulating phylloquinone and menaquinone concentrations have been seen in some subjects with reduced BMD[324,325] but not all.[326] A recent randomized controlled trial of 4015 Japanese subjects found no effect of vitamin D_2 on incidence of vertebral fracture, although there was evidence that vitamin K was effective in postmenopausal women with severe osteoporosis.[327] A review of the literature by Iwamoto et al found that any effect of vitamin K appears to be independent of bone mineral density.[328]

Although outright vitamin K deficiency is rare in adults, vitamin K deficiency in breastfed newborn infants remains a major worldwide cause of infant morbidity and mortality.[329] In the United States, injections of vitamin K for newborn infants are standard procedure.

Older assays overestimated the vitamin K content of foods, and surveys indicated that vitamin K content greatly exceeded requirements. Because recommendations for vitamin K have increased and dietary intake is lower than previously believed, it appears that many people may not meet vitamin K needs.

The AI for adult men and women is 120 μg and 90 μg, respectively. Data summarized by Booth and Suttie show that average daily vitamin K intake to be 150 μg for people >55 years of age and 80 μg for younger adults.[330] According to NHANES III data, average intake was 79 to 88 μg and 89 to 117 μg for adult men and women, respectively. Based on 14-day food records, Booth et al found that average intake is between 70 and 80 μg.[331] Green leafy vegetables are the major source of vitamin K, whereas animal products, fruits, and grains are extremely poor sources (Table 7-13). For example, just one serving of kale provides more than five times the RDA for vitamin K. In omnivore diets, green leafy vegetables contribute 40–50% of phylloquinone intake.[332,333] Soybean, cottonseed, canola, and olive oils are other good sources of vitamin K; 1 tbsp of soybean oil provides about a third of the RDA. Fermented soybean products are also good sources of vitamin K.

Fat enhances vitamin K absorption. Vitamin K from cooked spinach was only 4% as bioavailable as that from a supplement, but the addition of butter increased absorption threefold.[334] Vegetarians should easily be able to meet their vitamin K needs; very limited available data suggest this is the case.[335]

Vitamin K is generally not toxic. Even large amounts ingested over an extended period of time do not produce any overt signs of toxicity,[336] although administration of the synthetic vitamin K menadione can be toxic.[336] Also, the vitamin K status of patients receiving anticoagulant drugs (which inhibit the clotting action of vitamin K) should be carefully monitored, particularly if individuals make marked changes in their intake of foods high in vitamin K.

Table 7-13 Vitamin K Content of Foods

Food	Vitamin K Content
Vegetables, ½ cup cooked	
Asparagus	45
Broccoli	110
Brussels sprouts	109
Cabbage	81
Collard greens	418
Kale	531
Romaine lettuce, 1 cup raw	48
Spinach	444
Turnip greens	265
Miscellaneous	
Soybean oil, 1 tsp	8.3
Miso, 1 tbsp	15.0

Source: Data from USDA National Nutrient Database for Standard Reference, Release 22, 2009.

Case Study

Carolynn is a 57-year-old lacto-ovo vegetarian woman. Recent blood work showed that her intake of vitamin B_{12} is low. She also broke her wrist last year and is concerned about bone health.

Her 24-hour recall

Breakfast
   1 cup cooked oatmeal
   ½ cup 2% milk
   1 banana
   1 slice whole wheat bread
   1 tbsp peanut butter
   1 cup coffee with 2 tbsp nondairy creamer

Snack
   6 oz non-fat strawberry yogurt
   2 graham crackers

Lunch
   Sandwich:
      2 slices whole wheat bread
      2 oz vegetarian "turkey" slices

Sliced tomato
Lettuce
1 tbsp low-fat mayonnaise

Snack
   Apple
   ¼ cup soynuts

Dinner
   1 cup brown rice
   1 cup curried lentils
   1 cup steamed carrots
   ½ cup strawberry sorbet

Daily vitamin supplements: 1000 mg calcium, 1000 IU vitamin D, a multivitamin pill that contains 10 μg vitamin B_{12}.

What changes would you suggest to Carolynn's diet to reduce her risk for bone loss? Is she taking appropriate and sufficient supplements to meet vitamin B_{12} needs?

REFERENCES

1. Bor MV, von Castel-Roberts KM, Kauwell GP, et al. Daily intake of 4 to 7 microg dietary vitamin B-12 is associated with steady concentrations of vitamin B-12-related biomarkers in a healthy young population. *Am J Clin Nutr.* 2010;91(3):571–577.
2. Herbert V, Drivas G, Manusselis C, Mackler B, Eng J, Schwartz E. Are colon bacteria a major source of cobalamin analogues in human tissues? 24-hr human stool contains only about 5 micrograms of cobalamin but about 100 micrograms of apparent analogue (and 200 micrograms of folate). *Trans Assoc Am Physicians.* 1984;97:161–171.
3. Cooper B, Rosenblatt D. Inherited defects of vitamin B12 metabolism. *Annu Rev Nutr.* 1987;7:291–320.
4. De Meer K, Finglas PM, Molloy A, et al. Position paper: goals for folate and related vitamins in Europe and the developing world. *Eur J Clin Nutr.* 2005;34:187–193.
5. Pfeiffer CM, Johnson CL, Jain RB, et al. Trends in blood folate and vitamin B-12 concentrations in the United States, 1988–2004. *Am J Clin Nutr.* 2007;86(3):718–727.
6. Haan MN, Miller JW, Aiello AE, et al. Homocysteine, B vitamins, and the incidence of dementia and cognitive impairment: results from the Sacramento Area Latino Study on Aging. *Am J Clin Nutr.* 2007;85(2):511–517.
7. Smith AD, Refsum H. Vitamin B-12 and cognition in the elderly. *Am J Clin Nutr.* 2009;89(2):707S–711S.
8. Raman G, Tatsioni A, Chung M, et al. Heterogeneity and lack of good quality studies limit association between folate, vitamins B-6 and B-12, and cognitive function. *J Nutr.* 2007;137(7):1789–1794.

9. Su TC, Jeng JS, Wang JD, et al. Homocysteine, circulating vascular cell adhesion molecule and carotid atherosclerosis in postmenopausal vegetarian women and omnivores. *Atherosclerosis.* 2006;184(2):356–362.
10. Herbert V. Recommended dietary intakes (RDI) of vitamin B-12 in humans. *Am J Clin Nutr.* 1987;45(4):671–678.
11. Allen RH, Stabler SP, Savage DG, Lindenbaum J. Metabolic abnormalities in cobalamin (vitamin B12) and folate deficiency. *Faseb J.* 1993;7(14):1344–1353.
12. Louwman MW, van Dusseldorp M, van de Vijver FJ, et al. Signs of impaired cognitive function in adolescents with marginal cobalamin status. *Am J Clin Nutr.* 2000;72(3):762–769.
13. von Schenck U, Bender-Gotze C, Koletzko B. Persistence of neurological damage induced by dietary vitamin B-12 deficiency in infancy. *Arch Dis Child.* 1997;77:137–139.
14. Crane MG, Register UD, Lukens RH, Gregory R. Cobalamin (CBL) studies on two total vegetarian (vegan) families. *Veg Nutr.* 1998;2:87–92.
15. Miller DR, Specker BL, Ho ML, Norman EJ. Vitamin B-12 status in a macrobiotic community. *Am J Clin Nutr.* 1991;53(2):524–529.
16. Donaldson MS. Metabolic vitamin B(12) status on a mostly raw vegan diet with follow-up using tablets, nutritional yeast, or probiotic supplements. *Ann Nutr Metab.* 2000;44(5–6):229–234.
17. Tucker KL, Mahnken B, Wilson PW, Jacques P, Selhub J. Folic acid fortification of the food supply. Potential benefits and risks for the elderly population. *JAMA.* 1996;276(23):1879–1885.
18. Hirsch S, de la Maza P, Barrera G, Gattas V, Petermann M, Bunout D. The Chilean flour folic acid fortification program reduces serum homocysteine levels and masks vitamin B-12 deficiency in elderly people. *J Nutr.* 2002;132(2):289–291.
19. Selhub J, Morris MS, Jacques PF, Rosenberg IH. Folate-vitamin B-12 interaction in relation to cognitive impairment, anemia, and biochemical indicators of vitamin B-12 deficiency. *Am J Clin Nutr.* 2009;89(2):702S–706S.
20. Allen LH. How common is vitamin B-12 deficiency? *Am J Clin Nutr.* 2009;89(2):693S–696S.
21. Ford ES, Smith SJ, Stroup DF, Steinberg KK, Mueller PW, Thacker SB. Homocyst(e)ine and cardiovascular disease: a systematic review of the evidence with special emphasis on case-control studies and nested case-control studies. *Int J Epidemiol.* 2002;31(1):59–70.
22. Seshadri S, Beiser A, Selhub J, et al. Plasma homocysteine as a risk factor for dementia and Alzheimer's disease. *N Engl J Med.* 2002;346(7):476–483.
23. Omenn GS, Beresford SA, Motulsky AG. Preventing coronary heart disease: B vitamins and homocysteine. *Circulation.* 1998;97(5):421–424.
24. Mann NJ, Li D, Sinclair AJ, et al. The effect of diet on plasma homocysteine concentrations in healthy male subjects. *Eur J Clin Nutr.* 1999;53(11):895–899.
25. Mezzano D, Munoz X, Martinez C, et al. Vegetarians and cardiovascular risk factors: hemostasis, inflammatory markers and plasma homocysteine. *Thromb Haemost.* 1999;81(6):913–917.
26. Herrmann W, Schorr H, Obeid R, Geisel J. Vitamin B-12 status, particularly holotranscobalamin II and methylmalonic acid concentrations, and hyperhomocysteinemia in vegetarians. *Am J Clin Nutr.* 2003;78(1):131–136.
27. Misra A, Vikram NK, Pandey RM, et al. Hyperhomocysteinemia, and low intakes of folic acid and vitamin B12 in urban North India. *Eur J Nutr.* 2002;41(2):68–77.
28. Herrmann W, Schorr H, Purschwitz K, Rassoul F, Richter V. Total homocysteine, vitamin B(12), and total antioxidant status in vegetarians. *Clin Chem.* 2001;47(6):1094–1101.
29. Hung CJ, Huang PC, Lu SC, et al. Plasma homocysteine levels in Taiwanese vegetarians are higher than those of omnivores. *J Nutr.* 2002;132(2):152–158.
30. Bissoli L, Di Francesco V, Ballarin A, et al. Effect of vegetarian diet on homocysteine levels. *Ann Nutr Metab.* 2002; 46(2):73–79.
31. Huang YC, Chang SJ, Chiu YT, Chang HH, Cheng CH. The status of plasma homocysteine and related B-vitamins in healthy young vegetarians and nonvegetarians. *Eur J Nutr.* 2003;42(2):84–90.
32. Obeid R, Geisel J, Schorr H, Hubner U, Herrmann W. The impact of vegetarianism on some haematological parameters. *Eur J Haematol.* 2002;69(5–6):275–279.
33. Dhonukshe-Rutten RA, van Dusseldorp M, Schneede J, de Groot LC, van Staveren WA. Low bone mineral density and bone mineral content are associated with low cobalamin status in adolescents. *Eur J Nutr.* 2005;44(6):341–347.
34. Herbert V. Staging vitamin B-12 (cobalamin) status in vegetarians. *Am J Clin Nutr.* 1994;59(5 suppl):1213S–1222S.

35. Herrmann W, Geisel J. Vegetarian lifestyle and monitoring of vitamin B-12 status. *Clin Chim Acta*. 2002;326 (1–2):47–59.

36. Herbert V. The 1986 Herman award lecture. Nutrition science as a continually unfolding story: the folate and vitamin B-12 paradigm. *Am J Clin Nutr*. 1987;46(3):387–402.

37. Bjorke Monsen AL, Ueland PM. Homocysteine and methylmalonic acid in diagnosis and risk assessment from infancy to adolescence. *Am J Clin Nutr*. 2003;78(1):7–21.

38. Clarke R, Refsum H, Birks J, et al. Screening for vitamin B-12 and folate deficiency in older persons. *Am J Clin Nutr*. 2003;77(5):1241–1247.

39. Miller JW, Garrod MG, Rockwood AL, et al. Measurement of total vitamin B12 and holotranscobalamin, singly and in combination, in screening for metabolic vitamin B12 deficiency. *Clin Chem*. 2006;52(2):278–285.

40. Stanger O, Weger M. Interactions of homocysteine, nitric oxide, folate and radicals in the progressively damaged endothelium. *Clin Chem Lab Med*. 2003;41(11):1444–1454.

41. Antoniades C, Antonopoulos AS, Tousoulis D, Marinou K, Stefanadis C. Homocysteine and coronary atherosclerosis: from folate fortification to the recent clinical trials. *Eur Heart J*. 2009;30(1):6–15.

42. Toole JF, Malinow MR, Chambless LE, et al. Lowering homocysteine in patients with ischemic stroke to prevent recurrent stroke, myocardial infarction, and death: the Vitamin Intervention for Stroke Prevention (VISP) randomized controlled trial. *JAMA*. 2004;291(5):565–575.

43. Lonn E, Yusuf S, Arnold MJ, et al. Homocysteine lowering with folic acid and B vitamins in vascular disease. *N Engl J Med*. 2006;354(15):1567–1577.

44. Bazzano LA, Reynolds K, Holder KN, He J. Effect of folic acid supplementation on risk of cardiovascular diseases: a meta-analysis of randomized controlled trials. *JAMA*. 2006;296(22):2720–2726.

45. Albert A, Altabre C, Baro F, et al. Efficacy and safety of a phytoestrogen preparation derived from Glycine max (L.) Merr in climacteric symptomatology: a multicentric, open, prospective and non-randomized trial. *Phytomedicine*. 2002;9(2):85–92.

46. Balk EM, Raman G, Tatsioni A, Chung M, Lau J, Rosenberg IH. Vitamin B_6, B_{12}, and folic acid supplementation and cognitive function: a systematic review of randomized trials. *Arch Intern Med*. 2007;167(1):21–30.

47. Morris MS, Jacques PF, Selhub J. Relation between homocysteine and B-vitamin status indicators and bone mineral density in older Americans. *Bone*. 2005;37(2):234–242.

48. Cagnacci A, Baldassari F, Rivolta G, Arangino S, Volpe A. Relation of homocysteine, folate, and vitamin B_{12} to bone mineral density of postmenopausal women. *Bone*. 2003;33(6):956–959.

49. Sato Y, Honda Y, Iwamoto J, Kanoko T, Satoh K. Effect of folate and mecobalamin on hip fractures in patients with stroke: a randomized controlled trial. *JAMA*. 2005;293(9):1082–1088.

50. Yazdanpanah N, Zillikens MC, Rivadeneira F, et al. Effect of dietary B vitamins on BMD and risk of fracture in elderly men and women: the Rotterdam study. *Bone*. 2007;41(6):987–994.

51. Krivosikova Z, Krajcovicova-Kudlackova M, Spustova V, et al. The association between high plasma homocysteine levels and lower bone mineral density in Slovak women: the impact of vegetarian diet. *Eur J Nutr*. 2010;49(3):147–153.

52. Herrmann M, Widmann T, Colaianni G, Colucci S, Zallone A, Herrmann W. Increased osteoclast activity in the presence of increased homocysteine concentrations. *Clin Chem*. 2005;51(12):2348–2353.

53. Waldmann A, Koschizke JW, Leitzmann C, Hahn A. Homocysteine and cobalamin status in German vegans. *Public Health Nutr*. 2004;7(3):467–472.

54. Sanders TA, Ellis FR, Dickerson JW. Haematological studies on vegans. *Br J Nutr*. 1978;40(1):9–15.

55. Bar-Sella P, Rakover Y, Ratner D. Vitamin B12 and folate levels in long-term vegans. *Isr J Med Sci*. 1990;26:309–312.

56. Ellis FR, Montegriffo VM. Veganism, clinical findings and investigations. *Am J Clin Nutr*. 1970;23(3):249–255.

57. Dong A, Scott SC. Serum vitamin B12 and blood cell values in vegetarians. *Ann Nutr Metab*. 1982;26(4):209–216.

58. Millet P, Guilland JC, Fuchs F, Klepping J. Nutrient intake and vitamin status of healthy French vegetarians and nonvegetarians. *Am J Clin Nutr*. 1989;50(4):718–727.

59. Helman AD, Darnton-Hill I. Vitamin and iron status in new vegetarians. *Am J Clin Nutr*. 1987;45(4):785–789.

60. Haddad EH, Berk LS, Kettering JD, Hubbard RW, Peters WR. Dietary intake and biochemical, hematologic, and immune status of vegans compared with nonvegetarians. *Am J Clin Nutr*. 1999;70(3 suppl):586S–593S.

61. Hokin BD, Butler T. Cyanocobalamin (vitamin B-12) status in Seventh-day Adventist ministers in Australia. *Am J Clin Nutr*. 1999;70(3 suppl):576S–578S.

62. Herman SK, Parnell WH. The nutritional health of New Zealand vegetarian and non- vegetarian Seventh-day Adventists, selected vitamin, mineral and lipid levels. *NZ Med J.* 1998;111:91–94.

63. Kwok T, Cheng G, Woo J, Lai WK, Pang CP. Independent effect of vitamin B12 deficiency on hematological status in older Chinese vegetarian women. *Am J Hematol.* 2002;70(3):186–190.

64. Tungtrongchitr R, Pongpaew P, Prayurahong B, et al. Vitamin B12, folic acid and haematological status of 132 Thai vegetarians. *Int J Vitam Nutr Res.* 1993;63(3):201–207.

65. Areekul S, Churdchu K, Pungpapong V. Serum folate, vitamin B12 and vitamin B12 binding protein in vegetarians. *J Med Assoc Thai.* 1988;71(5):253–257.

66. Mehta BM, Rege DV, Satoskar RS. Serum vitamin B12, and folic acid activity in lactovegetarians and nonvegetarian healthy adult Indians. *Am J Clin Nutr.* 1964;15:77–84.

67. Specker BL, Miller D, Norman EJ, Greene H, Hayes KC. Increased urinary methylmalonic acid excretion in breast-fed infants of vegetarian mothers and identification of an acceptable dietary source of vitamin B-12. *Am J Clin Nutr.* 1988;47(1):89–92.

68. van Dusseldorp M, Schneede J, Refsum H, et al. Risk of persistent cobalamin deficiency in adolescents fed a macro-biotic diet in early life. *Am J Clin Nutr.* 1999;69(4):664–671.

69. Sanders TA, Ellis FR, Dickerson JW. Studies of vegans: the fatty acid composition of plasma choline phosphoglycer-ides, erythrocytes, adipose tissue, and breast milk, and some indicators of susceptibility to ischemic heart disease in vegans and omnivore controls. *Am J Clin Nutr.* 1978;31(5):805–813.

70. Crane MGS, C, Patchett S, Register UD. Vitamin B12 studies in total vegetarians (vegans). *J Nutr Med.* 1994; 4:419–430.

71. Solberg EE, Magnus E, Sander J, Loeb M. Vegetarians and vitamin B12. A controlled trial of vitamin B12 status in 63 lactovegetarians [in Norwegian]. *Tidsskr Nor Laegeforen.* 1994;114(22):2601–2602.

72. Majchrzak D, Singer I, Manner M, et al. B-vitamin status and concentrations of homocysteine in Austrian omni-vores, vegetarians and vegans. *Ann Nutr Metab.* 2006;50(6):485–491.

73. Quinlivan EP, McPartlin J, McNulty H, et al. Importance of both folic acid and vitamin B12 in reduction of risk of vascular disease. *Lancet.* 2002;359(9302):227–228.

74. Waldmann A, Koschizke JW, Leitzmann C, Hahn A. German vegan study: diet, life-style factors, and cardiovascular risk profile. *Ann Nutr Metab.* 2005;49(6):366–372.

75. Karabudak E, Kiziltan G, Cigerim N. A comparison of some of the cardiovascular risk factors in vegetarian and omnivorous Turkish females. *J Hum Nutr Diet.* 2007;21:13–22.

76. Chen CW, Lin YL, Lin TK, Lin CT, Chen BC, Lin CL. Total cardiovascular risk profile of Taiwanese vegetarians. *Eur J Clin Nutr.* 2008;62(1):138–144.

77. Yajnik CS, Lubree HG, Thuse NV, et al. Oral vitamin B_{12} supplementation reduces plasma total homocysteine con-centration in women in India. *Asia Pac J Clin Nutr.* 2007;16(1):103–109.

78. Koebnick C, Garcia AL, Dagnelie PC, et al. Long-term consumption of a raw food diet is associated with favorable serum LDL cholesterol and triglycerides but also with elevated plasma homocysteine and low serum HDL choles-terol in humans. *J Nutr.* 2005;135(10):2372–2378.

79. Fata FT, Herzlich BC, Schiffman G, Ast AL. Impaired antibody responses to pneumococcal polysaccharide in elderly patients with low serum vitamin B12 levels. *Ann Intern Med.* 1996;124(3):299–304.

80. Hesseltime CW, Smith M, Bradle R, Djien KS. Investigations of tempeh, an Indonesian food. *Dev Indian Microbiol.* 1963;4:275–280.

81. Van Veen AG, Steinkraus KH. Nutritive values and wholesomeness of fermented foods. *J Agric Food Chem.* 1970; 18:576–579.

82. Truesdell DD, Green NR, Acosta PB. Vitamin B12 activity in miso and tempeh. *J Food Sci.* 1977;52:493–494.

83. Areekul S, Cheeramakara C, Nitavapabskoon S, Pattanamatum S, Churdchue K, Chongsanguan M. The source and content of vitamin B12 in the tempehs. *J Med Assoc Thailand.* 1990;73:153–156.

84. van den Berg H, Dagnelie PC, van Staveren WA. Vitamin B12 and seaweed. *Lancet.* 1988;1:242–243.

85. Long A. Vitamin B12 for vegans. *BMJ.* 1977;2:191.

86. Jathar VS, Desphande LV, Kulkarni PR, Satoskar RS, Rege DV. Vitamin B12 like activity in leafy vegetables. *Indian J Biochem Biophys.* 1974;11:71–73.

87. Herbert V, Drivas G, Ghu M, Levitt D, Cooper B. Differential radioassays better measure cobalamin content of vitamins and "health foods" than do macrobiologic assays. Some products sold to vegetarians as rich vitamin B12

sources are not. The official United States Pharmacopeia (USP) method (L leichmanii) and E gracilis assay as vitamin B12 non-cobalamin corrinoids. *Blood.* 1983;62:(suppl 1):37A.

88. Herbert V, Drivas G. Spirulina and vitamin B12. *JAMA.* 1982;248:3096–3097.

89. Watanabe F, Katsura H, Takenaka S, et al. Pseudovitamin B(12) is the predominant cobamide of an algal health food, spirulina tablets. *J Agric Food Chem.* 1999;47(11):4736–4741.

90. Watanabe F. Vitamin B12 sources and bioavailability. *Exp Biol Med (Maywood).* 2007;232(10):1266–1274.

91. Dagnelie PC, van Staveren WA, van den Berg H. Vitamin B-12 from algae appears not to be bioavailable. *Am J Clin Nutr.* 1991;53(3):695–697.

92. Rauma AL, Torronen R, Hanninen O, Mykkanen H. Vitamin B-12 status of long-term adherents of a strict uncooked vegan diet ("living food diet") is compromised. *J Nutr.* 1995;125(10):2511–2515.

93. Miyamoto E, Yabuta Y, Kwak CS, Enomoto T, Watanabe F. Characterization of vitamin B12 compounds from Korean purple laver (Porphyra sp.) products. *J Agric Food Chem.* 2009;57(7):2793–2796.

94. Koyyalamudi SR, Jeong SC, Cho KY, Pang G. Vitamin B12 is the active corrinoid produced in cultivated white button mushrooms (Agaricus bisporus). *J Agric Food Chem.* 2009;57(14):6327–6333.

95. La Guardia M, Venturella G, Venturella F. On the chemical composition and nutritional value of pleurotus taxa growing on umbelliferous plants (apiaceae). *J Agric Food Chem.* 2005;53(15):5997–6002.

96. Carmel R, Karnaze DS, Weiner JM. Neurologic abnormalities in cobalamin deficiency are associated with higher cobalamin "analogue" values than are hematologic abnormalities. *J Lab Clin Med.* 1988;111(1):57–62.

97. Yamada K, Yamada Y, Fukuda M, Yamada S. Bioavailability of dried asakusanori (porphyra tenera) as a source of cobalamin (vitamin B12). *Int J Vitam Nutr Res.* 1999;69(6):412–418.

98. Halsted JA, Carroll J, Robert S. Serum and tissue concentration of vitamin B12 in certain pathologic states. *N Engl J Med.* 1959;260:575–580.

99. Mozafar A, Oertli JJ. Uptake of a microbially-produced vitamin (B12) by soybean roots. *Plant Soil.* 1992;139:23–30.

100. Armstrong BK. Absorption of vitamin B12 from the human colon. *Am J Clin Nutr.* 1968;21:298–299.

101. Albert MJ, Mathan VI, Baker SJ. Vitamin B12 synthesis by human small intestinal bacteria. *Nature.* 1980;283(5749):781–782.

102. Kapadia CR, Mathan VI, Baker SJ. Free intrinsic factor in the small intestine in man. *Gastroenterology.* 1976;70(5 Pt 1):704–706.

103. Bhat P, Shantakumari S, Rajan D, et al. Bacterial flora of the gastrointestinal tract in southern Indian control subjects and patients with tropical sprue. *Gastroenterology.* 1972;62(1):11–21.

104. Rose CS, Gyorgy P, Butler M, et al. Age differences in vitamin B6 status of 617 men. *Am J Clin Nutr.* 1976;29(8):847–853.

105. Fabian E, Majchrzak D, Dieminger B, Meyer E, Elmadfa I. Influence of probiotic and conventional yoghurt on the status of vitamins B1, B2 and B6 in young healthy women. *Ann Nutr Metab.* 2008;52(1):29–36.

106. Hardinge MG, Gibb DS, Oakley SD, Hardinge MO, Register UD. New dietary source of vitamin B12 [abstract]. *Fed Proc.* 1974;33:665.

107. Lampkin BC, Saunders EF. Nutritional vitamin B12 deficiency in an infant. *J Pediatr.* 1969;75:1053–1055.

108. Higginbottom MC, Sweetman L, Nyhan WL. A syndrome of methylmalonic aciduria, homocystinuria, megaloblastic anemia and neurologic abnormalities in a vitamin B12- deficient breast- fed infant of a strict vegetarian. *N Engl J Med.* 1978;299(7):317–323.

109. Davis JR Jr, Goldenring J, Lubin BH. Nutritional vitamin B12 deficiency in infants. *Am J Dis Child.* 1981;135(6):566–567.

110. Wrighton MC, Manson JL, Speed I, Robertson E, Chapman E. Brain damage in infancy and dietary vitamin B12 deficiency. *Med J Aust.* 1979;2:1–3.

111. Gambon RC, Lentze MJ, Rossi E. Megaloblastic anaemia in one of monozygous twins breast fed by their vegetarian mother. *Eur J Pediatr.* 1986;145(6):570–571.

112. Grahamn SM, Arvela OM, Wise GA. Long-term neurologic consequences of nutritional vitamin B12 deficiency in infants. *J Pediatr.* 1992;121:710–714.

113. Sklar R. Nutritional vitamin B12 deficiency in a breast-fed infant of a vegan-diet mother. *Clin Pediatr (Phila).* 1986;25(4):219–221.

114. Specker BL, Black A, Allen L, Morrow F. Vitamin B-12: low milk concentrations are related to low serum concentrations in vegetarian women and to methylmalonic aciduria in their infants. *Am J Clin Nutr*. 1990;52(6):1073–1076.

115. MacPhee AJ, Davidson GP, Leahy M, Beare T. Vitamin B12 deficiency in a breast-fed infant. *Arch Dis Child*. 1988;63:921–923.

116. Vitamin B12 deficiency in strict vegetarians. *N Engl J Med*. 1978;299(23):1319–1320.

117. Zmora E, Gorodischer R, Bar-Ziv J. Multiple nutritional deficiencies in infants from a strict vegetarian community. *Am J Dis Child*. 1979;133(2):141–144.

118. Ashkenazi S, Weitz R, Varsano I, Mimouni M. Vitamin B12 deficiency due to a strictly vegetarian diet in adolescence. *Clin Pediatr (Phila)*. 1987;26(12):662–663.

119. Shinwell ED, Gorodischer R. Totally vegetarian diets and infant nutrition. *Pediatrics*. 1982;70(4):582–586.

120. Lovblad K, Ramelli G, Remonda L, Nirkko AC, Ozdoba C, Schroth G. Retardation of myelination due to dietary vitamin B12 deficiency: cranial MRI findings. *Pediatr Radiol*. 1997;27(2):155–158.

121. Renault F, Verstichel P, Ploussard JP, Costil J. Neuropathy in two cobalamin-deficient breast-fed infants of vegetarian mothers. *Muscle Nerve*. 1999;22(2):252–254.

122. Grattan-Smith PJ, Wilcken B, Procopis PG, Wise GA. The neurological syndrome of infantile cobalamin deficiency: developmental regression and involuntary movements. *Mov Disord*. 1997;12(1):39–46.

123. Neurologic impairment in children associated with maternal dietary deficiency of cobalamin—Georgia, 2001. *MMWR Morb Mortal Wkly Rep*. 2003;52(4):61–64.

124. Allen LH. Impact of vitamin B-12 deficiency during lactation on maternal and infant health. *Adv Exp Med Biol*. 2002;503:57–67.

125. Baker SJ, Jacob E, Rajan KT, Swaminathan SP. Vitamin B12 deficiency in pregnancy and the puerperium. *Br Med J*. 1962;16:1658–1661.

126. Gingliani ERJ, Jorge SM, Goncalves AL. Serum vitamin B12 levels in parturients, in the intervillous space of the placenta and in full-term newborns and their interrelationships with folate levels. *Am J Clin Nutr*. 1985;41:330–335.

127. Ford C, Rendle M, Tracy M, Richardson V, Ford H. Vitamin B12 levels in human milk during the first nine months of lactation. *Int J Vit Nutr Res*. 1996;66:329.

128. Allen LH, Rosado JL, Casterline JE, et al. Vitamin B-12 deficiency and malabsorption are highly prevalent in rural Mexican communities. *Am J Clin Nutr*. 1995;62(5):1013–1019.

129. Danielson L, Enecksson E, Hagenfeldt L, Rasmussen EB, Tillberg E. Failure to thrive due to subclinical maternal pernicious anemia. *Acta Paediatr Scand*. 1988;77:310–311.

130. Johnson RP, Roloff JS. Vitamin B12 deficiency in an infant strictly breastfed by a mother with latent pernicious anemia. *J Pediatr*. 1982;100:917–919.

131. Carmel R. Pernicous anemia: the expected findings of very low serum cobalamin levels, anemia, and macrocytosis are often lacking. *Arch Intern Med*. 1988;148:1712–1714.

132. Lubby AL, Cooperman JM, Donnfeld AM. Observations on transfer of vitamin B12 from mother to fetus and newborn. *Am J Dis Child*. 1958;96:532–533.

133. Black AK, Allen LH, Pelto GH, de Mata MP, Chavez A. Iron, vitamin B-12 and folate status in Mexico: associated factors in men and women and during pregnancy and lactation. *J Nutr*. 1994;124(8):1179–1188.

134. Kuhne T, Bubl R, Baumgartner R. Maternal vegan diet causing a serious infantile neurological disorder due to vitamin B12 deficiency. *Eur J Pediatr*. 1991;150(3):205–208.

135. Davey GK, Spencer EA, Appleby PN, Allen NE, Knox KH, Key TJ. EPIC-Oxford: lifestyle characteristics and nutrient intakes in a cohort of 33,883 meat-eaters and 31,546 non meat-eaters in the UK. *Public Health Nutr*. 2003;6(3):259–269.

136. Tucker KL, Rich S, Rosenberg I, et al. Plasma vitamin B-12 concentrations relate to intake source in the Framingham Offspring study. *Am J Clin Nutr*. 2000;71(2):514–522.

137. Messina V, Melina V, Mangels AR. A new food guide for North American vegetarians. *J Am Diet Assoc*. 2003;103(6):771–775.

138. Delpre G, Sark P, Niv Y. Sublingual therapy for cobalamin supplementation. *Lancet*. 1999;354:740–741.

139. Slot WB, Merkus FW, Van Deventer SJ, Tytgat GN. Normalization of plasma vitamin B12 concentration by intranasal hydroxocobalamin in vitamin B12-deficient patients. *Gastroenterology*. 1997;113(2):430–433.

140. Joosten E, van den Berg A, Riezler R, et al. Metabolic evidence that deficiencies of vitamin B-12 (cobalamin), folate, and vitamin B-6 occur commonly in elderly people. *Am J Clin Nutr.* 1993;58(4):468–476.

141. Lindenbaum J, Rosenberg IH, Wilson PW, Stabler SP, Allen RH. Prevalence of cobalamin deficiency in the Framingham elderly population. *Am J Clin Nutr.* 1994;60(1):2–11.

142. Healton EB, Savage DG, Brust JC, Garrett TJ, Lindenbaum J. Neurologic aspects of cobalamin deficiency. *Medicine (Baltimore).* 1991;70(4):229–245.

143. Ba A. Metabolic and structural role of thiamine in nervous tissues. *Cell Mol Neurobiol.* 2008;28(7):923–931.

144. Institute of Medicine. *Dietary Reference Intakes for Thiamin, Riboflavin, Niacin, Vitamin B6, Folate, Vitamin B12, Pantothenic Acid, Biotin, and Choline.* Washington, DC: National Academy Press; 1998.

145. Subar AF, Krebs-Smith SM, Cook A, Kahle LL. Dietary sources of nutrients among US adults, 1989 to 1991. *J Am Diet Assoc.* 1998;98(5):537–547.

146. Hilker DM, Somogyi JC. Antithiamins of plant origin: their chemical nature and mode of action. *Ann N Y Acad Sci.* 1982;378:137–145.

147. Vimokesant S, Kunjara S, Rungruangsak K, Nakornchai S, Panijpan B. Beriberi caused by antithiamin factors in food and its prevention. *Ann N Y Acad Sci.* 1982;378:123–136.

148. Tayter M, Stanek KL. Anthropometric and dietary assessment of omnivore and lacto-ovo-vegetarian children. *J Am Diet Assoc.* 1989;89(11):1661–1663.

149. Janelle KC, Barr SI. Nutrient intakes and eating behavior scores of vegetarian and nonvegetarian women. *J Am Diet Assoc.* 1995;95(2):180–186, 1899, quiz 187–188.

150. U.S. Department of Agriculture. *Nationwide Food Consumption Survey. Continuing Survey of Food Intakes by Individuals: Women 19–50 Years and Their Children 1–5 Years, 4 Days, 1985.* Hyattsville, MD: Nutrition Monitoring Division, Human Nutrition Information Service; 1986. Report 85.4.

151. U.S. Department of Agriculture. *Nationwide Food Consumption Survey. Continuing Survey of Food Intakes by Individuals. Men 19–50 Years, 1 Day, 1988.* Hyattsville, MD: Nutrition Monitoring Division, Human Nutrition Information Service, US Department of Agriculture; 1986. Report 85.3.

152. http://www.ars.usda.gov/SP2UserFiles/Place/12355000/pdf/0506/Table_1_NIF_05.pdf.

153. Keys A, Henschel AF, Mickelson O, Brozak JM, Crawford JH. Physiological and biochemical functions in normal young men on a diet restricted in riboflavin. *J Nutr.* 1944;27:165–178.

154. Horwitt MK, Harvey CC, Hills OW, Liebert E. Correlation of urinary excretion of riboflavin with dietary intake and symptoms of ariboflavinosis. *J Nutr.* 1950;41:247–264.

155. Sterner RT, Price WR. Sterner RT, Price WR. Restricted riboflavin: within-subject behavioral effects in humans. *Am J Clin Nutr.* 1973;26:150–160.

156. Prasad PA, Bamji MS, Lakshmi AV, Satyanarayana K. Functional impact of riboflavin supplementation in urban school children. *Nutr Res.* 1990;10:275–281.

157. Tavares NR, Moreira PA, Amaral TF. Riboflavin supplementation and biomarkers of cardiovascular disease in the elderly. *J Nutr Health Aging.* 2009;13(5):441–446.

158. McNulty H, Dowey le RC, Strain JJ, et al. Riboflavin lowers homocysteine in individuals homozygous for the MTHFR 677C->T polymorphism. *Circulation.* 2006;113(1):74–80.

159. Draper A, Lewis J, Malhotra N, Wheeler E. The energy and nutrient intakes of different types of vegetarian: a case for supplements? [published erratum appears in *Br J Nutr.* 1993;70(3):812]. *Br J Nutr.* 1993;69(1):3–19.

160. Carlson E, Kipps M, Lockie A, Thomson J. A comparative evaluation of vegan, vegetarian and omnivore diets. *J Plant Foods.* 1985;6:89–100.

161. Hughes J, Sanders TAB. Riboflavin levels in the diet and breast milk of vegans and omnivores. *Proc Nutr Soc.* 1979; 38:95A.

162. Jones PH. Expert perspective: reducing cardiovascular risk in metabolic syndrome and type 2 diabetes mellitus beyond low-density lipoprotein cholesterol lowering. *Am J Cardiol.* 2008;102(12A):41L–47L.

163. Carter EGA, Carpenter KJ. The bioavailability for humans of bound niacin from wheat bran. *Am J Clin Nutr.* 1982;36:855–861.

164. Goldsmith GA. Experimental niacin deficiency. *J Am Diet Assoc.* 1956;32:312–316.

165. Jain SK. Vitamin B6 (pyridoxamine) supplementation and complications of diabetes. *Metabolism.* 2007;56(2):168–171.

166. Olsen A, Halkjaer J, van Gils CH, et al. Dietary intake of the water-soluble vitamins B1, B2, B6, B12 and C in 10 countries in the European Prospective Investigation into Cancer and Nutrition. *Eur J Clin Nutr.* 2009;63(suppl 4):S122–S149.

167. McCully KS. Homocysteine, folate, vitamin B6, and cardiovascular disease. *JAMA*. 1998;279(5):392–393.

168. Dalery K, Lussier-Cacan S, Selhub J, Davignon J, Latour Y, Genest J Jr. Homocysteine and coronary artery disease in French Canadian subjects: relation with vitamins B12, B6, pyridoxal phosphate, and folate. *Am J Cardiol*. 1995; 75(16):1107–1111.

169. Ellis JM, McCully KS. Prevention of myocardial infarction by vitamin B6. *Res Commun Mol Pathol Pharmacol*. 1995;89(2):208–220.

170. Kelly PJ, Shih VE, Kistler JP, et al. Low vitamin B6 but not homocyst(e)ine is associated with increased risk of stroke and transient ischemic attack in the era of folic acid grain fortification. *Stroke*. 2003;34(6):e51–e54.

171. Lowik MR, Schrijver J, van den Berg H, Hulshof KF, Wedel M, Ockhuizen T. Effect of dietary fiber on the vitamin B6 status among vegetarian and nonvegetarian elderly (Dutch nutrition surveillance system). *J Am Coll Nutr*. 1990;9(3):241–249.

172. Kretsch MJ, Sauberlich HE, Johnson HL, Skala JH. Effect of animal or plant protein composition on the vitamin B6 requirement of young women [abstract]. *Fed Proc*. 1982;21:227.

173. Kretsch MJ, Sauberlich HE, Skala JH, Johnson HL. Vitamin B-6 requirement and status assessment: young women fed a depletion diet followed by a plant- or animal-protein diet with graded amounts of vitamin B-6. *Am J Clin Nutr*. 1995;61(5):1091–1101.

174. Leklem JE, Miller LT, Perera AD, Pefers DE. Bioavailability of vitamin B-6 from wheat bread in humans. *J Nutr*. 1980;110(9):1819–1828.

175. Lindberg AS, Leklem JE, Miller LT. The effect of wheat bran on the bioavailability of vitamin B-6 in young men. *J Nutr*. 1983;113(12):2578–2586.

176. Greenwood DC, Cade JE, White K, Burley VJ, Schorah CJ. The impact of high non-starch polysaccharide intake on serum micronutrient concentrations in a cohort of women. *Public Health Nutr*. 2004;7(4):543–548.

177. Waldmann A, Dorr B, Koschizke JW, Leitzmann C, Hahn A. Dietary intake of vitamin B6 and concentration of vitamin B6 in blood samples of German vegans. *Public Health Nutr*. 2006;9(6):779–784.

178. Shultz TD, Leklem JE. Vitamin B-6 status and bioavailability in vegetarian women. *Am J Clin Nutr*. 1987; 46(4):647–651.

179. Brants HA, Lowik MR, Westenbrink S, Hulshof KF, Kistemaker C. Adequacy of a vegetarian diet at old age (Dutch Nutrition Surveillance System). *J Am Coll Nutr*. 1990;9(4):292–302.

180. Lowik MR, Schrijver J, Odink J, van den Berg H, Wedel M. Long-term effects of a vegetarian diet on the nutritional status of elderly people (Dutch Nutrition Surveillance System). *J Am Coll Nutr*. 1990;9(6):600–609.

181. Toohey ML, Harris MA, DeWitt W, Foster G, Schmidt WD, Melby CL. Cardiovascular disease risk factors are lower in African-American vegans compared to lacto-ovo- vegetarians [see comments]. *J Am Coll Nutr*. 1998;17(5): 425–434.

182. Shultz TD, Leklem JE. Nutrient intake and hormonal status of premenopausal vegetarian Seventh- day Adventists and premenopausal nonvegetarians. *Nutr Cancer*. 1983;4(4):247–259.

183. Donaldson M. Food and nutrient intake of Hallelujah vegetarians. *Nutr Food Sci*. 2001;31:293–303.

184. Larsson CL, Johansson GK. Dietary intake and nutritional status of young vegans and omnivores in Sweden. *Am J Clin Nutr*. 2002;76(1):100–106.

185. Marti-Carvajal AJ, Sola I, Lathyris D, Salanti G. Homocysteine lowering interventions for preventing cardiovascular events. *Cochrane Database Syst Rev*. 2009(4):CD006612.

186. Mason JB, Levesque T. Mason JB, Levesque T. Folate: effects on carcinogenesis and the potential for cancer chemoprevention. *Oncology*. 1996;10:1727–1736.

187. Giovannucci E, Rimm EB, Ascherio A, Stampfer MJ, Colditz GA, Willett WC. Alcohol, low-methionine-low folate diets and risk of colon cancer in men. *J Natl Cancer Inst*. 1995;87:265–273.

188. Bingham S. The fibre-folate debate in colo-rectal cancer. *Proc Nutr Soc*. 2006;65(1):19–23.

189. Houghton LA, Green TJ, Donovan UM, Gibson RS, Stephen AM, O'Connor DL. Association between dietary fiber intake and the folate status of a group of female adolescents. *Am J Clin Nutr* .1997;66(6):1414–1421.

190. Krause LJ, Forsberg CW, O'Connor DL. Feeding human milk to rats increases Bifidobacterium in the cecum and colon which correlates with enhanced folate status. *J Nutr*. 1996;126(5):1505–1511.

191. Krajcovicova-Kudlackova M, Blazicek P, Mislanova C, Valachovicova M, Paukova V, Spustova V. Nutritional determinants of plasma homocysteine. *Bratisl Lek Listy*. 2007;108(12):510–515.

192. Zempleni J, Wijeratne SS, Hassan YI. *Biotin Biofactors*. 2009;35(1):36–46.

193. Baugh CM, Malone JW, Butterworth CE Jr, Baugh CM, Malone JW, Butterworth CE Jr. Human biotin deficiency. A case of biotin deficiency induced by raw egg consumption in a cirrhotic patient. *Am J Clin Nutr.* 1968;21:173–182.

194. Lombard KA, Mock DM. Biotin nutritional status of vegans, lactoovovegetarians, and nonvegetarians. *Am J Clin Nutr.* 1989;50(3):486–490.

195. Tarr JB, Tamura T, Stokstad ELR. Availability of vitamin B6 and pantothenate in an average American diet in man. *Am J Clin Nutr.* 1981;34:1328–1337.

196. Srinivasan V, Christensen N, Wyse BW, Hansen RG. Pantothenic acid nutritional status in the elderly—institutionalized and noninstitutionalized. *Am J Clin Nutr.* 1981;34:1736–1742.

197. Hemilä H. Does vitamin C alleviate the symptoms of the common cold? A review of current evidence. *Scand J Infect Dis Suppl.* 1994;26:1–6.

198. Jariwalla RJ, Harakeh S. Antiviral and immunomodulatory activities of ascorbic acid. *Subcell Biochem.* 1996;25:213–231.

199. Heimer KA, Hart AM, Martin LG, Rubio-Wallace S. Examining the evidence for the use of vitamin C in the prophylaxis and treatment of the common cold. *J Am Acad Nurse Pract.* 2009;21(5):295–300.

200. Honarbakhsh S, Schachter M. Vitamins and cardiovascular disease. *Br J Nutr.* 2009;101(8):1113–1131.

201. Krajcovicova-Kudlackova M, Valachovicova M, Paukova V, Dusinska M. Effects of diet and age on oxidative damage products in healthy subjects. *Physiol Res.* 2008;57(4):647–651.

202. Szeto YT, Kwok TC, Benzie IF. Effects of a long-term vegetarian diet on biomarkers of antioxidant status and cardiovascular disease risk. *Nutrition.* 2004;20(10):863–866.

203. Outila TA, Mattila PH, Piironen VI, Lamberg-Allardt CJ. Bioavailability of vitamin D from wild edible mushrooms (*Cantharellus tubaeformis*) as measured with a human bioassay. *Am J Clin Nutr.* 1999;69(1):95–98.

204. Heaney RP, Abraham S, Dawson-Hughes B, et al. Peak bone mass. *Osteoporos Int.* 2000;11:985–1009.

205. Heaney RP. Vitamin D and calcium interactions: functional outcomes. *Am J Clin Nutr.* 2008;88(2):541S–544S.

206. Janssen HC, Samson MM, Verhaar HJ. Vitamin D deficiency, muscle function, and falls in elderly people. *Am J Clin Nutr.* 2002;75(4):611–615.

207. Bischoff-Ferrari HA, Dawson-Hughes B, Willett WC, et al. Effect of vitamin D on falls: a meta-analysis. *JAMA.* 2004;291(16):1999–2006.

208. Wang TJ, Pencina MJ, Booth SL, et al. Vitamin D deficiency and risk of cardiovascular disease. *Circulation.* 2008;117(4):503–511.

209. Pittas AG, Lau J, Hu FB, Dawson-Hughes B. The role of vitamin D and calcium in type 2 diabetes. A systematic review and meta-analysis. *J Clin Endocrinol Metab.* 2007;92(6):2017–2029.

210. Freedman DM, Looker AC, Chang SC, Graubard BI. Prospective study of serum vitamin D and cancer mortality in the United States. *J Natl Cancer Inst.* 2007;99(21):1594–1602.

211. Munger KL, Levin LI, Hollis BW, Howard NS, Ascherio A. Serum 25-hydroxyvitamin D levels and risk of multiple sclerosis. *JAMA.* 2006;296(23):2832–2838.

212. Oudshoorn C, Mattace-Raso FU, van der Velde N, Colin EM, van der Cammen TJ. Higher serum vitamin D3 levels are associated with better cognitive test performance in patients with Alzheimer's disease. *Dement Geriatr Cogn Disord.* 2008;25(6):539–543.

213. Dent CE, Smith R. Nutritional osteomalacia. *Q J Med.* 1969;38:195–209.

214. Institute of Medicine. *Dietary Reference Intakes for Calcium, Phosphorus, Magnesium, Vitamin D, and Fluoride.* Washington, DC: National Academy Press; 1997.

215. Holick MF. Vitamin D deficiency. *N Engl J Med.* 2007;357(3):266–281.

216. Glerup H, Mikkelsen K, Poulsen L, et al. Commonly recommended daily intake of vitamin D is not sufficient if sunlight exposure is limited. *J Intern Med.* 2000;247(2):260–268.

217. Nesby-O'Dell S, Scanlon KS, Cogswell ME, et al. Hypovitaminosis D prevalence and determinants among African American and white women of reproductive age: third National Health and Nutrition Examination Survey, 1988–1994. *Am J Clin Nutr.* 2002;76(1):187–192.

218. Murphy SP, Calloway DH. Nutrient intakes of women in NHANES II, emphasizing trace minerals, fiber, and phytate. *J Am Diet Assoc.* 1986;86(10):1366–1372.

219. Yetley EA. Assessing the vitamin D status of the US population. *Am J Clin Nutr.* 2008;88(2):558S–564S.

220. Specker BL, Valanis B, Hertzberg V, Edwards N, Tsang RC. Sunshine exposure and serum 25-hydroxyvitamin D concentrations in exclusively breast-fed infants. *J Pediatr.* 1985;107(3):372–376.

221. Sato Y, Iwamoto J, Kanoko T, Satoh K. Amelioration of osteoporosis and hypovitaminosis D by sunlight exposure in hospitalized, elderly women with Alzheimer's disease: a randomized controlled trial. *J Bone Miner Res.* 2005; 20(8):1327–1333.

222. Haddad JG. Vitamin D—solar rays, the Milky Way, or both? *N Engl J Med.* 1992;326(18):1213–1215.

223. Cosman F, Nieves J, Dempster D, Lindsay R. Vitamin D economy in blacks. *J Bone Miner Res.* 2007;22(suppl 2): V34–V38.

224. Poskitt EM, Cole TJ, Lawson DE. Diet, sunlight, and 25-hydroxy vitamin D in healthy children and adults. *BMJ.* 1979;1(6158):221–223.

225. Kumpusalo E, Karinpää A, Jauhiainen M, Laitinen Lappeteläinen R, Mäenpää PH. Multivitamin supplementation of adult omnivores and lactovegetarians: Circulating levels of vitamin A, D, and E, lipids, apolipoproteins and selenium. *Int J Vitam Nutr Res.* 1989;60:58–66.

226. Webb AR, Kline L, Holick MF. Influence of season and latitude on the cutaneous synthesis of vitamin D3: exposure to winter sunlight in Boston and Edmonton will not promote vitamin D3 synthesis in human skin. *J Clin Endocrinol Metab.* 1988;67(2):373–378.

227. Clemens TL, Adams JS, Henderson SL, Holick MF. Increased skin pigment reduces the capacity of skin to synthesise vitamin D3. *Lancet.* 1982;1(8263):74–76.

228. Matsuoka LY, Ide L, Wortsman J, MacLaughlin JA, Holick MF. Sunscreens suppress cutaneous vitamin D3 synthesis. *J Clin Endocrinol Metab.* 1987;64(6):1165–1168.

229. Holick MF, Matsuoka LY, Wortsman J. Regular use of sunscreen on vitamin D levels. *Arch Dermatol.* 1995;131(11): 1337–1339.

230. Matsuoka LY, Wortsman J, Hanifan N, Holick MF. Chronic sunscreen use decreases circulating concentrations of 25- hydroxyvitamin D. A preliminary study. *Arch Dermatol.* 1988;124(12):1802–1804.

231. Gesensway D. Vitamin D. *Ann Intern Med.* 2000;133(4):318.

232. Gilchrest BA. Sun exposure and vitamin D sufficiency. *Am J Clin Nutr.* 2008;88(2):570S–577S.

233. Hellebostad M, Markestad T, Seeger Halvorsen K. Vitamin D deficiency rickets and vitamin B12 deficiency in vegetarian children. *Acta Paediatr Scand.* 1985;74(2):191–195.

234. Fitzpatrick S, Sheard NF, Clark NG, Ritter ML. Vitamin D-deficient rickets: a multifactorial disease. *Nutr Rev.* 2000;58(7):218–222.

235. Pugliese MT, Blumberg DL, Hludzinski J, Kay S. Nutritional rickets in suburbia. *J Am Coll Nutr.* 1998;17(6):637–641.

236. Kreiter SR, Schwartz RP, Kirkman HN, Charlton PA, Calikoglu AS, Davenport ML. Nutritional rickets in African American breast-fed infants. *J Pediatr.* 2000;137(2):153–157.

237. Eugster EA, Sane KS, Brown DM. Minnesota rickets. Need for a policy change to support vitamin D supplementation. *Minn Med.* 1996;79(8):29–32.

238. Rovner AJ, O'Brien KO. Hypovitaminosis D among healthy children in the United States: a review of the current evidence. *Arch Pediatr Adolesc Med.* 2008;162(6):513–519.

239. Iq-bal SJ. Evidence of continuing deprivational vitamin D deficiency in Asians in the UK. *J Hum Nutr Diet.* 1994;7:47–52.

240. Dent CE, Round JM, Rowe DJ, Stamp TC. Effect of chapattis and ultraviolet irradiation on nutritional rickets in an Indian immigrant. *Lancet.* 1973;1(7815):1282–1284.

241. Cooke WT, Asquith P, Ruck N, Melikian V, Swan CH. Rickets, growth, and alkaline phosphatase in urban adolescents. *Br Med J.* 1974;2(914):293–297.

242. Hunt SP, O'Riordan JL, Windo J, Truswell AS. Vitamin D status in different subgroups of British Asians. *BMJ.* 1976;2(6048):1351–1354.

243. Pietrek J, Preece MA, Windo J, et al. Prevention of vitamin-D deficiency in Asians. *Lancet.* 1976;1(7970):1145–1148.

244. Dandona P, Mohiuddin J, Weerakoon JW, Freedman DB, Fonseca V, Healey T. Persistence of parathyroid hypersecretion after vitamin D treatment in Asian vegetarians. *J Clin Endocrinol Metab.* 1984;59(3):535–537.

245. Henderson JB, Dunnigan MG, McIntosh WB, Abdul-Motaal AA, Gettinby G, Glekin BM. The importance of limited exposure to ultraviolet radiation and dietary factors in the aetiology of Asian rickets: a risk-factor model. *Q J Med.* 1987;63(241):413–425.

246. Awumey EM, Mitra DA, Hollis BW, Kumar R, Bell NH. Vitamin D metabolism is altered in Asian Indians in the southern United States: a clinical research center study. *J Clin Endocrinol Metab*. 1998;83(1):169–173.
247. Chan J, Jaceldo-Siegl K, Fraser GE. Serum 25-hydroxyvitamin D status of vegetarians, partial vegetarians, and non-vegetarians: the Adventist Health Study-2. *Am J Clin Nutr*. 2009;89(5):1686S–1692S.
248. Outila TA, Lamberg-Allardt CJ. Ergocalciferol supplementation may positively affect lumbar spine bone mineral density of vegans [letter]. *J Am Diet Assoc*. 2000;100(6):629.
249. Robertson I, Ford JA, McIntosh WB, Dunnigan MG. The role of cereals in the aetiology of nutritional rickets: the lesson of the Irish National Nutrition Survey 1943–8. *Br J Nutr*. 1981;45(1):17–22.
250. Batchelor AJ, Compston JE. Reduced plasma half-life of radio-labelled 25-hydroxyvitamin D3 in subjects receiving a high-fibre diet. *Br J Nutr*. 1983;49(2):213–216.
251. Pettifor JM, Daniels ED. Vitamin D deficiency and nutritional rickets in children. In: Feldman D, Glorieux FH, Pike JW, eds. *Vitamin D*. San Diego, CA: Academic Press; 1997:663–678.
252. Dwyer JT, Dietz WH Jr, Hass G, Suskind R. Risk of nutritional rickets among vegetarian children. *Am J Dis Child*. 1979;133(2):134–140.
253. Roberts IF, West RJ, Ogilvie D, Dillon MJ. Malnutrition in infants receiving cult diets: a form of child abuse. *BMJ*. 1979;1(6159):296–298.
254. Dagnelie PC, Vergote FJ, van Staveren WA, van den Berg H, Dingjan PG, Hautvast JG. High prevalence of rickets in infants on macrobiotic diets. *Am J Clin Nutr*. 1990;51(2):202–208.
255. Lamberg-Allardt C, Karkkainen M, Seppanen R, Bistrom H. Low serum 25- hydroxyvitamin D concentrations and secondary hyperparathyroidism in middle-aged white strict vegetarians. *Am J Clin Nutr*. 1993;58(5):684–689.
256. Maierhofer WJ, Gray RW, Cheung HS, Lemann J Jr. Bone resorption stimulated by elevated serum 1,25-(OH)2-vitamin D concentrations in healthy men. *Kidney Int*. 1983;24(4):555–560.
257. American Academy of Pediatrics. The prophylactic requirement and the toxicity of vitamin D. *Pediatrics*. 1963;31: 512–525.
258. Department of Health and Human Services. Grade "A" pasteurized milk ordinance. In: 21 CFR 131.110, 1989:243.
259. Lightwood R. Idiopathic hypercalcaemia with failure to thrive: Nephrocalcinosis. *Proc R Soc Med*. 1952;45:401.
260. Clemens TL, O'Riordan JLH. Vitamin D. In: Becker KL, ed. *Principles and Practice of Endocrinology and Metabolism*. Philadelphia, PA: Lippincott; 1990:417–423.
261. Chen TC, Shao A, Heath H 3rd, Holick MF. An update on the vitamin D content of fortified milk from the United States and Canada. *N Engl J Med*. 1993;329(20):1507.
262. Holick MF, Shao Q, Liu WW, Chen TC. The vitamin D content of fortified milk and infant formula. *N Engl J Med*. 1992;326(18):1178–1181.
263. Tanner JT, Smith J, Dfibaugh P, et al. Survey of vitamin content of fortified milk. *J Assoc Off Anal Chem*. 1988; 71:607–610.
264. Jacobus CH, Holick MF, Shao Q, et al. Hypervitaminosis D associated with drinking milk. *N Engl J Med*. 1992; 326(18):1173–1177.
265. Holick MF, MacLaughlin JA, Doppelt SH. Regulation of cutaneous previtamin D3 photosynthesis in man: skin pigment is not an essential regulator. *Science*. 1981;211(4482):590–593.
266. Armas LA, Hollis BW, Heaney RP. Vitamin D2 is much less effective than vitamin D3 in humans. *J Clin Endocrinol Metab*. 2004;89(11):5387–5391.
267. Trang HM, Cole DE, Rubin LA, Pierratos A, Siu S, Vieth R. Evidence that vitamin D3 increases serum 25-hydroxyvitamin D more efficiently than does vitamin D2. *Am J Clin Nutr*. 1998;68(4):854–858.
268. Romagnoli E, Mascia ML, Cipriani C, et al. Short and long term variations in serum calciotrophic hormones after a single very large dose of ergocalciferol (vitamin D2) or cholecalciferol (vitamin D3) in the elderly. *J Clin Endocrinol Metab*. 2008;93(8):3015–3020.
269. Glendenning P, Chew GT, Seymour HM, et al. Serum 25-hydroxyvitamin D levels in vitamin D-insufficient hip fracture patients after supplementation with ergocalciferol and cholecalciferol. *Bone*. 2009;45(5):870–875.
270. Holick MF, Biancuzzo RM, Chen TC, et al. Vitamin D2 is as effective as vitamin D3 in maintaining circulating concentrations of 25-hydroxyvitamin D. *J Clin Endocrinol Metab*. 2008;93(3):677–681.
271. Rapuri PB, Gallagher JC. Effect of vitamin D supplement use on serum concentrations of total 25OHD levels in elderly women. *J Steroid Biochem Mol Biol*. 2004;89–90(1–5):601–604.

272. Gordon CM, Williams AL, Feldman HA, et al. Treatment of hypovitaminosis D in infants and toddlers. *J Clin Endocrinol Metab.* 2008;93(7):2716–2721.

273. Thacher TD, Obadofin MO, O'Brien KO, Abrams SA. The effect of vitamin D2 and vitamin D3 on intestinal calcium absorption in Nigerian children with rickets. *J Clin Endocrinol Metab.* 2009;94(9):3314–3321.

274. Wolf G. A historical note on the mode of vitamin A for the cure of night blindness. *Am J Clin Nutr.* 1978;31:290–292.

275. Food and Agriculture Organization (FAO). *Requirements of Vitamin A, Iron, Folate, and Vitamin B12. Report of a Joint FAO/World Health Organization Expert Consultation.* Rome, Italy: Food and Agriculture Organization (FAO Food and Nutrition Series 23); 1988.

276. Krinsky NI. Antioxidant functions of carotenoids. *Free Radic Biol Med.* 1989;7:617–635.

277. Micozzi MS, Brown ED, Edwards BK, et al. Plasma carotenoid response to chronic intake of selected foods and beta- carotene supplements in men. *Am J Clin Nutr.* 1992;55(6):1120–1125.

278. Castenmiller JJ, West CE, Linssen JP, van het Hof KH, Voragen AG. The food matrix of spinach is a limiting factor in determining the bioavailability of beta-carotene and to a lesser extent of lutein in humans. *J Nutr.* 1999;129(2):349–355.

279. de Pee S, West CE, Muhilal, Karyadi D, Hautvast JG. Lack of improvement in vitamin A status with increased consumption of dark-green leafy vegetables. *Lancet.* 1995;346(8967):75–81.

280. van het Hof KH, Tijburg LB, Pietrzik K, Weststrate JA. Influence of feeding different vegetables on plasma levels of carotenoids, folate and vitamin C. Effect of disruption of the vegetable matrix. *Br J Nutr.* 1999;82(3):203–212.

281. Fielding JM, Rowley KG, Cooper P, K OD. Increases in plasma lycopene concentration after consumption of tomatoes cooked with olive oil. *Asia Pac J Clin Nutr.* 2005;14(2):131–136.

282. Garcia AL, Koebnick C, Dagnelie PC, et al. Long-term strict raw food diet is associated with favourable plasma beta-carotene and low plasma lycopene concentrations in Germans. *Br J Nutr.* 2008;99(6):1293–1300.

283. Alexander D, Ball MJ, Mann J. Nutrient intake and haematological status of vegetarians and age-sex matched omnivores. *Eur J Clin Nutr.* 1994;48(8):538–546.

284. Rana SK, Sanders TAB. Taurine concentrations in the diet, plasma, urine and breast milk of vegans compared with omnivores. *Br J Nutr.* 1986;56:17–27.

285. Rider AA, Arthur RS, Calkins BM. Diet, nutrition intake, and metabolism in populations at high and low risk for colon cancer. Laboratory analysis of 3-day composite of food samples. *Am J Clin Nutr.* 1984;40(4 suppl):914–916.

286. Malter M, Schriever G, Eilber U. Natural killer cells, vitamins, and other blood components of vegetarian and omnivorous men. *Nutr Cancer.* 1989;12(3):271–278.

287. van Poppel G. Carotenoids and cancer: an update with emphasis on human intervention studies. *Eur J Cancer.* 1993;29A:1335–1344.

288. Rao AV, Agarwal S. Role of antioxidant lycopene in cancer and heart disease. *J Am Coll Nutr.* 2000;19(5):563–569.

289. Osganian SK, Stampfer MJ, Rimm E, Spiegelman D, Manson JE, Willett WC. Dietary carotenoids and risk of coronary artery disease in women. *Am J Clin Nutr.* 2003;77(6):1390–1399.

290. McCann SE, Freudenheim JL, Marshall JR, Graham S. Risk of human ovarian cancer is related to dietary intake of selected nutrients, phytochemicals and food groups. *J Nutr.* 2003;133(6):1937–1942.

291. Hankinson SE, Stampfer MJ, Seddon JM, et al. Nutrient intake and cataract extraction in women: a prospective study. *BMJ.* 1992;305(6849):335–339.

292. Taylor A, Jacques PF, Chylack LT Jr, et al. Long-term intake of vitamins and carotenoids and odds of early age-related cortical and posterior subcapsular lens opacities. *Am J Clin Nutr.* 2002;75(3):540–549.

293. Beatty S, Koh H, Phil M, Henson D, Boulton M. The role of oxidative stress in the pathogenesis of age-related macular degeneration. *Surv Ophthalmol.* 2000;45(2):115–134.

294. Mares-Perlman JA, Millen AE, Ficek TL, Hankinson SE. The body of evidence to support a protective role for lutein and zeaxanthin in delaying chronic disease. Overview. *J Nutr.* 2002;132(3):518S–524S.

295. Palozza P, Krinsky NI. b-Carotene and a-tocopherol are synergistic antioxidants. *Arch Biochem Biophys.* 1992;297:184–187.

296. Bendich A. Carotenoids and the immune response. *J Nutr.* 1989;119:112–115.

297. Micozzi MS, Brown ED, Taylor PR, Wolfe E. Carotenodermia in men with elevated carotenoid intake from foods and beta-carotene supplements. *Am J Clin Nutr.* 1988;48(4):1061–1064.

298. Institute of Medicine. *Dietary Reference Intakes for Vitamin C, Vitamin E, Selenium, and Carotenoids.* Washington, DC: National Academy Press; 2000.

299. Cross CE. Oxygen radicals and human disease. *Ann Intern Med.* 1987;107:526–545.

300. Stampfer MJ, Hennekens CH, Manson JE, Colditz GA, Rosner B, Willett WC. Vitamin E consumption and the risk of coronary disease in women. *N Engl J Med.* 1993;328(20):1444–1449.

301. Rimm EB, Stampfer MJ, Ascherio A, Giovannucci E, Colditz GA, Willett WC. Vitamin E consumption and the risk of coronary heart disease in men. *N Engl J Med.* 1993;328(20):1450–1456.

302. Sesso HD, Buring JE, Christen WG, et al. Vitamins E and C in the prevention of cardiovascular disease in men: the Physicians' Health Study II randomized controlled trial. *JAMA.* 2008;300(18):2123–2133.

303. Kushi LH, Folsom AR, Prineas RJ, Mink PJ, Wu Y, Bostick RM. Dietary antioxidant vitamins and death from coronary heart disease in postmenopausal women. *N Engl J Med.* 1996;334(18):1156–1162.

304. Gaziano JM, Glynn RJ, Christen WG, et al. Vitamins E and C in the prevention of prostate and total cancer in men: the Physicians' Health Study II randomized controlled trial. *JAMA.* 2009;301(1):52–62.

305. Lippman SM, Klein EA, Goodman PJ, et al. Effect of selenium and vitamin E on risk of prostate cancer and other cancers: the Selenium and Vitamin E Cancer Prevention Trial (SELECT). *JAMA.* 2009;301(1):39–51.

306. Lonn E, Bosch J, Yusuf S, et al. Effects of long-term vitamin E supplementation on cardiovascular events and cancer: a randomized controlled trial. *JAMA.* 2005;293(11):1338–1347.

307. Witting LA, Lee I. Dietary levels of vitamin E and polyunsaturated fatty acids and plasma vitamin E. *Am J Clin Nutr.* 1975;28:571–576.

308. Gey KF. Extra vitamin E beyond PUFA-dependent vitamin E requirement is supplied by olive oil and sunflower oil but not by soybean oil and other oils with insufficient a- tocopherol/PUFA ratio. *Int J Vitam Nutr Res.* 1995;65:61–64.

309. Pronczuk A, Kipervarg Y, Hayes KC. Vegetarians have higher plasma alpha-tocopherol relative to cholesterol than do nonvegetarians. *J Am Coll Nutr.* 1992;11(1):50–55.

310. Reddy S, Sanders TA. Lipoprotein risk factors in vegetarian women of Indian descent are unrelated to dietary intake. *Atherosclerosis.* 1992;95(2–3):223–229.

311. Sanders TA, Roshanai F. Platelet phospholipid fatty acid composition and function in vegans compared with age- and sex-matched omnivore controls. *Eur J Clin Nutr.* 1992;46(11):823–831.

312. Waldmann A, Koschizke JW, Leitzmann C, Hahn A. Dietary intakes and blood concentrations of antioxidant vitamins in German vegans. *Int J Vitam Nutr Res.* 2005;75(1):28–36.

313. Krajcovicova-Kudlackova M, Blazicek P, Babinska K, et al. Traditional and alternative nutrition—levels of homocysteine and lipid parameters in adults. *Scand J Clin Lab Invest.* 2000;60(8):657–664.

314. Bendich A, Machlin LJ. Safety of oral intake of vitamin E. *Am J Clin Nutr.* 1988;48(3):612–619.

315. Suttie JW. The importance of menaquinones in human nutrition. *Annu Rev Nutr.* 1995;15:399–417.

316. Lipsky JJ. Nutritional sources of vitamin K. *Mayo Clin Proc.* 1994;69:462–466.

317. Morley JE, Mooradian AD, Silver AJ, Heber D, Alfin-Slater RB. Nutrition in the elderly. *Ann Intern Med.* 1988; 109(11):890–904.

318. Hasell K, Baloch KH. Vitamin K deficiency in the elderly. *Gerontol Clin.* 1970;12:10–17.

319. Hodges SJ, Akesson K, Vergnaud P, Obrant K, Delmas PD. Circulating levels of vitamins K1 and K2 decreased in elderly women with hip fracture. *J Bone Miner Res.* 1993;8(10):1241–1245.

320. Feskanich D, Weber P, Willett WC, Rockett H, Booth SL, Colditz GA. Vitamin K intake and hip fractures in women: a prospective study. *Am J Clin Nutr.* 1999;69(1):74–79.

321. Booth SL, Tucker KL, Chen H, et al. Dietary vitamin K intakes are associated with hip fracture but not with bone mineral density in elderly men and women. *Am J Clin Nutr.* 2000;71(5):1201–1208.

322. Booth SL, Broe KE, Gagnon DR, et al. Vitamin K intake and bone mineral density in women and men. *Am J Clin Nutr.* 2003;77(2):512–516.

323. Craciun AM, Wolf J, Knapen MH, Brouns F, Vermeer C. Improved bone metabolism in female elite athletes after vitamin K supplementation. *Int J Sports Med.* 1998;19(7):479–484.

324. Kanai T, Takagi T, Masuhiro K, Nakamura M, Iwata M, Saji F. Serum vitamin K level and bone mineral density in post-menopausal women. *Int J Gynaecol Obstet.* 1997;56(1):25–30.

325. Tamatani M, Morimoto S, Nakajima M, et al. Decreased circulating levels of vitamin K and 25-hydroxyvitamin D in osteopenic elderly men. *Metabolism.* 1998;47(2):195–199.

326. Rosen HN, Maitland LA, Suttie JW, Manning WJ, Glynn RJ, Greenspan SL. Vitamin K and maintenance of skeletal integrity in adults. *Am J Med.* 1993;94(1):62–68.

327. Inoue T, Fujita T, Kishimoto H, et al. Randomized controlled study on the prevention of osteoporotic fractures (OF study): a phase IV clinical study of 15-mg menatetrenone capsules. *J Bone Miner Metab.* 2009;27(1):66–75.

328. Iwamoto J, Sato Y, Takeda T, Matsumoto H. High-dose vitamin K supplementation reduces fracture incidence in postmenopausal women: a review of the literature. *Nutr Res.* 2009;29(4):221–228.

329. Lane PA, Hathaway WE. Vitamin K in infancy. *J Pediatr.* 1985;106(3):351–359.

330. Booth SL, Suttie JW. Dietary intake and adequacy of vitamin K. *J Nutr.* 1998;128(5):785–788.

331. Booth SL, Webb DR, Peters JC. Assessment of phylloquinone and dihydrophylloquinone dietary intakes among a nationally representative sample of US consumers using 14-day food diaries. *J Am Diet Assoc.* 1999;99(9):1072–1076.

332. Booth SL, Pennington JA, Sadowski JA. Food sources and dietary intakes of vitamin K-1 (phylloquinone) in the American diet: data from the FDA Total Diet Study. *J Am Diet Assoc.* 1996;96(2):149–154.

333. Bolton-Smith C, Price RJ, Fenton ST, Harrington DJ, Shearer MJ. Compilation of a provisional UK database for the phylloquinone (vitamin K1) content of foods. *Br J Nutr.* 2000;83(4):389–399.

334. Gijsbers BL, Jie KS, Vermeer C. Effect of food composition on vitamin K absorption in human volunteers. *Br J Nutr.* 1996;76(2):223–229.

335. Lloyd T, Schaeffer JM, Walker MA, Demers LM. Urinary hormonal concentrations and spinal bone densities of premenopausal vegetarian and nonvegetarian women [published erratum appears in *Am J Clin Nutr.* 1992;56(5):954]. *Am J Clin Nutr.* 1991;54(6):1005–1010.

336. Owen CAJ. Pharmacology and toxicology of the vitamin K group. In: Sebrell WH, Harris RS, eds. *The Vitamins.* New York, NY: Academic Press; 1971:492–509.

CHAPTER 8

Phytochemicals

Recognition of the potential biologic importance of dietary phytochemicals has impacted the way health professionals view the diet and health relationship. The term *phytochemical* (plant chemical) really has no formal definition in the strictest sense but is commonly used to refer to any biologically active, nonnutritive component of plants. A number of other terms that are often used interchangeable with phytochemicals include *phytonutrients* and *nutraceuticals*. The latter was originally defined as any substance that is a food or part of a food and provides medical or health benefits, including the prevention and treatment of disease.[1] Nutraceuticals have also been defined as "those diet supplements that deliver a concentrated form of a presumed bioactive agent from a food, presented in a nonfood matrix, and used to enhance health in dosages that exceed those that could be obtained from normal food."[2] In contrast to phytochemicals, nutraceuticals include both nutrients and nonnutrients.

Although not discussed in this chapter, a few biologically active nonnutrients found in animal foods, called *zoochemicals,* such as conjugated linolenic acid, have also attracted interest and very recently, the term *cosmeceuticals* (topical cosmetic-pharmaceutical hybrids) has come into being and includes some phytochemicals. Phytochemicals have been referred to as the vitamins of the 21st century, and for this reason, the phytochemical age has been referred to as the *Second Golden Age of Nutrition.*[3,4] *The Golden Age* was that truly remarkable period in nutrition history from 1910 to 1940 when all of the vitamins were identified. Of course, phytochemicals are not essential nutrients. Furthermore, it can be argued that evidence in support of the role of phytochemicals in promoting health and reducing disease risk, especially risk of chronic diseases like heart disease and cancer, has not been as forthcoming as was anticipated back in the 1980s when this field began to emerge.

Nevertheless, dietitians are often called on to know something about phytochemicals just as they are expected to know about vitamins and minerals. This is a challenging and overwhelming task in some respects because the number of potentially biologically relevant phytochemicals far exceeds the relatively few essential vitamins and minerals (Table 8-1). In addition, the chemistry of the many different classes of phytochemicals and the ways in which they can affect cellular processes can be extremely complex. Furthermore, inadequate intake of vitamins and minerals leads to well-characterized symptoms and diseases, whereas there are no accepted phytochemical deficiency diseases. Phytochemicals are primarily of interest because of their postulated protection against a variety of chronic diseases. Establishing diet–chronic disease relationships is understandably difficult, which makes identifying the precise contribution of phytochemicals to health also very tricky. Another obstacle toward understanding the phytochemical field is that are no official treatises on which health professionals can rely, unlike essential nutrients for which official bodies such as the Institute of Medicine (IOM) regularly and comprehensively review the literature.

The rapidity with which the term *phytochemicals* became a nutrition buzzword and an established specialty area among nutritionists is impressive. As late as the early 1990s, only a small minority of nutritionists would have felt comfortable discussing this subject, and yet by decade's end, phytochemicals such as resveratrol from grapes and wine and lycopene from tomatoes seemed to be discussed as much as vitamins and minerals. In more recent years, the phytochemicals (catechins) in chocolate[5] and tea[6] have been the subject of much discussion in the media and professional literature.[7] Prior to 1990, those few phytochemicals that nutritionists did recognize were considered to be antinutrients or toxicants. These include, for example, glucosinolates (goitrogens) in cabbage, protease inhibitors (inhibit protein digestion) in legumes, phytic acid (inhibits mineral absorption) in whole grains, and phytoestrogens (isoflavones) (possible endocrine disruptors) in soybeans.

The presence of phytochemicals in plant foods is relevant to all dietary patterns but may be especially important to vegetarians. Because vegetarians consume more plant foods, they can be expected to have a higher intake of phytochemicals. The objective of this chapter is not to evaluate the health effects of individual phytochemicals because that would require an entire book, many of which exist, but to provide a conceptual framework for understanding phytochemicals and their impact on the field of nutrition.

Until recently, understanding the role of phytochemicals in health and disease was limited by the lack of bioavailability data. However, this void is quickly being filled as there now exists good data for several phytochemicals including carotenoids,[8–10] flavonoids such as quercetin,[11–15] and isoflavones from soybeans,[16–18] and progress on many others within just the past couple of years has been made. However, insight into phytochemical tissue concentrations, not surprisingly, has been much slower in coming. If the phytochemical in question does not make it to the tissue in question in relevant concentrations, then theoretical discussions about potential benefits are meaningless. Relative to the serum, tissue concentrations can be equal to, lower, or higher.[19,20] Furthermore, a complete understanding of endogenous metabolism, not just bioavailability, is needed because in some instances, it may be a metabolite of the parent phytochemical found in a food that is the active or most biologically active molecule.[21] The huge interindividual differences in the metabolism of phytochemicals that exist may explain some of the inconsistency often found in the clinical literature with regard to health effects.

Another obstacle that is beginning to be overcome is the lack of comprehensive phytochemical databases.[22–28] In fact, the U.S. Department of Agriculture has available online databases of the isoflavone, carotenoid, and proanthocyanidin content of foods. Epidemiologic studies obviously depend on the accuracy of these databases. Despite the progress that has been made, when considering that plant variety, harvesting conditions, processing techniques, and many other factors

Table 8-1 Phytochemicals in Foods

Phytochemical	Reference	Good Sources*
Carotenoids		
Alpha-carotene	(19)	Pumpkin (5850 μg in ½ cup, canned)
		Carrot (2836 μg in 1 medium, raw)
Beta-carotene	(19)	Sweet potato (10,816 μg in 1 medium)
		Pumpkin (8467 μg in ½ cup, canned)
		Carrot (5390 μg in 1 medium, raw)
Beta-cryptoxanthin	(19)	Red pepper (2626 μg in 1 medium)
		Tangerine juice (1660 μg in 1 cup)
		Papaya (533 μg in ½ cup cubes)
Lycopene	(19)	Pasta sauce (19,988 μg in ½ cup)
		Watermelon (13,922 μg in 1 wedge)
		Tomato soup (13,104 μg in 1 cup, prepared)
Lutein + zeaxanthin	(19)	Kale (10,269 μg in ½ cup, cooked)
		Collard greens (7686 μg in ½ cup, cooked)
		Turnip greens (6339 μg in ½ cup, cooked)
Coumestan		
Coumesterol	(15,16)	Pinto beans (1087 μg in ½ cup)
		Mung bean sprouts (1040 μg in ½ cup)
		Alfalfa sprouts (752 μg in ½ cup)
Flavonoids		
Apigenin	(16)	Celery (3660 μg in 1 medium stalk)
Kampferol	(16)	Kale (8225 μg in ½ cup, cooked)
		Black tea (3792 μg in 8 oz)
		Green tea (2856 μg in 8 oz)
Luteolin	(16)	Celery (720 μg in 1 medium stalk)
Myrcetin	(16)	Cranberries (3696 μg in ½ cup)
		Fava beans (2210 μg in ½ cup)
		Green tea (2038 μg in 8 oz)
Procyanidin	(11)	Chocolate bar (164.7 mg in 1.3 oz bar)
		Apple (147.1 mg in 1 medium)
Quercetin	(16)	Onions (35,640 μg in ½ cup, raw)
		Cranberries (8428 μg in ½ cup)
		Vegetable soup (7498 μg in 1 cup)

(continued)

Table 8-1 Phytochemicals in Foods *(Continued)*

Phytochemical	Reference	Good Sources*
Isoflavones		
Biochanin A	(15,16)	Snow peas (2979 µg in ½ cup, raw)
		Garbanzo beans (1394 µg in ½ cup)
		Kidney beans (361 µg in ½ cup)
Daidzein	(15,16,†)	Soybeans (23,177 µg in ½ cup, cooked)
		Soynuts (22,377 µg in ¼ cup)
		Tempeh (14,600 µg in ½ cup)
Formononetin	(15)	Clover sprouts (643 µg in ½ cup)
		Alfalfa sprouts (624 µg in ½ cup)
		Licorice, black (448 µg in 1 oz)
Genistein	(†)	Soynuts (28,328 µg in ¼ cup)
		Soybeans (23,831 µg in ½ cup)
		Tempeh (20,626 µg in ½ cup)
Glycitein	(†)	Soynuts (5745 µg in ¼ cup)
		Tempeh (1743 µg in ½ cup)
		Soymilk (1344 µg in 8 oz)
Total isoflavones	(†)	Soynuts (55.2 mg in ¼ cup)
		Soybeans (47 mg in ½ cup, cooked)
		Tempeh (36.1 mg in ½ cup)
Lignans and Lignan Precursors		
Matairesinol	(16)	Flaxseed (65.2 µg in 1 tb)
Secoisolariciresinol	(16)	Flaxseed (27,096 µg in 1 tb)
Total lignans	(16)	Flaxseed (1707 µg in 1 tb)
		Soybeans (742 µg in ½ cup, cooked)
Phytosterols		
Beta-sitosterol	(16)	Green tea (529 mg in 8 oz)
		Black tea (505 mg in 8 oz)
Campesterol	(16)	Soybeans (19.8 mg in ½ cup, cooked)
		Corn, safflower, or sunflower oil (15.4 mg in 1 tb)
		Orange (15.4 mg in 1 medium)
Stigmasterol	(16)	Soybeans (34.4 mg in ½ cup, cooked)
		Kidney beans (27.3 mg in ½ cup, cooked)

*Good sources are examples of commonly used foods that have the highest amounts of a specific phytochemical in a serving.
†USDA-Iowa State University Database on the Isoflavone Content of Foods, Release 1.2-2000; available at http://www.nal.usda.gov/fnic/foodcomp/Data/isoflav/isoflav.html.

affect phytochemical content, like they do nutrient content, at best only a rough approximation of intake is possible. Still, even with these limitations, the current databases allow high and low consumers of different phytochemicals to be effectively separated.

PHYTOCHEMICALS, SECONDARY METABOLITES, AND PHYTOALEXINS

Although the concept of phytochemicals is relatively new to nutritionists, both botanists and plant chemists were well aware of phytochemicals because many are secondary metabolites. The primary metabolites in plants—amino acids, chlorophyll, nucleotides, and membrane lipids—are all identified as having direct roles in the processes of plant growth and development. In contrast, secondary metabolites cannot be directly linked to processes such as photosynthesis, respiration, solute transport, translocation, and nutrient assimilation and for this reason were, until fairly recently, thought to be waste products.

However, it gradually became apparent that, whereas primary metabolites were common to all plants, specific secondary metabolites were common to specific plants or plant species and that these secondary metabolites protected the plant against a variety of environmental insults. For this reason, many phytochemicals are classified as phytoalexins—chemicals that defend plants against a variety of insults such as attack by insects, extreme temperatures, or drought—and whose concentration increases dramatically in response to environmental stress. Phytoalexins are produced by the plant for their benefit but appear to benefit humans who consume the plants as well.

The scientific field most intimately connected to phytochemicals is pharmacognosy. Pharmacognosists identify plant components that can be used by the pharmaceutical industry as a basis for drug development. Historically, plants and plant extracts have been used to cure ailments. Hippocrates used white willow, which contains salicylic acid, the active ingredient in aspirin, to treat the aches and pains of his patients.[29] That early tradition continues today because plants still function as a key source of pharmaceuticals. Incredibly, of the 520 new drugs approved between 1983 and 1994 by the U.S. Food and Drug Administration and like entities in other countries, 30 came directly from natural product sources and 173 were either semisynthetic and derived from a natural product source or synthetically modified on a natural product patent.[30] The use of plants in folklore medicine and their contribution to the pharmaceutical industry explains why food has been referred to as a macro-drug taken three times per day. Plants from around the world continue to function as a source of new drugs.[31–35]

HISTORY OF PHYTOCHEMICALS

In some sense, 1982 may be viewed as the year the importance of phytochemicals first began to make its way into mainstream nutrition consciousness. In that year, the National Academy of Sciences, in their landmark report "Diet, Nutrition and Cancer," noted the possibility that phytochemicals in cruciferous vegetables might reduce cancer risk.[36] The emphasis on phytochemicals in cruciferous vegetables was largely due to the pioneering work of Dr. Lee Wattenberg from the University of Minnesota, who was among the first to recognize the ways in which phytochemicals might protect against cancer.[37]

Of course, it is now clear that the phytochemical content of cruciferous vegetables is no more or less impressive than many other plant foods and that the impact of phytochemicals on disease risk extends beyond cancer. In fact, in 1997, the American Heart Association published a position paper on phytochemicals and coronary heart disease.[38] Further, phytochemical supplementation has been shown to increase the effectiveness of a Mediterranean-style, low glycemic load diet on parameters associated with the metabolic syndrome and cardiovascular disease.[39] Phytochemicals such as isoflavones in soybeans have attracted attention for their possible skeletal[40] and coronary benefits[41] (Chapter 10). The proposed physiologic effects of phytochemicals are as diverse as those of vitamins and minerals.

The concept of phytochemicals led directly to the development of *functional foods*, which continues to one of the fastest growing segments of the food industry.[42] In the United States, sales are between $20 billion and $30 billion a year, which represents about 5% of the overall U.S. food market. Recent estimates for sector growth range from 8.5% to as much as 20% per year, ahead of the overall industry, where growth is estimated at 1–4% per year.[43]

But before functional foods there were designer foods. In 1989, the National Cancer Institute launched the "Designer Foods Program," a multiyear, multimillion-dollar program with the goal of developing or designing foods rich in phytochemicals that would lower cancer risk.[44,45] The term *designer foods* has largely been replaced by the term *functional foods*, referring to any food or ingredient that has a positive impact on an individual's health, physical performance, or state of mind, in addition to its nutritive value.[46] A shortened definition is "foods that provide health benefits beyond basic nutrition."[47] The IOM limits functional foods to those in which the concentrations of one or more ingredients have been manipulated or modified to enhance their contribution to a healthful diet.[48] According to the American Dietetic Association (ADA), functional foods include whole foods and fortified, enriched, or enhanced foods that "have a potentially beneficial effect on health when consumed as part of a varied diet on a regular basis, at effective levels."[49] The first ADA position paper on functional foods was published in 1995[50] and the most recent in 2009.[49] In reality this term has lost (not that it ever had much) nearly all of its meaning because there are seemingly few plant foods (and even animal foods) that do not fit this category.[51]

The ADA position paper lists as functional foods low-fat foods, oatmeal, calcium-enriched foods, all vegetables and fruits, psyllium-containing products, whole grain breads, high-fiber cereals, beverages with antioxidants, beverages with herbal additives, snack foods with echinacea, grapes, grape juice, phytosterol-enriched margarines, soy, tea, fish, beef, dairy, lamb, fermented dairy products, eggs, garlic, and many others. Given just how unrestrictive the category of functional foods is, it arguably makes more sense simply to refer to the few foods that do not qualify as functional foods (e.g., sugar, refined grains, and oils) as dysfunctional foods and everything else as just plain foods.

CLASSIFYING PHYTOCHEMICALS

For simplicity's sake, phytochemicals are divided below into three different categories that include most of the phytochemicals. They are phenolic compounds, isoprenoids, and protein-amino acid based and/or sulfur-containing compounds. By far, most phytochemicals are phenolics.

Phenolic Phytochemicals

Phenolics are derivatives of benzene (cyclic derivatives in the case of polyphenols) with one or more hydroxyl groups associated with their ring structure. There are reportedly 8000 phenolic structures, ranging from simple molecules, such as phenolic acids (e.g., gallic, vanillic, and syringic) to highly polymerized compounds such as tannins, which are found in tea.[52] The phenolics can be divided into 16 different categories, but the most important class of phenolic compounds is the flavonoids, which can be divided into 13 different classes. More than 5000 flavonoids have been identified.[52]

Isoprenoid

Isoprenoids, also called terpenoids, is one of the largest groups of secondary metabolites and therefore form the basis for many nutraceuticals. This group includes the carotenoids, tocopherols, tocotrienols, and saponins. In nature, approximately 600 carotenoids have been identified; but only about 20 of these are commonly found in foods.[53]

The principal building block molecule of these compounds is isoprene. Repeating isoprene units give rise to 10-carbon monoterpenes, such as limonene and perillyl alcohol, which are found in the oil of citrus peels and may possess anticancer activity;[54] 20-carbon diterpenes, such as kahweol and cafestol,[55,56] which are found in coffee; and 30-carbon triterpenes, such as the phytosterols that lower serum cholesterol;[57–59] and saponins, which are found in legumes[60,61] and ginseng.[62]

Amino Acid and Sulfur-Based Compounds

This group includes polypeptides, amino acids, and nitrogenous and sulfur amino acid derivatives. One amino acid of particular interest is arginine, which may increase nitric oxide synthesis, which enhances arterial relaxation.[63–65] Probably the most studied phytochemicals in this group are the glucosinolates, which are found in cruciferous vegetables, such as broccoli, cabbage, brussels sprouts, and in rapeseed oil and mustard seed. There are 10 to 12 primary glucosinolates. Two of the more well-studied glucosinolates are sulforaphane,[66–69] which is an antioxidant and may reduce breast cancer risk by affecting carcinogen or xenobiotic metabolism and regulating genes that control cell growth,[70,71] and indole-3-carbinol, which may also decrease risk of estrogen-dependent cancers, perhaps by favorably affecting estrogen metabolism[72–75] and hormone-independent cancers, through mechanisms unrelated to the estrogen receptor.[76]

Also prominent among this group are the allyl sulfur compounds found in allium vegetables, such as garlic, onions, leeks, and chives. Major allyl compounds found in garlic include allicin (diallyl trisulfide), allixin (S-allyl cysteine), and allyl mercaptan (S-allylmercaptocysteine). Garlic has a prominent role in folklore medicine and has been investigated for its role in reducing stomach cancer risk[77–80] and lowering cholesterol,[81–83] although the evidence is equivocal in both cases.

PHYTOCHEMICALS: MECHANISMS OF ACTION

There are numerous ways in which nutraceuticals exert biological effects, but several primary mechanisms have emerged, especially in regard to the risk of the major chronic diseases. These are (1) antioxidant effects, (2) effects on xenobiotic metabolism, (3) hormonal effects (estrogenic and antiestrogenic), (4) effects on signal transduction (cell regulation) pathways, and (5) anti-inflammatory and immune stimulatory effects. The following discussion focuses primarily on the first three areas. It is important to recognize in considering this discussion that there may be additive and synergistic combinations of phytochemicals and phytochemicals and nutrients[84] and that the effects of these interactions are not easy to predict from studies using isolated compounds.[85]

Free Radicals and Antioxidants

Tragic insight into the importance of free radical damage occurred during the 1940s when there was an unexplained increase in the incidence of eye damage, sometimes resulting in complete blindness, among infants born prematurely. In 1954, the cause was identified as the high oxygen concentrations in incubators used for premature babies, which resulted in oxidative damage to the eye. Because free radical damage is linked to a variety of diseases, especially cancer and heart disease, antioxidant intake is often associated with a reduced risk of chronic diseases.[86] This having been said, the role of antioxidants in reducing disease risk is uncertain. The disappointing results from clinical trials evaluating the effects of vitamin E (a major antioxidant) on heart disease risk provide many examples of this uncertainty.[87]

There are many causes of free radicals, including electromagnetic radiation from the environment, cigarette smoking, and metabolism of certain drugs via the P450 system. Furthermore, some molecules in the body naturally react with oxygen causing free radical formation. But one of the most important causes is energy production. Electrons regularly escape from the electron transport system (ETS) leading to constant generation of free radicals.[88,89] Furthermore, ETS-related free radical generation appears to increase with age, and the balance between pro-oxidants and antioxidants seems to be a critical factor in determining overall health.[90]

A common attribute among the flavonoid phytochemicals is that they all possess at least some antioxidant activity. This is because of their chemical structure. All flavonoids are comprised of a phenol ring to which is attached a hydroxyl group; it is this structure that accounts for their antioxidant activity.[91–93] Many flavonoids are good scavengers of free radicals due to the high reactivities of their hydroxyl groups. But there are as many as six different mechanisms by which flavonoids exert antioxidant activity.[94]

Research demonstrating the antioxidant effects of fruits and vegetables has found that vitamin C accounts for only a small part of this activity, clearly indicating the contribution of phytochemicals.[95–97] The antioxidant activity of one apple was found to be equivalent to that of 1500 mg of vitamin C,[98] and the antioxidant activity of 1 pound of fresh strawberries was estimated to be equivalent to that of 2.3 g of vitamin C or 3 g of vitamin E.[99] One analysis showed that the leading vegetable sources of antioxidant activities against the peroxyl radicals were green pepper, spinach, purple onion, broccoli, beet, and cauliflower.[93]

Xenobiotic Metabolism and the Cytochrome P450 System

Dietary carcinogens as well as endogenous steroids (estrogen, vitamin D, etc.) are metabolized through a system of enzymes referred to as the cytochrome P450 system, which is located in many tissues but especially the liver and intestine. One of the primary responsibilities of this system is to detoxify and eliminate carcinogens from the body.[100] The P450 system is composed of two primary phases that includes many enzymes and isoenzymes. Importantly, the activity of the P450 system is greatly affected by diet, especially by phytochemicals. It should be noted, however, that in some cases, the P450 system can actually activate carcinogens thereby increasing their carcinogenicity.[101] The glucosinolates in cruciferous vegetables are especially known for their effects on the P450 system.[102–104] The most efficient elimination of carcinogens is thought to occur when the second phase of the P450 system is enhanced to a greater extent than the first. In recent years evidence has shown that there are genetic polymorphisms regarding the enzymes involved in the P450 system and that these polymorphisms are associated with cancer risk.[105] That is, how you metabolize the many carcinogens to which you are exposed can determine in part your susceptibility to their harmful effects.

Estrogens and Antiestrogens

As long ago as 1954, Bradbury and White[106] identified 53 plants with estrogenic activity; many more have been identified since then.[106,107] Not surprisingly, the estrogenic activity of phytoestrogens is quite weak relative to the primary female sex hormone, 17β-estradiol. However, serum levels of phytoestrogens in response to the ingestion of phytoestrogen-containing foods can be an order of magnitude higher than endogenous estrogens. Thus it is not unreasonable to expect phytoestrogens to exert biologic effects.

The most studied group of phytoestrogens is the isoflavones, which are found in nutritionally significant amounts only in soybeans, although very minor amounts are found in many foods and in some alcoholic beverages.[108,109] Flax contains lignans, another group of phytoestrogens attracting attention.[110,111] But there is also an assortment of phytochemicals with weak estrogenic activity, including many of the flavonoids, such as quercetin in apples, tea, and onions, and resveratrol in grapes and wine.[112–114] Coumestans, which are found in alfalfa,[115] and glucosinolates, which are found in cruciferous vegetables,[116] also have weak estrogenic activity.

Estrogen receptors are located throughout the body; therefore the effects of phytoestrogens may be widespread. Estrogen has been postulated to reduce risk of coronary heart disease and osteoporosis, and perhaps to delay age-related declines in cognitive function and prevent Alzheimer's disease.[117] However, the disappointing results from the Women's Health Initiative Trial as well as other trials and epidemiologic studies have seriously called into question our understanding of the role of estrogen in health and disease.[118–121] Although estrogen therapy clearly reduces fracture risk for example, some of the other proposed benefits have not only not been supported by the clinical studies, but results have shown the opposite may in fact be true. For example, there is concern that for at least some women, estrogen exposure may increase risk of heart disease[122] and impair cognition.[123] It is important to recognize, however, that the health effects of estrogen noted in the clinical studies and randomized trials are based on specific hormone preparations. Much remains to be learned about the physiologic effects resulting from the use of the different hormone preparations now available, both when estrogens are used alone and when used in conjunction with different progestins, the latter of which must be taken to prevent endometrial cancer in women who have a uterus.[124]

In any event, phytoestrogens cannot be equated with the hormone estrogen, and in some instances phytoestrogens are classified as selective estrogen receptor modulators or mixed estrogen agonists/antagonists. This indicates that phytoestrogens in theory can exert estrogenic effects in some tissues and antiestrogenic or no effects in others.[125] Whether a given phytoestrogen exerts biologic activity in vivo and whether that activity is antiestrogenic or estrogenic can depend on many factors including serum and tissue phytoestrogen concentrations, type and relative amount of estrogen receptors in a given tissue, cofactors within a cell, and the hormonal milieu in which the phytoestrogen is placed. The important point is that although some insight about the possible physiologic effects of phytoestrogens can be gained from knowledge about estrogen, conclusions about the former can only be based on direct experimentation.

Signal Transduction

Cell proliferation and differentiation are regulated by cascades of enzyme activation, most of which involve protein phosphorylation. Such cascades of enzyme activation are generally known as signal transduction pathways.[126] Phytochemicals that can affect signal transduction and thus, in turn, cell proliferation and differentiation, are especially important. These processes are in some ways at the core of most pathologies including bone loss,[127] arterial plaque formation,[128] and, most importantly, cancer.[129,130] Phytochemicals that affect signal transduction in vivo hold the potential to have wide-sweeping effects. However, much of the evidence in support of the effects of phytochemicals on signal transduction comes from in vitro and animal studies.[131]

Other Mechanisms

There are many additional mechanisms by which phytochemicals may exert biologic effects in vivo. For example, several dietary components including allyl sulfur compounds in garlic may have physiologically relevant immunomodulatory effects.[132,133] Similarly, flavonoids have been shown to have a variety of effects on several different cell types of the immune system.[134-136] And the immune system may also be affected by dietary phytoestrogens.[137] A number of different classes of phytochemicals may also exert anti-inflammatory effects,[136,138] which is especially significant because inflammatory processes may be involved in the etiology of both cancer[139,140] and coronary heart disease.[141]

Finally, the rate-limiting step in arachidonate metabolism is mediated by enzymes known as cyclooxygenases (COXs). These enzymes lead to the biosynthesis of hormones such as prostaglandins, prostacyclins, and thromboxanes, which are involved in many inflammatory reactions.[142] Several of the phytochemicals, such as quercetin, have been shown to inhibit COX activity.[143,144] Of course, one reason for the interest in omega-3 fatty acids is because of their possible anti-inflammatory effects.[145,147]

PHYTOCHEMICAL INTAKE

As noted, one reason it is difficult to quantify phytochemical intake accurately is because the phytochemical content of a food differs according to the variety in question and the environmental conditions under which the plant was grown. For example, there is a fourfold difference in flavonoid and phenolic acid content among different varieties of apples[148] and a comparable range for quercetin content between red and yellow onions.[149] Similarly, the isoflavone content of soybeans can vary fourfold.[150] Nevertheless, as previously discussed, phytochemical databases do exist, and within the past few years several estimates of phytochemical intake have been published. Certainly, intake is substantial and almost certainly nutritionally relevant. In Japan, a survey of 1500 women found phytochemical intake averaged about 150 mg per day; women in the 90th percentile consumed three times more phytochemicals than the mean.[151] A small study in Mexico found that women consumed about 200 mg of selected phytochemicals per day.[152]

Using consumption levels typical of the United States, Vinson et al[153] calculated that the total intake of phenols from vegetables (garlic, legumes, and potatoes were included among the 23 vegetables considered) was 218 mg/d. This estimate is impressive considering the low intake of vegetables in the United States. Phenol intake exceeds the recommended intake levels for vitamins C and E, and β-carotene combined, and some phenols are more potent antioxidants than vitamins C and E.[154] Also, neither tea nor chocolate were included in this estimate. Average 40-gram servings of milk chocolate and dark chocolate provide 394 mg and 951 mg, respectively, of polyphenol antioxidants—mostly catechins. Tea is also a rich source of catechins.

Scalbert and Williamson[155] suggested that the estimate by Vinson et al[153] was likely exaggerated because their value may have inadvertently included some vitamin C. Nevertheless, a person consuming one large apple, a small serving of dark chocolate, a cup of black tea, and glass of red wine would consume >500 mg of phenols. And this is without the consumption of legumes, garlic, or flax. Furthermore, their estimate did not include the intake of phytosterols, phytic acid, and saponins, which could easily add another 200 to 400 mg,[156] 1000 to 2000 mg,[157] and 200 mg,[158] respectively. Although no good data exist on vegetarian intake, their often higher intakes of beans, which are high in polyphenols and saponins, and whole grains, which are very high in phenols,[159] suggest their phytochemical intake is almost certainly higher than that of nonvegetarians (Exhibit 8-1). The ADA position paper on vegetarian diets suggests vegetarian phytochemical intake is higher than that of nonvegetarians and offers this as one reason for the lower rate of certain diseases among the former.[160]

PRACTICAL IMPLICATIONS

Despite the enthusiasm, the extent to which typical intakes of phytochemicals affect disease risk is unknown. Much of the enthusiasm for the beneficial effects of phytochemicals comes from the inverse association between fruit and vegetable intake and risk of several chronic diseases including cancer, heart disease, stroke, hypertension, diverticulitis, and chronic obstructive pulmonary disease, rather than direct data on phytochemicals per se.[161] However, despite the large amount of investigation, the protective effects of fruits and vegetables, in regard to breast cancer,[162] colorectal cancer,[163] and perhaps lung cancer,[164] have been questioned. It is notable that in their comprehensive review of the scientific literature published in 2007, the American Institute for Cancer Research/World Research Cancer Fund concluded that the evidence that fruit and vegetable intake reduces cancer risk is weaker today than it was in 1997. Some have postulated that high fruit and vegetable intake is simply a marker for an overall healthy lifestyle and is not protective in and of itself.[165]

Exhibit 8-1 Comparison of Polyphenols in Sample Vegetarian and Nonvegetarian Menus

Food Vegetarian	Total phenols (mg*)
Orange juice, 4 oz	90
Black tea, 6 oz	180
Cereal (1 oz) with bran (0.3 oz)	50
Milk	—
Kidney bean burrito:	
Kidney beans, ½ cup	667
Chopped tomatoes, ¼ cup	17
Apple, 1 large	470
Carrot sticks, 8	12
Dark chocolate, 1 oz	252
Pinto beans, 1 cup	1181
Sweet potato, 1 medium, baked	85
Corn, 1 medium ear	106
Salad:	
Lettuce, 3 oz	23
Tomato, ¼ cup	17
Onion, 2 slices	18
Cherries, ½ cup	320
TOTAL	**3488**

Food Nonvegetarian	Total phenols (mg*)
Orange juice, 4 oz	90
Black tea, 6 oz	180
Cereal (1 oz) with bran (0.3 oz)	50
Milk	—
Bologna sandwich	—
Apple, 1 large	470
Carrot sticks, 8	12
Dark chocolate, 1 oz	252
Baked chicken, 4 oz	—
Mashed potato, 1 cup	57
Green beans, ½ cup	20
Salad:	
Lettuce, 3 oz	23
Tomato, ¼ cup	17
Onion, 2 slices	18
Cherries, ½ cup	320
TOTAL	**1509**

*Values based on phenols assayed with the Folin-Ciocalteu colorimetric assay except for cherry and wheat bran, which used chromatographic estimates.[117,119]
Sources: LeBlanc ES, Janowsky J, Chan BK, Nelson HD. Hormone replacement therapy and cognition: systematic review and meta-analysis. *JAMA* 2001;285:1489–1499; Yaffe K. Hormone therapy and the brain: deja vu all over again? *JAMA* 2003;289:2717-2719.

Of course, the key lesson from the study of phytochemicals is that plant foods are more than fiber, macronutrients, and vitamins and minerals. To quote from a paper published in the *Journal of the American Dietetic Association* two decades ago, "It is no longer appropriate to evaluate foods solely on the basis of their nutrient and fiber content."[3] It is likely a collective effect of phytochemicals contributes positively to human health. Increasing the overall intake of phytochemicals requires increasing the consumption of plant foods. As mentioned earlier, studies using isolated phytochemicals do not consider the possible additive and synergistic effects that occur among phytochemicals or between phytochemicals and nutrients within the same food or among different foods. Consequently, a consensus is beginning to emerge that ignoring these additive and synergistic effects, what is commonly referred to as the reductionist approach to nutrition, underestimates the true contribution of overall dietary pattern to health.[166,167] For a review of this topic, see Messina et al.[168]

Still, it is important not to let enthusiasm about the postulated health benefits of phytochemicals overshadow the importance of nutrients and other known chronic disease risk factors. In the Nurses' Health Study, for example, the risk of having a heart attack was decreased by >80% in women who regularly exercised, had normal blood pressure and cholesterol, took folate, were of normal weight, and did not smoke.[169] Furthermore, the cutoffs used for these lifestyle measures were not optimal, indicating that these factors were even more influential.

REFERENCES

1. The Foundation for Innovative Medicine. The nutraceuticals initiative: a proposal for economic and regulatory reform. *Food Technol.* 1992;6:77.
2. Zeizel S. Regulation of 'nutraceuticals.' *Science.* 1999;285:1853–1855.
3. Messina M, Messina V. Increasing use of soyfoods and their potential role in cancer prevention. *J Am Diet Assoc.* 1991;91:836–840.
4. Messina M, Messina V. Nutritional implications of dietary phytochemicals. In: American Institute for Cancer Research, ed. *Dietary Phytochemicals in Cancer Prevention and Treatment.* New York: Plenum Press; 1996.
5. Spadafranca A, Martinez Conesa C, Sirini S, Testolin G. Effect of dark chocolate on plasma epicatechin levels, DNA resistance to oxidative stress and total antioxidant activity in healthy subjects. *Br J Nutr.* 2010:103(7):1008–1014.
6. Butt MS, Sultan MT. Green tea: nature's defense against malignancies. *Crit Rev Food Sci Nutr.* 2009;49:463–473.
7. Lee KW, Kim YJ, Lee HJ, Lee CY. Cocoa has more phenolic phytochemicals and a higher antioxidant capacity than teas and red wine. *J Agric Food Chem.* 2003;51:7292–7295.
8. van het Hof KH, de Boer BC, Tijburg LB, et al. Carotenoid bioavailability in humans from tomatoes processed in different ways determined from the carotenoid response in the triglyceride-rich lipoprotein fraction of plasma after a single consumption and in plasma after four days of consumption. *J Nutr.* 2000;130:1189–1196.
9. van Lieshout M, West CE, van Breemen RB. Isotopic tracer techniques for studying the bioavailability and bioefficacy of dietary carotenoids, particularly beta-carotene, in humans: a review. *Am J Clin Nutr.* 2003;77:12–28.
10. Maiani G, Caston MJ, Catasta G, et al. Carotenoids: actual knowledge on food sources, intakes, stability and bioavailability and their protective role in humans. *Mol Nutr Food Res.* 2009;53(suppl 2):S194–S218.
11. Boyle SP, Dobson VL, Duthie SJ, Hinselwood DC, Kyle JA, Collins AR. Bioavailability and efficiency of rutin as an antioxidant: a human supplementation study. *Eur J Clin Nutr.* 2000;54:774–782.
12. Walle T, Otake Y, Walle UK, Wilson FA. Quercetin glucosides are completely hydrolyzed in ileostomy patients before absorption. *J Nutr.* 2000;130:2658–2661.
13. Ross JA, Kasum CM. Dietary flavonoids: bioavailability, metabolic effects, and safety. *Annu Rev Nutr.* 2002;22:19–34.

14. Rasmussen SE, Breinholt VM. Non-nutritive bioactive food constituents of plants: bioavailability of flavonoids. *Int J Vitam Nutr Res.* 2003;73:101–111.

15. Prasain JK, Barnes S. Metabolism and bioavailability of flavonoids in chemoprevention: current analytical strategies and future prospectus. *Mol Pharm.* 2007;4:846–864.

16. Xu X, Wang HJ, Murphy PA, Hendrich S. Neither background diet nor type of soy food affects short-term isoflavone bioavailability in women. *J Nutr.* 2000;130:798–801.

17. Setchell KD, Brown NM, Desai PB, et al. Bioavailability, disposition, and dose-response effects of soy isoflavones when consumed by healthy women at physiologically typical dietary intakes. *J Nutr.* 2003;133:1027–1035.

18. Chanteranne B, Branca F, Kaardinal A, et al. Food matrix and isoflavones bioavailability in early post menopausal women: a European clinical study. *Clin Interv Aging.* 2008;3:711–718.

19. Clinton SK, Emenhiser C, Schwartz SJ, et al. cis-trans lycopene isomers, carotenoids, and retinol in the human prostate. *Cancer Epidemiol Biomarkers Prev.* 1996;5:823–833.

20. Morton MS, Matos-Ferreira A, Abranches-Monteiro L, et al. Measurement and metabolism of isoflavonoids and lignans in the human male. *Cancer Lett.* 1997;114:145–151.

21. Setchell KD, Brown NM, Lydeking-Olsen E. The clinical importance of the metabolite equol—a clue to the effectiveness of soy and its isoflavones. *J Nutr.* 2002;132:3577–3584.

22. Horn-Ross PL, Barnes S, Lee M, et al. Assessing phytoestrogen exposure in epidemiologic studies: development of a database (United States). *Cancer Causes Control.* 2000;11:289–298.

23. Pillow PC, Duphorne CM, Chang S, et al. Development of a database for assessing dietary phytoestrogen intake. *Nutr Cancer.* 1999;33:3–19.

24. Hammerstone JF, Lazarus SA, Schmitz HH. Procyanidin content and variation in some commonly consumed foods. *J Nutr.* 2000;130:2086S–2092S.

25. Le Marchand L, Murphy SP, Hankin JH, Wilkens LR, Kolonel LN. Intake of flavonoids and lung cancer. *J Natl Cancer Inst.* 2000;92:154–160.

26. USDA-NCC Carotenoid Database for U.S. Foods—1998. http://www.nal.usda.gov/fnic/foodcomp/Data/car98/car98.html.

27. Hakim IA, Hartz V, Graver E, Whitacre R, Alberts D. Development of a questionnaire and a database for assessing dietary d-limonene intake. *Public Health Nutr.* 2002;5:939–945.

28. Watanabe S, Zhuo XG, Kimira M. Food safety and epidemiology: new database of functional food factors. *Biofactors.* 2004;22:213–219.

29. Barbour J. Aspirin starts 2nd century as a wonder drug. *Los Angeles Times.* January 26, 1992:A3.

30. De Smet PAGM. The role of plant-derived drugs and herbal medicines in healthcare. *Drugs.* 1997;54:801–840.

31. Balbani AP, Silva DH, Montovani JC. Patents of drugs extracted from Brazilian medicinal plants. *Expert Opin Ther Pat.* 2009;19:461–473.

32. Xie H, Huo KK, Chao Z, Pan SL. Identification of crude drugs from Chinese medicinal plants of the genus Bupleurum using ribosomal DNA ITS sequences. *Planta Med.* 2009;75:89–93.

33. Pillay P, Maharaj VJ, Smith PJ. Investigating South African plants as a source of new antimalarial drugs. *J Ethnopharmacol.* 2008;119:438–454.

34. Soh PN, Benoit-Vical F. Are West African plants a source of future antimalarial drugs? *J Ethnopharmacol.* 2007;114:130–140.

35. Gurib-Fakim A. Medicinal plants: traditions of yesterday and drugs of tomorrow. *Mol Aspects Med.* 2006;27:1–93.

36. The Committee on Diet NaC; Assembly of Life Sciences; National Academy of Sciences, *Diet, nutrition, and cancer.* Washington, DC: National Academy Press; 1982.

37. Wattenberg LW. Inhibition of neoplasia by minor dietary constituents. *Cancer Res.* 1983;43:2448s–2453s.

38. Howard BV, Kritchevsky D. Phytochemicals and cardiovascular disease. A statement for healthcare professionals from the American Heart Association. *Circulation.* 1997;95:2591–2593.

39. Lerman RH, Minich DM, Darland G, et al. Enhancement of a modified Mediterranean-style, low glycemic load diet with specific phytochemicals improves cardiometabolic risk factors in subjects with metabolic syndrome and hypercholesterolemia in a randomized trial. *Nutr Metab (Lond).* 2008;5:29.

40. Marini H, Minutoli L, Polito F, et al. Effects of the phytoestrogen genistein on bone metabolism in osteopenic postmenopausal women: a randomized trial. *Ann Intern Med.* 2007;146:839–847.

41. Messina M, Lane B. Soy protein, soybean isoflavones, and coronary heart disease risk: Where do we stand? *Future Lipidology*. 2007;2:55–74.

42. Meyer A. The 1998 top 100 R & D survey. *Food Proc*. 1998;59:32–40.

43. PricewaterhouseCoopers LLP. Leveraging growth in the emerging functional foods industry: trends and market opportunities. 2009 PricewaterhouseCoopers LLP. August 2009.

44. Hiebert H. Designer foods for healthier diets. An interview with Herbert F. Pierson. In: Burlington M, ed. Spectrum, Decision Resources, Inc.; 1991.

45. Caragay AH. Cancer-preventive foods and ingredients. *Food Technol*. 1992;April:65–68.

46. Hardy G. Nutraceuticals and functional foods: introduction and meaning. *Nutrition*. 2000;16:688–697.

47. Position of the American Dietetic Association: functional foods. *J Am Diet Assoc*. 1999;99:1278–1285.

48. Committee on Opportunities in the Nutrition and Food Sciences. Food and Nutrition Board IoM. *Opportunities in the Nutrition and Food Sciences: Research Challenges and the Next Generation of Investigators*. Washington, DC: National Academy Press; 1994.

49. Hasler CM, Brown AC. Position of the American Dietetic Association: functional foods. *J Am Diet Assoc*. 2009; 109:735–746.

50. Position of the American Dietetic Association: phytochemicals and functional foods. *J Am Diet Assoc*. 1995;95:493–496.

51. Robertfroid MB. A European consensus of scientific concepts of functional foods. *Nutrition*. 2000;16:689–691.

52. Harborne JB. *The Flavonoids: Advances in Research Since 1986*. London: Chapman and Hall; 1993.

53. Olson JA. Biological actions of carotenoids. *J Nutr*. 1989;119:94–95.

54. Sahin MB, Perman SM, Jenkins G, Clark SS. Perillyl alcohol selectively induces G0/G1 arrest and apoptosis in Bcr/Abl-transformed myeloid cell lines. *Leukemia*. 1999;13:1581–1591.

55. De Roos B, Meyboom S, Kosmeijer-Schuil TG, Katan MB. Absorption and urinary excretion of the coffee diterpenes cafestol and kahweol in healthy ileostomy volunteers. *J Intern Med*. 1998;244:451–460.

56. Huber WW, Scharf G, Nagel G, Prustomersky S, Schulte-Hermann R, Kaina B. Coffee and its chemopreventive components Kahweol and Cafestol increase the activity of O6-methylguanine-DNA methyltransferase in rat liver—comparison with phase II xenobiotic metabolism. *Mutat Res*. 2003;522:57–68.

57. Law M. Plant sterol and stanol margarines and health. *BMJ*. 2000;320:861–864.

58. St-Onge MP, Jones PJ. Phytosterols and human lipid metabolism: efficacy, safety, and novel foods. *Lipids*. 2003;38:367–375.

59. Demonty I, Ras RT, van der Knaap HC, et al. Continuous dose-response relationship of the LDL-cholesterol-lowering effect of phytosterol intake. *J Nutr*. 2009;139(2):271–284.

60. Yoshiki Y, Kudou S, Okubo K. Relationship between chemical structures and biological activities of triterpenoid saponins from soybean. *Biosci Biotechnol Biochem*. 1998;62:2291–2299.

61. Rochfort S, Panozzo J. Phytochemicals for health, the role of pulses. *J Agric Food Chem*. 2007;55:7981–7994.

62. Brown NM, Lamartiniere CA. Genistein regulation of transforming growth factor-alpha, epidermal growth factor (EGF), and EGF receptor expression in the rat uterus and vagina. *Cell Growth Differ*. 2000;11:255–260.

63. Wu G, Meininger CJ, Knabe DA, Bazer FW, Rhoads JM. Arginine nutrition in development, health and disease. *Curr Opin Clin Nutr Metab Care*. 2000;3:59–66.

64. Lekakis JP, Papathanassiou S, Papaioannou TG, et al. Oral L-arginine improves endothelial dysfunction in patients with essential hypertension. *Int J Cardiol*. 2002;86:317–323.

65. Lucotti P, Monti L, Setola E, et al. Oral L-arginine supplementation improves endothelial function and ameliorates insulin sensitivity and inflammation in cardiopathic nondiabetic patients after an aortocoronary bypass. *Metabolism*. 2009;58:1270–1276.

66. Fahey JW, Talalay P. Antioxidant functions of sulforaphane: a potent inducer of phase II detoxication enzymes. *Food Chem Toxicol*. 1999;37:973–979.

67. Solowiej E, Kasprzycka-Guttman T, Fiedor P, Rowinski W. Chemoprevention of cancerogenesis—the role of sulforaphane. *Acta Pol Pharm*. 2003;60:97–100.

68. Steinkellner H, Rabot S, Freywald C, et al. Effects of cruciferous vegetables and their constituents on drug metabolizing enzymes involved in the bioactivation of DNA- reactive dietary carcinogens. *Mutat Res*. 2001;480–481:285–297.

69. Lampe JW. Sulforaphane: from chemoprevention to pancreatic cancer treatment? *Gut*. 2009;58:900–902.

70. Jo EH, Kim SH, Ahn NS, et al. Efficacy of sulforaphane is mediated by p38 MAP kinase and caspase-7 activations in ER-positive and COX-2-expressed human breast cancer cells. *Eur J Cancer Prev.* 2007;16:505–510.

71. Telang U, Brazeau DA, Morris ME. Comparison of the effects of phenethyl isothiocyanate and sulforaphane on gene expression in breast cancer and normal mammary epithelial cells. *Exp Biol Med (Maywood).* 2009;234:287–295.

72. Bell MC, Crowley-Nowick P, Bradlow HL, et al. Placebo-controlled trial of indole-3-carbinol in the treatment of CIN. *Gynecol Oncol.* 2000;78:123–129.

73. Meng Q, Goldberg ID, Rosen EM, Fan S. Inhibitory effects of indole-3-carbinol on invasion and migration in human breast cancer cells. *Breast Cancer Res Treat.* 2000;63:147–152.

74. Frydoonfar HR, McGrath DR, Spigelman AD. The effect of indole-3-carbinol and sulforaphane on a prostate cancer cell line. *ANZ J Surg.* 2003;73:154–156.

75. Auborn KJ, Fan S, Rosen EM, et al. Indole-3-carbinol is a negative regulator of estrogen. *J Nutr.* 2003;133: 2470S–2475S.

76. Choi HS, Cho MC, Lee HG, Yoon DY. Indole-3-carbinol induces apoptosis through p53 and activation of caspase-8 pathway in lung cancer A549 cells. *Food Chem Toxicol.* 2010;48(3):883–890.

77. Fleischauer AT, Poole C, Arab L. Garlic consumption and cancer prevention: meta-analyses of colorectal and stomach cancers. *Am J Clin Nutr.* 2000;72:1047–1052.

78. Das S. Garlic—a natural source of cancer preventive compounds. *Asian Pac J Cancer Prev.* 2002;3:305–311.

79. Thomson M, Ali M. Garlic [*Allium sativum*]: a review of its potential use as an anticancer agent. *Curr Cancer Drug Targets.* 2003;3:67–81.

80. Nagini S. Cancer chemoprevention by garlic and its organosulfur compounds—panacea or promise? *Anticancer Agents Med Chem.* 2008;8:313–321.

81. Stevinson C, Pittler MH, Ernst E. Garlic for treating hypercholesterolemia. A metaanalysis of randomized clinical trials. *Ann Intern Med.* 2000;133:420–429.

82. Alder R, Lookinland S, Berry JA, Williams M. A systematic review of the effectiveness of garlic as an anti-hyperlipidemic agent. *J Am Acad Nurse Pract.* 2003;15:120–129.

83. Maslin D. Effects of garlic on cholesterol: not down but not out either. *Arch Intern Med.* 2008;168:111–112; author reply 2–3.

84. Ma WW, Xiang L, Yu HL, et al. Neuroprotection of soyabean isoflavone coadministration with folic acid against beta-amyloid 1–40-induced neurotoxicity in rats. *Br J Nutr.* 2009;102:502–505.

85. Liu RH. Health benefits of fruit and vegetables are from additive and synergistic combinations of phytochemicals. *Am J Clin Nutr.* 2003;78:517S–520S.

86. Gate L, Paul J, Ba GN, Tew KD, Tapiero H. Oxidative stress induced in pathologies: the role of antioxidants. *Biomed Pharmacother.* 1999;53:169–180.

87. Jialal I, Devaraj S. Scientific evidence to support a vitamin E and heart disease health claim: research needs. *J Nutr.* 2005;135:348–353.

88. Traber MG. Vitamin E, oxidative stress and 'healthy ageing.' *Eur J Clin Invest.* 1997;27:822–824.

89. Van Remmen H, Jones DP. Current thoughts on the role of mitochondria and free radicals in the biology of aging. *J Gerontol A Biol Sci Med Sci.* 2009;64:171–174.

90. Jacob RA, Burri BJ. Oxidative damage and defense. *Am J Clin Nutr.* 1996;63:985S–990S.

91. Cao G, Sofic E, Prior RL. Antioxidant and prooxidant behavior of flavonoids: structure activity relationships. *Free Radic Biol Med.* 1997;22:749–760.

92. Potapovich AI, Kostyuk VA. Comparative study of antioxidant properties and cytoprotective activity of flavonoids. *Biochemistry (Mosc).* 2003;68:514–519.

93. Georgetti SR, Casagrande R, Di Mambro VM, Azzolini AE, Fonseca MJ. Evaluation of the antioxidant activity of different flavonoids by the chemiluminescence method. *AAPS PharmSci.* 2003;5:E20.

94. DiSilvestro RA. Flavonoids as antioxidants. In: Wildman R. E.C., ed. *Handbook of Nutraceuticals and Functional Foods.* Boca Raton, FL: CRC Press; 2001.

95. Wang H, Cao G, Prior RL. Total antioxidant capacity of fruits. *J Agric Food Chem.* 1996;44:701–705.

96. Kalt W, Forney CF, Martin A, Prior RL. Antioxidant capacity, vitamin C, phenolics, and anthocyanins after fresh storage of small fruits. *J Agric Food Chem.* 1999;47:4638–4644.

97. Heinonen M, Meyer AS, Frankel EN. Antioxidant activity of berry phenolics on human low-density lipoprotein and liposome oxidation. *J Agric Food Chem*. 1998;46:4107–4112.

98. Eberhardt MV, Lee CY, Liu RH. Antioxidant activity of fresh apples. *Nature*. 2000;405:903–904.

99. Guo C, Cao G, Sofic E, Prior RL. High-performance liquid chromatography coupled with coulmetric array detection of electroactive components in fruits and vegetables. Relationship to oxygen radical absorbance capacity. *J Agric Food Chem*. 1997;45:1787–1796.

100. Anderson KE, Kappas A. Dietary regulation of cytochrome P450. *Annu Rev Nutr*. 1991;11:141–167.

101. Surh V-J. Cancer chemoprevention by dietary phytochemicals: a mechanistic viewpoint. *The Cancer J*. 1997;11:1–8.

102. Staack R, Kingston S, Wallig MA, Jeffery EH. A comparison of the individual and collective effects of four glucosinolate breakdown products from brussels sprouts on induction of detoxification enzymes. *Toxicol Appl Pharmacol*. 1998;149:17–23.

103. Fahey JW, Zhang Y, Talalay P. Broccoli sprouts: an exceptionally rich source of inducers of enzymes that protect against chemical carcinogens. *Proc Natl Acad Sci U S A*. 1997;94:10367–10372.

104. Yoxall V, Kentish P, Coldham N, Kuhnert N, Sauer MJ, Ioannides C. Modulation of hepatic cytochromes P450 and phase II enzymes by dietary doses of sulforaphane in rats: implications for its chemopreventive activity. *Int J Cancer*. 2005;117:356–362.

105. Bozina N, Bradamante V, Lovric M. Genetic polymorphism of metabolic enzymes P450 (CYP) as a susceptibility factor for drug response, toxicity, and cancer risk. *Arh Hig Rada Toksikol*. 2009;60:217–242.

106. Bradbury RB, White DR. Estrogen and related substances in plants. In: Harris RS, Marrian GF, Thimann KV, eds. *Vitam Horm*. New York: Academic Press; 1954:207–230.

107. Verdeal K, Ryan DS. Naturally-occurring estrogens in plant foodstuffs—a review. *J Food Protection*. 1979;42:577–583.

108. Promberger A, Dornstauder E, Fruhwirth C, Schmid ER, Jungbauer A. Determination of estrogenic activity in beer by biological and chemical means. *J Agric Food Chem*. 2001;49:633–640.

109. Franke AA, Custer LJ, Cerna CM, Narala K. Rapid HPLC analysis of dietary phytoestrogens from legumes and from human urine. *Proc Soc Exp Biol Med*. 1995;208:18–26.

110. Tou JC, Thompson LU. Exposure to flaxseed or its lignan component during different developmental stages influences rat mammary gland structures. *Carcinogenesis*. 1999;20:1831–1835.

111. Tou JC, Chen J, Thompson LU. Dose, timing, and duration of flaxseed exposure affect reproductive indices and sex hormone levels in rats. *J Toxicol Environ Health A*. 1999;56:555–570.

112. Gehm BD, McAndrews JM, Chien PY, Jameson JL. Resveratrol, a polyphenolic compound found in grapes and wine, is an agonist for the estrogen receptor. *Proc Natl Acad Sci U S A*. 1997;94:14138–14143.

113. Li X, Phillips FM, An HS, et al. The action of resveratrol, a phytoestrogen found in grapes, on the intervertebral disc. *Spine (Phila Pa 1976)*. 2008;33:2586–2595.

114. Liu ZH, Kanjo Y, Mizutani S. A review of phytoestrogens: their occurrence and fate in the environment. *Water Res*. 2010;44(2):567–577.

115. Kurzer MS, Xu X. Dietary phytoestrogens. *Annu Rev Nutr*. 1997;17:353–381.

116. Ju YH, Carlson KE, Sun J, et al. Estrogenic effects of extracts from cabbage, fermented cabbage, and acidified brussels sprouts on growth and gene expression of estrogen-dependent human breast cancer (MCF-7) cells. *J Agric Food Chem*. 2000;48:4628–4634.

117. LeBlanc ES, Janowsky J, Chan BK, Nelson HD. Hormone replacement therapy and cognition: systematic review and meta-analysis. *JAMA*. 2001;285:1489–1499.

118. Shumaker SA, Legault C, Thal L, et al. Estrogen plus progestin and the incidence of dementia and mild cognitive impairment in postmenopausal women: the Women's Health Initiative Memory Study: a randomized controlled trial. *JAMA*. 2003;289:2651–2662.

119. Yaffe K. Hormone therapy and the brain: déjà vu all over again? *JAMA*. 2003;289:2717–2719.

120. Grady D, Yaffe K, Kristof M, Lin F, Richards C, Barrett-Connor E. Effect of postmenopausal hormone therapy on cognitive function: the Heart and Estrogen/progestin Replacement Study. *Am J Med*. 2002;113:543–548.

121. Marsden J. Hormone replacement therapy and female malignancy: what has the Million Women Study added to our knowledge? *J Fam Plann Reprod Health Care*. 2007;33:237–243.

122. Fugh-Berman A, Scialli AR. Gynecologists and estrogen: an affair of the heart. *Perspect Biol Med*. 2006;49:115–130.

123. Hogervorst E, Bandelow S. Brain and cognition. Is there any case for improving cognitive function in menopausal women using estrogen treatment? *Minerva Ginecol.* 2009;61:499–515.

124. Utian WH, Archer DF, Bachmann GA, et al. Estrogen and progestogen use in postmenopausal women: July 2008 position statement of The North American Menopause Society. *Menopause.* 2008;15:584–602.

125. Oseni T, Patel R, Pyle J, Jordan VC. Selective estrogen receptor modulators and phytoestrogens. *Planta Med.* 2008;74:1656–1665.

126. Blenis J. Signal transduction via the MAP kinases: proceed at your own RSK. *Proc Natl Acad Sci U S A.* 1993; 90:5889–5892.

127. Yoon HK, Chen K, Baylink DJ, Lau KH. Differential effects of two protein tyrosine kinase inhibitors, tyrphostin and genistein, on human bone cell proliferation as compared with differentiation. *Calcif Tissue Int.* 1998;63:243–249.

128. Dubey RK, Gillespie DG, Imthurn B, Rosselli M, Jackson EK, Keller PJ. Phytoestrogens inhibit growth and MAP kinase activity in human aortic smooth muscle cells. *Hypertension.* 1999;33:177–182.

129. Pixley F, Mann J. Dietary factors in the aetiology of gall stones: a case control study. *Gut.* 1988;29:1511–1515.

130. Kundu JK, Surh YJ. Breaking the relay in deregulated cellular signal transduction as a rationale for chemoprevention with anti-inflammatory phytochemicals. *Mutat Res.* 2005;591:123–146.

131. Dalu A, Haskell JF, Coward L, Lamartiniere CA. Genistein, a component of soy, inhibits the expression of the EGF and ErbB2/Neu receptors in the rat dorsolateral prostate. *Prostate.* 1998;37:36–43.

132. Salman H, Bergman M, Bessler H, Punsky I, Djaldetti M. Effect of a garlic derivative (alliin) on peripheral blood cell immune responses. *Int J Immunopharmacol.* 1999;21:589–597.

133. Colic M, Savic M. Garlic extracts stimulate proliferation of rat lymphocytes in vitro by increasing IL-2 and IL-4 production. *Immunopharmacol Immunotoxicol.* 2000;22:163–181.

134. Middleton E Jr. Effect of plant flavonoids on immune and inflammatory cell function. *Adv Exp Med Biol.* 1998;439: 175–182.

135. Johnson VJ, He Q, Osuchowski MF, Sharma RP. Physiological responses of a natural antioxidant flavonoid mixture, silymarin, in BALB/c mice: III. Silymarin inhibits T-lymphocyte function at low doses but stimulates inflammatory processes at high doses. *Planta Med.* 2003;69:44–49.

136. Mao TK, van de Water J, Keen CL, Schmitz HH, Gershwin ME. Modulation of TNFalpha secretion in peripheral blood mononuclear cells by cocoa flavonols and procyanidins. *Dev Immunol.* 2002;9:135–141.

137. Ahmed SA. The immune system as a potential target for environmental estrogens (endocrine disrupters): a new emerging field. *Toxicology.* 2000;150:191–206.

138. Chan MM, Ho CT, Huang HI. Effects of three dietary phytochemicals from tea, rosemary and turmeric on inflammation-induced nitrite production. *Cancer Lett.* 1995;96:23–29.

139. Vainio H, Morgan G. Cyclo-oxygenase 2 and breast cancer prevention. Non- steroidal anti- inflammatory agents are worth testing in breast cancer. *BMJ.* 1998;317:828.

140. Vainio H, Morgan G. Non-steroidal anti-inflammatory drugs and the chemoprevention of gastrointestinal cancers. *Scand J Gastroenterol.* 1998;33:785–789.

141. Danesh J, Whincup P, Walker M, et al. Low grade inflammation and coronary heart disease: prospective study and updated meta-analyses. *BMJ.* 2000;321:199–204.

142. Taketo MM. Cyclooxygenase-2 inhibitors in tumorigenesis (Part II). *J Natl Cancer Inst.* 1998;90:1609–1620.

143. Mutoh M, Takahashi M, Fukuda K, et al. Suppression by flavonoids of cyclooxygenase-2 promoter-dependent transcriptional activity in colon cancer cells: structure-activity relationship. *Jpn J Cancer Res.* 2000;91:686–691.

144. Vincent HK, Bourguignon CM, Taylor AG. Relationship of the dietary phytochemical index to weight gain, oxidative stress and inflammation in overweight young adults. *J Hum Nutr Diet.* 23:20–29.

145. Tull SP, Yates CM, Maskrey BH, et al. Omega-3 fatty acids and inflammation: novel interactions reveal a new step in neutrophil recruitment. *PLoS Biol.* 2009;7:e100–e177.

146. Ebrahimi M, Ghayour-Mobarhan M, Rezaian S, et al. Omega-3 fatty acid supplements improve the cardiovascular risk profile of subjects with metabolic syndrome, including markers of inflammation and auto-immunity. *Acta Cardiol.* 2009;64:321–327.

147. Weylandt KH, Nadolny A, Kahlke L, et al. Reduction of inflammation and chronic tissue damage by omega-3 fatty acids in fat-1 transgenic mice with pancreatitis. *Biochim Biophys Acta.* 2008;1782:634–641.

148. Amiot MJ, Tacchini M, Aubert S, Nicolas J. Phenolic composition and browning susceptibility of various apple cultivars at maturity. *J Food Sci.* 1992;57:958–962.

149. Tsushida T, Svzuki M. Content of flavonol glucosides and some properties of enzymes metabolizing the glucosides in onion. 3. Flavonoid in fruits and vegetables. *J Jpn Soc Food Sci Technol.* 1996;43:642–649.

150. Wang H-J, Murphy PA. Isoflavone composition of American and Japanese soybeans in Iowa: effects of variety, crop year, and location. *J Agric Food Chem.* 1994;42:1674–1677.

151. Melby MK, Murashima M, Watanabe S. Phytochemical intake and relationship to past health history in Japanese women. *Biofactors.* 2004;22:265–269.

152. Galvan-Portillo MV, Wolff MS, Torres-Sanchez LE, Lopez-Cervantes M, Lopez- Carrillo L. Assessing phytochemical intake in a group of Mexican women. *Salud Publica Mex.* 2007;49:126–131.

153. Vinson JA, Hao Y, Su X, Zubik L. Phenol antioxidant quantity and quality in foods: vegetables. *J Agric Food Chem.* 1998;46:3630–3634.

154. Vinson JA. Plant flavonoids, especially tea flavonols, are powerful antioxidants using an in vitro oxidation model for heart disease. *J Agric Food Chem.* 1998;43:2800–2802.

155. Scalbert A, Williamson G. Dietary intake and bioavailability of polyphenols. *J Nutr.* 2000;130:2073S–2085S.

156. Cerqueira MT, Fry MM, Connor WE. The food and nutrient intakes of the Tarahumara Indians of Mexico. *Am J Clin Nutr.* 1979;32:905–915.

157. Harland BF, Peterson M. Nutritional status of lacto-ovo vegetarian Trappist monks. *J Am Diet Assoc.* 1978;72:259–264.

158. Ridout CL, Wharf SG, Price KR, Johnson IT, Fenwick GR. UK mean daily intakes of saponins—intestine permeabilizing factors in legumes. *Food Sci Nutr.* 1988;42F:111–116.

159. Hudson EA, Dinh PA, Kokubun T, Simmonds MS, Gescher A. Characterization of potentially chemopreventive phenols in extracts of brown rice that inhibit the growth of human breast and colon cancer cells. *Cancer Epidemiol Biomarkers Prev.* 2000;9:1163–1170.

160. Craig WJ, Mangels AR. Position of the American Dietetic Association: vegetarian diets. *J Am Diet Assoc.* 2009; 109:1266–1282.

161. Van Duyn MA, Pivonka E. Overview of the health benefits of fruit and vegetable consumption for the dietetics professional: selected literature. *J Am Diet Assoc.* 2000;100:1511–1521.

162. Smith-Warner SA, Spiegelman D, Yaun SS, et al. Intake of fruits and vegetables and risk of breast cancer: a pooled analysis of cohort studies. *JAMA.* 2001;285:769– 776.

163. Michels KB, Edward G, Joshipura KJ, et al. Prospective study of fruit and vegetable consumption and incidence of colon and rectal cancers. *J Natl Cancer Inst.* 2000;92:1740–1752.

164. Feskanich D, Ziegler RG, Michaud DS, et al. Prospective study of fruit and vegetable consumption and risk of lung cancer among men and women. *J Natl Cancer Inst.* 2000;92:1812–1823.

165. Nestle M. Fruits and vegetables: protective or just fellow travelers? *Nutr Rev.* 1996;54:255–257.

166. Jacobs DRJ, Murtaugh MA. It's more than an apple a day: an appropriately processed, plant-centered dietary pattern may be good for your health. *Am J Clin Nutr.* 2000;72:899–900.

167. American Institute for Cancer Research. Cancer expert faults reductionist thinking in diet-cancer research. *Today's Dietitian.* 2000:18–19.

168. Messina M, Lampe JW, Birt DF, et al. Reductionism and the narrowing nutrition perspective: time for reevaluation and emphasis on food synergy. *J Am Diet Assoc.* 2001;101:1416–1419.

169. Stampfer MJ, Hu FB, Manson JE, Rimm EB, Willett WC. Primary prevention of coronary heart disease in women through diet and lifestyle. *N Engl J Med.* 2000;343:16–22.

CHAPTER 9

Soyfoods

Soyfoods have made major inroads into the mainstream during the past 10 years in large part because of consumer belief that independent of their nutrient content, these foods may confer health benefits such as reducing risk of cancer and heart disease. According to a nationally representative survey published in 2009, 32% of Americans reported using soy products at least once per month and 84% consider soy products to be healthy; the latter represents a substantial increase from the 59% reported in 1997.[1] Soymilk is the most commonly consumed soy product, with nearly a quarter of Americans reporting they drink it regularly. For comparison, in 1999, 18% of consumers reported that they had tried soymilk. Emerging soyfoods are also capturing consumer interest as well. For example, the percentage of Americans trying edamame (green soybeans or sweet beans) increased more than fivefold during the past decade. Not surprisingly given consumer awareness and interest, dietitians indicate they desire training about soyfoods.[2]

Foods made from the soybean have been consumed for centuries in many Asian countries and for decades by Western vegetarians, being prized as much for their protein content as for their versatility. Soyfoods also appeal to those interested in eating a plant-based diet for ethical and environmental reasons, the latter of which is gaining scientific support.[3] There is little question that soyfoods are nutritious and that the many meat and dairy-based substitutes made from soybeans make adopting a vegetarian diet easier.

However, the role of soyfoods in an overall healthy diet has become somewhat of a confusing issue in recent years. In part, this is simply because of the sheer volume of research that has been conducted; approximately 2000 soy-related peer-reviewed papers are published annually. Correctly interpreting this research is challenging because it requires understanding the strengths and weaknesses of an extensive variety of experimental models and designs. Much of the research involving soy has focused on one particular constituent: isoflavones. The presence of isoflavones in soybeans largely accounts for claims that soyfoods reduce risk of certain chronic diseases as well as concerns that these foods may be contraindicated for some individuals.

This chapter provides the background necessary to address the most frequently asked questions about the health consequences of soy consumption. Because isoflavones are the subject of so much research, extensive discussion of these soybean constituents is provided first.

ISOFLAVONES

Isoflavones are a subclass of the rather ubiquitous flavonoids, but by comparison they have a much more limited distribution in nature. The primary dietary sources of isoflavones are soybeans and soyfoods. In the literature it is common to find statements that many legumes, fruits, and vegetables contain isoflavones. Although these statements are technically correct, they are unintentionally misleading because the amounts in most of these foods are so small as to almost certainly be physiologically irrelevant.[4] In contrast to phytoalexins (substances that are formed by host tissue in response to physiologic stimuli, infectious agents, or their products and that accumulate to levels that inhibit the growth of microorganisms), isoflavones are constitutive and are thus always present in significant quantities in soybeans because one of their primary functions is to stimulate nodulation genes in soil bacteria belonging to the genus *Rhizobium*.[5] Rhizobia have the ability to induce the formation of nodules on soybean roots, required for the reduction of atmospheric nitrogen to ammonia, which the soybean can then use as a source of nitrogen for growth.

Isoflavone Content of Soyfoods

In total, there are 12 different soybean isoflavone isomers (Table 9-1). These are the three aglycons genistein (4′,5,7-trihydroxyisoflavone), daidzein (4′,7-dihydroxyisoflavone), and glycitein (7,4′-dihydroxy-6-methoxyisoflavone), their respective β-glycosides genistin, daidzin, and glycitin, and three β-glucosides each esterified with either malonic or acetic acid (Figures 9-1 and 9-2). Typically, there is somewhat more genistin/genistein than daidzein/daidzin in soybeans and soyfoods, whereas glycitein/glycitin makes up only 5–10% of the total isoflavone content.[6] In soybeans and in nonfermented soyfoods, isoflavones are present primarily as their glycosides (<2% is present as the aglycone), whereas in fermented soy products, the isoflavones are present to a greater extent in their aglycone form due to microorganism-induced fermentation and hydrolysis of the parent compounds.

A general rule of thumb for estimating the isoflavone content of a *traditional* Asian soyfood is to multiply the grams of protein in that food by 3.5 mg (isoflavone amounts refer to the aglycone equivalent weight as that is the active form).[7] Thus one serving (e.g., 3 to 4 oz. of tofu or 1 cup (250 ml) soy beverage) of a traditional soyfood provides approximately 25 mg isoflavones. Isoflavones are relatively heat stable; baking or frying at high temperature alters total isoflavone content very little or not at all; however, the processing of the soybean into many of the Westernized soyfoods can cause significant isoflavone loss. Thus the 3.5 mg/g protein rule will not apply. For example, the average isoflavone content of isolated soy proteins (ISP) is about 1 mg/g. Similarly, the isoflavone content of the most common type of soy protein concentrate, which is alcohol washed and the source of protein in many soy-based meat substitutes, is only 5–20% of the isoflavone content of the soybean itself. The U.S. Department of Agriculture (USDA), in conjunction with Iowa State University, operates an online database (http://www.nal.usda.gov/fnic/foodcomp/Data/isoflav/isoflav.html) that provides the isoflavone content of foods.

Table 9-1 Chemical and Common Names and Molecular Weights (MW) of the 12 Isoflavone Isomers Found in Soybeans

Food (USDA IDN)	Genistein units	Daidzein units	Glycitein units	Total Iso units	Min units	Max units	Protein/ 100g	Kcal/ 100g	mg isol/ g protein
Tofu									
Firm (16126)	134	94	21	247	79	346	8.0	77	3.1
Firm (99085)	162	128	24	314	NA	NA	NA	NA	NA
Regular (16427)	136	90	20	236	51	337	8.1	76	2.9
Silken, firm (16162)	156	111	24	279	238	320	6.9	62	4.0
Extra firm (99084)	128	80	19	227	NA	NA	NA	NA	NA
Extra firm (99083)	125	82	20	226	202	251	NA	NA	NA
Natto (16113)	290	219	82	589	464	870	17.7	212	3.3
Soymilk (16120)	61	45	6	97	13	211	2.8	33	3.5
Miso (16112)	246	161	29	426	227	892	11.8	206	3.6
Tempeh (16114)	249	176	21	435	69	625	18.5	193	2.3
Soybeans, raw, US food grade (16108)	737	466	109	1283	362	2209	36.5	416	3.5
Soybeans, cooked (16109)	277	270	NA	547	NA	NA	16.6	173	3.3
Soybeans, raw, Japan (99092)	648	345	139	1185	688	2389	NA	NA	NA
Soybeans, raw, Korea (99093)	723	727	NA	1450	458	2317	NA	NA	NA
Soybeans, raw, Taiwan (99040)	315	282	NA	598	NA	NA	NA	NA	NA

(continued)

Table 9-1 Chemical and Common Names and Molecular Weights (MW) of the 12 Isoflavone Isomers Found in Soybeans (Continued)

Food (USDA IDN)	Genistein units	Daidzein units	Glycitein units	Total Iso units	Min units	Max units	Protein/ 100g	Kcal/ 100g	mg iso/ g protein
Soybeans, green, cooked (11451)	69	69	NA	138	NA	NA	12.4	141	1.1
Soybean curd, fermented (99034)	224	143	23	390	NA	NA	NA	NA	NA
Soymilk skin (Foo jook/ yuba, cooked) (99096)	325	182	NA	507	NA	NA	NA	NA	NA
Soymilk skin (Foo jook/ yuba, raw) (99053)	1048	799	184	1939	1217	2661	NA	NA	NA
Isolate soy protein (16122)	596	336	94	1027	456	1992	80.7	338	1.3
Soy protein concentrate									
Water washed (99060)	556	430	52	1021	612	1670	NA	NA	NA
Alcohol washed (16121)	53	68	16	125	21	318	58.1	332	0.22
Soyflour									
Full fat (16115)	968	712	162	1779	598	2648	34.5	436	5.2
Defatted (16117)	712	575	76	1312	737	1681	47.0	329	2.8

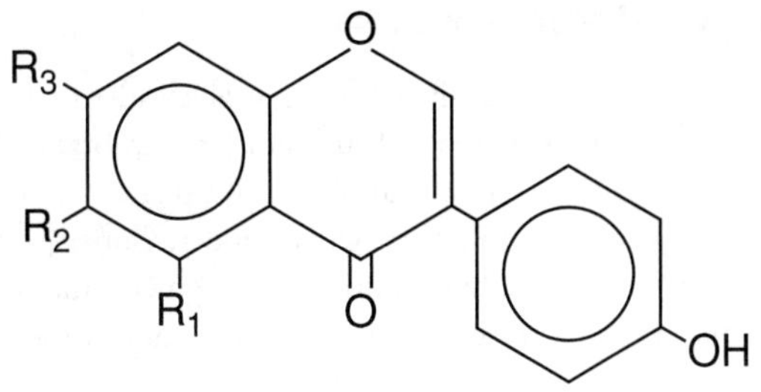

Figure 9-1 Chemical structures of soybean isoflavone aglycones.

Isoflavone Aglycones	R$_1$	R$_2$	R$_3$
Daidzein	H	H	OH
Genistein	OH	HO	H
Glycitein	H	OCH$_3$	OH

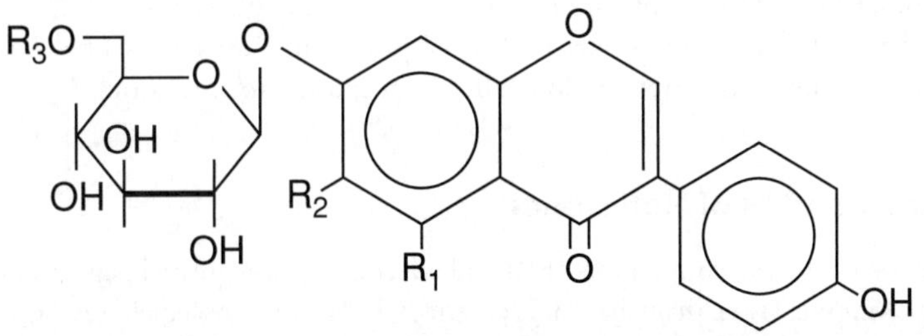

Figure 9-2 Chemical structures of soybean isoflavone glycosides.

Isoflavone Glycosides	R$_1$	R$_2$	R$_3$
Daidzin	H	H	OH
Malonyl daidzin	H	H	COCH$_2$COOH
Acetyl daidzin	H	H	COCH$_2$
Genistin	OH	H	OH
Malonyl genistin	OH	H	COCH$_2$COOH
Acetyl genistin	OH	H	COCH$_2$
Glycitin	H	OCH$_3$	H
Malonyl glycitin	H	OCH$_3$	COCH$_2$COOH
Acetyl glycitin	H	OCH$_3$	COCH$_3$

Isoflavone Absorption and Metabolism

The absorption of isoflavones present in the intestine as glycosides first requires hydrolysis to the aglycone, a reaction that occurs via the action of brush border membrane glucosidases and bacterial glucosidases. During passage across the enterocyte, significant phase 2 metabolism occurs with conjugation to glucuronic acid to form the isoflavone-glucuronides. Consequently, isoflavones circulate in plasma mostly in the conjugated form, bound primarily to glucuronic acid; <4% circulate in the free form. Plasma isoflavone levels increase in relation to the amount ingested, although some evidence, but not all, suggests there is a curvilinear relationship between the area under the plasma curve and isoflavone dose.[8,9] Isoflavones undergo enterohepatic circulation; nevertheless, most of the isoflavones absorbed are excreted from the body within 24 hours after a single ingestion.

Daidzein is metabolized primarily to the isoflavan equol and *O*-desmethylangolensin, whereas genistein is metabolized to dihydrogenistein and a number of other oxidative metabolites. It is widely recognized, however, that there is a huge interindividual variation in isoflavone metabolism. In response to the ingestion of the same amount of isoflavones, there can be dramatically different circulating levels of the parent isoflavones and their metabolites among individuals.[10] The conversion of daidzein to equol, which is accomplished by intestinal bacteria, may be particularly significant because it has been proposed that equol is an especially beneficial compound and that those individuals possessing equol-synthesizing bacteria are more likely to benefit from soyfood consumption.[11] Importantly, only approximately 50% of Asians and 25% of Westerners possess these bacteria; evidence indicates that equol-producing status is essentially a lifelong attribute with the exception of a temporary loss following exposure to antibiotics.[12]

Physiologic Properties of Isoflavones

Isoflavones bind to estrogen receptors (ER) and affect estrogen-regulated gene products, although their binding affinity is lower than that of 17β-estradiol, the primary female sex hormone. For this reason, isoflavones are classified as phytoestrogens. It is, however, probably more accurate to refer to the estrogen-like, rather than estrogenic, properties of isoflavones because isoflavones are much different from the hormone estrogen. Furthermore, because of their preferential binding to and transactivation of ERβ in comparison to ERα, isoflavones are also commonly referred to as selective estrogen receptor modulators (SERMs) (mixed estrogen agonists/antagonists).[13] SERMs such as the breast cancer drug tamoxifen and anti-osteoporotic drug raloxifene have estrogen-like effects in some tissues but either no effects or antiestrogenic effects in other tissues in which ERs are present.[13] Not surprisingly, research shows that isoflavones affect the expression of many genes differently than estrogen.[14]

Even categorizing isoflavones as SERMs does not fully describe the potential mechanisms by which isoflavones exert physiologic effects because they (especially genistein) may affect signal transduction pathways by inhibiting the activity of enzymes (e.g., tyrosine protein kinase, mitogen-activated kinase, DNA topoisomerase, etc.) and regulating cellular factors that control the growth and differentiation of cells.[15] There is debate about the relevance of these estrogen-independent effects because they are observed in vitro at concentrations that exceed circulating levels obtainable in vivo. However, there are impressive examples in both animals[16] and humans[17] indicating they are.

Finally, it would be remiss to also not mention that isoflavones are frequently classified as endocrine disruptors, chemicals that alter the function of the endocrine system and potentially cause adverse health effects.[18] Consequently, isoflavones have become controversial, although as discussed later, the human safety-related data are very reassuring. In considering potential adverse effects, it is important to recognize that the metabolism of isoflavones by rodents and monkeys, two species in which untoward health effects of isoflavones have been observed and on which the endocrine disruptor classification is based, differs markedly from humans, making extrapolations of the findings difficult.[19] Furthermore, these effects often occur in response to amounts of isoflavones that greatly exceed that to which humans are exposed.

ASIAN SOY INTAKE

The lower rates of certain chronic diseases in soyfood-consuming countries[20,21] contributed to the initial enthusiasm for investigating the role of soy in reducing chronic disease risk.[22] Consequently, Asian soyfood intake can serve as one guide for Western intake. Unfortunately, estimates of Asian soy intake have frequently been misrepresented in both the online and print media. There is no reason for any confusion or misunderstanding regarding this issue because intake data are widely available in the peer-reviewed literature. These data come from studies in which validated food frequency questionnaires designed to comprehensively assess soy intake were administered to thousands of individuals.

A comprehensive review[7] published in 2006 that included five studies involving older adults in Japan,[23–27] found soy protein intake in women ranged from a low of 6.0 g/d[26] to a high of 10.5 g/d,[25] whereas the range in men was 8.0 g/d[27] to 11.3 g/d.[25] Soyfoods contributed from 6.5[26]–12.8%[25] of total protein intake. These data are consistent with a large amount of more recently published data.[28–31] Survey data also indicate that mean isoflavone intake ranges from about 25 to 50 mg/d.[7,28–30] For comparison, one serving of a traditional soyfood provides anywhere from about 7 g (1 cup soymilk) to as much as 15 g (3 to 4 ounces of some types of tofu) protein per serving.

Interestingly, according to food disappearance data from the Food and Agricultural Organization, per capita soy protein intake has remained constant during the past 40 years in Japan. However, as a percentage of total protein intake, it has decreased from about 13% to 10%.[7] This is because of the increased protein content (mostly from animal sources) of the Japanese diet. Because soy intake is decreasing among younger Japanese, absolute per capita intake may slowly begin to decline.

In comparison to Japan, soy intake of Hong Kong is about only half as much.[32] Korean intake appears to be between that of Japan and Hong Kong.[33] In mainland China, estimating intake is more difficult because the population has a very heterogeneous dietary behavior varying according to geographic region. There are excellent data from Shanghai, however, where soy intake appears to be higher than in other parts of China. The Shanghai Men's Health Study (SMHS) and the Shanghai Women's Health Study (SHWS) are prospective epidemiologic studies each involving approximately 50,000 subjects.[34–36] These studies indicate that daily mean soy protein and isoflavone intakes are similar to Japan[34,35] or somewhat higher.[36] For example, in the SMHS, for soy protein and isoflavones, the mean $\pm$ standard error of the mean were 12.5 and 7.94 g/d, respectively, and 36.2 and 24.4 mg/d, respectively.[36]

There are also excellent data on the upper range of soy intake in Shanghai. In a report from the SHWS, about 10% of women reportedly consumed about 20 g of soy protein and about 85 mg/d isoflavones, whereas about 2% consumed $\geq$25 g/d soy protein (mean isoflavone intake in this group was 145 mg/d).[34] In another report from Shanghai, among those women consuming a more plant- rather than meat-based diet, fourth quartile soy protein intake was 17 g/d.[37] Finally, in a study involving almost 3000 Shanghai men, the overall and fourth quartile soy protein intake means were 7.82 and 16.34 g/d, respectively.[38] These upper intake data are consistent with that reported in some but not all Japanese studies. For example, in a case-control study involving 1400 participants, Akhter et al[29] found that the mean fourth quartile ($N = 174$) isoflavone intake was 78.5 mg/d (estimated soy protein intake, approximately 20 g).

The major soy products consumed in Shanghai are soymilk and tofu, whereas in Japan, about 90% of soy is consumed via four foods. About half of Japanese intake is in the form of the fermented foods such as miso and natto, and half is from unfermented products such as tofu and dried soybeans.

NUTRITIONAL COMPOSITION OF SOYBEANS AND SOYFOODS

Protein

When expressed on a caloric basis, legumes are generally between 20% and 30% protein, whereas soybeans are about 35% protein.[39,40] Not surprisingly, therefore, soyfoods are excellent sources of protein; whole soybeans and many traditional soyfoods, such as tofu and tempeh, provide 10 to 14 g per serving (Table 9-2). As previously noted, many meat substitutes and beverages are made using soy protein products. These include ISP, soy protein concentrates, and soy flour, which by definition are at least 90%, 65%, and 50% protein, respectively. Foods such as cereals, beverages, and energy bars, which are based on these products, can provide as much as 10 to 20 g of protein per serving.

Soy protein products typically have a protein digestibility corrected amino acid score (PDCAAS) (Chapter 3) >0.9, which is similar to that of meat and milk protein.[41,42] Consequently, consuming the recommended dietary allowance (RDA, 0.8 mg/kg body weight [bw]) for protein entirely in the form of soy will meet the biologic requirement for amino acids. Modest differences in PDCAASs among soy products stem from differences in digestibility (e.g., whole soybeans are more poorly digested than tofu) and amino acid changes that occur during processing.

The high PDCAAS of soy protein is not surprising because the concentration of the sulfur amino acids (SAA), methionine and cysteine, which are the limiting amino acids in legumes, is approximately 27 mg/g protein, which exceeds the biologic requirement of 26 mg/g protein for 1- to 2-year-olds (SAA requirements decrease slightly with age).[43] The digestibility of most soy products, the other component along with amino acid content that determines protein quality, is quite good, usually >90%.[44]

As noted in Chapter 3, there is discussion in the literature about the need to change the manner in which protein digestibility is assessed, from digestibility at the fecal level to digestibility at the ileal level.[43,45] The effect of any such change on the PDCAAS of soy protein has yet to be formerly determined.[46,47] There are also criticisms of the PDCAAS independent of digestibility.[48,49] Nevertheless, a variety of assays, including nitrogen balance studies in humans, support the high quality of soy protein.[50,51] Formal recognition of the high quality of soy protein came in the form of a ruling by the USDA allowing soy protein to replace 100% of meat protein in the Federal School Lunch Program.[52] To qualify for complete substitution, a protein must have a PDCAAS that is at least 80% that of milk protein.

Table 9-2 Isoflavone, Caloric, and Protein Content of Selected Soyfoods* per 100 Grams Edible Portion

Food (USDA No.)	Isoflavones (mg)	Protein (g)	Kcal	mg isoflavones/ g protein
Tofu				
Firm (16126)	24.7	8.2	70	3.0
Regular (16427)	23.6	8.1	76	2.9
Silken, firm (16162)	27.9	6.9	62	4.0
Natto (16113)	58.9	17.7	212	3.3
Soymilk (16120)	9.7	3.8	54	2.5
Miso (16112)	42.6	11.7	199	3.6
Tempeh (16114)	43.5	18.5	193	2.3
Soynuts (16111) dry roasted	128.4	39.6	451	3.2
Soybeans, cooked (16109)	54.7	16.6	173	3.3
Soybeans, green, cooked (11451)	13.8	12.3	141	
Isolated soy protein (16122)	102.7	80.7	338	1.3
Soy protein concentrate†				
Acid washed (99060)/16420	102.1	58.1	331	1.8
Alcohol washed (16121)	12.5	58.1	331	0.22
Soy flour				
Full fat (16115)	177.9	34.5	436	5.2
Defatted (16117)	131.2	47.0	330	2.8

*Note: The isoflavone and protein contents of soy products within the same category vary markedly according to the manner in which they are processed. Also, the isoflavone content of the same product can vary markedly over time due to processing changes and to the variation in the isoflavone content of soybeans from one variety to another and from one year to another.
†99060 is referred to as aqueous washed soy protein concentrate in the isoflavone database and 16420 as acid washed in the USDA National Nutrient Database for Standard Reference.
Source: Data from USDA National Nutrient Database for Standard Reference, Release 22, 2009 and USDA-Iowa State University Database on Isoflavone Content of Foods, Release 1.3–2002.

Fat

Soybeans derive approximately 40% of their calories from fat (Table 9-1) which is much higher than all other commonly consumed legumes, which are generally <10% fat.[39] For this reason, most traditional soyfoods, such as tofu and soymilk, are quite high in fat on a caloric basis. The predominant fatty acid in soy oil, as in many vegetable oils, is the essential fatty acid linoleic acid (an omega-6 fatty acid), which accounts for about 55% of the total fat content. Over the years some concerns have arisen that too much of this fatty acid could raise coronary heart disease (CHD) risk by increasing inflammation. However, the American Heart Association recently rejected concerns about the proinflammatory properties of omega-6 fats and concluded that that these fatty acids play a critically important role in heart-healthy diets.[53]

Unlike most other vegetable oils (the primary exceptions are flax, walnut, and canola oils), soy oil also contains significant amounts (7–8% of total fatty acids) of the essential fatty acid, α-linolenic acid. Although soyfoods can be good plant sources of this short-chain omega-3 fatty acid, many soy products, such as those using ISP and soy protein concentrates, which are nearly fat free, and defatted soymilks and defatted flours such as textured vegetable protein (TVP) are not. Not surprisingly, the α-linolenic acid content of soy oil is markedly reduced (by 50–80%) by partial hydrogenation.[54,55]

There is considerable interest in the coronary benefits of omega-3 fatty acids,[56,57] and although α-linolenic acid does not possess the same properties as the long-chain omega-3 fatty acids (eicosapentaenoic acid [EPA] and docosahexaenoic acid [DHA]) found in cold-water fish, evidence suggests that α-linolenic acid has direct coronary benefits.[58,59] However, there is not only debate on this point,[60] but recently Jenkins et al[61] questioned the evidence that EPA and DHA are useful in the prevention of cardiovascular disease; they also highlighted the environmental threat posed by an increase in fish consumption.

Carbohydrate

In contrast to other beans, there is essentially no complex carbohydrate in soybeans because approximately half of the soybean carbohydrate is fiber and half is the oligosaccharides raffinose and stachyose.[62] In many traditional soyfoods, such as soymilk and tofu, the fiber is largely removed during processing. Soy fiber is a mixture of cellulosic and noncellulosic structural components of the internal plant cell wall and has many of the same attributes as other soluble fibers, although it has not been studied extensively.[63]

Bean consumption often leads to flatulence[64,65] as a result of the intestinal metabolism of the oligosaccharides.[66,67] The oligosaccharide content of beans is roughly 25 to 50 mg/g (dry wt), but soybeans have a higher oligosaccharide content than most legumes (60 mg/g of defatted meal).[62,68,69] It is possible to remove substantial amounts of oligosaccharides (up to 60%) and to markedly reduce flatulence by removing the water in which beans are boiled one or more times.[70] Also, consuming fermented soyfoods, such as tempeh and miso, in which the sugars have already undergone bacterial metabolism or products from which the oligosaccharides have largely been removed (e.g., tofu and ISP) during processing leads to much less flatulence.

However, there may be some beneficial effects associated with oligosaccharide consumption because of their prebiotic properties. A prebiotic is defined as "a non-digestible food ingredient that beneficially affects the host selectively by stimulating the growth and/or activity of one or a limited number of bacteria in the colon."[71] Because of their growth-promoting effect on bifidobacteria, soybean oligosaccharides have been hypothesized to promote the health of the colon, increase longevity, and decrease colon cancer risk.[72–76] Bifidobacteria compete with less desirable bacteria found in the colon such as *Clostridium perfringens*.

Studies have shown that soybean oligosaccharides increase the bifidobacteria population 2- to 10-fold in human subjects.[75] The soybean oligosaccharides are commercially available in Japan,[77] and one group of Japanese researchers actually suggested that soybean oligosaccharides be used as a substitute for common table sugar.[78] Research also suggests that soy carbohydrate may slow digestibility, lower insulin responses, and help to control hyperglycemia.[79]

Finally, there is quite a bit of interest in utilizing okara, which is a by-product of soymilk production.[80,81] It contains mostly crude fiber composed of cellulose, hemicellulose, and lignin, about 25% protein, 10–15% oil, but little starch or simple carbohydrates.[82] Okara has been used to make a wide range of products including burgers, baked products, candy, and rice cakes.[80,83,84]

Vitamins

The vitamin content of soybeans is unremarkable in comparison to other legumes (Table 9–2). Like most beans, soybeans are good sources of folate and other B vitamins. However, because of the high vitamin K (phylloquinone) content of soy oil, soyfoods are often included on lists of foods that should be avoided by patients on anticoagulants such as warfarin. Consuming vitamin K in amounts greater than average for a given patient can result in warfarin resistance, whereas consuming below average intakes can lead to warfarin sensitivity and unexpected bleeding.[85] The average adult vitamin K intake in the United States is between 80 and 150 μg/d.[86]

According to the USDA, the vitamin K content (μg/100 g) of soy oil, canola oil, olive oil, and corn oil is 184, 71, 60, and 2, respectively.[87] However, the vitamin K content of raw soybeans, dry roasted soybeans, soymilk, and regular tofu is reported to be only 47, 37, 3, and 2 μg/100 g, respectively. Because 100 g each of tofu and soymilk would be expected to contain approximately 5 g and 2 g of fat, respectively, the reported vitamin K content of these foods, based on the amount in soy oil, appears to be somewhat low. Kamao et al[88] reported values for soy oil, Japanese hard tofu, Japanese soft tofu, and deep fried bean curd of 234, 12, 12, and 62 μg/100 g, respectively. Even these somewhat higher values would not preclude soyfoods from being part of a diet consumed by patients taking warfarin for the prevention of thromboembolism.

The one exception may be natto, a fermented soyfood that has a very high vitamin K content (860 μg/100 g) and has been shown to interfere with warfarin therapy.[89,90] In addition to its vitamin K content, natto contains living *Bacillus subtilis*, which continues to synthesize vitamin K in the intestine for several days after natto has been eaten.[91] This having been said, research shows that if natto is boiled, which removes the bacteria and may partially inactivate vitamin K, the substantial increases in circulating vitamin K levels that occur in response to untreated natto are not observed.[92] Still, as of yet, the effects of boiled natto on prothrombin time in patients on warfarin has not been determined. One case report indicated that soymilk intake interfered with the efficacy of warfarin, but the reason for this is not clear.[93] Consequently, at this point, it is premature to conclude soymilk is problematic for warfarin patients.

Finally, it is important for patients taking warfarin to meet the vitamin K requirements.[94] Once a warfarin dose has been set, patients can avoid any complications resulting from variations in vitamin K intake by continuing to follow their normal dietary patterns. Thus all soyfoods with the exception of natto can fit into the diet of patients on anticoagulant therapy, but patients should avoid inconsistent consumption of large amounts of soy.

Minerals

The content and availability of minerals from soyfoods is an important issue because these foods are frequently used in place of animal foods, many of which are good sources of iron and zinc, and, in the case of dairy foods, calcium. Concerns about the impact of soy on iron and zinc status is primarily only germane to vegetarians because relatively little red meat is needed to meet daily zinc requirements for these minerals.[95] The degree to which calcium is absorbed from calcium-fortified soymilk is especially important for vegans. In regard to mineral content, it is noteworthy that legumes including soy are good sources of potassium, which is recognized as a problem nutrient in the United States because adult intake is approximately only half the dietary reference intake.[96] One serving of soybeans and other soyfoods provides approximately as much potassium as a cup of cow's milk.

Iron

Compared to other legumes, soybeans are relatively high in iron. The iron content (mg) of 100 g of cooked legumes is as follows: soybeans (5.1), lentils (3.3), black beans (2.1), pinto beans (2.6), kidney beans (2.9), and navy beans (2.5). One serving (½ cup) of soybeans provides 4.4 mg of iron, about 40% of the recommended dietary allowance (RDA) for men and postmenopausal women and about 25% for premenopausal women. However, concern has arisen over a possible detrimental effect of soyfood consumption on iron status because of the poor iron bioavailability from soy products. In the USDA ruling allowing soy protein to replace meat and milk protein in the Federal School Lunch Program, a decision was made not to require iron and zinc fortification of soy protein based on the premise that students were consuming a nonvegetarian diet that included some sources of highly bioavailable iron.[52] Obviously, this premise does not apply to vegetarians.

In single-meal studies, both soy protein and phytic acid in soybeans inhibit iron absorption from soyfoods, whereas vitamin C has been shown to markedly enhance absorption.[97,98] For vitamin C to enhance iron absorption in vivo, it must be present in the intestine with iron.[99] However, in general, the pronounced effect of vitamin C on iron absorption noted in acute studies is not as apparent as judged by iron status in long-term studies as discussed in Chapter 6.[100] Older research indicated iron absorption from soybeans and traditional soyfoods was similar to or somewhat better than from legumes and other plant foods.[101–103] Interestingly, although fermentation leads to the hydrolysis of phytate, the extent to which fermentation of soy products affects iron absorption is unclear.[102–108]

Most importantly, new research suggests iron bioavailability from soybeans has been greatly underestimated.[109] This research, the key to which is the improved methodology used to assess absorption, indicates that iron absorption from soy is excellent. The reason is that most of the iron in soy is in the form of ferritin. Although there is some debate about the bioavailability of ferritin iron,[110] two clinical studies in women show soybean ferritin iron to be highly bioavailable, essentially being equal to the absorption of iron from $FeSO_4$.[109,111] Ferritin is a large protein that reversibly concentrates iron as a solid mineral, thereby making the mineral more bioavailable. Soybean varieties differ markedly in their ferritin concentration, which suggests iron bioavailability from different soybean varieties may differ.[112] If future research confirms the high bioavailability of soybean ferritin iron, it will require a complete reevaluation of how soyfoods are viewed as sources of iron.

In long-term studies, partial substitution of soy protein for meat protein does not compromise iron status. For example, in a 6-month study that included both adults and children, iron status was unaffected by the daily consumption of beef extended with soy protein, although many measures of iron status are relatively insensitive.[113] Also, although older men undergoing resistive training for 12 weeks who were randomly assigned to consume a beef-containing diet had an increased hematologic profile compared to men assigned to a vegetarian diet in which approximately 50% of the protein was derived from soy, the profile of the latter was well within the clinical normal range.[114]

A recently presented study designed specifically to examine the effect of soyfoods on mineral status also provides very reassuring results that mineral status is not detrimentally affected by the inclusion of soyfoods. In this randomized placebo-controlled trial, young premenopausal women consumed either two to three servings of soyfoods daily or two to three servings of foods that were matched for type of soyfood (i.e., hamburgers in place of soy burgers, cow's milk in place of soymilk). Results showed there were no statistically significant effects of soy on serum hemoglobin and iron, or transferrin saturation (see Messina et al[115] for a description of this study).

In addition to the clinical work, several epidemiologic studies have examined the impact of soyfood consumption on iron status. For example, one report indicated that the iron status of Chinese Buddhist lacto-ovo vegetarian women residing in Taiwan who consumed a diet in which 17.5% of the iron was derived from soyfoods was considerably worse than that of nonvegetarian women; 31% and 13% of the vegetarians and nonvegetarians, respectively, were considered anemic.[116] However, the superior iron status of the nonvegetarians was likely because 35% of their iron was derived from animal products rather than because less of their iron was derived from soy. Furthermore, and surprisingly, nonvegetarians consumed 40% more vitamin C than vegetarians. Also, although vegetarian iron intake was higher than nonvegetarian intake (15.6 mg vs 11.8 mg/d), both groups consumed less iron than the U.S. RDA.

Finally, in contrast to the preceding discussion are the results from a cross-sectional household survey of 2849 men and women ≥ 20 years of age (mean age: 47.0 ± 14.5 years), from a nationally representative random sample in Jiangsu province (China).[117] In this study, tofu intake was assessed by food frequency questionnaire. Mean hemoglobin values increased by quartiles of tofu intake (men: 14.1, 14.0, 14.5, and 14.8 mg/dl; women: 12.4, 12.5, 12.6, and 13.3 g/dl), and the prevalence of anemia decreased concomitantly. Comparing first and fourth quartiles of tofu intake, the prevalence of anemia was 23.9% versus 10.7% in men, and 38.1% versus 16.8% in women. In multivariate analyses, the odds ratio (OR) of anemia for men in the fourth compared to the first quartile of tofu intake was 0.30 (95% confidence interval [CI], 0.17 to 0.50], and the corresponding OR for women was 0.31 (95% CI, 0.20 to 0.47).

Zinc

In contrast to iron, soybeans are not high in zinc relative to the RDA, nor do they contain significantly more zinc than other legumes. The zinc content (mg) of 100 g of different cooked legumes is as follows: soybeans (1.2), pinto beans (1.1), kidney beans (1.1), lentils (1.3), navy beans (1.1), and black beans (1.1). One-half cup of cooked soybeans provides $<10\%$ of the zinc RDA for adults. It is important to recognize when considering meeting zinc requirements that zinc status is much more difficult to assess than iron status.

Partial replacement of meat protein with soy protein has been shown to only modestly inhibit zinc absorption if at all.[118–121] For example, Greger at al[120] found no difference in zinc retention over a 30-day period among adolescent girls when soy protein was substituted for 30% of meat protein in the school lunch program. Zinc bioavailability from an equal mixture of ISP and milk was 47%, which was not different from the zinc bioavailability from milk (51%).[122] However, zinc bioavailability from ISP was only 37%. Other research also indicates zinc absorption from soy to be similar or about 25% lower than zinc absorption from animal foods.[119,121,123,124]

As is the case for iron, both the phytic acid and protein in soy inhibit zinc absorption, although in the case of zinc the effects are much more modest.[124–126] For example, zinc absorption in young (23 to 43 years of age) and elderly (71 to 78 years of age) men from dephytinized and half dephytinized (130 mg/200 ml) soymilk was significantly greater than from regular nondephytinized (260 mg/200 ml) soymilk.[127] Similarly, in healthy males ($N = 10$), serum zinc levels over a 4-hour period were markedly reduced in response to the consumption of nondephytinized ground soybeans and tofu, in comparison to dephytinized tofu and ground soybeans.[128] Lo et al[129] concluded that the phytate-to-zinc molar ratios should be <10 to optimize zinc absorption from ISP. Fermentation of soybean flour with *Aspergillus usamii* has been shown to reduce phytic acid content and, at least in rats and chicks, improve zinc bioavailability.[130–132]

Finally, there are the results from two studies that examined zinc status in response to soyfood intake. In one, when premenopausal women ($N = 9$) were fed similar diets that differed primarily only as to whether they contained tofu (280 g) or cheese (80 g), no differences in zinc balance were noted.[133] The tofu and cheese each provided approximately 28% of the total zinc intake during the 3-week feeding periods. In the other previously mentioned study, the consumption of two to three servings of soyfoods daily did not adversely affect urinary and serum zinc levels in premenopausal women.[115]

In conclusion, zinc bioavailability from soy products has not been as well studied as has iron bioavailability, although the data suggest zinc absorption from soy is lower than from animal products. Further, relative to the RDA, soy is not very high in zinc.

Calcium

The calcium content (mg) of 100 g of cooked legumes is as follows: soybeans (102), pinto beans (48), kidney beans (28), lentils (19), navy beans (70), and black beans (27). Soybeans are very high in calcium relative to other legumes, although one serving (½ cup) of cooked soybeans provides just 88 mg, or only from 6% to 11% of the RDA for adult women. Furthermore, whereas the calcium content of 100 g of tofu not precipitated with calcium is about 103 mg, 1 cup of unfortified soymilk contains only about 40 to 60 mg of calcium. However, nearly all soymilk sold in the United States is fortified with calcium and vitamin D.

Calcium bioavailability from soyfoods has been studied for more than 70 years. The first report, which was published in 1932, involved only three subjects but indicated that calcium bioavailability from tofu was similar to that from dairy milk.[134] Although soybeans are high in both oxalate and phytic acid—two components that strongly inhibit calcium absorption—calcium bioavailability from soy is surprisingly good.[135] The relatively high calcium bioavailability from soy is rather remarkable given that calcium bioavailability from legumes is generally $<20\%$[136] and that the oxalate-to-calcium ratio in soy is similar to rhubarb and about twice as high as in spinach.[137] Calcium absorption from rhubarb and spinach is only about 9%[138] and 5%,[139] respectively.

In 1991, Heaney et al[140] published a seminal paper on calcium bioavailability from soybeans. Using two different strains of soybeans, they found that in healthy premenopausal women, calcium absorption from high-phytate soybeans, low-phytate soybeans, and 2% fat dairy milk was 31.0%, 41.4%, and 37.7%, respectively. The difference between the soybean strains was statistically significant, indicating that soy phytate does reduce calcium absorption. Almost a decade later, Heaney et al[141] found that in healthy men, calcium absorption from intrinsically labeled calcium-fortified soymilk was about 75% that of calcium absorption from cow's milk (0.237 vs 0.306; $P < 0.01$). The calcium salt used in that study was tricalcium phosphate (TCP). Because TCP in different food matrices was found to be absorbed as well as calcium from dairy milk, Heaney et al[141] concluded that the lower calcium absorption from soymilk was due to factors in soy, not to the TCP.

In 2005, the TCP findings were replicated by research from Purdue University. Zhao et al[142] found that the bioavailability of calcium from calcium-fortified soymilk depends on the type of supplemental calcium used. Calcium absorption from soymilk fortified with TCP was about 25% lower than from cow's milk.[142] However, when calcium carbonate was used as the fortificant in soymilk, absorption was essentially identical to that seen with cow's milk. Calcium carbonate is the fortificant used in most soymilk sold in the United States. Furthermore, according to Zhao et al,[142] because of the high amounts of TCP added, the amount of calcium available to the body from both types of calcium-fortified soymilks is similar to that from cow's milk. In general agreement with the findings from Zhao et al,[142] Weaver et al[143] found no difference in the absorption of calcium from tofu fortified with calcium sulfate or calcium chloride, in comparison to calcium absorption from dairy milk.

Finally, questions have been raised about the solubility of calcium in soymilk. Some research indicates that, even with vigorous shaking, the calcium in soymilk comes out of the solution.[144] However, although some sedimentation occurs in certain soymilks, for most of the soymilk sold in the United States, this sediment is resuspended with mild shaking.

CHRONIC DISEASE PREVENTION AND TREATMENT

Coronary Heart Disease

Cholesterol Reduction

In 1995, a meta-analysis of the clinical data, which included 38 different comparisons, found that soy protein reduced low-density lipoprotein cholesterol (LDL-C) by approximately 13%.[145] This reduction was independent of the fatty acid content of the diets and at that time was larger than that reported for any other single nonpharmacologic treatment. In fact, because statins were not yet widely used in clinical practice, the effect of soy protein was essentially equal to that of the available cholesterol-lowering medications.

Some data suggest that cholesterol reduction is a result of the upregulation of hepatic LDL receptors by the peptides formed upon digestion of soy protein.[146,147] Researchers also continue to explore whether isoflavones in soybeans impact the cholesterol-lowering effects of soy protein.[148]

In 1999, the U.S. Food and Drug Administration (FDA) approved a health claim for soy protein and CHD based on its cholesterol-lowering effects.[149] In total, >100 clinical trials investigating the hypocholesterolemic effects of soy protein have been published. However, despite the health claim, questions have recently been raised about the efficacy of soy protein.[150] In fact, the FDA announced in December 2007 its intention to reevaluate evidence in support of the claim, although the stated reason for this reevaluation was not because of concerns that the evidence no longer supported the claim but because so much new research had been published since the claim was initially approved.

This having been said, the current estimates of the degree to which soy protein reduces LDL-C are much lower than initially reported. Meta-analyses and reviews published between 2004 and 2007, including ones by the American Heart Association[150] and the federal Agency for Healthcare Research and Quality,[151] have concluded that soy protein lowers LDL-C 3–5%,[152] which is similar to the effects of soluble fiber.[153] These estimates agree with a recently presented analysis that covered the relevant literature published since 1978 (see Messina et al[154] for a brief description of this research).

The reasons for the lowered estimates are not entirely known, although compared to earlier studies, those published after the 1995 meta-analysis involved subjects with lower baseline cholesterol levels and used somewhat lower amounts of soy protein. Also, many of the earliest studies that showed very large reductions in cholesterol reportedly used a soy protein processed differently than the products used in most other studies, although these earlier studies also involved very hypercholesterolemic individuals.[155] In any event, the extent to which each of these factors influences the cholesterol-lowering effects of soy is unclear.

From a public health perspective, even reducing LDL-C by 3–5% is meaningful. Over time, each 1% decrease in LDL-C reduces CHD risk and/or mortality by as much as 2–5%.[156,157] Furthermore, the advantage of incorporating soyfoods into heart-healthy diets extends beyond the direct effect of soy protein on cholesterol levels. When soyfoods displace more traditional sources of protein in Western diets, overall saturated fat intake is reduced, polyunsaturated fat intake is increased, and blood cholesterol levels will be lowered.[158,159] Not surprisingly, comprehensive dietary approaches that have resulted in reductions in LDL-C ranging from 20–30% have relied heavily on soyfoods; the high-quality of soy protein and its hypocholesterolemic effects combined with the favorable fatty acid profile of soyfoods make these foods especially attractive in such diets.[160]

It is noteworthy that in response to the ingestion of soy protein, meta-analyses have also found that in addition to lowering LDL-C, there are very modest increases (1–3%) in high-density-ipoprotein cholesterol (HDL-C) and modest decreases (5–10%) in triglyceride levels. Each 1% or 1 mg increase in HDL lowers CHD risk by 2–3%.[161–163] Although there is debate about whether an elevated triglyceride level is an independent predictor of CHD risk,[164] evidence suggests that the role of fasting triglyceride levels in the etiology of CHD has been underestimated.[165,166]

Finally, the amount of soy protein needed to lower cholesterol is uncertain. The threshold intake required for cholesterol reduction is generally considered to be 25 g/d, and it is the amount established by the FDA. In large part, this figure has been adopted because few trials used <25 g, although there is evidence suggesting that lower amounts are also efficacious.[167]

Lipid-Independent Effects

There is epidemiologic evidence that soyfoods exert coronary benefits independent of their effect on blood cholesterol levels. For example, after controlling for a wide variety of CHD risk factors, a prospective study involving nearly 65,000 postmenopausal women from Shanghai found that soy protein intake was associated with an 86% reduction in the risk of nonfatal myocardial infarction.[168] In agreement, a cross-sectional study involving 406 Chinese adults ages 40 to 65 years (134 males, 272 females) without confirmed relevant diseases found that soyfood intake was inversely related to bifurcation intima-media thickness, although the association was more apparent in men than women.[169] Also, a prospective study involving 40,462 Japanese participants (40 to 59 years old, without cardiovascular disease or cancer at baseline) found that when comparing women with frequent (≥5 times per week) versus infrequent (≤2 times per week) soy consumption, the multivariable hazard ratios were 0.64, 0.55, and 0.31 for risk of the incidence of cerebral infarction, myocardial infarction, and CHD mortality, respectively.[170]

In support of the epidemiologic studies are various clinical studies that show soyfoods, soy protein, or soybean isoflavones favorably affect a number of biologic measures that impact heart disease risk. The proposed hypotensive effects of soyfoods are particularly intriguing. A recent meta-analysis found that soyfoods reduced systolic and diastolic blood pressure by about 6 and 4 mm Hg, respectively, although these data were based on only five studies.[171] Other biologic processes and measures related to heart disease that may be favorably affected by various soy components include endothelial function, systematic arterial compliance, LDL-oxidation and LDL particle size.[172] It is likely that the isoflavones in soybeans are responsible for the effects on endothelial function.

Despite the encouraging results from some clinical studies, the very inconsistent findings overall do not allow conclusions about the effects of soy on these lipid-independent risk factors to be drawn, with the exception of endothelial function. Recent studies do provide possible explanations for some of the inconsistency, however. For example, endothelial dysfunction, which is regarded as an independent CHD risk factor, was found to be improved by isoflavones primarily only among subjects whose endothelial function was impaired at baseline.[173,174] Similarly, the anti-inflammatory effects of isoflavones may be observed only in subjects at risk of CHD who have elevated levels of inflammatory markers.[175] The clinical studies in which effects of different soy products on biologic measures of CHD risk were examined involved subjects at both normal and elevated risk. Thus the differences in baseline subject characteristics may account for some of the overall inconsistent clinical results.

Cancer

The role of soyfoods in reducing cancer risk has been rigorously investigated for 20 years since the US National Cancer Institute first funded research in this area.[176] Initially, and still today, most of this research focused on cancer of the breast, in part because of the historically low breast cancer incidence rates in soyfood-consuming countries.[20] There has also been much investigation of the role of soy in reducing risk of prostate cancer, the rates of which are also low in Asian countries.[20] Because these two cancers have been investigated most intensely, only they are discussed here. However, it is noteworthy that genistein inhibits the growth of a wide range of both hormone-dependent and -independent cancer cells in vitro.[15] The in vitro concentrations required to inhibit cancer cell growth are typically much higher than serum isoflavone levels, but the animal data suggest the in vitro anticancer effects may still be relevant.[177,178] In fact, there is some evidence indicating the in vitro data underestimate the in vivo anticancer activity of isoflavones.[179]

Like all foods, the soybean contains many biologically active components including phytate, protease inhibitors, fatty acids, phytosterols, lunasin, and saponins. Many of these have been investigated for their chemopreventive properties; however, most evidence suggests that if, in fact, soy intake is protective against cancer, it is because of the presence of isoflavones.

Breast Cancer

A published meta-analysis in 2008 by Wu et al[180] that included only those studies with a relatively complete assessment of dietary soy exposure in the targeted populations, and appropriate consideration for potential confounders in the statistical analysis of the data found there was a significant trend of decreasing risk with increasing soyfood intake. Compared to the lowest level of soyfood intake (≤5 mg isoflavones per day), risk was intermediate (OR: 0.88; 95% CI, 0.78 to 0.98) among those with modest (about 10 mg isoflavones per day) intake and lowest (OR: 0.71; 95% CI, 0.60 to 0.85) among those with high intake (≥20 mg isoflavones per day). However, as recently reviewed by Messina and Wu[181] and Messina and Hilakivi-Clarke,[182] evidence suggests that to derive protection against breast cancer, soy consumption has to occur during childhood and/or adolescence.

All four epidemiologic studies[183–186] that examined this hypothesis reported protective effects with reductions in risk ranging from 28% to 60%, whereas, as discussed later, the clinical studies show adult exposure does not affect markers of breast cancer risk (see Messina and Wood[187]). In addition, in young rats, genistein exposure for just a few weeks reduces chemically induced mammary cancer by half, whereas exposure only during adulthood has no effect.[188,189] Interestingly, adult exposure further reduces mammary tumor development in rats given genistein also when young.

Exposure to genistein causes breast tissue differentiation and reduces the number of terminal end buds, the anatomic structure within the rodent mammary gland that is the likely site of tumor development.[188,190] There is evidence that these kinds of changes are also important in humans.[191] The notion that early isoflavone exposure is protective against later development of breast cancer is consistent with the school of thought that maintains early life events—such as becoming pregnant at a young age—profoundly impact breast cancer risk.[191–195]

Prostate Cancer

In 2009, Yan and Spitznagel[196] systematically reviewed 15 epidemiologic studies on soy consumption and 9 on isoflavones in association with prostate cancer risk. The soy intake data yielded a combined relative risk (RR)/OR of 0.74 ($P = 0.01$). When separately analyzed, studies on nonfermented and fermented soyfoods yielded a combined RR/OR of 0.70 ($P = 0.01$) and 1.02 ($P = 0.92$), respectively. The isoflavone studies yielded a combined RR/OR of 0.88 ($P = 0.09$); however, when analyzed separately, the combined RR/OR for studies involving Asian and Western populations were 0.52 ($P = 0.01$) and 0.99 ($P = 0.91$), respectively. Research in animals supports these findings[197,198] as does a second analysis of the epidemiologic data also published in 2009.[199] The lack of benefit observed in Western studies can be attributed to the low soy intake among the populations studied. Despite the ability to identify statistically significant associations between soy/isoflavone intake and health outcomes in epidemiologic studies involving typical Western populations, it is likely that because of the negligible intake these associations do not have a causal basis.[200]

In addition to helping prevent the development of prostate cancer, there is speculative but intriguing animal and human evidence suggesting soy may also be useful for stopping its spread. Prostate cancer, like many cancers, is lethal only when tumors metastasize from the site of origin to vital organs. A recent study reported that levels of an enzyme that allow cells to invade tissues was markedly reduced in prostate cancer patients given genistein.[17] In agreement, adding isoflavones to the diet of mice inhibited prostate tumor metastasis to the lung, the primary site of metastasis in this animal model, by 96%.[201]

Finally, to examine the potential role of soy in reducing prostate cancer risk, numerous investigators have focused on the impact of isoflavone-rich products on levels of prostate-specific antigen (PSA). PSA is the most common clinical test for the detection of prostate cancer and is a measure by which treatment efficacy can be assessed.[202] In men with prostate tumors, serum PSA concentration is proportional to prostate tumor volume,[203] and successful treatments for prostate cancer lower PSA levels.[204–212]

The evidence that soy or isoflavones affect PSA levels is mixed. In a review published in 2006, no effects were noted in healthy subjects with low PSA levels.[213] However, the lack of effect on PSA does not necessarily contradict the animal[214] or epidemiologic data[215] supportive of protective effects of soy because recent clinical data indicate that, in healthy men with low PSA levels, it is possible to reduce prostate cancer risk without affecting PSA.[216] In contrast to the results in healthy men, four of the eight trials involving prostate cancer patients that were included in the previously mentioned review showed isoflavones slowed the rise in PSA levels, although no study showed an absolute decrease in PSA.[213] In support of these findings are recent studies showing soy increases the PSA doubling time.[217,218] These data, along with the preliminary evidence mentioned earlier about inhibiting metastasis, hold open the possibility that soyfoods may be useful in the treatment of prostate cancer.

Osteoporosis

In response to declining estrogen levels, women can lose substantial amounts of bone mass in the decade following menopause, which markedly increases their fracture risk.[219] Estrogen therapy has been definitively shown to reduce postmenopausal bone loss and hip fracture risk by approximately a third.[220] Initial speculation that soyfoods might promote bone health in postmenopausal women was based on the estrogen-like effects of isoflavones and early research showing that the synthetic isoflavone, ipriflavone, exerted skeletal benefits.[221]

The first clinical trial to investigate the impact of an isoflavone-rich product on bone mineral density (BMD) in postmenopausal women was published in 1998.[222] Since then, more than 25 trials have done so (for reviews, see references), although many involved small numbers of subjects and were conducted for relatively short durations.[223,224] Bone trials should ideally be at least 2 years in length. The results of the clinical research are quite mixed. Although recently published meta-analyses of the data concluded that isoflavones inhibit bone breakdown[225] and increase both bone formation[225] and BMD in postmenopausal women,[226] a more rigorously conducted meta-analysis failed to provide support for the skeletal benefits of isoflavones.[227]

Among the many clinical trials, one of the longest and largest (304 subjects over a period of 2 years) found that postmenopausal osteopenic Italian women in the placebo group lost approximately 6% of their BMD at the spine and hip, whereas those women in the genistein group (54 mg/d provided as a supplement) gained approximately this much bone at both skeletal sites.[228] The amount of genistein administered to the subjects is found in approximately four servings of soyfoods. Although intended to last only 2 years, among those subjects that agreed to continue for a third year, the differences between groups was even more striking.[229] These results concur with those from a 2-year study but that was much smaller in size.[230]

However, the results of this Italian study stand in stark contrast to several recently conducted trials. For example, a 1-year study involving women from three European countries failed to show that isoflavone supplements (110 mg/d) inhibit bone loss in early postmenopausal women.[231] In agreement, another 1-year trial failed to show that either isoflavone supplements or isoflavone-rich soy protein affected bone loss in postmenopausal women.[232] Similarly, a just-published 2-year study found soy protein, regardless of isoflavone content, failed to prevent bone loss in postmenopausal women, although this study had a large dropout rate and many women were non-compliant with the intervention.[233] Finally, and most importantly, a large 3-year trial that used two different doses (80 and 120 mg/d) of isoflavone supplements found that only in response to the high dose was there a suggestion of even modest benefit.[234] These results agree with those from a trial that utilized a novel methodology to examine the effects of estrogen and a variety of phytoestrogen supplements on bone resorption; only at very high doses—doses exceeding typical isoflavone exposure from soyfoods—was there any evidence of antiresorptive effects.[235]

In contrast to the clinical data are the results from the only two prospective epidemiologic studies to evaluate the relationship between soy intake and fracture risk. In both, risk was reduced by approximately one third when women in the highest soy intake quintile or quartile were compared to women in the first. This degree of protection is similar to that noted for estrogen therapy.[220] In one of the prospective studies, approximately 1800 fractures of all types occurred in the 24,000 postmenopausal Shanghai women who were followed for 4.5 years.[236] In the other, there were almost 700 hip fractures (the only site studied) among the 35,000 postmenopausal Singaporean women during the 7-year follow-up period.[237]

As to why the Italian study produced such striking results in comparison to the other clinical trials just cited is unclear. But it is noteworthy that the genistein used in that study was in the aglycone form, whereas in all other trials, isoflavones were in the glycoside form. It remains to be determined whether this difference influences efficacy, but it is an intriguing possibility. As to why the two epidemiologic studies show such pronounced protective effects in contrast to the clinical studies also remains to be determined. In the former, isoflavone intake occurred via the consumption of traditional soyfoods, whereas the clinical studies have generally used soy extracts, although there is no evidence this difference matters with respect to skeletal effects. It may also be that the effects noted in the epidemiologic studies result from lifelong intake as opposed to the relatively short-term intervention periods begun in adulthood in the clinical studies, although again, there is no direct evidence supporting this suggestion. Finally, it could simply be that the epidemiologic studies are identifying a "a healthy user effect." Perhaps, soy consumers lead a bone-healthy lifestyle. In any event, only the results from clinical trials can be used as a basis for conclusions about the possible skeletal benefits of soyfoods.

Therefore, at this point, it is clear that no conclusions about the possible skeletal benefits of soyfoods can be made. Still, soyfoods provide high-quality protein,[51] which may be important for bone health,[238] and some soyfoods are good sources of calcium and also vitamin D.[142] Thus soyfoods can still be part of a bone-healthy diet, but whether isoflavones offer a direct skeletal benefit remains to be determined.

Alleviation of Menopausal Symptoms

Hot flashes are the most common reason given by women for seeking treatment for menopausal symptoms. For most women who experience them, hot flashes begin prior to menopause and are severe and frequent in about 10–15% of these women.[239] Although hot flashes usually subside after 6 months to 2 years,[240] many women report having them for up to 20 years after menopause.[241]

In 1992, Adlercreutz and colleagues[242] suggested that the low prevalence of hot flashes reported by Japanese menopausal women might be at least partially due to their high consumption of soyfoods. Speculation was that the estrogen-like effects of isoflavones might mitigate the drop in estrogen levels—one trigger for hot flashes—that occurs when women enter menopause. It is noteworthy that some recent data suggest Japanese women are actually less likely to report having hot flashes than Western women.

More than 50 hot flash trials evaluating the efficacy of isoflavone-containing products have been conducted. Over the past few years, several reviews and analyses of these data have been published but with mixed conclusions. For example, a meta-analysis published in 2006 by Howes and colleagues[243] that included 11 trials found that isoflavones were modestly efficacious, whereas a more recent review by the Cochrane Collaboration[244] stated that there were no definitive data allowing such a conclusion to be reached, although five of the nine studies evaluated reported that the soy isoflavone intervention significantly alleviated hot flash frequency and/or severity. Similar conclusions were reached by Jacobs et al[245] in their recent review.

It can be argued that even the inconsistent data are sufficiently encouraging to justify health professionals recommending the use of isoflavones because benefit can be subjectively determined, and the overall improvement (including placebo response) in many studies in response to isoflavones is about a 50% reduction in the severity and frequency of hot flashes. This magnitude of response is likely to be viewed quite favorably by women seeking nonhormonal alternatives to estrogen for menopausal symptom relief.[246]

Several explanations for the mixed data have been proposed including the variation in baseline hot flash frequency (i.e., some work suggests initial hot flash frequency is related to efficacy),[247] interindividual differences in isoflavone metabolism, and the differing genistein content of the intervention products.[248] There are two primary types of commercially available supplements that have been used in the clinical setting; these vary widely in isoflavone profile. One has a profile similar to that found in soyfoods (i.e., it is high in genistein and low in glycitein), whereas the other is low in genistein and high in glycitein.

In an attempt to provide some clarity about the effects of isoflavones on the alleviation of hot flashes, a team of investigators including those from the National Institutes of Health in Japan and the University of Minnesota conducted a systematic review and meta-analysis of the literature, although only studies evaluating the effects of isoflavone supplements derived from soybeans were considered.[249] The overall results showed that supplements with an isoflavone profile similar to that in soybeans consistently alleviated hot flashes. In comparison to the placebo, hot flash frequency and severity was reduced by about 20% and 30%, respectively. Thus the evidence clearly warrants health professionals recommending that women wanting a nonhormonal alternative to estrogen for the treatment of hot flashes try isoflavones and soyfoods.

Renal Function

The impact of dietary protein on overall renal function and glomerular filtration rate (GFR) has been recognized for more than two decades; for this reason protein restriction has been viewed as one approach to preventing further decline in renal function in renal disease patients.[250,251] It is unlikely that the type or amount of protein has clinically relevant effects on kidney function in healthy individuals. For example, in the Nurses' Health Study, over an 11-year follow-up period, high protein intake was not significantly associated with change in estimated GFR in middle-aged women with normal renal function, whereas in women with mild renal insufficiency, GFR decreased 1.69 ml/min per 1.73 m^2 per 10-g increase in protein intake. Thus the authors of this study concluded that high total protein intake, particularly high intake of nondairy animal protein, may accelerate renal function decline in women with mild renal insufficiency.[251]

Current recommendations for predialysis patients include, depending on the functioning of the kidney, a reduction in protein intake to no more than 0.6 to 0.8 g/kg bw,[252,253] which is only about 50% of usual U.S. adult protein intake.[254] With the rising numbers of people at risk of developing chronic kidney disease (between 1988–1994 and 1999–2004, the prevalence of chronic kidney disease increased by 30%[255]) as a result of the increasing prevalence of diabetes, data suggesting that soy protein may favorably affect renal function relative to animal proteins have attracted attention.[256–263] For general reviews on this topic, see Bernstein et al[264] and Anderson.[265]

Unlike animal protein, soy protein appears not to increase postprandial GFR or renal blood flow.[256, 266–268] Also, some research indicates that soy protein, when substituted for animal protein, decreases urinary protein levels (a measure of kidney function) in individuals with chronic renal disease and in patients with diabetes.[269–273] Parenthetically, recent data suggest that soyfoods may also be useful for dialysis patients[274–277] and may have advantages for renal transplant patients.[278]

In conclusion, there are intriguing data suggesting soy protein may favorably affect renal function in individuals at risk for developing renal disease. More research is needed, however, before definitive conclusions are possible.

CONTROVERSIES

As noted at the outset, in recent years concerns have arisen that soyfoods might be contraindicated for some individuals. Most concerns are based on the estrogen-like effects of isoflavones. But others are not, such as the impact of soyfoods on mineral status, which has already been addressed. Somewhat ironically, in some cases concerns have arisen in areas where there is also evidence of benefit, such as the impact of soyfood intake on the prognosis of breast cancer patients. Whenever possible in the treatment of these issues, in the text that follows, the human data have been emphasized.

Soy Infant Formula

Despite its long history of use, soy infant formula (SIF) has become controversial in recent years due primarily to the naturally high isoflavone content of the soybean. This issue is only briefly discussed here because both the American Academy of Pediatrics (AAP) and the U.S. National Toxicology Program (NTP) Center for the Evaluation of Risks to Human Reproduction recently evaluated SIF. In 2008, the AAP acknowledged that SIF produces normal growth and development and stated that "although studied by numerous investigators in various species, there is no conclusive evidence from animal, adult human, or infant populations that dietary soy isoflavones may adversely affect human development, reproduction, or endocrine function."[279] In 2009, the conclusion of the 14-member panel of independent scientists that examined SIF at the request of the NTP reached the conclusion that there was "minimal concern" (the five levels of concern are negligible concern, minimal concern, some concern, concern, and serious concern) about safety. Two panel members dissented from this consensus opinion, one in favor of "negligible concern" and the other in support of "some concern." Importantly, the AAP expressed in writing their opinion that the risk associated with SIF should be considered negligible.

Within the next couple of years it is likely that valuable insights into the health effects of SIF will be gained. Currently underway is the Beginnings Study, a longitudinal cohort consisting of infants who were fed SIF, cow milk–based formula (CMF) or breast milk (BM). The aim of the study is to enroll 200 infants per group and to follow them until at least 6 years of age. Preliminary results from this study were published in 2009.[280] In this study, breast buds, uterus, ovaries, prostate, and testicular volumes in 40 BM-fed, 41 CMF-fed, and 39 SIF-fed infants at age 4 months were measured ultrasonically. There were no significant feeding group effects in anthropometric or body composition overall, and among girls there were no feeding group differences in breast bud or uterine volume, although CMF-fed infants had greater ($P < 0.05$) mean ovarian volume and greater ($P < 0.01$) numbers of ovarian cysts per ovary than did BF infants. These preliminary results are reassuring but are based on very small numbers. More definite data from this study will soon be available.

Cognitive Function

The role of estrogen in the etiology of Alzheimer's disease and in the prevention of age-related cognitive decline has become less clear in recent years, but the possibility that estrogen therapy improves cognitive function spurred investigation of the cognitive benefits of isoflavones. However, two epidemiologic studies raised concern about possible detrimental effects.

One was a prospective study (begun in 1965 as the Honolulu Heart Study), published in 2000, that found tofu consumption was associated with impaired cognitive function in Japanese men and women residing in Hawaii.[281] More recently, an Indonesian cross-sectional study among mainly Javanese and Sudanese elderly ($N = 719$; age range, 52 to 98 years) found that worse memory, as measured using a word-learning test sensitive to dementia, was associated with high tofu consumption (measured by food frequency questionnaire), whereas high tempeh consumption was independently related to better memory, particularly in participants >68 years of age.[282] The analyses were controlled for age, sex, education, site, and intake of other foods. In both studies, isoflavones were thought to be responsible for the observed effects. In contrast to these two studies, however, are the results of a cross-sectional study conducted in Hong Kong involving 3999 men and women ≥65 years that found isoflavone intake was unrelated to cognitive function.[283] Dietary intake was assessed using a 7-day food frequency questionnaire, and cognitive function was assessed by the cognitive part of the Community Screening Instrument for Dementia.

In evaluating these epidemiologic data, it is important to recognize the limitations of the Hawaiian and Indonesian studies. In the former, the intake of only 26 foods was assessed, questions about tofu intake were not consistent over the course of the follow-up period, and cognitive function was a secondary end point added near the end of the study. In regard to the Indonesian study, the results are unusual in that two isoflavone-rich soyfoods had opposite effects. The authors of this study suggested the high folate content of tempeh but not tofu was responsible for the differing findings. However, for several reasons, a more likely explanation, also discussed by the authors, is that tofu but not tempeh contained formaldehyde, a known toxin shown to adversely affect memory in rodents[284] and urinary levels of which are markedly elevated in dementia patients.[285] In Indonesia, tofu production is a cottage industry and despite attempts to prevent its use, formaldehyde is sometimes used as a preservative.

The three epidemiologic studies are clearly an insufficient basis for drawing conclusions about the effects of isoflavones on cognitive function. Even if the epidemiologic evidence was more persuasive, definitive conclusions could still not be made because this requires data from clinical trials. Since 2001, at least eight different trials have been published; most of these have involved postmenopausal women.[286] These data provide some reason for optimism and certainly justify continued research in this area. Most trials found benefits in one or more aspects of cognition, but the data are not internally consistent, with studies often showing benefits in different aspects of cognitive function. At this point, the evidence related to cognitive function does not provide a basis for or against using soyfoods.

Thyroid Function

In in vitro studies and in rats, isoflavones have been shown to partially inactivate thyroid peroxidase, an enzyme required for the synthesis of thyroid hormones.[287] However, despite inhibiting enzyme activity, soy-containing diets allow normal thyroid function in rats[288] even though they are extremely sensitive to thyroid insults.[289] Furthermore, and most importantly, a comprehensive review of the literature published in 2006 found that the clinical evidence clearly indicates that isoflavone exposure has no effect on thyroid function in euthyroid individuals.[290] Studies published subsequent to this review support this conclusion.[291–293] In many of these studies, isoflavone exposure was considerably higher than typical for Japanese adults consuming a traditional diet.

There are, however, two relevant clinical situations related to soy and thyroid function yet to be evaluated. One involves individuals with subclinical hypothyroidism, which represents about 5% of the general adult population but a higher percentage among individuals >60 years of age.[294] This condition is defined as having normal levels of the two primary thyroid hormones, thyroxine and triiodothyronine, but elevated levels of thyroid-stimulating hormone.[295] There is no evidence that soyfoods pose a problem for subclinical hypothyroid patients, but research specifically addressing this issue has not been conducted, although there are plans to do so.

The second situation involves individuals whose iodine intake is marginal or inadequate. Due to ethical concerns, it is unlikely that a clinical trial evaluating the effects of soy in such individuals could be conducted. In the United States, iodine intake is generally quite good.[296] But this is not the case in many parts of the world.[297] From a clinician's perspective, when individuals whose iodine intake is inadequate are identified, the appropriate recommendation is not to avoid soyfoods but to increase iodine intake.

Fertility and Feminization

Although the large Asian populations seemingly argue against any antifertility effects, isoflavones have been shown to cause infertility in some animal species, such as the captive cheetah in North American zoos[298] and sheep in Western Australia grazing on a type of clover rich in isoflavones.[299–301] However, problems in the former arose because felines are poorly able to glucuronidate phenolic compounds, a major step in the bodily elimination of isoflavones—a good example of differences in isoflavone metabolism between animals and humans—which, as a result, would lead to extremely high circulating levels of total and aglycone isoflavones.[11,302,303] In the case of the sheep, serum levels of equol, a bacterially synthesized metabolite of the soybean isoflavone daidzein, far exceeded anything approaching human levels simply because daily isoflavone intake was estimated to be several grams[304] versus the 40 mg common to Asian populations.[7]

More relevant to infertility concerns is the finding of a multivariate analysis from a pilot epidemiologic study involving 99 infertile men that subjects in the highest soyfoods intake category had, on average, 41 million sperm/ml less than men who did not eat soyfoods ($P = 0.02$).[305] It is not clear that these findings have implications for fertility, however, because the inverse relation between soyfood intake and sperm concentration was more pronounced in the high end of the distribution. Furthermore, there were several weaknesses of this research that raise questions about the validity of the findings. For example, other than soy intake, no assessment of diet was made. In addition, much of the decrease in sperm concentration seems to have occurred because ejaculate volume increased. In fact, the total number of sperm was unaffected. It seems unlikely that soy intake could increase ejaculate volume.

Most importantly, the clinical data do not support this epidemiologic finding. Three clinical studies,[115,306,307] one of which is available only as an abstract (see Messina et al[115] for description), and one case report[308] have examined the impact of isoflavone exposure on sperm and semen parameters, and none have reported adverse effects even though isoflavone exposure ranged from that typical for Japanese men to 10 times this amount. In fact, in the case report, sperm concentration normalized in an individual with oligospermia after isoflavone treatment.[308] This led to a successful pregnancy and to the authors of this report suggesting isoflavones could be a treatment for low sperm count.

In animals in which sperm and semen parameters had been adversely affected by isoflavones, circulating testosterone levels decreased dramatically. In contrast, a recent meta-analysis found that neither soy nor isoflavones affect circulating testosterone levels in men.[309] Similarly, there is essentially no clinical evidence that isoflavone exposure increases estrogen levels in men.[310] These hormone-related findings should help to allay concerns about both fertility and feminization.

Finally, soy and isoflavone intake has only minor and likely clinically insignificant effects on reproductive hormones in pre- and postmenopausal women.[311] Although soy may increase the length of the menstrual cycle by approximately 1 day, ovulation is only delayed and not prevented.

Breast Cancer Patients

The estrogen-like effects of isoflavones form the theoretical basis for concern that soyfoods might be contraindicated for women at increased risk of breast cancer and for breast cancer patients with estrogen-sensitive tumors.[312–316] Isoflavones bind to estrogen receptors, stimulate the growth of human ER-positive breast cancer cells in vitro, and, in certain types of experimental rodent models, stimulate the growth of existing estrogen-responsive mammary tumors.[317,318] However, not all rodent models show that soy stimulates the growth of existing mammary tumors,[319] and even in rodent models where stimulation occurs, whole soyfoods do not have this effect.[320] More importantly, the human data suggest that isoflavones, regardless of the source or form in which they are delivered, do not exert stimulatory effects on breast tissue.

In none of the four clinical trials, three involving postmenopausal and one premenopausal women in which researchers took breast tissue biopsies before and after exposure to isoflavones, were effects on cell proliferation noted.[321–324] Increased cell proliferation is generally regarded as a risk factor for cancer. Isoflavone exposure also has no effect on breast tissue density (increased density is a marker of cancer risk).[325–328] In contrast to the lack of effects of isoflavones, estrogen plus progestin hormone therapy, which increases breast cancer risk,[220] increases both breast tissue density and breast cell proliferation.[329,330]

Finally, three prospective epidemiologic studies provide important insight into the soy and breast cancer relationship. The findings from these studies are not only reassuring in regard to safety but even suggestive of benefit. In one, neither soy nor isoflavone intake was related to the disease-free survival of Chinese breast cancer patients over the 5.2-year follow-up period.[331] In this study, of the 1001 patients for whom data on receptor status were available, approximately 63% were ER-positive. The limitation of this study is that soy intake was assessed prior to diagnosis.

In the second study, data from the Shanghai Breast Cancer Survival Study, a population-based cohort study of breast cancer survivors were analyzed to investigate the effect of soy intake after diagnosis on breast cancer prognosis.[332] During the median follow-up period of approximately 3.9 years, women in the highest quartile of soy protein intake were about 30% less likely to die from breast cancer or suffer a recurrence. In this study high soy intake was as protective as tamoxifen use. In an editorial accompanying this article, the authors remarked that "Patients with breast cancer can be assured that enjoying a soy latte or indulging in pad thai with tofu causes no harm and, when consumed in plentiful amounts, may reduce risk of disease recurrence."[333]

A third study, which was conducted in the United States, involved 1954 breast cancer survivors who were followed for 6.3 years. During this time, there were 282 breast cancer recurrences. Suggestive trends for a reduced risk of cancer recurrence were observed with increasing quintiles of isoflavone intake compared to no intake among postmenopausal women and among tamoxifen users.[334] Interestingly, the benefit of soyfood intake on survival was more pronounced among women with ER-positive breast cancer.

The clinical and epidemiologic findings just described are certainly consistent with the position of the American Cancer Society that breast cancer patients can safely consume up to three servings of traditional soyfoods daily.[335] However, because none of the data can be considered definitive, breast cancer patients should always discuss any dietary changes with their healthcare provider.

Allergy

Soy protein, as is the case for essentially all food proteins, can cause allergic reactions in sensitive individuals. Soy protein is one of the eight foods responsible for approximately 90% of all food-induced allergic reactions in the United States.[336] But these foods are not equally allergenic, and allergy to soy protein is actually relatively rare.[337] A recent U.S. nationally representative telephone survey found that only approximately 1 of 2500 adults reported having doctor-diagnosed allergies to soy protein.[338] The rate is undoubtedly higher in children because children are more likely to have food allergies. However, most children outgrow soy allergies early in life.[339] This having been said, because small amounts of soy protein are often added to a wide variety of foods for functional purposes (moisture retention, texture improvement, etc.), those individuals who are allergic to soy must be quite diligent in their efforts to avoid exposure.

INTAKE RECOMMENDATIONS

Legumes are an underutilized food source in the United States despite their being included in the Dietary Guidelines in both the meat and bean group and the vegetable group. Data from the National Health and Nutrition Examination Survey 1999–2002 revealed that only 7.9% of the adult population consumed beans, peas, or lentils on any given day.[340] Soyfoods represent a convenient way to meet the legume recommendation, and for this reason alone their consumption can be encouraged. Furthermore, they are essentially unique dietary sources of isoflavones. However, there are many different legumes from which to choose, and no food should play too large a role in the diet.

If median Asian soy intake is used as a guide, than approximately 10 g of soy protein and about 30 to 35 mg/d isoflavones could be recommended. However, as discussed, for a variety of end points, a considerable number of epidemiologic studies show that among Asians, higher soy and isoflavone intakes are associated with lower disease risks. Thus a persuasive argument can be made that using these higher values makes more sense than the mean or median intakes. (Certainly the mean U.S. intake of many nutrients is less than optimal.) Furthermore, clinical studies that have reported health benefits have used amounts that equal or exceed even these higher values.

Recently, Biesalski et al[341] defined the physiologic intake of a dietary compound as a daily consumption that is no more than two to three times the average intake of that compound in a respective population. If one accepts this definition, then an upper intake of about four servings of soyfoods per day for adults, or approximately 100 mg isoflavones and 25 g soy protein, the latter figure matching the amount set by the FDA for cholesterol reduction, still falls within this category. There is no clinical evidence to suggest exceeding this level is harmful, but there is also no historical precedent for doing so. For most adult Americans, consuming 25 g soy protein would mean that soyfoods would provide about 30% of total protein intake.[342] For young children, whose overall caloric and protein intake is reduced (the latter by at least a third) in comparison to adults, a downward adjustment in soy makes sense. Thus, as a general rule, for young people two servings of soyfoods per day seem reasonable.

REFERENCES

1. United Soybean Board. *16th Annual Consumer Attitudes About Nutrition. 2009 National Report.* St. Louis, MO: United Soybean Board; 2000.
2. Lee YK, Georgiou C, Raab C. The knowledge, attitudes, and practices of dietitians licensed in Oregon regarding functional foods, nutrient supplements, and herbs as complementary medicine. *J Am Diet Assoc.* 2000;100:543–548.
3. Friel S, Dangour AD, Garnett T, et al. Public health benefits of strategies to reduce greenhouse-gas emissions: food and agriculture. *Lancet.* 2009;374:2016–2025.
4. Franke AA, Custer LJ, Wang W, Shi CY. HPLC analysis of isoflavonoids and other phenolic agents from foods and from human fluids. *Proc Soc Exp Biol Med.* 1998;217:263–273.
5. Long SR. Rhizobium-legume nodulation: life together in the underground. *Cell.* 1989;56:203–214.
6. Murphy PA, Barua K, Hauck CC. Solvent extraction selection in the determination of isoflavones in soy foods. *J Chromatogr B Analyt Technol Biomed Life Sci.* 2002;777:129–138.
7. Messina M, Nagata C, Wu AH. Estimated Asian adult soy protein and isoflavone intakes. *Nutr Cancer.* 2006;55: 1–12.
8. Setchell KD, Brown NM, Desai PB, et al. Bioavailability, disposition, and dose-response effects of soy isoflavones when consumed by healthy women at physiologically typical dietary intakes. *J Nutr.* 2003;133:1027–1035.
9. Setchell KD, Faughnan MS, Avades T, et al. Comparing the pharmacokinetics of daidzein and genistein with the use of 13C-labeled tracers in premenopausal women. *Am J Clin Nutr.* 2003;77:411–419.
10. Wiseman H, Casey K, Bowey EA, et al. Influence of 10 wk of soy consumption on plasma concentrations and excretion of isoflavonoids and on gut microflora metabolism in healthy adults. *Am J Clin Nutr.* 2004;80:692–699.
11. Setchell KD, Brown NM, Lydeking-Olsen E. The clinical importance of the metabolite equol—a clue to the effectiveness of soy and its isoflavones. *J Nutr.* 2002;132:3577–3584.
12. Lampe JW. Is equol the key to the efficacy of soy foods? *Am J Clin Nutr.* 2009;89:1664S–1667S.
13. Oseni T, Patel R, Pyle J, Jordan VC. Selective estrogen receptor modulators and phytoestrogens. *Planta Med.* 2008; 74:1656–1665.
14. Naciff JM, Jump ML, Torontali SM, et al. Gene expression profile induced by 17alpha-ethynyl estradiol, bisphenol A, and genistein in the developing female reproductive system of the rat. *Toxicol Sci.* 2002;68:184–199.
15. Sarkar FH, Li Y. Soy isoflavones and cancer prevention. *Cancer Invest.* 2003;21:744–757.
16. Zhou JR, Gugger ET, Tanaka T, Guo Y, Blackburn GL, Clinton SK. Soybean phytochemicals inhibit the growth of transplantable human prostate carcinoma and tumor angiogenesis in mice. *J Nutr.* 1999;129:1628–1635.
17. Xu L, Ding Y, Catalona WJ, et al. MEK4 function, genistein treatment, and invasion of human prostate cancer cells. *J Natl Cancer Inst.* 2009;101:1141–1155.
18. Amaral Mendes JJ. The endocrine disrupters: a major medical challenge. *Food Chem Toxicol.* 2002;40:781–788.
19. Gu L, House SE, Prior RL, et al. Metabolic phenotype of isoflavones differ among female rats, pigs, monkeys, and women. *J Nutr.* 2006;136:1215–1221.
20. Pisani P, Bray F, Parkin DM. Estimates of the world-wide prevalence of cancer for 25 sites in the adult population. *Int J Cancer.* 2002;97:72–81.
21. Menotti A, Lanti M, Kromhout D, et al. Forty-year coronary mortality trends and changes in major risk factors in the first 10 years of follow-up in the seven countries study. *Eur J Epidemiol.* 2007;22:747–754.
22. Messina M, Messina V. Increasing use of soyfoods and their potential role in cancer prevention. *J Am Diet Assoc.* 1991; 91:836–840.

23. Nagata C, Shimizu H, Takami R, Hayashi M, Takeda N, Yasuda K. Soy product intake is inversely associated with serum homocysteine level in premenopausal Japanese women. *J Nutr.* 2003;133:797–800.
24. Nagata C, Takatsuka N, Kawakami N, Shimizu H. Association of diet with the onset of menopause in Japanese women. *Am J Epidemiol.* 2000;152:863–867.
25. Nagata C, Takatsuka N, Kawakami N, Shimizu H. A prospective cohort study of soy product intake and stomach cancer death. *Br J Cancer.* 2002;87:31–36.
26. Takata Y, Maskarinec G, Franke A, Nagata C, Shimizu H. A comparison of dietary habits among women in Japan and Hawaii. *Public Health Nutr.* 2004;7:319–326.
27. Nagata C, Takatsuka N, Kurisu Y, Shimizu H. Decreased serum total cholesterol concentration is associated with high intake of soy products in Japanese men and women. *J Nutr.* 1998;128:209–213.
28. Nagata C, Nakamura K, Oba S, Hayashi M, Takeda N, Yasuda K. Association of intakes of fat, dietary fibre, soya isoflavones and alcohol with uterine fibroids in Japanese women. *Br J Nutr.* 2009;101:1427–1431.
29. Akhter M, Inoue M, Kurahashi N, Iwasaki M, Sasazuki S, Tsugane S. Dietary soy and isoflavone intake and risk of colorectal cancer in the Japan public health center-based prospective study. *Cancer Epidemiol Biomarkers Prev.* 2008;17:2128–2135.
30. Nanri A, Mizoue T, Takahashi Y, et al. Soy product and isoflavone intakes are associated with a lower risk of type 2 diabetes in overweight Japanese women. *J Nutr.* 2010;140:580–586.
31. Shimazu T, Inoue M, Sasazuki S, et al. Isoflavone intake and risk of lung cancer: a prospective cohort study in Japan. *Am J Clin Nutr.* 2010;9:456–464.
32. Ho SC, Chan SG, Yip YB, Chan CS, Woo JL, Sham A. Change in bone mineral density and its determinants in pre- and perimenopausal Chinese women: the Hong Kong Perimenopausal Women Osteoporosis Study. *Osteoporos Int.* 2008;19:1785–1796.
33. Kim MK, Kim JH, Nam SJ, Ryu S, Kong G. Dietary intake of soy protein and tofu in association with breast cancer risk based on a case-control study. *Nutr Cancer.* 2008;60:568–576.
34. Yang G, Shu XO, Jin F, et al. Longitudinal study of soy food intake and blood pressure among middle-aged and elderly Chinese women. *Am J Clin Nutr.* 2005;81:1012–1017.
35. Yang G, Shu XO, Li H, et al. Prospective cohort study of soy food intake and colorectal cancer risk in women. *Am J Clin Nutr.* 2009;89:577–583.
36. Lee SA, Wen W, Xiang YB, et al. Assessment of dietary isoflavone intake among middle-aged Chinese men. *J Nutr.* 2007;137:1011–1016.
37. Cui X, Dai Q, Tseng M, Shu XO, Gao YT, Zheng W. Dietary patterns and breast cancer risk in the Shanghai breast cancer study. *Cancer Epidemiol Biomarkers Prev.* 2007;16:1443–1448.
38. Pan Y, Anthony M, Watson S, Clarkson TB. Soy phytoestrogens improve radial arm maze performance in ovariectomized retired breeder rats and do not attenuate benefits of 17beta-estradiol treatment. *Menopause.* 2000;7:230–235.
39. USDA Nutrient Database for Standard Reference, Release 13. 1999. Nutrient Data Laboratory Home Page, http://www.nal.usda.gov/fnic/foodcomp.
40. Phillips RD. Starchy legumes in human nutrition, health and culture. *Plant Foods Hum Nutr.* 1993;44:195–211.
41. Sarwar G, Peace RW, Botting HG. Corrected relative net protein ratio (CRNPR) method based on differences in rat and human requirements for sulfur amino acids. *J Am Oil Chem Soc.* 1985;68:68:689–693.
42. Sarwar G. The protein digestibility-corrected amino acid score method overestimates quality of proteins containing antinutritional factors and of poorly digestible proteins supplemented with limiting amino acids in rats. *J Nutr.* 1997;127:758–764.
43. World Health Organization. *Protein and Amino Acid Requirements in Human Nutrition.* World Technical Series 935. Report of a Joint WHO/FAO/UNU Expert Consultation. Geneva, Switzerland: United Nations University; 2007.
44. Gilani GS, Sepehr E. Protein digestibility and quality in products containing antinutritional factors are adversely affected by old age in rats. *J Nutr.* 2003;133:220–225.
45. Fuller MF, Tome D. In vivo determination of amino acid bioavailability in humans and model animals. *J AOAC Int.* 2005;88:923–934.
46. Mariotti F, Mahe S, Benamouzig R, et al. Nutritional value of [15N]-soy protein isolate assessed from ileal digestibility and postprandial protein utilization in humans. *J Nutr.* 1999;129:1992–1997.

47. Gaudichon C, Bos C, Morens C, et al. Ileal losses of nitrogen and amino acids in humans and their importance to the assessment of amino acid requirements. *Gastroenterology.* 2002;123:50–59.
48. Millward DJ, Layman DK, Tome D, Schaafsma G. Protein quality assessment: impact of expanding understanding of protein and amino acid needs for optimal health. *Am J Clin Nutr.* 2008;87:1576S–1581S.
49. Schaafsma G. The Protein Digestibility-Corrected Amino Acid Score (PDCAAS)—a concept for describing protein quality in foods and food ingredients: a critical review. *J AOAC Int.* 2005;88:988–994.
50. Young VR. Soy protein in relation to human protein and amino acid nutrition. *J Am Diet Assoc.* 1991;91:828–835.
51. Rand WM, Pellett PL, Young VR. Meta-analysis of nitrogen balance studies for estimating protein requirements in healthy adults. *Am J Clin Nutr.* 2003;77:109–127.
52. U.S. Department of Agriculture. Modification of the Vegetable Protein Products Requirements for the National School Lunch Program, School Breakfast Program, Summer Food Service Program and Child and Adult Care Food Program. *Fed Regist.* 2000;7 CFR Parts 210, 215, 220, 225 and 226:12429–12442.
53. Harris WS, Mozaffarian D, Rimm E, et al. Omega-6 fatty acids and risk for cardiovascular disease. A Science Advisory From the American Heart Association Nutrition Subcommittee of the Council on Nutrition, Physical Activity, and Metabolism; Council on Cardiovascular Nursing; and Council on Epidemiology and Prevention. *Circulation.* 2009;119:902–907.
54. Laine DC, Snodgrass CM, Dawson EA, Ener MA, Kuba K, Frantz ID. Lightly hydrogenated soy oil versus other vegetable oils as a lipid- lowering dietary constituent. *Am J Clin Nutr.* 1982;35:683–690.
55. Applewhite TH. Nutritional effects of hydrogenated soya oil. *J Am Oil Chem Soc.* 1981;58:260–269.
56. Marckmann P. Fishing for heart protection. *Am J Clin Nutr.* 2003;78:1–2.
57. Lichtenstein AH, Appel LJ, Brands M, et al. Diet and lifestyle recommendations revision 2006: a scientific statement from the American Heart Association Nutrition Committee. *Circulation.* 2006;114:82–96.
58. Brouwer IA, Katan MB, Zock PL. Dietary alpha-linolenic acid is associated with reduced risk of fatal coronary heart disease, but increased prostate cancer risk: a meta-analysis. *J Nutr.* 2004;134:919–922.
59. Holguin F, Tellez-Rojo MM, Lazo M, et al. Cardiac autonomic changes associated with fish oil vs soy oil supplementation in the elderly. *Chest.* 2005;127:1102–1107.
60. Whelan J. Dietary stearidonic acid is a long chain (n-3) polyunsaturated fatty acid with potential health benefits. *J Nutr.* 2009;139:5–10.
61. Jenkins DJ, Sievenpiper JL, Pauly D, Sumaila UR, Kendall CW, Mowat FM. Are dietary recommendations for the use of fish oils sustainable? *CMAJ.* 2009;180:633–637.
62. Karr-Lilienthal LK, Grieshop CM, Spears JK, Fahey GC Jr. Amino acid, carbohydrate, and fat composition of soybean meals prepared at 55 commercial U.S. soybean processing plants. *J Agric Food Chem.* 2005;53:2146–2150.
63. Slavin J. Nutritional benefits of soy protein and soy fiber. *J Am Diet Assoc.* 1991;91:816–819.
64. Steggerda FR, Richards EA, Rackis JJ. Effects of various soybean products on flatulence in the adult man. *Proc Soc Exp Biol Med.* 1966;121:1235–1239.
65. Steggerda FR, Dimmick JF. Effects of bean diets on concentration of carbon dioxide in flatus. *Am J Clin Nutr.* 1966;19:120–124.
66. Rackis JJ, Sessa DJ, Steggerda FR, Shimizu T, Anderson T, Pearl SL. Soybean factors relating to gas production by intestinal bacteria. *J Food Sci.* 1970;35:634–639.
67. Rackis JJ, Honig DH, Sessa DJ, Steggerda FR. Flavor and flatulence factors in soybean protein products. *J Agric Food Chem.* 1970;18:977–982.
68. Carlsson N-G, Karlsson H, Sandberg A-S. Determination of oligosaccharides in foods, diets, and intestinal contents by high-temperature gas chromatography and gas chromatography/mass spectrometry. *J Agric Food Chem.* 1992;40:2404–2412.
69. Kuo TM, VanMiddlesworth JF, Wolf WJ. Content of raffinose oligosaccharides and sucrose in various plant seeds. *J Agric Food Chem.* 1988;36:32–36.
70. Anderson RL, Rackis JJ, Tallent WH. Biologically active substances in soy products. In: Wilcke HL, Hopkins DT, Waggle DH, eds. *Soy Protein and Human Nutrition.* New York, NY: Academic Press; 1979.
71. Gibson GR, Roberfroid MB. Dietary modulation of the human colonic microbiota: introducing the concept of prebiotics. *J Nutr.* 1995;125:1401–1412.
72. Mitsuoka T. Recent trends in research on intestinal flora. *Bifidobacteria Microflora.* 1982;1:3–24.

73. Benno Y, Endo K, Mizutani T, Namba Y, Komori T, Mitsuoka T. Comparison of fecal microflora of elderly persons in rual and urban areas of Japan. *Applied Environ Microbiol.* 1989;55:1100–1105.
74. Koo M, Rao AV. Long-term effect of Bifidobacteria and Neosugar on precursor lesions of colonic cancer in CF1 mice. *Nutr Cancer.* 1991;16:249–257.
75. Hayakawa K, Mizutani J, Wada K, Masa T, Yoshihara I, Mitsuoka T. Effects of soybean oligosaccharides on human faecal flora. *Microbial Ecol Health Dis.* 1990;3:292–303.
76. Schrezenmeir J, de Vrese MM. Probiotics, prebiotics, and synbiotics—approaching a definition. *Am J Clin Nutr.* 2001;73:361S-364S.
77. Cummings JH, Macfarlane GT, Englyst HN. Prebiotic digestion and fermentation. *Am J Clin Nutr.* 2001;73: 415S–420S.
78. Hata Y, Yamamoto M, Nakajima K. Effects of soybean oligosaccharides on human digestive organs: estimate of fifty percent effective dose and maximum non-effective dose based on diarrhea. *J Clin Biochem Nutr.* 1991;10:135–144.
79. Hill RC, Burrows CF, Bauer JE, Ellison GW, Finke MD, Jones GL. Texturized vegetable protein containing indigestible soy carbohydrate affects blood insulin concentrations in dogs fed high fat diets. *J Nutr.* 2006;136: 2024S–2027S.
80. Katayama M, Wilson LA. Utilization of okara, a byproduct from soymilk production, through the development of soy-based snack food. *J Food Sci.* 2008;73:S152–S157.
81. Jimenez-Escrig A, Tenorio MD, Espinosa-Martos I, Ruperez P. Health-promoting effects of a dietary fiber concentrate from the soybean byproduct okara in rats. *J Agric Food Chem.* 2008;56:7495–7501.
82. O'Toole DK. Characteristics and use of okara, the soybean residue from soy milk production—a review. *J Agric Food Chem.* 1999;47:363–371.
83. Xie M, Huff H, Hsieh F, Mustapha A. Puffing of okara/rice blends using a rice cake machine. *J Food Sci.* 2008;73: E341–E348.
84. Genta HD, Genta ML, Alvarez NV, Santana MS. Production and acceptance of a soy candy. *J Food Engineering.* 2002; 53:199–202.
85. Lubetsky A, Dekel-Stern E, Chetrit A, Lubin F, Halkin H. Vitamin K intake and sensitivity to warfarin in patients consuming regular diets. *Thromb Haemost.* 1999;81:396–399.
86. Booth SL, Suttie JW. Dietary intake and adequacy of vitamin K. *J Nutr.* 1998;128:785–788.
87. U.S. Department of Agriculture; Agricultural Research Service. USDA National Nutrient Database for Standard Reference, Release 22. Nutrient Data Laboratory home page, http://www.ars.usda.gov/ba/bhnrc/ndl.
88. Kamao M, Suhara Y, Tsugawa N, et al. Vitamin K content of foods and dietary vitamin K intake in Japanese young women. *J Nutr Sci Vitaminol (Tokyo).* 2007;53:464–470.
89. Kudo T. Warfarin antagonism of natto and increase in serum vitamin K by intake of natto. *Artery.* 1990;17:189–201.
90. Sakata T, Kario K, Asada S, et al. Increased activated factor VII levels caused by intake of natto, a Japanese vitamin K-rich food prepared from fermented soybean. *Blood Coagul Fibrinolysis.* 1997;8:533–534.
91. Kaneki M, Hedges SJ, Hosoi T, et al. Japanese fermented soybean food as the major determinant of the large geographic difference in circulating levels of vitamin K2: possible implications for hip-fracture risk. *Nutrition.* 2001;17:315–321.
92. Homma K, Wakana N, Suzuki Y, et al. Treatment of natto, a fermented soybean preparation, to prevent excessive plasma vitamin K concentrations in patients taking warfarin. *J Nutr Sci Vitaminol (Tokyo).* 2006;52:297–301.
93. Cambria-Kiely JA. Effect of soy milk on warfarin efficacy. *Ann Pharmacother.* 2002;36:1893–1896.
94. Booth SL, Charnley JM, Sadowski JA, Saltzman E, Bovill EG, Cushman M. Dietary vitamin K1 and stability of oral anticoagulation: proposal of a diet with constant vitamin K1 content. *Thromb Haemost.* 1997;77:504–509.
95. Johnson JM, Walker PM. Zinc and iron utilization in young women consuming a beef-based diet. *J Am Diet Assoc.* 1992;92:1474–1478.
96. Hajjar IM, Grim CE, George V, Kotchen TA. Impact of diet on blood pressure and age-related changes in blood pressure in the US population: analysis of NHANES III. *Arch Intern Med.* 2001;161:589–593.
97. Lynch SR, Dassenko SA, Cook JD, Juillerat MA, Hurrell RF. Inhibitory effect of a soybean-protein–related moiety on iron absorption in humans. *Am J Clin Nutr.* 1994;60:567–572.
98. Hurrell RF, Juillerat MA, Reddy MB, Lynch SR, Dassenko SA, Cook JD. Soy protein, phytate, and iron absorption in humans. *Am J Clin Nutr.* 1992;56:573–578.

99. Hallberg L. Bioavailability of dietary iron in man. *Annu Rev Nutr.* 1981;1:1:123–147.

100. Hunt JR, Gallagher SK, Johnson LK. Effect of ascorbic acid on apparent iron absorption by women with low iron stores. *Am J Clin Nutr.* 1994;59:1381–1385.

101. Lynch SR, Beard JL, Dassenko SA, Cook JD. Iron absorption from legumes in humans. *Am J Clin Nutr.* 1984; 40:42–47.

102. Garcia-Casal MN, Layrisse M, Solano L, et al. Vitamin A and beta-carotene can improve nonheme iron absorption from rice, wheat and corn by humans. *J Nutr.* 1998;128:646–650.

103. Macfarlane BJ, van der Riet WB, Bothwell TH, et al. Effect of traditional oriental soy products on iron absorption. *Am J Clin Nutr.* 1990;51:873–880.

104. Lynch SR, Husaini S, Dassenko SA, Beard JL, Cook JD. A soybean product with improved iron bioavailability for humans. *Am J Clin Nutr.* 1984;39:664.

105. Brune M, Rossander-Hulten L, Hallberg L, Gleerup A, Sandberg AS. Iron absorption from bread in humans: inhibiting effects of cereal fiber, phytate and inositol phosphates with different numbers of phosphate groups. *J Nutr.* 1992;122:442–449.

106. Huisheng Q, Jilin Y, Weiping Y, et al. The effect of fermented soy food in preventing iron deficiency anemia in children. *Acta Nutrimenta Sinica.* 1989;11:295–298.

107. Cook JD, Morck TA, Lynch SR. The inhibitory effect of soy products on nonheme iron absorption in man. *Am J Clin Nutr.* 1981;34:2622–2629.

108. Derman DP, Ballot D, Bothwell TH, et al. Factors influencing the absorption of iron from soya-bean protein products. *Br J Nutr.* 1987;57:345–353.

109. Murray-Kolb LE, Welch R, Theil EC, Beard JL. Women with low iron stores absorb iron from soybeans. *Am J Clin Nutr.* 2003;77:180–184.

110. Lonnerdal B. Soybean ferritin: implications for iron status of vegetarians. *Am J Clin Nutr.* 2009;89:1680S–1685S.

111. Lonnerdal B, Bryant A, Liu X, Theil EC. Iron absorption from soybean ferritin in nonanemic women. *Am J Clin Nutr.* 2006;83:103–107.

112. Beard JL, Burton JW, Theil EC. Purified ferritin and soybean meal can be sources of iron for treating iron deficiency in rats. *J Nutr.* 1996;126:154–160.

113. Bodwell CE, Miles CW, Morris E, Prather ES, Mertz W, Canary JJ. Long-term consumption of beef extended with soy protein by men, women and children: II. Effects on iron status. *Plant Foods Hum Nutr.* 1987;37:361–376.

114. Wells AM, Haub MD, Fluckey J, Williams DK, Chernoff R, Campbell WW. Comparisons of vegetarian and beef-containing diets on hematological indexes and iron stores during a period of resistive training in older men. *J Am Diet Assoc.* 2003;103:594–601.

115. Messina M, Watanabe S, Setchell KD. Report on the 8th International Symposium on the Role of Soy in Health Promotion and Chronic Disease Prevention and Treatment. *J Nutr.* 2009;139:796S–802S.

116. Shaw NS, Chin CJ, Pan WH. A vegetarian diet rich in soybean products compromises iron status in young students. *J Nutr.* 1995;125:212–219.

117. Shi Z, Hu X, Yuan B, et al. Strong negative association between intake of tofu and anemia among Chinese adults in Jiangsu, China. *J Am Diet Assoc.* 2008;108:1146–1153.

118. Sandstrom B, Andersson H, Kivisto B, Sandberg AS. Apparent small intestinal absorption of nitrogen and minerals from soy and meat-protein-based diets. A study on human ileostomy subjects. *J Nutr.* 1986;116:2209–2218.

119. Sandstrom B, Kivisto B, Cederblad A. Absorption of zinc from soy protein meals in humans. *J Nutr.* 1987;117:321–327.

120. Greger JL, Abernathy RP, Bennett OA. Zinc and nitrogen balance in adolescent females fed varying levels of zinc and soy protein. *Am J Clin Nutr.* 1978;31:112–116.

121. Sandstrom B, Cederblad A. Zinc absorption from composite meals. II. Influence of the main protein source. *Am J Clin Nutr.* 1980;33:1778–1783.

122. Young VR, Janghorbani M. Soy protein in human diets in relation to bioavailability of iron and zinc. *Cereal Chem.* 1981;58:12–17.

123. Davidsson L, Almgren A, Sandstrom B, Juillerat M, Hurrell RF. Zinc absorption in adult humans: the effect of protein sources added to liquid test meals. *Br J Nutr.* 1996;75:607–613.

124. Lonnerdal B, Cederblad A, Davidsson L, Sandstrom B. The effect of individual components of soy formula and cows' milk formula on zinc bioavailability. *Am J Clin Nutr.* 1984;40:1064–1070.

125. Davidsson L, Ziegler EE, Kastenmayer P, van Dael P, Barclay D. Dephytinisation of soyabean protein isolate with low native phytic acid content has limited impact on mineral and trace element absorption in healthy infants. *Br J Nutr*. 2004;91:287–294.

126. Etcheverry P, Hawthorne KM, Liang LK, Abrams SA, Griffin IJ. Effect of beef and soy proteins on the absorption of non-heme iron and inorganic zinc in children. *J Am Coll Nutr*. 2006;25:34–40.

127. Couzy F, Mansourian R, Labate A, Guinchard S, Montagne DH, Dirren H. Effect of dietary phytic acid on zinc absorption in the healthy elderly, as assessed by serum concentration curve tests. *Br J Nutr*. 1998;80:177–182.

128. Cranwell K, Liebman M. Effect of soybean fiber and phytate on serum zinc response. *Nutr Res*. 1989;9:127–132.

129. Lo GS, Settle SL, Steinke FH, Hopkins DT. Effect of phytate:zinc molar ratio and isolated soybean protein on zinc bioavailability. *J Nutr*. 1981;111:2223–2235.

130. Hirabayashi M, Matsui T, Yano H. Fermentation of soybean flour with *Aspergillus usamii* improves availabilities of zinc and iron in rats. *J Nutr Sci Vitaminol (Tokyo)*. 1998;44:877–886.

131. Hirabayashi M, Matsui T, Yano H. Fermentation of soybean meal with *Aspergillus usamii* improves zinc availability in rats. *Biol Trace Elem Res*. 1998;61:227–234.

132. Hirabayashi M, Matsui T, Yano H, Nakajima T. Fermentation of soybean meal with *Aspergillus usamii* reduces phosphorus excretion in chicks. *Poult Sci*. 1998;77:552–556.

133. Liebman M, Landis W. Calcium and zinc balances of premenopausal women consuming tofu- compared to cheese-containing diets. *Nutr Res*. 1989;9:5–14.

134. Adolph WH, Chen SC. The utilization of calcium in soy bean diets. *J Nutr*. 1932;5:379–385.

135. Fredlund K, Isaksson M, Rossander-Hulthen L, Almgren A, Sandberg AS. Absorption of zinc and retention of calcium: dose-dependent inhibition by phytate. *J Trace Elem Med Biol*. 2006;20:49–57.

136. Weaver CM, Plawecki KL. Dietary calcium: adequacy of a vegetarian diet. *Am J Clin Nutr*. 1994;59:1238S–1241S.

137. Chai W, Liebman M. Effect of different cooking methods on vegetable oxalate content. *J Agric Food Chem*. 2005; 53:3027–3030.

138. Weaver CM, Heaney RP, Nickel KP, Packard PI. Calcium bioavailability from high oxalate vegetables: Chinese vegetables, sweet potatoes and rhubarb. *J Food Sci*. 1997;63:524–525.

139. Heaney RP, Weaver CM, Recker RR. Calcium absorbability from spinach. *Am J Clin Nutr*. 1988;47:707–709.

140. Heaney RP, Weaver CM, Fitzsimmons ML. Soybean phytate content: effect on calcium absorption. *Am J Clin Nutr*. 1991;53:745–747.

141. Heaney RP, Dowell MS, Rafferty K, Bierman J. Bioavailability of the calcium in fortified soy imitation milk, with some observations on method. *Am J Clin Nutr*. 2000;71:1166–1169.

142. Zhao Y, Martin BR, Weaver CM. Calcium bioavailability of calcium carbonate fortified soymilk is equivalent to cow's milk in young women. *J Nutr*. 2005;135:2379–2382.

143. Weaver CM, Heaney RP, Connor L, Martin BR, Smith DL, Nielsen E. Bioavailability of calcium from tofu vs. milk in premenopausal women. *J Food Sci*. 2002;68:3144–3147.

144. Heaney RP, Rafferty K. The settling problem in calcium-fortified soybean drinks. *J Am Diet Assoc*. 2006;106:1753; author reply 5.

145. Anderson JW, Johnstone BM, Cook-Newell ME. Meta-analysis of the effects of soy protein intake on serum lipids. *N Engl J Med*. 1995;333:276–282.

146. Cho SJ, Juillerat MA, Lee CH. Cholesterol lowering mechanism of soybean protein hydrolysate. *J Agric Food Chem*. 2007;55:10599–10604.

147. Manzoni C, Duranti M, Eberini I, et al. Subcellular localization of soybean 7S globulin in HepG2 cells and LDL receptor up-regulation by its alpha' constituent subunit. *J Nutr*. 2003;133:2149–2155.

148. Zhuo XG, Melby MK, Watanabe S. Soy isoflavone intake lowers serum LDL cholesterol: a meta-analysis of 8 randomized controlled trials in humans. *J Nutr*. 2004;134:2395–2400.

149. Food labeling: health claims; soy protein and coronary heart disease. *Fed Regist*. 1999;64(206):57699–57733.

150. Sacks FM, Lichtenstein A, Van Horn L, Harris W, Kris-Etherton P, Winston M. Soy protein, isoflavones, and cardiovascular health: an American Heart Association Science Advisory for professionals from the Nutrition Committee. *Circulation*. 2006;113:1034–1044.

151. Balk E, Chung M, Chew P, et al. *Effects of Soy on Health Outcomes*. Evidence Report/Technology Assessment No. 126 (prepared by Tufts-New England Medical Center Evidence-based Practice Center under Contract No. 290–02–0022). AHRQ Publication No. 05-E024–2. Rockville, MD: Agency for Healthcare Research and Quality; July 2005.

152. Zhan S, Ho SC. Meta-analysis of the effects of soy protein containing isoflavones on the lipid profile. *Am J Clin Nutr.* 2005;81:397–408.

153. Brown L, Rosner B, Willett WW, Sacks FM. Cholesterol-lowering effects of dietary fiber: a meta-analysis. *Am J Clin Nutr.* 1999;69:30–42.

154. Messina M, Watanabe S, Setchell KD. Report on the 8th International Symposium on the Role of Soy in Health Promotion and Chronic Disease Prevention and Treatment. *J Nutr.* 2009;139:796S–802S.

155. Sirtori CR, Gianazza E, Manzoni C, Lovati MR, Murphy PA. Role of isoflavones in the cholesterol reduction by soy proteins in the clinic. *Am J Clin Nutr.* 1997;65:166–167.

156. Law MR, Wald NJ, Thompson SG. By how much and how quickly does reduction in serum cholesterol concentration lower risk of ischaemic heart disease? *BMJ.* 1994;308:367–372.

157. Law MR, Wald NJ, Wu T, Hackshaw A, Bailey A. Systematic underestimation of association between serum cholesterol concentration and ischaemic heart disease in observational studies: data from the BUPA study. *BMJ.* 1994;308:363–366.

158. Wu Z, Rodgers RP, Marshall AG. Characterization of vegetable oils: detailed compositional fingerprints derived from electrospray ionization fourier transform ion cyclotron resonance mass spectrometry. *J Agric Food Chem.* 2004; 52:5322–5328.

159. Hayes KC. Dietary fatty acids, cholesterol, and the lipoprotein profile. *Br J Nutr.* 2000;84:397–399.

160. Jenkins DJ, Kendall CW, Faulkner D, et al. A dietary portfolio approach to cholesterol reduction: combined effects of plant sterols, vegetable proteins, and viscous fibers in hypercholesterolemia. *Metabolism.* 2002;51:1596–1604.

161. Boden WE. High-density lipoprotein cholesterol as an independent risk factor in cardiovascular disease: assessing the data from Framingham to the Veterans Affairs High-Density Lipoprotein Intervention Trial. *Am J Cardiol.* 2000;86:19L–22L.

162. Gotto AM Jr. High-density lipoprotein cholesterol and triglycerides as therapeutic targets for preventing and treating coronary artery disease. *Am Heart J.* 2002;144:S33–S42.

163. Grover SA, Kaouache M, Joseph L, Barter P, Davignon J. Evaluating the incremental benefits of raising high-density lipoprotein cholesterol levels during lipid therapy after adjustment for the reductions in other blood lipid levels. *Arch Intern Med.* 2009;169:1775–1780.

164. Cullen P. Evidence that triglycerides are an independent coronary heart disease risk factor. *Am J Cardiol.* 2000; 86:943–949.

165. Bansal S, Buring JE, Rifai N, Mora S, Sacks FM, Ridker PM. Fasting compared with nonfasting triglycerides and risk of cardiovascular events in women. *JAMA.* 2007;298:309–316.

166. Nordestgaard BG, Benn M, Schnohr P, Tybjaerg-Hansen A. Nonfasting triglycerides and risk of myocardial infarction, ischemic heart disease, and death in men and women. *JAMA.* 2007;298:299–308.

167. Messina M. Potential public health implications of the hypocholesterolemic effects of soy protein. *J Nutr.* 2003; 19:280–281.

168. Zhang X, Shu XO, Gao YT, et al. Soy food consumption is associated with lower risk of coronary heart disease in Chinese women. *J Nutr.* 2003;133:2874–2878.

169. Zhang B, Chen YM, Huang LL, et al. Greater habitual soyfood consumption is associated with decreased carotid intima-media thickness and better plasma lipids in Chinese middle-aged adults. *Atherosclerosis.* 2008;198:403–411.

170. Kokubo Y, Iso H, Ishihara J, Okada K, Inoue M, Tsugane S. Association of dietary intake of soy, beans, and isoflavones with risk of cerebral and myocardial infarctions in Japanese populations: the Japan Public Health Center-based (JPHC) study cohort I. *Circulation.* 2007;116:2553–2562.

171. Hooper L, Kroon PA, Rimm EB, et al. Flavonoids, flavonoid-rich foods, and cardiovascular risk: a meta-analysis of randomized controlled trials. *Am J Clin Nutr.* 2008;88:38–50.

172. Messina M, Lane B. Soy protein, soybean isoflavones, and coronary heart disease risk: where do we stand? *Future Lipidol.* 2007;2:55–74.

173. Chan YH, Lau KK, Yiu KH, et al. Reduction of C-reactive protein with isoflavone supplement reverses endothelial dysfunction in patients with ischaemic stroke. *Eur Heart J.* 2008;29:2800–2807.

174. Li SH, Liu XX, Bai YY, et al. Effect of oral isoflavone supplementation on vascular endothelial function in postmenopausal women: a meta-analysis of randomized placebo- controlled trials. *Am J Clin Nutr.* 2010;91:480–486.

175. Fuchs D, Vafeiadou K, Hall WL, et al. Proteomic biomarkers of peripheral blood mononuclear cells obtained from postmenopausal women undergoing an intervention with soy isoflavones. *Am J Clin Nutr.* 2007;86:1369–1375.

176. Messina M, Barnes S. The role of soy products in reducing risk of cancer. *J Natl Cancer Inst.* 1991;83:541–546.

177. Dalu A, Blaydes B, Bryant C, Latendresse J, Weis C, Barry Delclos K. Estrogen receptor expression in the prostate of rats treated with dietary genistein. *J Chromatogr B Analyt Technol Biomed Life Sci.* 2002;777:249.

178. Dalu A, Haskell JF, Coward L, Lamartiniere CA. Genistein, a component of soy, inhibits the expression of the EGF and ErbB2/Neu receptors in the rat dorsolateral prostate. *Prostate.* 1998;37:36–43.

179. Zhou JR, Yu L, Zhong Y, Blackburn GL. Soy phytochemicals and tea bioactive components synergistically inhibit androgen-sensitive human prostate tumors in mice. *J Nutr.* 2003;133:516–521.

180. Wu AH, Yu MC, Tseng CC, Pike MC. Epidemiology of soy exposures and breast cancer risk. *Br J Cancer.* 2008;98:9–14.

181. Messina M, Wu AH. Perspectives on the soy-breast cancer relation. *Am J Clin Nutr.* 2009;89:1673S–1679S.

182. Messina M, Hilakivi-Clarke L. Early intake appears to be the key to the proposed protective effects of soy intake against breast cancer. *Nutr Cancer.* 2009;61:792–798.

183. Shu XO, Jin F, Dai Q, et al. Soyfood intake during adolescence and subsequent risk of breast cancer among Chinese women. *Cancer Epidemiol Biomarkers Prev.* 2001;10:483–488.

184. Wu AH, Yu MC, Tseng CC, Stanczyk FZ, Pike MC. Dietary patterns and breast cancer risk in Asian American women. *Am J Clin Nutr.* 2009;89:1145–1154.

185. Korde LA, Wu AH, Fears T, et al. Childhood soy intake and breast cancer risk in Asian American women. *Cancer Epidemiol Biomarkers Prev.* 2009;18:1050–1059.

186. Lee SA, Shu XO, Li H, et al. Adolescent and adult soy food intake and breast cancer risk: results from the Shanghai Women's Health Study. *Am J Clin Nutr.* 2009;89:1920–1926.

187. Messina MJ, Wood CE. Soy isoflavones, estrogen therapy, and breast cancer risk: analysis and commentary. *Nutr J.* 2008;7:17.

188. Lamartiniere CA, Zhao YX, Fritz WA. Genistein: mammary cancer chemoprevention, in vivo mechanisms of action, potential for toxicity and bioavailability in rats. *J Women's Cancer.* 2000;2:11–19.

189. Peng JH, Zhang F, Zhang HX, Fan HY. Prepubertal octylphenol exposure up-regulate BRCA1 expression, down-regulate ERalpha expression and reduce rat mammary tumorigenesis. *Cancer Epidemiol.* 2009;33:51–55.

190. Rowlands JC, Hakkak R, Ronis MJ, Badger TM. Altered mammary gland differentiation and progesterone receptor expression in rats fed soy and whey proteins. *Toxicol Sci.* 2002;70:40–45.

191. Russo J, Lareef H, Tahin Q, Russo IH. Pathways of carcinogenesis and prevention in the human breast. *Eur J Cancer.* 2002;38(suppl 6):S31–S32.

192. Russo J, Mailo D, Hu YF, Balogh G, Sheriff F, Russo IH. Breast differentiation and its implication in cancer prevention. *Clin Cancer Res.* 2005;11:931s–936s.

193. Russo J, Russo IH. The role of estrogen in the initiation of breast cancer. *J Steroid Biochem Mol Biol.* 2006;102:89–96.

194. Russo J, Balogh GA, Russo IH. Full-term pregnancy induces a specific genomic signature in the human breast. *Cancer Epidemiol Biomarkers Prev.* 2008;17:51–66.

195. Chlebowski RT, Anderson GL, Lane DS, et al. Predicting risk of breast cancer in postmenopausal women by hormone receptor status. *J Natl Cancer Inst.* 2007;99:1695–1705.

196. Yan L, Spitznagel EL. Soy consumption and prostate cancer risk in men: a revisit of a meta-analysis. *Am J Clin Nutr.* 2009;89:1155–1163.

197. Hikosaka A, Asamoto M, Hokaiwado N, et al. Inhibitory effects of soy isoflavones on rat prostate carcinogenesis induced by 2-amino-1-methyl-6-phenylimidazo[4,5-b]pyridine (PhIP). *Carcinogenesis.* 2004;25:381–387.

198. Mentor-Marcel R, Lamartiniere CA, Eltoum IA, Greenberg NM, Elgavish A. Dietary genistein improves survival and reduces expression of osteopontin in the prostate of transgenic mice with prostatic adenocarcinoma (TRAMP). *J Nutr.* 2005;135:989–995.

199. Hwang YW, Kim SY, Jee SH, Kim YN, Nam CM. Soy food consumption and risk of prostate cancer: a meta-analysis of observational studies. *Nutr Cancer.* 2009;61:598–606.

200. Messina M. Western soy intake is too low to produce health effects. *Am J Clin Nutr.* 2004;80:528–529.

201. Lakshman M, Xu L, Ananthanarayanan V, et al. Dietary genistein inhibits metastasis of human prostate cancer in mice. *Cancer Res.* 2008;68:2024–2032.
202. Hernandez BY, McDuffie K, Franke AA, Killeen J, Goodman MT. Reports: plasma and dietary phytoestrogens and risk of premalignant lesions of the cervix. *Nutr Cancer.* 2004;49:109–124.
203. Stamey TA, Yang N, Hay AR, McNeal JE, Freiha FS, Redwine E. Prostate-specific antigen as a serum marker for adenocarcinoma of the prostate. *N Engl J Med.* 1987;317:909–916.
204. Agarwal PK, Oefelein MG. Testosterone replacement therapy after primary treatment for prostate cancer. *J Urol.* 2005;173:533–536.
205. Stock RG, Cahlon O, Cesaretti JA, Kollmeier MA, Stone NN. Combined modality treatment in the management of high-risk prostate cancer. *Int J Radiat Oncol Biol Phys.* 2004;59:1352–1359.
206. Wang LG, Mencher SK, McCarron JP, Ferrari AC. The biological basis for the use of an anti-androgen and a 5-alpha-reductase inhibitor in the treatment of recurrent prostate cancer: case report and review. *Oncol Rep.* 2004;11:1325–1329.
207. Fontana D, Mari M, Martinelli A, et al. 3-month formulation of goserelin acetate ('Zoladex' 10.8-mg depot) in advanced prostate cancer: results from an Italian, open, multicenter trial. *Urol Int.* 2003;70:316–320.
208. Small EJ, Baron AD, Fippin L, Apodaca D. Ketoconazole retains activity in advanced prostate cancer patients with progression despite flutamide withdrawal. *J Urol.* 1997;157:1204–1207.
209. Picus J, Schultz M. Docetaxel (Taxotere) as monotherapy in the treatment of hormone- refractory prostate cancer: preliminary results. *Semin Oncol.* 1999;26:14–18.
210. Petrylak DP, Macarthur RB, O'Connor J, et al. Phase I trial of docetaxel with estramustine in androgen-independent prostate cancer. *J Clin Oncol.* 1999;17:958–967.
211. Savarese D, Taplin ME, Halabi S, Hars V, Kreis W, Vogelzang N. A phase II study of docetaxel (Taxotere), estramustine, and low-dose hydrocortisone in men with hormone-refractory prostate cancer: preliminary results of cancer and leukemia group B Trial 9780. *Semin Oncol.* 1999;26:39–44.
212. Sinibaldi VJ, Carducci MA, Moore-Cooper S, Laufer M, Zahurak M, Eisenberger MA. Phase II evaluation of docetaxel plus one-day oral estramustine phosphate in the treatment of patients with androgen independent prostate carcinoma. *Cancer.* 2002;94:1457–1465.
213. Messina M, Kucuk O, Lampe JW. An overview of the health effects of isoflavones with an emphasis on prostate cancer risk and prostate-specific antigen levels. *J AOAC Int.* 2006;89:1121–1134.
214. Messina M. Emerging evidence on the role of soy in reducing prostate cancer risk. *Nutr Rev.* 2003;61:117–131.
215. Yan L, Spitznagel EL. Soy consumption and prostate cancer risk in men: a revisit of a meta-analysis. *Am J Clin Nutr.* 2009;89:1155–1163.
216. Meyer F, Galan P, Douville P, et al. Antioxidant vitamin and mineral supplementation and prostate cancer prevention in the SU.VI.MAX trial. *Int J Cancer.* 2005;116:182–186.
217. Pendleton JM, Tan WW, Anai S, et al. Phase II trial of isoflavone in prostate specific antigen recurrent prostate cancer after previous local therapy. *BMC Cancer.* 2008;8:132.
218. Kwan W, Duncan G, Van Patten C, Liu M, Lim J. A phase II trial of a soy beverage for subjects without clinical disease with rising prostate-specific antigen after radical radiation for prostate cancer. *Nutr Cancer.* 2010;62:198–207.
219. Finkelstein JS, Brockwell SE, Mehta V, et al. Bone mineral density changes during the menopause transition in a multi-ethnic cohort of women. *J Clin Endocrinol Metab.* 2008;93:861–868.
220. Writing Group for the Women's Health Initiative Investigators. Risks and benefits of estrogen plus progestin in healthy postmenopausal women: principal results from the Women's Health Initiative randomized controlled trial. *JAMA.* 2002;288:321–333.
221. Brandi ML, Gennari C. Ipriflavone: new insights into its mechanisms of action on bone remodeling. *Calcif Tissue Int.* 1993;52:151–152.
222. Potter SM, Baum JA, Teng H, Stillman RJ, Shay NF, Erdman JW Jr. Soy protein and isoflavones: their effects on blood lipids and bone density in postmenopausal women. *Am J Clin Nutr.* 1998;68:1375S–1379S.
223. Atmaca A, Kleerekoper M, Bayraktar M, Kucuk O. Soy isoflavones in the management of postmenopausal osteoporosis. *Menopause.* 2008;15:748–757.
224. Messina M, Ho S, Alekel DL. Skeletal benefits of soy isoflavones: a review of the clinical trial and epidemiologic data. *Curr Opin Clin Nutr Metab Care.* 2004;7:649–658.

225. Ma DF, Qin LQ, Wang PY, Katoh R. Soy isoflavone intake inhibits bone resorption and stimulates bone formation in menopausal women: meta-analysis of randomized controlled trials. *Eur J Clin Nutr.* 2008;62:155–161.

226. Ma DF, Qin LQ, Wang PY, Katoh R. Soy isoflavone intake increases bone mineral density in the spine of menopausal women: meta-analysis of randomized controlled trials. *Clin Nutr.* 2008;27:57–64.

227. Liu J, Ho SC, Su YX, Chen WQ, Zhang CX, Chen YM. Effect of long-term intervention of soy isoflavones on bone mineral density in women: a meta-analysis of randomized controlled trials. *Bone.* 2009;44:948–953.

228. Marini H, Minutoli L, Polito F, et al. Effects of the phytoestrogen genistein on bone metabolism in osteopenic post-menopausal women: a randomized trial. *Ann Intern Med.* 2007;146:839–847.

229. Marini H, Bitto A, Altavilla D, et al. Breast safety and efficacy of genistein aglycone for postmenopausal bone loss: a follow-up study. *J Clin Endocrinol Metab.* 2008;93:4787–4796.

230. Lydeking-Olsen E, Beck-Jensen JE, Setchell KD, Holm-Jensen T. Soymilk or progesterone for prevention of bone loss: a 2 year randomized, placebo-controlled trial. *Eur J Nutr.* 2004;43:246–257.

231. Brink E, Coxam V, Robins S, Wahala K, Cassidy A, Branca F. Long-term consumption of isoflavone-enriched foods does not affect bone mineral density, bone metabolism, or hormonal status in early postmenopausal women: a randomized, double-blind, placebo controlled study. *Am J Clin Nutr.* 2008;87:761–770.

232. Kenny AM, Mangano KM, Abourizk RH, et al. Soy proteins and isoflavones affect bone mineral density in older women: a randomized controlled trial. *Am J Clin Nutr.* 2009;90:234–242.

233. Vupadhyayula PM, Gallagher JC, Templin T, Logsdon SM, Smith LM. Effects of soy protein isolate on bone mineral density and physical performance indices in postmenopausal women—a 2-year randomized, double-blind, placebo-controlled trial. *Menopause.* 2009;16:320–328.

234. Alekel DL, Van Loan MD, Koehler KJ, et al. The soy isoflavones for reducing bone loss (SIRBL) study: a 3-y randomized controlled trial in postmenopausal women. *Am J Clin Nutr.* 2010;91:218–230.

235. Weaver CM, Martin BR, Jackson GS, et al. Antiresorptive effects of phytoestrogen supplements compared with estradiol or risedronate in postmenopausal women using (41)Ca methodology. *J Clin Endocrinol Metab.* 2009; 94:3798–3805.

236. Zhang X, Shu XO, Li H, et al. Prospective cohort study of soy food consumption and risk of bone fracture among postmenopausal women. *Arch Intern Med.* 2005;165:1890–1895.

237. Koh WP, Wu AH, Wang R, et al. Gender-specific associations between soy and risk of hip fracture in the Singapore Chinese Health Study. *Am J Epidemiol.* 2009;170:901–909.

238. Darling AL, Millward DJ, Torgerson DJ, Hewitt CE, Lanham-New SA. Dietary protein and bone health: a systematic review and meta-analysis. *Am J Clin Nutr.* 2009;90:1674–1692.

239. Kronenberg F. Hot flashes: epidemiology and physiology. *Ann N Y Acad Sci.* 1990;592:52–86; discussion 123–133.

240. Berg G, Gottwall T, Hammar M, Lindgren R, Gottgall T. Climacteric symptoms among women aged 60–62 in Linkoping, Sweden, in 1986. *Maturitas.* 1988;10:193–199.

241. Rodstrom K, Bengtsson C, Lissner L, Milsom I, Sundh V, Bjorkelund C. A longitudinal study of the treatment of hot flushes: the population study of women in Gothenburg during a quarter of a century. *Menopause.* 2002;9:156–161.

242. Adlercreutz H, Hamalainen E, Gorbach S, Goldin B. Dietary phyto-oestrogens and the menopause in Japan. *Lancet.* 1992;339:1233.

243. Howes LG, Howes JB, Knight DC. Isoflavone therapy for menopausal flushes: a systematic review and meta-analysis. *Maturitas.* 2006;55:203–211.

244. Lethaby A, Brown J, Marjoribanks J, Kronenberg F, Roberts H, Eden J. Phytoestrogens for vasomotor menopausal symptoms. *Cochrane Database Syst Rev.* 2007(4):CD001395.

245. Jacobs A, Wegewitz U, Sommerfeld C, Grossklaus R, Lampen A. Efficacy of isoflavones in relieving vasomotor menopausal symptoms—a systematic review. *Mol Nutr Food Res.* 2009;53:1084–1097.

246. Butt DA, Deng LY, Lewis JE, Lock M. Minimal decrease in hot flashes desired by postmenopausal women in family practice. *Menopause.* 2007;14:203–207.

247. Messina M, Hughes C. Efficacy of soyfoods and soybean isoflavone supplements for alleviating menopausal symptoms is positively related to initial hot flush frequency. *J Med Food.* 2003;6:1–11.

248. Williamson-Hughes PS, Flickinger BD, Messina MJ, Empie MW. Isoflavone supplements containing predominantly genistein reduce hot flash symptoms: a critical review of published studies. *Menopause.* 2006;13:831–839.

249. Kurzer MS. Soy isoflavones reduce postmenopausal hot flush frequency and severity: results of a systematic review and meta-analysis of randomized controlled trials. Paper presented at: Efficacy and Safety of Isoflavones for Postmenopausal Women; May 13–14, 2009; Milan, Italy.

250. Brenner BM, Meyer TW, Hostetter TH. Dietary protein intake and the progressive nature of kidney disease: the role of hemodynamically mediated glomerular injury in the pathogenesis of progressive glomerular sclerosis in aging, renal ablation, and intrinsic renal disease. *N Engl J Med.* 1982;307:652–659.

251. Knight EL, Stampfer MJ, Hankinson SE, Spiegelman D, Curhan GC. The impact of protein intake on renal function decline in women with normal renal function or mild renal insufficiency. *Ann Intern Med.* 2003;138:460–467.

252. Kopple JD. National kidney foundation K/DOQI clinical practice guidelines for nutrition in chronic renal failure. *Am J Kidney Dis.* 2001;37:S66–S70.

253. Franz MJ, Wheeler ML. Nutrition therapy for diabetic nephropathy. *Curr Diab Rep.* 2003;3:412–417.

254. Smit E, Nieto FJ, Crespo CJ, Mitchell P. Estimates of animal and plant protein intake in US adults: results from the Third National Health and Nutrition Examination Survey, 1988–1991. *J Am Diet Assoc.* 1999;99:813–820.

255. Coresh J, Selvin E, Stevens LA, et al. Prevalence of chronic kidney disease in the United States. *JAMA.* 2007; 298:2038–2047.

256. Kontessis P, Jones S, Dodds R, et al. Renal, metabolic and hormonal responses to ingestion of animal and vegetable proteins. *Kidney Int.* 1990;38:136–144.

257. D'Amico G, Gentile MG. Effect of dietary manipulation on the lipid abnormalities and urinary protein loss in nephrotic patients. *Miner Electrolyte Metab.* 1992;18:203–206.

258. Kontessis PA, Bossinakou I, Sarika L, et al. Renal, metabolic, and hormonal responses to proteins of different origin in normotensive, nonproteinuric type I diabetic patients. *Diabetes Care.* 1995;18:1233.

259. Guijarro C, Keane WF. Lipid-induced glomerular injury. *Nephron.* 1994;67:1–6.

260. Fried LF, Orchard TJ, Kasiske BL. Effect of lipid reduction on the progression of renal disease: a meta-analysis. *Kidney Int.* 2001;59:260–269.

261. Anderson JW, Blake JE, Turner J, Smith BM. Effects of soy protein on renal function and proteinuria in patients with type 2 diabetes. *Am J Clin Nutr.* 1998;68:1347S–1353S.

262. Soroka N, Silverberg DS, Greemland M, et al. Comparison of a vegetable-based (soya) and an animal-based low-protein diet in predialysis chronic renal failure patients. *Nephron.* 1998;79:173–180.

263. Teixeira SR, Tappenden KA, Carson L, et al. Isolated soy protein consumption reduces urinary albumin excretion and improves the serum lipid profile in men with type 2 diabetes mellitus and nephropathy. *J Nutr.* 2004;134:1874–1880.

264. Bernstein AM, Treyzon L, Li Z. Are high-protein, vegetable-based diets safe for kidney function? A review of the literature. *J Am Diet Assoc.* 2007;107:644–650.

265. Anderson JW. Beneficial effects of soy protein consumption for renal function. *Asia Pac J Clin Nutr.* 2008;17(suppl 1): 324–328.

266. Pecis M, de Azevedo MJ, Gross JL. Chicken and fish diet reduces glomerular hyperfiltration in IDDM patients. *Diabetes Care.* 1994;17:665–672.

267. Nakamura H, Takasawa M, Kashara S, et al. Effects of acute protein loads of different sources on renal function of patients with diabetic nephropathy. *Tohoku J Exp Med.* 1989;159:153–162.

268. Kitazato H, Fujita H, Shimotomai T, et al. Effects of chronic intake of vegetable protein added to animal or fish protein on renal hemodynamics. *Nephron.* 2002;90:31–36.

269. Chan AY, Cheng ML, Keil LC, Myers BD. Functional response of healthy and diseased glomeruli to a large, protein-rich meal. *J Clin Invest.* 1988;81:245–254.

270. D'Amico G, Gentile MG. Influence of diet on lipid abnormalities in human renal disease. *Am J Kidney Dis.* 1993; 22:151–157.

271. Barsotti G, Navalesi R, Giampietro O, et al. Effects of a vegetarian, supplemented diet on renal function, proteinuria, and glucose metabolism in patients with 'overt' diabetic nephropathy and renal insufficiency. *Contrib Nephrol.* 1988;65:87–94.

272. Azadbakht L, Esmaillzadeh A. Soy-protein consumption and kidney-related biomarkers among type 2 diabetics: a crossover, randomized clinical trial. *J Ren Nutr.* 2009;19:479–486.

273. Azadbakht L, Atabak S, Esmaillzadeh A. Soy protein intake, cardiorenal indices, and C- reactive protein in type 2 diabetes with nephropathy: a longitudinal randomized clinical trial. *Diabetes Care.* 2008;31:648–654.

274. Chen ST, Chen JR, Yang CS, Peng SJ, Ferng SH. Effect of soya protein on serum lipid profile and lipoprotein concentrations in patients undergoing hypercholesterolaemic haemodialysis. *Br J Nutr.* 2006;95:366–371.

275. Chen ST, Ferng SH, Yang CS, Peng SJ, Lee HR, Chen JR. Variable effects of soy protein on plasma lipids in hyperlipidemic and normolipidemic hemodialysis patients. *Am J Kidney Dis.* 2005;46:1099–1106.

276. Fanti P, Asmis R, Stephenson TJ, Sawaya BP, Franke AA. Positive effect of dietary soy in ESRD patients with systemic inflammation—correlation between blood levels of the soy isoflavones and the acute-phase reactants. *Nephrol Dial Transplant.* 2006;21:2239–2246.

277. Imani H, Tabibi H, Atabak S, Rahmani L, Ahmadinejad M, Hedayati M. Effects of soy consumption on oxidative stress, blood homocysteine, coagulation factors, and phosphorus in peritoneal dialysis patients. *J Ren Nutr.* 2009; 19:389–395.

278. Cupisti A, Ghiadoni L, D'Alessandro C, et al. Soy protein diet improves endothelial dysfunction in renal transplant patients. *Nephrol Dial Transplant.* 2007;22:229–234.

279. Bhatia J, Greer F. Use of soy protein-based formulas in infant feeding. *Pediatrics.* 2008;121:1062–1068.

280. Gilchrist JM, Moore MB, Andres A, Estroff JA, Badger TM. Ultrasonographic patterns of reproductive organs in infants fed soy formula: comparisons to infants fed breast milk and milk formula. *J Pediatr.* 2010;156:215–220.

281. White LR, Petrovitch H, Ross GW, et al. Brain aging and midlife tofu consumption. *J Am Coll Nutr.* 2000;19:242–255.

282. Hogervorst E, Sadjimim T, Yesufu A, Kreager P, Rahardjo TB. High tofu intake is associated with worse memory in elderly indonesian men and women. *Dement Geriatr Cogn Disord.* 2008;26:50–57.

283. Woo J, Lynn H, Lau WY, et al. Nutrient intake and psychological health in an elderly Chinese population. *Int J Geriatr Psychiatry.* 2006;21:1036–1043.

284. Lu Z, Li CM, Qiao Y, Yan Y, Yang X. Effect of inhaled formaldehyde on learning and memory of mice. *Indoor Air.* 2008;18:77–83.

285. Tong Z, Zhang J, Luo W, et al. Urine formaldehyde level is inversely correlated to mini mental state examination scores in senile dementia. *Neurobiol Aging.* 2009; October 29 (Epub ahead of print).

286. Zhao L, Brinton RD. WHI and WHIMS follow-up and human studies of soy isoflavones on cognition. *Expert Rev Neurother.* 2007;7:1549–1564.

287. Doerge D, Chang H. Inactivation of thyroid peroxidase by soy isoflavones, in vitro and in vivo. *J Chromatogr B Analyt Technol Biomed Life Sci.* 2002;777:269.

288. Divi RL, Chang HC, Doerge DR. Anti-thyroid isoflavones from soybean: isolation, characterization, and mechanisms of action. *Biochem Pharmacol.* 1997;54:1087–1096.

289. Poirier LA, Doerge DR, Gaylor DW, et al. An FDA review of sulfamethazine toxicity. *Regul Toxicol Pharmacol.* 1999;30:217–222.

290. Messina M, Redmond G. Effects of soy protein and soybean isoflavones on thyroid function in healthy adults and hypothyroid patients: a review of the relevant literature. *Thyroid.* 2006;16:249–258.

291. Bosland MC, Zeleniuch-Jacquotte A, Melamed J, et al. Design and accrual of a randomized, placebo-controlled clinical trial with soy protein isolate in men at high risk for PSA failure after radical prostatectomy. Paper presented at: American Urological Association Annual Meeting, April 25–30, 2009; Chicago, IL. Abstract 1861.

292. Sharma P, Wisniewski A, Braga-Basaria M, et al. Lack of an effect of high dose isoflavones in men with prostate cancer undergoing androgen deprivation therapy. *J Urol.* 2009;182:2265–2272.

293. Ryan-Borchers T, Boon C, Park JS, McGuire M, Fournier L, Beerman K. Effects of dietary and supplemental forms of isoflavones on thyroid function in healthy postmenopausal women. *Topics Clinical Nutr.* 2008;23:13–22.

294. Villar HC, Saconato H, Valente O, Atallah AN. Thyroid hormone replacement for subclinical hypothyroidism. *Cochrane Database Syst Rev.* 2007(3):CD003419.

295. Aoki Y, Belin RM, Clickner R, Jeffries R, Phillips L, Mahaffey KR. Serum TSH and total T4 in the United States population and their association with participant characteristics: National Health and Nutrition Examination Survey (NHANES 1999–2002). *Thyroid.* 2007;17:1211–1223.

296. Caldwell KL, Miller GA, Wang RY, Jain RB, Jones RL. Iodine status of the U.S. population, National Health and Nutrition Examination Survey 2003–2004. *Thyroid.* 2008;18:1207–1214.

297. Delange F, de Benoist B, Burgi H. Determining median urinary iodine concentration that indicates adequate iodine intake at population level. *Bull World Health Organ.* 2002;80:633–636.

298. Setchell KD, Gosselin SJ, Welsh MB, et al. Dietary estrogens—a probable cause of infertility and liver disease in captive cheetahs. *Gastroenterology.* 1987;93:225–233.
299. Bennetts HW, Underwood EJ, Shier FL. A specific breeding problem of sheep on subterranean clover pastures in Western Australia. *Aust J Agric Res.* 1946;22:131–138.
300. Bradbury RB, White DR. Estrogen and related substances in plants. In: Harris RS, Marrian GF, Thimann KV, eds. *Vitam Horm.* New York, NY: Academic Press; 1954:207–230.
301. Lundh TJ-O, Petterson HL, Martinsson KA. Comparative levels of free and conjugated plant estrogens in blood plasma of sheep and cattle fed estrogenic silage. *J Agric Food Chem.* 1990;38:1530–1534.
302. Rowland I, Faughnan M, Hoey L, Wahala K, Williamson G, Cassidy A. Bioavailability of phyto-oestrogens. *Br J Nutr.* 2003;89(suppl 1):S45–S58.
303. Rowland IR, Wiseman H, Sanders TA, Adlercreutz H, Bowey EA. Interindividual variation in metabolism of soy isoflavones and lignans: influence of habitual diet on equol production by the gut microflora. *Nutr Cancer.* 2000; 36:27–32.
304. Urpi-Sarda M, Morand C, Besson C, et al. Tissue distribution of isoflavones in ewes after consumption of red clover silage. *Arch Biochem Biophys.* 2008;476:205–210.
305. Chavarro JE, Toth TL, Sadio SM, Hauser R. Soy food and isoflavone intake in relation to semen quality parameters among men from an infertility clinic. *Hum Reprod.* 2008;23:2584–2590.
306. Mitchell JH, Cawood E, Kinniburgh D, Provan A, Collins AR, Irvine DS. Effect of a phytoestrogen food supplement on reproductive health in normal males. *Clin Sci (Lond).* 2001;100:613–618.
307. Beaton LK, McVeigh BL, Dillingham BL, Lampe JW, Duncan AM. Soy protein isolates of varying isoflavone content do not adversely affect semen quality in healthy young men. *Fertil Steril.* 2009; October 9 (Epub ahead of print).
308. Casini ML, Gerli S, Unfer V. An infertile couple suffering from oligospermia by partial sperm maturation arrest: can phytoestrogens play a therapeutic role? A case report study. *Gynecol Endocrinol.* 2006;22:399–401.
309. Hamilton-Reeves JM, Vazquez G, Duval SJ, Phipps WR, Kurzer MS, Messina MJ. Clinical studies show no effects of soy protein or isoflavones on reproductive hormones in men: results of a meta-analysis. *Fertil Steril.* 2009; June 11 (Epub ahead of print).
310. Messina M. Soybean isoflavone exposure does not have feminizing effects on men: a critical examination of the clinical evidence. *Fertil Steril.* In press.
311. Hooper L, Ryder JJ, Kurzer MS, et al. Effects of soy protein and isoflavones on circulating hormone concentrations in pre- and post-menopausal women: a systematic review and meta-analysis. *Hum Reprod Update.* 2009;15:423–440.
312. Bouker KB, Hilakivi-Clarke L. Genistein: Does it prevent or promote breast cancer? *Environ Health Perspect.* 2000;108:701–708.
313. Messina MJ, Loprinzi CL. Soy for breast cancer survivors: a critical review of the literature. *J Nutr.* 2001;131: 3095S–3108S.
314. Affenito SG, Kerstetter J. Position of the American Dietetic Association and Dietitians of Canada: women's health and nutrition. *J Am Diet Assoc.* 1999;99:738–751.
315. American College of Obstetricians and Gynecologists. Use of botanicals for management of menopausal symptoms. *ACOG Practice Bulletin.* 2001;28:1–11.
316. American Cancer Society Workshop on Nutrition and Physical Activity for Cancer Survivors. Nutrition during and after cancer treatment: a guide for informed choices by cancer survivors. *CA Cancer J Clin.* 2001;51:153–187.
317. Ju YH, Allred CD, Allred KF, Karko KL, Doerge DR, Helferich WG. Physiological concentrations of dietary genistein dose-dependently stimulate growth of estrogen-dependent human breast cancer (MCF-7) tumors implanted in athymic nude mice. *J Nutr.* 2001;131:2957–2962.
318. Allred CD, Ju YH, Allred KF, Chang J, Helferich WG. Dietary genistin stimulates growth of estrogen-dependent breast cancer tumors similar to that observed with genistein. *Carcinogenesis.* 2001;22:1667–1673.
319. Kang X, Jin S, Zhang Q. Antitumor and antiangiogenic activity of soy phytoestrogen on 7,12-dimethylbenz[alpha] anthracene-induced mammary tumors following ovariectomy in Sprague-Dawley rats. *J Food Sci.* 2009;74: H237–H242.
320. Allred CD, Allred KF, Ju YH, Goeppinger TS, Doerge DR, Helferich WG. Soy processing influences growth of estrogen-dependent breast cancer tumors. *Carcinogenesis.* 2004;25:1649–1657.

321. Sartippour MR, Rao JY, Apple S, et al. A pilot clinical study of short-term isoflavone supplements in breast cancer patients. *Nutr Cancer.* 2004;49:59–65.

322. Palomares MR, Hopper L, Goldstein L, Lehman CD, Storer BE, Gralow JR. Effect of soy isoflavones on breast proliferation in postmenopausal breast cancer survivors. *Breast Cancer Res Treatment.* 2004;88(suppl 1):4002.

323. Cheng G, Wilczek B, Warner M, Gustafsson JA, Landgren BM. Isoflavone treatment for acute menopausal symptoms. *Menopause.* 2007;14:468–473.

324. Hargreaves DF, Potten CS, Harding C, et al. Two-week dietary soy supplementation has an estrogenic effect on normal premenopausal breast. *J Clin Endocrinol Metab.* 1999;84:4017–4024.

325. Maskarinec G, Williams AE, Carlin L. Mammographic densities in a one-year isoflavone intervention. *Eur J Cancer Prev.* 2003;12:165–169.

326. Maskarinec G, Franke AA, Williams AE, et al. Effects of a 2-year randomized soy intervention on sex hormone levels in premenopausal women. *Cancer Epidemiol Biomarkers Prev.* 2004;13:1736–1744.

327. Atkinson C, Warren RM, Sala E, et al. Red-clover-derived isoflavones and mammographic breast density: a double-blind, randomized, placebo-controlled trial. *Breast Cancer Res.* 2004;6:R170–R179.

328. Messina M, McCaskill-Stevens W, Lampe JW. Addressing the soy and breast cancer relationship: review, commentary, and workshop proceedings. *J Natl Cancer Inst.* 2006;98:1275–1284.

329. Boyd NF, Lockwood GA, Martin LJ, Byng JW, Yaffe MJ, Tritchler DL. Mammographic density as a marker of susceptibility to breast cancer: a hypothesis. *IARC Sci Publ.* 2001;154:163–169.

330. Boyd NF, Martin LJ, Li Q, et al. Mammographic density as a surrogate marker for the effects of hormone therapy on risk of breast cancer. *Cancer Epidemiol Biomarkers Prev.* 2006;15:961–966.

331. Boyapati SM, Shu XO, Ruan ZX, et al. Soyfood intake and breast cancer survival: a followup of the Shanghai Breast Cancer Study. *Breast Cancer Res Treat.* 2005;92:11–17.

332. Shu XO, Zheng Y, Cai H, et al. Soy food intake and breast cancer survival. *JAMA.* 2009;302:2437–2443.

333. Ballard-Barbash R, Neuhouser ML. Challenges in design and interpretation of observational research on health behaviors and cancer survival. *JAMA.* 2009;302:2483–2484.

334. Guha N, Kwan ML, Quesenberry CP Jr, Weltzien EK, Castillo AL, Caan BJ. Soy isoflavones and risk of cancer recurrence in a cohort of breast cancer survivors: the Life After Cancer Epidemiology study. *Breast Cancer Res Treat.* 2009;118:395–405.

335. Doyle C, Kushi LH, Byers T, et al. Nutrition and physical activity during and after cancer treatment: an american cancer society guide for informed choices. *CA Cancer J Clin.* 2006;56:323–353.

336. Frias J, Song YS, Martinez-Villaluenga C, Gonzalez de Mejia E, Vidal-Valverde C. Immunoreactivity and amino acid content of fermented soybean products. *J Agric Food Chem.* 2008;56:99–105.

337. Cordle CT. Soy protein allergy: incidence and relative severity. *J Nutr.* 2004;134:1213S–1219S.

338. Vierk KA, Koehler KM, Fein SB, Street DA. Prevalence of self-reported food allergy in American adults and use of food labels. *J Allergy Clin Immunol.* 2007;119:1504–1510.

339. Aaronov D, Tasher D, Levine A, Somekh E, Serour F, Dalal I. Natural history of food allergy in infants and children in Israel. *Ann Allergy Asthma Immunol.* 2008;101:637–640.

340. Mitchell DC, Lawrence FR, Hartman TJ, Curran JM. Consumption of dry beans, peas, and lentils could improve diet quality in the US population. *J Am Diet Assoc.* 2009;109:909–913.

341. Biesalski HK, Dragsted LO, Elmadfa I, et al. Bioactive compounds: safety and efficacy. *Nutrition.* 2009;25:1206–1211.

342. Fulgoni VL 3rd. Current protein intake in America: analysis of the National Health and Nutrition Examination Survey, 2003–2004. *Am J Clin Nutr.* 2008;87:1554S–1557S.

CHAPTER 10

Food Guides for Vegetarians

A HISTORY OF FOOD GUIDES

The first food guide, introduced by the U.S. Department of Agriculture (USDA) in 1916, included five groups: vegetables and fruits; meat, fish, and milk; cereals; simple sweets; and butter and wholesome fats. Although there was limited knowledge about the newly discovered vitamins at this time, nutritionists well understood the importance of these new nutrients. In 1918, McCollum coined the phrase *protective foods* for foods rich in calcium, vitamin A, and ascorbic acid. He suggested that daily food habits should address the consumption of these nutrients specifically and recommended daily consumption of a quart of milk, a large serving of greens or pot-herbs, and at least two salads with raw fruits and vegetables. There was little concern about harmful effects of overnutrition, as was evident in McCollum's advice to "Eat what you want after you have eaten what you should."[1]

The first recommended dietary allowances (RDAs) were announced over the radio in 1941. With this kind of specific information about nutrient needs available, several new food guides were developed by various government agencies. Eating well and keeping fit were viewed as patriotic duties. The Office of Defense, Health and Welfare Services introduced eight new food groups in 1942 and attached a wartime slogan to the new guide: "US Needs Us Strong—Eat Nutritional Food." The objective of the new nutritional program was to seek "full health returns from the nation's food resources . . . for victory."[2] Indeed, the link between nutrition and the war effort was a real one because a report published at the time noted that "a third of all men rejected by Selective Service were disqualified for reasons of physical disability and defects related to malnutrition."[3] This food guide also gave special consideration to the food shortages brought on by the war by including alternative choices in certain groups.

The guide that was to become the standard until the mid-1950s was introduced in 1943 and billed as the National Wartime Nutrition Guide.[1] It was based on seven food groups: leafy green and yellow vegetables; citrus fruits; potatoes and other vegetables; milk and milk products; meat, poultry, fish, eggs, dried beans, and peanuts; cereals, breads, and flours; and butter and margarine. This food guide was presented via a Wheel of Good Eating to indicate that no group was more important than any other. This was the nation's nutrition education model until 1955.

In 1956, the Basic Four Food Groups guide was introduced. Widely embraced for its simplicity and ease of use, it was employed with relatively few changes by nutrition educators until the Food Guide Pyramid was introduced in 1992. Foods were grouped as follows: meat, milk, vegetables and fruits, and breads and cereals. In 1979, the guide was revised into the Daily Food Guide, which used the same groups but expanded the number of servings of grains, fruits, and vegetables and added a group that included fats, sweets, and alcohol. In view of the increasing body of data on the harmful effects of dietary overconsumption, however, the Daily Food Guide became a nutritional anachronism long before it was discarded. Criticisms included the fact that meat and dairy foods were visually overemphasized in the guide and that it allowed, or even encouraged, the consumption of too much fat and cholesterol. The Daily Food Guide continued in use even though other government guidelines (the Dietary Guidelines) were urging Americans to reduce consumption of fat and cholesterol.

Both the Basic Four Food Groups and the Daily Food Guide were somewhat adaptable to lacto-ovo vegetarian diets. Vegetarians could use the guide exactly as it was, choosing "alternatives" from the meat, fish, and poultry group. One problem was that the alternative choices were limited to eggs, beans, and peanut butter. Also, serving sizes for legumes were too large. For example, a 3-oz piece of chicken could be replaced by 1½ cups of cooked beans, providing significantly greater food volume and more calories. Because there were no alternatives to dairy foods in the milk group, neither the Basic Four Food Groups nor the Daily Food Guide was useful for vegans.

In 1992, the USDA released the Food Guide Pyramid. Although its release was steeped in controversy, the nutrition profession largely hailed it as a marked improvement over former plans. The pyramid visually reinforced the idea that plant foods need to be emphasized in a healthy diet. It also promoted the consumption of animal foods in amounts that may be greater than is advised for optimal health, however.

A revised guide, called MyPyramid, was introduced by the USDA in 2005. It includes a new symbol to represent the importance of physical activity and presents recommendations in common household measures of ounces and cups, rather than servings. MyPyramid provides more individualized guidelines via a Web site, www.mypyramid.gov. Although the guide does emphasize plant foods, it is not particularly useful to vegetarians and is not usable by vegans.

DEVELOPING FOOD GUIDES FOR VEGETARIANS

In a 1981 issue of the *Journal of Nutrition Education*, Food and Drug Administration nutritionist Jean Pennington wrote, "A food guide is an instrument which converts the professional's scientific knowledge of food composition and nutrient requirements for health into a practical plan for food selection by those without training in nutrition."[4]

Challenges in developing such a guide exist for any type of dietary pattern. At best, a food guide can only provide general guidelines to increase the likelihood that a consumer will choose a healthy diet. Diets of individuals using the same food guide may differ in quality depending on individual food preferences, habits, and choices within food groups. A food guide cannot act as a foolproof means of ensuring adequate nutrient intake and of avoiding dietary excesses. For example, food guides for omnivores have not been completely successful in guaranteeing diets that fall within recommendations for fat, cholesterol, and fiber intake.

A number of food guides for vegetarians have been developed over the past several decades. In the past, food guides for vegetarians have often used the USDA food guide pyramid as a blueprint. However, this guide is not necessarily a useful staring point because vegetarian diets differ from standard American eating patterns in a number of significant ways. In addition, guidelines for vegans have often focused on the replacement of cow's milk with fortified soymilk. This practice does not reflect the way many vegans eat and does not allow for the variety of ways in which calcium needs can be met.

A food guide for vegetarians should:

- Meet the needs of people following different types of vegetarian diets. Most food guides have focused specifically on either lacto-ovo or vegan populations. Or they have been targeted to lacto-ovo vegetarians with only limited options for vegans.
- Be adaptable to the needs of children and of pregnant and lactating women. It should aim to guide consumers toward planning diets that meet the most recent recommendations for nutrient intake from the Institute of Medicine.
- Give specific attention to nutrients that have sometimes been marginal in vegetarian diets.
- Emphasize variety and include the wide variety of foods available to vegetarians.

Figure 10-1 shows a food guide that was developed for North American vegetarians and was designed to achieve the goals just listed. In a departure from traditional food guides that have largely focused on dairy foods or dairy substitutes, such as soymilk, as primary calcium choices, this one does not contain a dairy group. Dairy foods are instead grouped with other protein-rich foods such

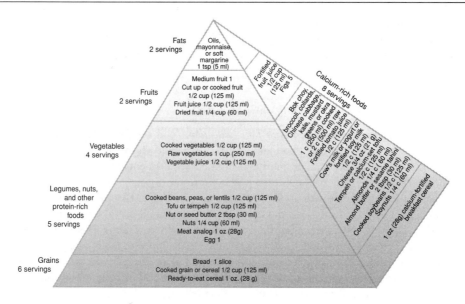

Figure 10-1 Vegetarian food guide pyramid.

Tips for meal planning:

1. Choose a variety of foods.
2. The number of servings in each group is for minimum daily intakes. Choose more foods from any of the groups to meet energy needs.
3. A serving from the calcium-rich food group provides approximately 10% of adult daily requirements. Choose eight or more servings per day. These also count toward servings from the other food groups in the guide. For example, ½ cup of fortified fruit juice counts as a calcium-rich food and also counts toward servings from the fruit group.
4. For the best balance of fats in your diet, olive and canola oils are the optimum choices for cooking.
5. Servings of nuts and seeds may be used in place of servings from the fats group.
6. Be sure to get adequate vitamin D from daily sun exposure or through fortified foods and supplements. Cow's milk and some brands of soymilk, juice, and breakfast cereals are fortified with vitamin D.
7. Include at least three good food sources of vitamin B_{12} in your diet every day. These include 1 tablespoon of Red Star Vegetarian Support Formula nutritional yeast, 1 cup fortified soymilk, ½ cup cow's milk, ¾ cup yogurt, 1 large egg, 1 ounce fortified breakfast cereal, 1½ ounce of fortified meat analog. If you don't eat these foods regularly, take a daily vitamin B_{12} supplement of 6 to 10 µg or a weekly B_{12} supplement of 2000 µg.
8. If you include sweets or alcohol in your diet, consume these foods in moderation. Get most of your daily calories from the foods in the Vegetarian Food Guide.

One-Day Menu for Lacto-Ovo or Vegan Based on Minimum Servings from the Vegetarian Food Guide

| | Food Group Servings | | | | | |
Menu	Grains	Legumes/ Nuts/Dairy	Vegetables	Fruits	Fats	Calcium-Rich Foods

Breakfast
  1 cup oatmeal
  1 slice whole wheat bread w/1 tsp margarine
  ½ cup skim milk or fortified soymilk
  1 cup calcium-fortified orange juice
	3	1		2	1	3

Snack ½ cup low-fat soy yogurt with ¼ cup granola	½	1				1
Lunch 2 cups vegetable soup (includes 1 cup vegetables and ½ cup kidney beans) with 1 tbsp nutritional yeast and croutons	½	1	2			

Snack
  1 apple
  2 tbsp almond butter
		1		1		1

Dinner
  1 cup rice
  Stir-fry with ½ cup calcium-set tofu and 1 cup bok choy and broccoli in 1 tsp canola oil
	2	1	2		1	3

Total servings from food groups	6	5	4	3	2	8

as beans and nuts. The addition of a calcium-rich food group that overlaps with each of the other food groups illustrates the concept that calcium is available from a wide variety of foods, including healthful foods that are fortified with this nutrient. This allows the guide to be used by both lacto-ovo vegetarians and vegans as well as those who might be transitioning to a vegan diet.

Servings of calcium-rich foods in this guide provide approximately 10–15% (100–150 mg) of the adult adequate intake for calcium. This allows consumers to meet requirements using a variety of foods in realistic serving sizes and promotes the concepts of variety and moderation. It encourages lacto-ovo vegetarians to explore sources of calcium in addition to dairy foods.

A set of meal-planning guidelines is an important part of this tool because it directs consumers toward meeting needs for vitamin B_{12} and vitamin D, which are available primarily through fortified foods and supplements.

Adaptations of this guide for pregnant and lactating women, children and teens can be found in Chapters 11, 13, and 14.

FOOD GUIDE GROUPINGS

The Food Guide for North American Vegetarians is built around five food groups.[5]

Grains

Whole grains are emphasized, although refined grains are included. Refined grains can play an important role in the diets of children or others who may have difficulty meeting calorie needs.

Foods included are all breads, corn and flour tortillas, dry cereals, cooked cereals, cooked grains such as rice, quinoa, and wheat berries, and pasta. Foods from this group contribute fiber, protein, iron, B vitamins, and, when whole grains are used, some trace nutrients. These foods tend to be low in fat, but this is not always the case. Also, fortified dry cereals can make significant contributions to nutrient intake because many are fortified with vitamin D, vitamin B_{12}, calcium, iron, and other nutrients. Breakfast cereals can also be high in sugar and fat, however. It is a good idea to suggest to vegetarians that they read labels of cereals for further nutrition information, however, because fortification can change over time and different brands of similar cereals contain different nutrients.

One of the easiest ways to increase consumption from this group is to increase the number of servings of bread, a food that requires no preparation and is portable and generally well liked. Clients should be encouraged to make all meals grain based. That is, grains should become "center of the plate" choices, a concept that is important for planning healthy menus in both vegetarian and omnivore diets. Exploring ethnic cuisine can help clients introduce more grains into meals.

Grains can be prepared in simple but appealing ways by cooking them in vegetable broth or by using apple juice for part of the cooking liquid and by tossing the grains with herbs, chopped dried fruits, or nuts.

Breakfasts provide a good opportunity for clients to consume more grains as well because staples of this meal include cereals, breads, muffins, pancakes, and French toast. Lunch ideas that make good use of whole grains include sandwiches, cold pasta or rice salads, and soups with pasta, rice, or barley. Snacks can also be grain based. Good snack ideas include popcorn, bread, muffins, graham crackers, oatmeal cookies, bagels, and pretzels.

Vegetables

This group comprises all vegetables including those that are botanically fruits (e.g., avocado and plantain). Leafy green vegetables are the calcium-rich foods in this group. Although they are somewhat common in the cuisine of southern Americans, African Americans, and Asian Americans, leafy green vegetables, excepting spinach, have not been an especially popular vegetable choice in this country. When counseling new vegetarians, it can be helpful to provide recipes or cooking hints for these vegetables.

Sea vegetables (alaria, dulse, kelp, nori, and wakame) are also included in this group. Again, these vegetables, which are common in the cuisine of some Asian countries, are still considered an unusual food choice, even among some vegetarians. Because macrobiotic diets make wide use of sea vegetables, macrobiotic cookbooks can serve as good resources for ways to incorporate more of these foods into the diet. Sea vegetables contribute fiber, protein, and a variety of micronutrients depending on choices within the group. Sea vegetables are generally served as an ingredient in soups or stir-fries rather than as a vegetable side dish.

To boost vegetable intake with fairly simple preparation, clients can consume a serving of raw vegetables each day and include at least one salad per day in their menus. When dark green leafy vegetables are purchased as tender young greens, they can be consumed raw in salads. Cooked vegetables can be flavored with salad dressing, herb vinegars, or Parmesan cheese. If clients do not care for the strong taste of some of the green leafy vegetables, these flavors can be tempered with more bland ingredients by blending them with a cream sauce made with soymilk or cow's milk. They can also be torn into small pieces and added to tomato-based dishes, stews, or vegetable soups.

Fruits

This group includes all whole fresh fruits, fruit juices, dried fruits, and canned or frozen fruits. Some foods are botanically fruits (avocado, plantain, tomatoes, and peppers), but because of their nutrient composition and the fact that they are traditionally viewed as vegetables, they are placed in the vegetable group. Fruits contribute vitamins C and A, and some B vitamins and minerals. Dried fruits can contribute significant iron.

Fruit juice is especially popular with young children and can often displace other nutritious foods. Where possible, all vegetarians should be encouraged to make more use of whole fruits rather than fruit juice. Stewed or cooked mashed fruits can be an excellent option for older people or young children who have problems chewing.

Legumes, Nuts, Seeds, and Other Protein-Rich Foods

This group includes a variety of foods that are among the best sources of protein in vegetarian diets. Many also provide vitamins and minerals, including iron and zinc. Foods in this group that are good sources of calcium include calcium-set tofu, fortified soymilk, almonds, dairy products, cooked soybeans, and soynuts.

Legumes, including soy products, are used extensively in many parts of the world and are common to a number of international cuisines, including Indian, Latin American, and African cooking. They play a minor role in the diets of most Americans, however, and are generally served

as baked beans or in bean soups. In vegetarian diets legumes tend to play an important supporting role in the diet.

Canned beans are a good choice for those who have limited time to prepare these long-cooking
foods, although a pressure cooker can greatly speed their preparation. Chapter 17 includes instructions for cooking beans to reduce gas production. Where flatulence and discomfort persist, clients
can be encouraged to make greater use of legumes that are less gas producing, such as lentils or split
peas. Also, gradual introduction of small amounts of legumes often leads to better tolerance.

New vegetarians in particular may find it a challenge to introduce more legumes into their
diet. Familiar dishes such as chili, baked beans, and lentil soup can provide good starting points
for introducing more legumes into family meals. Beans can also be added to salads and vegetable
soups. Exploration of ethnic dishes, such as dal (a curried lentil dish), hummus, and pasta fagioli,
can provide clients with new ideas for eating more beans. Well-cooked beans can be pureed with
olive oil and herbs to create sandwich spreads or dips.

Soyfoods are included in the legume food group and provide an easy way for clients to add
versatility to meals and to consume more legumes. Chapter 17 includes suggestions for using tofu
and textured soy protein in meals. Other soyfoods include soymilk, tempeh, and fresh green soybeans (edamame).

Meat analogs are simulated or "faux" meat products, often made from soy protein or gluten
(wheat protein) but sometimes from other legumes or from vegetables. Products are available to
simulate burgers, hot dogs, sausages, chicken patties, sandwich meats, meat loaf, ground beef,
chicken breasts, and many other popular meats. The nutrient content of analogs varies greatly.
They tend to be high in protein and vary greatly in fat content; some are fat free. Many are also
very high in sodium. Cheese analogs are also available, although their contribution to nutrient
intakes tends to be much lower.

Dairy products in this group include all forms of cow's milk (whole, low fat, non-fat, and
buttermilk) and its derivatives (yogurt, kefir, and cheese). These foods contribute significant
amounts of calcium, protein, vitamin D, and riboflavin but may also provide considerable amounts
of fat and saturated fat. Lacto-ovo vegetarians may choose to meet some of their nutrient needs
using these foods, but they should be encouraged to explore a wide range of protein- and calcium-
rich plant foods as well.

Regular soymilk is a good source of protein and B vitamins. When soymilk is fortified, it is an
excellent source of calcium and can also provide vitamin D, riboflavin, and vitamin B_{12}. Fortification varies considerably, however, and many brands supply some, but not all of these nutrients.
Soymilks also are available in different flavors.

Because of concerns about allergies to both soymilk and cow's milk protein, and in an effort to
broaden the range of products available to vegans, there are a number of other milks on the market including those made from rice, almonds, hazelnuts, hempseed, coconut, and oats. Some
brands are fortified with both calcium and vitamin D, but all are considerably lower in protein
than either soymilk or cow's milk. Unless these foods are supplemented, they make minimal contributions to nutrient intake.

Nuts, seeds, and their butters contribute protein, fiber, iron, calcium, and trace minerals.
Because nuts and seeds have been linked to reduced risk for chronic disease and are an excellent
source of micronutrients, they can play an important role in vegetarian diets. They can be an

especially valuable source of nutrients and calories for children. In addition to their more common use as sandwich spreads, nut and seed butters can be thinned and seasoned for use as sauces over grains and vegetables. Chopped nuts and seeds can be added to cooked grains or vegetables or sprinkled over salads.

Fats

Fats are generally included in food guides as an option for adults and as an important contributor of calories for children. They include vegetable oils, mayonnaise, salad dressings, margarine, butter, soy or dairy cream cheese, and sour cream. These foods contribute calories to the diet and can offer vitamin E and essential fatty acids. Some foods in this group, such as walnuts and flax seed, canola and soy oils, provide alpha-linolenic acid.

Supplemental Foods

Two supplemental foods that do not fit into any of the food groups are included in the meal planning guidelines. Blackstrap molasses is a valuable addition to the vegan diet in particular because it is rich in calcium. One level tablespoon contains 200 mg of calcium. Nutritional yeast is inactive yeast grown on a nutrient-rich culture. Its actual nutrient content depends on the culture. Nutritional yeast that is grown on a vitamin B_{12}-rich culture is especially valuable in the diets of vegans. The brand that is most likely to be a reliable source of B_{12} is Red Star brand Vegetarian Support Formula. This nutritional yeast is also a good source of other B vitamins, iron, and potassium.

Case Study

Denise is a 28-year-old woman who has been a lacto-ovo vegetarian for 5 years and a vegan for the past 6 months. She has recently complained of feeling tired and is concerned that her diet may not be adequate.

Here is her 24-hour recall:

Breakfast:
  1 cup bran flakes with ½ cup fortified almond milk
  1 slice whole wheat toast with 2 tbsp strawberry jam
  1 cup orange juice
  1 multivitamin supplement with iron

Snack:
  1 cup soy yogurt with a few tablespoons of granola

Lunch:
  1 cup lentil soup
  Apple
  2 small homemade oatmeal cookies

continued

Snack
  ½ cup trail mix
  Banana

Dinner:
  1 cup pasta with ½ cup marinara sauce
  2 cups salad made with iceberg and romaine lettuce, 2 tbsp Italian salad dressing
  ½ cup nondairy ice cream with ½ cup blueberries

For discussion:

Based on the Vegetarian Food Guide, is Denise's diet providing adequate calcium, vitamin D, vitamin B$_{12}$, and protein?

Using the food guide, what menu changes would you suggest to improve the quality of her diet?

REFERENCES

1. Hertzler AA, Anderson HL. Food guides in the United States. *J Am Diet Assoc.* 1974;64:19–28.
2. Office of Defense, Health and Welfare Services. US Needs Us Strong—Eat Nutritional Food. Washington, DC: Government Printing Office; Office of Defense, Health and Welfare Services publication 0-457183; 1942.
3. Office of Defense, Health and Welfare Services. *How Industry Can Cooperate with the National Nutrition Plan.* Washington, DC: Information Services; 1943.
4. Pennington JT. Considerations for a new food guide. *J Nutr Educ.* 1981;13:53–55.
5. Messina V, Melina V, Mangels AR. A new food guide for North American vegetarians. *Can J Diet Pract Res.* 2003; 64(2):82–86.

PART III

Vegetarian Diets
Throughout the Life Cycle

CHAPTER **11**

Pregnancy and Lactation

The requirements for most nutrients increase with pregnancy and lactation. Energy needs increase also but to a lesser extent, so that some attention to dietary needs and food choices that highlight nutrient-dense foods is important for all pregnant and lactating women. Vegetarian diets can be planned to meet energy and nutrient needs of pregnant and lactating women.[1] A rigorous evidence analysis conducted by the American Dietetic Association's Evidence Analysis Library concluded that "limited research on non-US populations indicates that there are no significant health differences in babies born to nonvegan vegetarian mothers vs. nonvegetarians."[2] No research on outcomes of vegan pregnancies was identified.[2] In addition, use of a vegetarian diet during pregnancy may offer significant advantages including a reduced risk of excessive weight gain.[3]

ENERGY NEEDS AND WEIGHT GAIN IN PREGNANCY

Estimates of the average energy cost of pregnancy in well-nourished women are close to 77,000 kcal over the 280 days of pregnancy.[4] During pregnancy, energy needs increase due in part to the energy costs of new tissue deposition in the fetus, placenta, uterus, breasts, and other areas (Table 11-1), and in part due to an increased Basal Energy Expenditure (BEE).[5] Only a minor increase in energy needs is seen in the first trimester because of a very small increase in BEE and little weight gain. An increase of 340 kcal/d above pre-pregnancy energy recommendations is suggested in the second trimester and an increase of 452 kcal/d is recommended in the third trimester.[6] For a woman whose pre-pregnancy estimated energy requirement was 2200 kcal, this represents a 15% increase (second trimester) or a 20% increase (third trimester) in energy needs. The increased need for some nutrients is much greater than this, however. For example, the recommended dietary allowances (RDAs) for pregnant women for folate and iron are 50% higher than for nonpregnant women. Therefore, when pregnant women eat to appetite, they may easily meet energy needs but will not necessarily meet nutrient needs unless some attention is given to choosing nutrient-dense foods.

Appropriate weight gain during pregnancy will sustain both the fetus and the placenta and promote growth in maternal tissues that support the pregnancy and provide stored energy for

301

Table 11-1 Theoretical Protein, Fat, and Weight Gain and Energy Deposition of the Products of Pregnancy

Product	Protein Gain (g)	Fat Gain (g)	Total Energy Deposition (kcal)	Weight (kg)
Fetus	440	40	6644	3.4
Placenta	100	4	598	0.6
Amniotic Fluid	3	0	17	0.8
Uterus	166	4	968	0.7
Breasts	81	12	568	0.7
Blood	135	20	946	1.3
Maternal stores		3345	31,778	3.4
Extracellular fluid				1.7
Total	925	3425	41,519	12.6

Source: Adapted from Hytten FE. Weight gain in pregnancy. In: Hytten FE, Chamberlain G, eds. *Clinical Physiology in Obstetrics*. Oxford, UK: Blackwell Scientific; 1991:173–203.

lactation. Weight gain recommendations in pregnancy vary, depending on the woman's weight prior to pregnancy, her needs for growth if she is still an adolescent, and whether or not it is a singleton pregnancy; therefore energy requirements vary as well. Table 11-2 shows current weight gain recommendations.

In healthy, normal-weight women carrying one fetus, weight gain ideally follows a pattern of 1.1 to 4.4 lb in total for the first trimester of pregnancy and then 0.8 to 1 lb per week thereafter.[7] Weight gain goals (for both total and weekly weight gains) for adolescents, especially young adolescents, may need to be higher than those in Table 11-2. In twin pregnancy, provisional weight gain goals for women of normal pre-pregnant weight are 37 to 54 lb.[7]

Weight Gain in Pregnant Vegetarians

Because of the low-fat, high-fiber content of many vegetarian diets, the energy density (kilocalories per gram) of these vegetarian diets is lower than that of omnivore diets. Weight gain of pregnant vegan and lacto-ovo vegetarians is generally adequate, however, and infants of vegetarian women are of normal weight. For example, average weight gain in vegan women living on the Farm, a vegetarian community in western Tennessee, was 5 lb greater than for the reference population.[8] Interestingly, the longer a woman had been on a vegan diet, the greater her weight gain. Similarly, in a British study, although weight gain during pregnancy was not reported, birth weights of infants born to vegan mothers were almost identical to those of infants of nonvegetarian mothers.[9] A study comparing Asian vegetarian and nonvegetarian women living in India and in England showed no differences in maternal weight gain or in infant birth weight.[10] Finally, studies in the United States and Britain found that birth weights of infants born to lacto-ovo vegetarian women were similar to those of infants born to nonvegetarian mothers;[11–14] maternal weight gain was also similar in the one study in which those values were reported.[11]

Table 11-2 Recommendations for Weight Gain during Pregnancy

Pre-Pregnancy BMI (kg/m²)	Recommended Weight Gain (lb)	Recommended Weight Gain (kg)
<18.5 (underweight)	28–40	12.5–18
18.5–24.9 (normal weight)	25–35	11.5–16
25–29.9 (overweight)	15–25	7–11.5
≥30 (obese)	11–20	5–9

Source: Adapted from Rasmussen KM, Yaktine AL. *Weight Gain During Pregnancy: Reexamining the Guidelines.* Washington, DC: Institute of Medicine, National Research Council; 2009.

In contrast to these findings, inadequate weight gain resulting in small offspring has been seen in some macrobiotic populations and has been attributed to low energy intake.[15,16] Macrobiotics often eat a diet that is much more restrictive than that of nonmacrobiotic vegetarians. Consistent with this, Shull et al[17] found that, although overall birth weight of infants of vegetarian mothers was similar to that of the reference population, macrobiotic vegetarian mothers gave birth to infants with markedly lower birth weights.

For women who have difficulty meeting calorie needs and sustaining an ideal weight gain, it is important to identify foods that are calorie rich but high in nutrients. Because adequate calories are of paramount importance, judicious use of added fats, even where they do not add nutritional value to the diet, can be appropriate. Therefore, use of salad dressings, spreads such as margarine, or small amounts of oil for cooking can be encouraged. Foods that are rich in both calories and nutrients include soy products, nuts, seeds, nut and seed butters, avocados, and legumes. Because the high fiber content of vegetarian diets can produce satiety on fewer calories, using some refined products such as fruit juices and refined enriched grains can help meet energy needs.

MEETING NUTRIENT NEEDS OF PREGNANCY ON A VEGETARIAN DIET

Table 11-3 compares the RDAs for protein, vitamins, and minerals for nonpregnant, pregnant, and lactating women.

Protein

Protein synthesis increases during pregnancy to support expansion of the maternal blood volume, uterus, and breasts and to produce fetal and placental proteins. The net result is a deposition of around 454 g (1 lb) of protein in the fetus and slightly more protein in the maternal tissues.[6] During the first trimester, protein requirements are similar to those prior to pregnancy. The requirement for protein is averaged over the second and third trimesters, resulting in a protein RDA of 1.1 g/kg per day or 25 additional grams of protein per day in the second and third trimesters.[6] In twin pregnancy, during the second and third trimesters, protein recommendations are 50 g/d higher than those for nonpregnant women, although these recommendations are based on very limited data.[6]

The RDA of 71 g of protein represents close to a 50% increase over nonpregnant recommendations. Because the average protein intake of nonpregnant women in the United States is about

Table 11-3 Comparison of RDAs for Nonpregnant, Pregnant, and Lactating Women Age 19 and Older

Nutrient	Nonpregnant	Pregnant	Lactating
Protein (g)	46	71	71
Vitamin A (μg)	700	770	1300
Vitamin D (μg)*	5	5	5
Vitamin E (mg)	15	15	19
Vitamin K (μg)*	90	90	90
Vitamin C (mg)	75	85	120
Folic acid (μg)	400	600	500
Niacin (mg)	14	18	17
Riboflavin (mg)	1.1	1.4	1.6
Thiamin (mg)	1.1	1.4	1.4
Vitamin B_6 (mg)	1.3	1.9	2.0
Vitamin B_{12} (μg)	2.4	2.6	2.8
Calcium (mg)*	1000	1000	1000
Phosphorus (mg)	700	700	700
Iodine (μg)	150	220	290
Magnesium (mg)	310–320	350–360	310–320
Iron (mg)†	32	49	16
Zinc (mg)‡	8	11	12
Selenium (μg)	55	60	70

*Adequate Intake (AI).
†Reflects the RDA for vegetarians that is 1.8 times higher than the values established for omnivores.
‡May be as much as 50% higher for vegetarians.

70 g, most women can meet protein needs in pregnancy with little change in dietary habits other than increasing energy intake to support weight gain. Because inadequate protein intake is correlated with a higher incidence of low birth weight,[18] dietitians should assess the protein content of pregnant women's diets and make recommendations for increasing protein intake if needed. Lacto-ovo vegetarian women typically consume diets composed of between 12% and 14% of calories from protein. If this diet was continued in pregnancy, it generally would be adequate to meet the RDA for protein, but the lower range of those intakes could be near or slightly below the RDA. Vegan women consume diets with between 10% and 12% of calories from protein. These diets could still be adequate to meet the RDA for pregnancy if energy intake was high enough. Attention to good sources of protein such as soy products, dried beans, whole grains, and nuts and nut butters can make it possible to meet protein recommendations. Menus based on the food guide in Table 11-4 provide protein intakes that are close to the RDA.

Table 11-4 Food Guide for Pregnant and Breastfeeding Vegetarians

Food Group	Number of Servings per Day*	
	Pregnant Women	*Breastfeeding Women*
Grains	6	6
Legumes, nuts, and other protein-rich foods	7	8
Vegetables	4	4
Fruits	2	2
Fats	2	2
Calcium-rich foods	8	8

*Suggested minimum number of servings to meet needs for key nutrients like protein. Most women need additional servings and/or added fats to maintain adequate weight gain in pregnancy or to prevent excess weight loss in lactation. See Chapter 10 for additional information on foods in each food group and serving sizes.
Source: Adapted from Messina V, Melina V, Mangels AR. A new food guide for North American vegetarians. *J Am Diet Assoc.* 2003;103:771–775.

Docosahexaenoic Acid and Alpha-Linolenic Acid

In the last trimester of pregnancy, the fetus accumulates 50 to 60 mg of omega-3 fatty acids, most of which is docosahexaenoic acid (DHA).[19] This DHA accumulates in the infant's brain and retinal tissues.[20] Maternal intake and stores are used to meet the need for DHA. Infants of vegetarian mothers have been reported to have lower cord plasma DHA than infants of nonvegetarians, although the functional significance of this is not known.[14,21] Beneficial effects of higher maternal intakes of DHA during pregnancy include improved infant visual acuity at 4 months of age (although no effect was seen at 6 months),[22] a small but statistically significant increase in gestational length,[23] and more mature infant attentional function in the first year.[24]

Some concern has been expressed that pregnancy depletes maternal DHA stores.[19,25] This may be an issue for vegans and vegetarians who do not eat foods fortified with DHA regularly because vegan diets contain little or no DHA and vegetarian diets rarely contain significant amounts of DHA. (See Chapter 4 for more information about DHA.) Pregnant vegetarians have lower blood concentrations of DHA than nonvegetarians.[14]

Increased intake of alpha-linolenic acid (ALA), another omega-3 fatty acid, has been suggested to improve the DHA status of pregnant women. ALA can be converted to DHA. The conversion rate of ALA to DHA is somewhat higher in pregnant women than in nonpregnant women or men, but the rate is still very low.[26,27] Provision of ALA supplements to pregnant women did not increase maternal or infant DHA levels.[28] It appears unlikely that ALA can substitute for DHA in pregnancy in terms of improving DHA status.[29]

A vegetarian DHA supplement derived from microalgae[30] can be used to improve maternal DHA status. This supplement appears effective in lactation,[31] but its use has not been reported in pregnancy. Although there is no RDA for DHA, an expert panel has recommended an intake of 300 mg/d of DHA in pregnancy.[32]

ALA is an essential fatty acid. The AI for ALA in pregnancy is 1.4 g/d.[6] Foods rich in ALA include canola oil, flaxseed oil, and flaxseeds. Reduction of dietary linoleic acid and trans-fatty acids appear to enhance the synthesis of DHA from ALA.[19,33,34]

Iron

In pregnancy, iron is needed for the manufacture of hemoglobin in maternal and fetal red blood cells. A full-term infant has about 245 mg of iron in its blood and stores. An additional 75 mg is found in the placenta, about 500 mg is necessary for expansion of the mother's blood volume, obligatory basal losses account for 250 mg, and maternal blood loss at delivery averages 150 to 250 mg.[35] The net cost of pregnancy is 700 to 800 mg of iron because iron used to increase the red blood cell mass is returned to stores after pregnancy and because of the absence of menstruation during pregnancy.[36]

Generally, maternal iron stores are used to meet the needs of the fetus so that even infants born to iron-deficient mothers are unlikely to be anemic unless maternal anemia is severe. Both iron from maternal stores and dietary iron appear to be preferentially transferred to the fetus in women with marginal iron status.[37] This transfer reduces the risk of anemia in the infant, but the combined transfer of iron from maternal stores and from the mother's diet can lead to depletion of maternal stores. Maternal iron deficiency can lead to a reduction in iron stores in the infant and is also associated with increased risk of premature delivery, low birth weight, and maternal mortality.[38,39]

Several factors promote iron sufficiency in pregnancy. Lack of menstruation saves about 160 mg of iron over the 36 weeks of pregnancy. Iron absorption increases, to as much as 25% compared with 10–20% in nonpregnant women.[35] More relevant to vegetarians, nonheme iron absorption may be as high as 40–60% in the second trimester.[40] The iron requirement of pregnancy is still high enough, however, that the diet needs to be especially iron rich.

Iron supplements are commonly prescribed for pregnant women. The Centers for Disease Control and Prevention recommend that pregnant women receive a low-dose (30 mg) iron supplement throughout pregnancy along with use of iron-rich foods.[36] Additional iron is recommended for women with low hemoglobin levels. The World Health Organization (WHO) recommends daily iron supplementation of 60 mg/d for 6 months or, if 6 months of treatment cannot be achieved during the pregnancy, either continue supplementation during the postpartum period or increase the dosage to 120 mg/d during pregnancy.[41] Even for women who enter pregnancy with adequate iron stores, iron supplements improve iron status during pregnancy and appear to provide some protection against iron deficiency in subsequent pregnancy.[38] It is extremely difficult for pregnant vegetarians to meet the iron RDA of 48.6 mg/d[35] without the use of supplements.

Iron deficiency is a common concern among pregnant women and may or may not occur more frequently in vegetarians than in the general population.[8,13] One study of pregnant lacto-ovo vegetarians showed iron intake without supplements to average close to 17 mg/d, whereas nonvegetarians had slightly lower intakes, averaging 15 mg/d; both groups used iron supplements to increase their iron intake to 37 mg/d (vegetarians) and 48 mg/d (nonvegetarians).[42] In a study of Tennessee vegan women, rates of anemia among pregnant women who were not using supplements were low; in fact, the incidence of anemia actually increased when supplements were used.[8]

Another study found that iron intakes of lacto-ovo vegetarians averaged only 13.8 mg/d without supplements but 57.1 mg/d with supplemental iron.[13] Iron stores are often lower in vegetarians, which may make them theoretically more vulnerable to iron deficiency during pregnancy.

The use of iron-rich foods should be stressed in the diets of all pregnant women. Vegetarian women should include a wide variety of whole and enriched grains, legumes, soy products, nuts, seeds, dried fruits, and vegetables in their diet. Consuming a source of vitamin C with each meal can improve iron absorption.[43] For optimal absorption, iron supplements should not be taken with dairy products, tea, coffee, whole grain cereals, legumes, or calcium supplements. Iron supplements should be taken between meals to reduce interference with zinc absorption.[44]

Calcium

Current recommendations do not call for an increased calcium intake during pregnancy, provided calcium intake was adequate prior to pregnancy.[45] Although calcium needs are higher due to fetal skeletal formation, efficiency of calcium absorption increases markedly in pregnancy and precludes a need for increased dietary calcium requirements. Besides increased calcium absorption, other adaptations in maternal calcium metabolism are seen in pregnancy, including increased bone turnover and increased urinary calcium excretion.[46] Dietary calcium intake does not appear to influence pregnancy-associated changes in calcium and bone metabolism.[47] Despite pregnancy-related increases in calcium absorption, women with low calcium intakes (<500 mg/d) lose significant amounts of calcium from their bones and may be at risk of compromised bone density.[48] In addition, low maternal calcium intakes have been associated with a reduced bone mineral content in neonates.[49]

Lacto-ovo vegetarian women tend to have calcium intakes that meet current recommendations of 1000 mg/d.[42,50] Despite the high calcium content of many plant foods, the calcium intake of vegans is often substantially lower than that of omnivores and lacto-ovo vegetarians. Because adequate calcium intakes are important in pregnancy, vegan women should be able to identify several good sources of calcium that can be included in their diet every day. Many practitioners suggest daily use of fortified soymilk as a convenient way to meet calcium needs. Where clients prefer not to use soymilk or do not use it daily, a list of calcium-rich foods can help in planning diets that meet needs. (See again Table 11-4, which includes a food group of calcium-rich foods.)

It is also important to remember that calcium absorption from some plant foods is superior to that from milk. Therefore, the amount of calcium absorbed may meet biologic needs even when total calcium consumed is lower than recommendations. If only foods with poorly absorbed calcium are chosen, the opposite will be true.

Vitamin D

Historically, severe osteomalacia has caused pelvic deformities significant enough to prevent normal delivery, but it was not until the 1920s that vitamin D deficiency was found to be the cause. Although severe cases of osteomalacia are now rare, women with inadequate vitamin D status can give birth to infants with tetany and congenital rickets.[51,52]

Vitamin D deficiency has been reported in vegetarians, particularly Asian vegetarians,[53–57] and in comparison with omnivores, vitamin D intake is lower in vegans and somewhat lower in lacto-ovo vegetarians.[58–62] Also, lower circulating levels of vitamin D have been seen in Asian vegetarians,[53,63–69] although in some cases where vegetarian vitamin D intake was lower than in nonvegetarians, no differences in serum levels of vitamin D were observed.[70,71] In most people, even in the winter, the concentration of vitamin D in the serum is not determined by current vitamin D intake but rather by the amount of exposure to solar radiation during the previous summer.[72]

Vitamin D recommendations are not increased in pregnancy because the relatively small quantities transferred to the fetus do not appear to affect maternal vitamin D status.[45] It is possible to meet vitamin D requirements through sun exposure, but this may not be a realistic option for many women. Exogenous sources of the vitamin are sometimes required. The best way to provide dietary vitamin D is nearly always with fortified foods. For vegetarians, fortified foods can include some brands of soymilk, cow's milk, some cheeses, some cereals, and some meat analogs. Chapter 7 provides more information about fortified foods. A daily intake of 10 μg (400 IU) of vitamin D, as is commonly seen in prenatal supplements, is not excessive.[45] The current RDA for vitamin D in pregnancy is 5 μg/d (200 IU/d); intakes of ≥2000 IU/d have been proposed.[73]

Vitamin B$_{12}$

The fetus accumulates 0.1 to 0.2 μg/d of vitamin B$_{12}$ throughout pregnancy.[74] Apparently, maternal stores of vitamin B$_{12}$ are not available to the fetus, so only newly absorbed vitamin B$_{12}$ is readily transported across the placenta.[75,76] Infants may be born with low stores of vitamin B$_{12}$ if maternal B$_{12}$ levels are low.[77] Low stores of vitamin B$_{12}$ followed by negligible dietary intake if the infant is breastfed and the mother's diet is deficient in vitamin B$_{12}$ can result in a severe vitamin B$_{12}$ deficiency in as short a time as 2 months after birth. Maternal vitamin B$_{12}$ deficiency has also been associated with an increased risk of preterm birth.[78] Low maternal serum vitamin B$_{12}$ levels in vegetarian women have also been associated with elevated serum free β-human chorionic gonadotropin levels leading to an elevated false-positive rate in screening for Down syndrome.[79]

All pregnant vegetarians should consume a reliable daily source of vitamin B$_{12}$ throughout pregnancy. The RDA for pregnancy is 2.6 μg/d,[74] although at least one study has found that at least 3.0 μg/d are needed in pregnancy to maintain maternal serum vitamin B$_{12}$ levels.[80]

Milk and eggs can provide considerable amounts of vitamin B$_{12}$ in the diets of lacto-ovo vegetarians. In one study, an average of 74.2% of the vitamin B$_{12}$ in pregnant lacto-ovo vegetarians' diets was from dairy products.[80] Vegans can easily meet needs if fortified foods or supplements are used. Table 7-1 provides information about the vitamin B$_{12}$ content of foods eaten by vegetarians. Chapter 7 provides more information about vitamin B$_{12}$.

Zinc

Zinc is involved extensively in cell differentiation and replication and thus plays an important role in prenatal development. Poor maternal zinc status has been associated with low birth weight, congenital anomalies, prolonged labor, and preterm delivery.[81–84] Approximately 100 mg of additional zinc is needed in pregnancy.[85] This additional need can be met through a combination of increased dietary intake and an increase in zinc absorption.[84]

The RDA for zinc in pregnancy is 13 mg/d for those ≤18 years of age and 11 mg/d for those ≥19 years.[35] Zinc intake is generally quite a bit lower than the RDA among Western pregnant women, with a reported mean dietary intake of 9.2 mg.[86] The mean total zinc intake, including supplements, is 21.8 mg.[86] Studies of vegetarian pregnancy report mean intakes of 12.6 mg,[11] 10.5 mg,[12] 8.0 mg,[13] and 7.6 mg[87] with the lowest zinc intakes seen in Hindu lacto-ovo vegetarians. Although Hindu lacto-ovo vegetarians had low zinc intakes, even in the few subjects who consumed <5 mg/d, the birth weights of infants were normal.[88]

Assessment of zinc status is difficult, especially during pregnancy when plasma zinc concentration declines in proportion to the increase in plasma volume.[89,90] Plasma zinc in pregnant vegetarians has been reported to be similar to that in pregnant omnivores.[10–12, 91]

Although zinc intakes of vegetarian women are often similar to those of nonvegetarians, intakes are below the RDA, and zinc absorption is likely to be lower from a vegetarian diet due to the presence of inhibitors of zinc absorption such as phytate and fiber. Also, the use of iron supplements, which is common in pregnancy, can adversely affect zinc status.[92–94] Pregnant vegetarians need to emphasize zinc-rich foods in the diet and may consider the use of a 25 mg/d zinc supplement if their diet is high in phytates, if they smoke, abuse alcohol, or have an acute stress such as an infection or trauma.[84] Zinc supplementation (15 mg/d) has been recommended when >30 mg of supplemental iron is taken; a 2-mg copper supplement should be given when a zinc supplement is used.[95] Chapter 6 provides a list of vegetarian foods that are rich in zinc.

Folate

Adequate folate intake in the periconceptional period of about 1 month before to 6 weeks after conception appears to be important in reducing the risk of having a fetus with a neural tube defect.[74,96] The Institute of Medicine recommends that women capable of becoming pregnant consume 400 μg of folate daily from supplements, fortified foods, or both in addition to consuming food folate from a varied diet.[74] Although food folate would seem to be as effective as supplements of folic acid or fortified foods in reducing the risk of having an infant with a neural tube defect, research has not been conducted to determine this adequately. Therefore, use of supplements or fortified foods seems warranted.[74] Prenatal supplements containing folic acid are one way to meet recommendations for folic acid. Since January 1998, all enriched cereals, flours, and grain products in the United States including breads, pasta, and rice have been fortified with 140 μg folic acid/100 g.[97]

The RDA for folate in pregnancy is 600 μg/d of dietary folate equivalents (DFE).[74] Low blood folate levels during pregnancy are associated with increased risk of preterm delivery, low birth weight, and growth retardation.[98]

The recommendations for folate are expressed as DFE to account for differences in bioavailability of food folate and synthetic folic acid as found in fortified foods and supplements. The DFE is calculated as follows:

$$\text{DFE} = \text{food folate} + (1.7 \times \text{synthetic folic acid})^{74}$$

Thus a vegetarian woman consuming 300 μg/d of folate from foods such as orange juice and dark green leafy vegetables, 240 μg/d of folic acid from enriched bread, pasta, and breakfast cereal, and 400 μg/d of folic acid from a prenatal supplement would have a DFE of:

$$300 + [1.7 \times (240 + 400)] = 1388 \text{ DFE}$$

Although the tolerable Upper Limit (UL) for folate in pregnancy is 1000 μg/d for women ≥19 years of age, the UL does not apply to food folate but only to synthetic forms from fortified foods or supplements. There are no data that indicate that food folate can "mask" vitamin B_{12}-deficiency anemia.[74,99]

Lacto-ovo vegetarian women whose diets are high in vegetables (mean: 277 g/d) appear to have higher intakes of folate and a lower risk of folate deficiency in pregnancy than do nonvegetarians.[91] Although many vegetarians do have diets that are high in folate, vegetarians who eat few fruits, vegetables, or enriched breads and cereals may need guidance to meet folate needs.

Iodine

Iodine requirements are higher in pregnancy to provide adequate iodine for the synthesis of fetal thyroid hormones. Inadequate iodine intakes increase the risk of congenital anomalies, mental retardation, stillbirth, and other poor outcomes.[95] Iodine intakes in the United States are lower than in the past due in part to changes in the production of bread and milk and to frequent use of noniodized salt in food production facilities. Iodine deficiency was found in 6.9% of pregnant women.[100] Vegetarians who do not use iodized salt may be at an increased risk of developing iodine deficiency because of the generally low iodine levels in plant foods.[101–103]

Iodized salt represents an important source of iodine. Three quarters of a teaspoon of iodized salt provides enough iodine to meet the 220 μg/d RDA for pregnancy. Because many people prefer not to use this amount of salt, an iodine supplement may be needed. The iodine content of prenatal supplements used by clients should be assessed; not all prenatal supplements contain iodine. The American Thyroid Association recommends that pregnant women living in the United States and Canada take a prenatal vitamin containing 150 μg of supplemental iodine daily.[104]

Sea vegetables are another source of iodine, although their content is variable and some sea vegetables provide large amounts of iodine.[105] Excessive maternal iodine intake (levels >2300 μg/d) have been linked to hypothyroidism in neonates[106] and to postpartum thyroiditis.[107]

MEAL-PLANNING GUIDELINES

A number of food guides have been developed to help pregnant vegetarians meet nutrient needs. As is true at all stages of the life cycle, these can serve only as a general guide. Calorie needs vary among women depending on many factors.

A meal pattern of three meals and several snacks per day can help many women meet their calorie needs. As the third trimester progresses, many women feel some discomfort after large meals, so frequent small meals are advised. This may be especially valuable for vegetarians, whose diets are higher in fiber and therefore produce a greater feeling of fullness. Exhibit 11-1 shows two menus for pregnancy featuring three meals and three snacks.

Although a woman experiencing a first-time pregnancy may have the time and energy to prepare a variety of meals throughout the day, women with small children and/or those who work full time outside of the home may have little time and energy for meal preparation. Dietitians can help pregnant clients plan meals and snacks that take little time and should encourage clients to use convenience foods if time is a factor. There are many that are suitable for vegetarians. Exhibit 11-2 provides some ideas for fast meals and snacks.

Exhibit 11-1 Sample Menus for Pregnancy

Meal	Day 1	Day 2
Breakfast	1 ounce fortified ready-to-eat cereal with ½ cup fortified soymilk and ½ cup sliced strawberries;	½ cup scrambled calcium-set tofu with onions and mushrooms, 1 cup calcium-fortified orange juice, 2 slices whole wheat toast with 1 tsp margarine
Snack	¼ cup soynuts with ¼ cup raisins	5 dried figs, ¼ cup almonds
Lunch	1 cup vegetarian baked beans, 1 corn muffin, carrot and celery sticks	Sandwich with 2 ounces of veggie deli slices, shredded lettuce, and tomato slices; ½ cup grapes
Snack	½ cup calcium-fortified juice with ½ cup tofu salad and crackers	½ cup hummus (made with 2 tbsp tahini) and crackers
Dinner	1 cup spaghetti with ½ cup sauce and ½ cup chickpeas, 1 cup steamed kale, whole wheat roll with margarine	Stir-fry with 2 cups bok choy, broccoli, and Chinese cabbage, ½ cup tofu, and 1 cup rice; ½ cup sliced pineapple
Snack	Crackers with 2 tbsp almond butter, ½ cup calcium-fortified soymilk	1 cup fortified soymilk with 2 graham crackers

Exhibit 11-2 Suggestions for Fast Meals and Snacks

- Bagel with almond butter and a piece of fruit
- Canned vegetable soup, salad, bread
- Rice pilaf using a packaged mix tossed with steamed frozen mixed vegetables
- Cereal with soymilk or cow's milk and sliced fresh fruit
- Bran muffin and fruit juice
- Trail mix and fruit juice
- Spaghetti with prepared sauce
- Textured vegetable protein with meatless Sloppy Joe sauce served over hamburger buns
- Bean burritos using canned or dehydrated beans and chopped tomatoes

USE OF SOY PRODUCTS IN PREGNANCY

During pregnancy, isoflavones from soy products in the maternal diet appear to be transferred to the fetus. There is a high correlation between the level of isoflavones in maternal serum and in cord blood.[108] Although isoflavones can modify estrogen metabolism, no significant correlation was seen between cord blood isoflavone levels and levels of estradiol, estriol, or testosterone, suggesting that isoflavones do not affect estrogen metabolism in utero.[108]

The levels of isoflavones that occur in utero do not appear to be associated with any health problems in infants.[109,110] Several reports have found that a birth defect of the penis, hypospadias, occurred more frequently in infants whose mothers followed a vegetarian diet or did not eat meat or fish during pregnancy[111,112] although other studies have reported no correlation between maternal vegetarian diet and incidence of hypospadias.[113] Although some have attributed these results to use of soy, several studies have reported no significant association between use of soymilk and other soy products and development of hypospadias.[111,114]

At this point, there seems to be no reason to avoid soy in pregnancy as a part of a varied diet. Based on soy consumption in countries where soy is a regular part of the diet, an upper limit of two to three servings per day of soy appears reasonable.

VEGETARIAN MULTIVITAMIN-MINERAL SUPPLEMENTS

A variety of vegetarian prenatal vitamin-mineral supplements have been developed. Composition varies and may include levels of some vitamins that are much higher than the Dietary Reference Intakes (DRIs). In addition, some products are low in calcium and iodine, two nutrients that may be low in vegetarian or vegan diets.[115] Vitamin-mineral supplements do not replace a nutrient dense diet but can provide significant levels of some nutrients whose intake levels can be low even in otherwise adequate diets.

ADOLESCENT PREGNANCY

The frequency of perinatal complications is higher among adolescents than among adult women with the highest rates of complications seen in young adolescents (<15 years of age). Good nutrition, proper prenatal care, and improved health habits can all serve to reduce the risk of complications in adolescent pregnancy.[116] Because the median age of menarche in the United States is 12.43 years[117] and growth usually continues for 4 years after menarche, pregnant adolescents <17 years need to meet the high nutritional needs of both pregnancy and their own growth and development.

Estimated energy requirements for adolescent girls range between 1700 and 2900 kcal/d depending on activity level.[6] Just as for pregnant adults, an additional 340 kcal/d are recommended in the second trimester and 452 kcal/d in the third trimester.[6] Energy needs are somewhat difficult to determine, however, because growth rates and calorie needs vary considerably throughout adolescence. It is more helpful to monitor weight gain during the pregnancy. Weight gain goals for the adolescent should be based on body mass index (BMI) prior to pregnancy (Table 11-2). To produce babies with normal birth weights, young adolescents (<15 years) appear to cease linear growth during pregnancy as well as reducing their resting energy expenditure.[118] Postpartum, these adolescents should receive information about nutritionally adequate diets that will support their further growth.

Adolescents frequently have inadequate diets due to a variety of factors, including lack of knowledge, poor food choices, and time constraints. These poor eating habits may continue during pregnancy unless the adolescent becomes aware of the importance of adequate nutrition during pregnancy and makes significant dietary changes. Energy intakes are frequently below recommendations in adolescent pregnancy as are intakes of iron, folate, calcium, vitamins D and E, and magnesium.[119,120] For information about good sources of minerals, see Chapters 5 and 6; for vitamins, Chapter 7.

DRIs provide specific nutrient recommendations for pregnant adolescents. For some nutrients, such as vitamin D, the B vitamins, and vitamin E, recommendations for pregnant teens are no higher than those for older pregnant women. Recommendations for calcium are 30% higher.[45] Because teenage girls commonly do not meet the RDA for iron, supplements are typically advised for pregnant teens. Supplemental zinc (15 mg/d) is indicated when >30 mg of supplemental iron is taken; a 2-mg copper supplement should be given when a zinc supplement is used.[95]

Birth rates for U.S. teens 15 to 19 years were 41.1 per 1000 women in this age group in 2004.[121] Dietitians who counsel pregnant women are likely to encounter pregnant teenagers who are vegetarians. Pregnancy is on the rise among the adolescent population, and vegetarianism is increasingly popular with this age group as well. Lacto-ovo vegetarian diets can meet the calorie and nutrient needs of pregnant adolescents with ease. Vegan diets can also supply all the nutrients to support a healthy pregnancy. The satiety value of the high-fiber vegan diet and the lower fat content, however, may require that some attention be given to meeting energy and nutrient needs.

There are no data on the pregnancy outcome of pregnant vegetarian teens. Pregnancy outcome in well-nourished vegetarian adult women is at least as good as in nonvegetarian adult women, however, and growth of nonpregnant vegetarian teens is comparable to that of omnivore teens. Based on these relationships, it is a fair assumption that pregnancy outcome among vegetarian adolescents should be comparable to that of nonvegetarian adolescents.

POTENTIAL COMPLICATIONS OF PREGNANCY

Pregnancy-Induced Hypertension

Pregnancy-induced hypertension (PIH), encompassing preeclampsia and eclampsia, is a set of symptoms that include elevated blood pressure, edema, and proteinuria. Women who are especially at risk include older women, women carrying more than one fetus, and women with a history of preeclampsia. If preeclampsia progresses to eclampsia, the result can be convulsions, coma, and maternal and fetal death.

The etiology of preeclampsia remains elusive. It is more likely to occur in women who had hypertension before pregnancy as well as women with obesity, diabetes, and kidney disease.

The role of calcium in preeclampsia is being investigated. An evidence-based review concluded that the relationship between calcium and PIH and preeclampsia was highly unlikely.[122] A large multicenter trial found that calcium supplementation of pregnant women with an average calcium intake of approximately 1100 mg/d did not significantly reduce the incidence or severity of preeclampsia.[123] Calcium supplementation of women with inadequate intake appears to reduce risk.[124]

Elevated maternal plasma homocysteine levels, possibly due to folate or vitamin B_{12} deficiency, have been associated with increased risk of preeclampia.[98,125] Interestingly, one study has shown a remarkable reduction in risk among vegetarians. Of 775 vegan pregnancies, there was only one case of preeclampsia.[8] Because preeclampsia occurs in about 5–10% of all pregnancies in the general population, the rate among these vegans was about 2% of the rate seen in the general population.[8] In a smaller study, however, there were no differences in the incidence of PIH between vegans and controls.[9] Women whose diets are high in vegetables, fruits, rice, and vegetables oils have a decreased risk of preeclampsia compared to women whose diets are high in processed foods, sweets, and salty snacks.[126] These results suggest that there may be benefits associated with a whole foods-based vegetarian diet in pregnancy.

Gestational Diabetes

Gestational diabetes is a temporary condition that occurs during pregnancy and generally disappears after delivery. It occurs in 3–8% of pregnancies in the United States. Gestational diabetes is a more extreme case of the insulin resistance that is typical in pregnancy, which is due to activity of placental hormones. Complications of gestational diabetes include macrosomia, hypoglycemia in the newborn, respiratory distress syndrome in the newborn, preterm deliveries, and an increased rate of caesarean deliveries.

Goals for gestational diabetes identified by the American Dietetic Association's Nutrition Practice Guidelines are as follows:[127]

- To achieve and maintain normoglycemia
- To provide sufficient calories to promote appropriate weight gain and avoid maternal ketosis
- To provide adequate nutrition for maternal and infant health

Carbohydrates are typically limited to 40–45% of total calories with emphasis on complex carbohydrates with a low glycemic response such as whole grains, dry beans, and lentils. At least 175 g of carbohydrate per day should be consumed to provide adequate glucose for the fetal brain and to prevent ketosis. Use of three meals and two to four snacks is recommended to help control blood glucose levels.[127] Careful planning may be needed to achieve carbohydrate goals in women on vegetarian diets who may be accustomed to higher carbohydrate intakes. A higher than usual intake of protein and of unsaturated fat may be needed to meet energy needs.

Food-Borne Illness

Food-borne illness during pregnancy can have serious consequences. Listeriosis can cause premature birth, stillbirth, or an infection in the neonate.[128] Vegetarians do not eat some foods associated with listeriosis such as hot dogs, luncheon meats, or deli meats. Pregnant lacto-ovo vegetarians should be advised to avoid soft cheeses such as feta, Brie, Camembert, blue-veined cheeses, and Mexican-style cheeses such as "queso blanco fresco" and to avoid unpasteurized milk and products made with unpasteurized milk to reduce risk of listeriosis.[129] In addition, the U.S. Dietary Guidelines recommend that pregnant women avoid unpasteurized juices and raw sprouts to reduce risk of food-borne illness.[130]

COMMON CONDITIONS OF PREGNANCY

Dietitians are frequently called on to help clients manage temporary conditions of pregnancy.

Nausea

Commonly referred to as morning sickness, nausea of early pregnancy can occur at any time of the day. An empty stomach can exacerbate nausea; thus many women experience nausea first thing in the morning. Although nausea typically disappears by the end of the fourth month of pregnancy, it can persist throughout pregnancy. Nausea of pregnancy is linked to the presence of progesterone and estrogens in the stomach.

In addition to the discomfort of the mother, the most serious consequence of nausea of pregnancy is that women often do not feel like eating, or the variety of foods they are comfortable eating may be limited. The dietitian can help clients plan food intake in such a way that it will ease the symptoms of morning sickness and maximize the nutritional quality of the diet to the greatest extent possible under the circumstances. The following suggestions may be helpful:

- *Avoid an empty stomach.* Increased acid in the stomach and the possibility of low blood glucose can exacerbate nausea. Frequent small meals help the pregnant woman keep something in her stomach and maintain normal levels of blood glucose.
- *Keep food near the bed.* Eating immediately upon waking may stave off morning sickness in some women. Dry foods such as crackers or bread may be best tolerated.
- *Eat healthy foods that are well tolerated.* The pregnant woman may experience many food aversions, so that the number of foods tolerated may be limited, but by concentrating on the foods she is able to tolerate, it is often possible to plan a diet that will meet both calorie and nutrient needs. Many women will find starchy, sweet, and salty foods to be best tolerated. Good suggestions in these categories include whole grain breads, bagels, crackers, muffins, stewed fruits, dried fruits, vegetable juices, dry cereals, miso broth, and mashed potatoes. Although some foods tend to be tolerated better than others, this can vary considerably among women. Conventional wisdom can aid the dietitian in generating a list of suggested foods, but it is important to listen to the client's own ideas about what appeals to her. Many foods that are staples in some vegetarian diets, such as soymilk, leafy green vegetables, and legumes, may not appeal to the woman with morning sickness. The consumption of these foods should be encouraged on the days when the woman does feel good, and more acceptable ways in which they can be included in the diet should be considered. For example, although a serving of steamed kale may not be tolerated, a small amount of kale in a cup of miso broth may be acceptable.
- *Avoid liquids with meals.* The mixture of solid foods with liquids can increase nausea in some women.

Constipation

Constipation is common in the last trimester of pregnancy but can occur at any time. It is partly due to increased levels of the hormone progesterone, which slows muscle contractions. Also, the pressure of the growing uterus on the intestines can interfere with elimination. The constipating effects of iron supplements and, in some women, reduced physical activity as pregnancy progresses also contribute to constipation. Vegetarians may have an advantage because they eat high-fiber diets. Other ways to relieve constipation include moderate exercise (such as walking) and drinking plenty of liquids.

Heartburn

Heartburn results when stomach acid is released into the esophagus. It is common in pregnancy for two reasons. First, progesterone causes the esophageal sphincter to relax, allowing acid to pass into the esophagus more easily. Second, as the uterus presses on the stomach, it creates pressure, allowing more acid to pass into the esophagus. The following strategies can help ease heartburn in pregnancy:

- Eat smaller, more frequent meals to avoid feelings of overfullness.
- Remain upright after eating.
- Engage in moderate exercise, such as walking, after a meal.
- Avoid fatty foods, carbonated beverages, and acidic foods.
- Eat slowly.

Leg Cramps

Many women experience leg cramps in pregnancy, especially in the last trimester. Leg cramps frequently occur at night and may contribute to disrupted sleeping patterns. Both calcium and magnesium have been used to treat leg cramps in pregnancy. Some evidence indicates that magnesium reduces the incidence of leg cramps; calcium does not appear to be effective.[131] Lacto-ovo vegetarians appear to have higher mean magnesium intakes than nonvegetarians and to have a reduced frequency of calf cramps during the third trimester of pregnancy.[132] Whole grains, dried beans, soy products, nuts, and green leafy vegetables provide significant amounts of magnesium.

VEGETARIANS AND LACTATION

There are many reasons why breastfeeding should be promoted, from the standpoint of both the mother and the infant. Chapter 12 provides more information about benefits of breastfeeding.

The nutritional composition of milk is affected by the woman's diet to variable degrees. Nutrients that are most sensitive to the mother's intake are most of the B vitamins and vitamins A, C, and D.[133,134] The levels of other nutrients, including protein, vitamin K, sodium, calcium, phosphorus, magnesium, iron, zinc, and copper, remain constant regardless of the mother's diet (see Table 11-5). Concentrations of selenium in human milk show geographic variations that reflects soil selenium levels.[135]

The milk of vegetarian mothers is nutritionally adequate, and breastfed infants of well-nourished vegetarian women grow and develop normally.[1,136] An analysis of the milk of a group of macrobiotic women showed slightly decreased levels of calcium, magnesium, and vitamin B_{12} but no significant differences in energy or protein levels.[137]

Generally, the mineral content of milk does not vary with maternal diet.[133] Specifically, no differences were reported in levels of iron, copper, zinc, sodium, potassium, calcium, magnesium, and lactose or in total fat in the milk of vegetarians and omnivores, although in this study both groups used supplements.[138]

Meeting Nutrient and Energy Needs of Lactation with a Vegetarian Diet

Nutritional needs of lactating women are similar to those of pregnant women. The nutritional cost of milk synthesis and of providing nutrients for a growing infant means that breastfeeding women require more calories and higher amounts of some nutrients than do nonpregnant, nonlactating women.

Table 11-5 Effects of Maternal Dietary Changes on Nutrient Composition of Breast Milk

Nutrient Levels That Change with Changes in Maternal Diet	Nutrient Levels That Do Not Change with Changes in Maternal Diet
Thiamin	Sodium
Riboflavin	Calcium
Niacin	Phosphorus
Pantothenic acid	Magnesium
Vitamin B$_{12}$	Iron
Vitamin C	Zinc
Vitamin A	Copper
Vitamin D	Fluoride
Manganese	Protein
Vitamin K	
Vitamin E	
Biotin	
Vitamin B$_6$	
Selenium	
Folate	
Iodine	

Energy Needs in Lactation

Energy requirements in the first 6 months of lactation are about 500 calories above the needs of a nonpregnant, nonlactating woman. although many women partially meet energy needs by mobilization of tissue stores.[6] An average postpartum weight loss of 0.8 kg/mo is equivalent to 170 kcal/d resulting in an Estimated Energy Requirement (EER) of 330 kcal/d for the first 6 months of lactation.[6] The EER for the second 6 months of lactation is 400 kcal/d assuming weight loss has ceased and milk production has decreased to approximately 600 ml/d.[6] Thus energy recommendations in lactation are similar to those in pregnancy.

Protein

Protein recommendations for lactation are based on milk nitrogen output and the efficiency of dietary protein utilization. This results in a protein RDA of 1.1 g/kg per day or 25 g/d of additional protein, identical to the RDA for pregnancy.[6]

Fat and Cholesterol

Generally, breast milk has about 50% of calories from fat, but in women with low body fat, milk fat concentration may be lower.[139,140] The total fat content of the milk of vegetarian mothers is similar to that of omnivores.[141] Fatty acid content varies according to the type of dietary fat consumed, however.[142–144] The saturated fat content of vegetarians' milk reflects the lower saturated fat content of the maternal diet.[141] A study of four British vegans found that their breast milk contained less eicosapentaenoic acid (EPA) and saturated fat and more linoleic and linolenic acid than that of the general population.[145] The milk of macrobiotic vegans is also higher in linoleic and linolenic acid than that of omnivores.[137,146]

Fat composition will vary only to a limited degree, however. There appears to be an upper limit to how much fat can be removed from the mother's blood and passed into milk; above this level, the primary source of fatty acids is mammary synthesis.[141] The cholesterol content of breast milk is not sensitive to maternal diet and ranges from 10 to 20 mg/dl; daily infant consumption is about 100 mg.

Docosahexaenoic Acid

Levels of docosahexaenoic acid (DHA) in breast milk from vegan women appear to be lower than levels in lacto-ovo vegetarians and nonvegetarians[147,148] but higher than in unfortified infant formula.[149] DHA plays a role in vision and mental development.[24,150–152] Although observational studies link higher DHA intakes to improved cognition or visual function, there are few randomized trials of DHA supplementation in human lactation that demonstrate beneficial effects for the infant.[24,153]

Because DHA is found primarily in fish, vegans do not consume it but depend on endogenous synthesis from the omega-3 fatty acid ALA. Both term and preterm infants can synthesize DHA from ALA,[154–156] so increased levels of breast milk ALA could promote DHA synthesis in breastfed infants. The rate of conversion of ALA to DHA is very limited. Although flaxseed oil supplements (20 g/d) have been shown to increase breast milk levels of ALA and EPA, no increase was seen in milk DHA levels.[157] This may have been due to limited conversion of ALA to DHA and the short duration of supplementation. Despite these results, in order to meet recommendations for ALA, lactating vegan and vegetarian women should be advised to include sources of ALA in their diet (ground flaxseed, flaxseed oil, canola oil, walnuts).

Microalgae-derived DHA given to lactating women has been shown to increase plasma phospholipid DHA levels in their breastfed infants.[31] This form of DHA does not contain animal products and is available as a supplement as well as in fortified foods such as soymilk, olive oil, and energy bars. Although there is no DRI for DHA, one expert panel has recommended an intake of 300 mg/d in lactation.[32] (Chapter 4 provides more information about ALA and DHA sources.)

Vitamin D

There is no evidence that lactating women require more vitamin D than nonlactating women, so recommendations are not increased in lactation.[45] Adequate intakes are important, however, and lactating women who do not use foods fortified with vitamin D and who have limited sunlight exposure or regularly use sunscreen should use a vitamin D supplement providing 5 μg (200 IU)/d.[45] The current dietary reference intake of 200 IU/d may be too low, however, to maintain a desirable serum 25(OH)D level in women.[158]

Because of the typically low concentration of vitamin D in human milk, supplemental vitamin D is recommended for breastfed infants. Milk vitamin D levels can be increased by high-dose maternal vitamin D supplementation, which improves the vitamin D status of both the mother and the infant.[158] Oral vitamin D_2 supplements of 2000 IU/d or 60,000 IU/mo for 3 months in lactating women appear to be safe and effective in increasing their serum 25(OH)D levels; higher doses may be needed when sunlight exposure is limited to achieve optimal vitamin D status.[159] A maternal intake of 4000 IU/d of a combination of vitamin D_2 (3600 IU) and vitamin D_3 (400 IU in prenatal vitamin) has been shown to effectively increase both maternal and infant status;[158] a maternal supplement of 6400 IU/d of vitamin D_3 resulted in infant 25(OH)D levels that were equivalent to those seen in infants receiving supplemental vitamin D directly.[160] Chapter 12 provides information about vitamin D needs of breastfed infants.

Vitamin B_{12}

In lactation, maternal vitamin B_{12} intake appears to be more important than maternal stores in determining breast milk levels of vitamin B_{12}.[161–163] Specker et al[164] reported that in infants breastfed by vegetarian mothers, levels of methylmalonic acid (MMA) were not related to the length of time that the mother had been a vegetarian, although maternal levels of serum vitamin B_{12} decreased the longer she had been a vegetarian. MMA levels increase in response to a deficiency of vitamin B_{12} because the vitamin B_{12}-requiring enzyme methylmalonyl coenzyme A mutase is required for the normal metabolism of MMA.[165] Consequently, it was suggested that only newly absorbed vitamin B_{12} is transported across the placenta or into breast milk. In contrast, however, a later study by Specker et al[166] found that breast milk vitamin B_{12} levels decreased the longer a woman had followed a vegetarian diet. This suggests that, for breastfeeding at least, storage forms of B_{12} do pass into breast milk. Other studies have shown that, when maternal serum vitamin B_{12} levels are low, breast milk vitamin B_{12} levels will also be low, resulting in inadequate vitamin intake in infants.[161–163,167,168] Lactation may also deplete maternal vitamin B_{12} stores.[169] Breastfed infants of mothers who had inadequate intakes of vitamin B_{12} have been reported to be developmentally delayed, suffer from failure to thrive, and, in some cases, experience seizures.[170] As long as the availability of vitamin B_{12} from maternal stores remains controversial, it is prudent to recommend that all lactating vegetarians consume at least four servings of vitamin B_{12}-rich foods (see Chapter 10 for more information about these foods) daily or use a daily vitamin B_{12} supplement.

Taurine and Carnitine

The milk of vegans is lower in the amino acid taurine compared with the milk of omnivores,[171] but values overlap considerably between the groups. Carnitine content of breast milk from non-vegetarians is variable[172] and appears to be independent of maternal dietary carnitine content.[173] Because maternal stores appear to contribute to breast milk carnitine content and vegetarians apparently synthesize an adequate amount of carnitine, breast milk carnitine concentrations of vegetarians would be expected to be adequate.

Selenium

Selenium levels and glutathione peroxidase activity were significantly greater in the breast milk of vegetarians in comparison to that of nonvegetarians in one study, which may provide the infant with an extra measure of protection against free radical–induced oxidative damage.[174] Selenium intake of both groups were similar, suggesting that some factor in the vegetarian diet enhanced selenium absorption or that the molecular form of selenium in foods chosen by vegetarians was more bioavailable.[175]

Zinc

Lactating women need to absorb approximately 1.5 to 2 mg more zinc daily than do nonpregnant, nonlactating women.[176] If there were no changes in zinc absorption or retention, women would need to double their intake to meet this need.[177] A study from China suggests that lactating women with low dietary zinc intakes (7.6 mg/d) and a low dietary phytate level (923 mg/d) had increased zinc absorption and conservation of endogenous fecal zinc so that the level of milk zinc was relatively high.[178] Lactating vegetarians whose diets are low in zinc may benefit from selecting foods that are relatively low in phytate and high in zinc.

Calcium

Human milk contains approximately 264 mg/L of calcium during the first 6 months of lactation.[179] This represents a transfer of close to 200 mg/d from mother to infant. Maternal dietary calcium intake has little effect on milk calcium content;[180,181] nor does calcium absorption increase significantly during lactation.[45,182,183] An increased rate of calcium mobilization from the maternal skeleton, independent of calcium intake, is seen in lactation and this, combined with decreased urinary calcium excretion, provides calcium for milk production.[45,46] The loss of calcium from the maternal skeleton has been shown to be recovered at some sites following onset of menses[184] or after weaning.[182]

Because skeletal calcium loss does not appear to be prevented by increased dietary calcium, the recommended level of calcium intake for lactating women is not different from that for nonlactating women of the same age.[45] One study has shown that lactating adolescents who had a dietary calcium intake of at least 1600 mg/d had no bone loss between 2 and 16 weeks postpartum, whereas lactating adolescents with a calcium intake of 900 mg/d had a 10% decrease in bone mineral content.[185] Due to uncertainties about this study, including the reported extremely high rate of bone loss, calcium recommendations for lactating adolescents are not different from nonlactating adolescents.[45]

Iodine

When iodine needs are met, the breast milk content of iodine is between 75 and 200 μg/d.[186] To meet iodine needs of both the infant and the lactating mother, the RDA for iodine in lactation has been set at 290 μg/d.[35] The American Thyroid Association[104] recommends that lactating women receive 150 μg/d of supplemental iodine. Continued use of a prenatal supplement containing iodine can help to meet recommendations for iodine. Additional iodine from iodized salt, sea vegetables, or an iodine supplement may be needed, depending on the iodine content of the prenatal supplement.

Other Nutrients

Requirements for vitamin E, vitamin C, riboflavin, vitamin B_6, vitamin B_{12}, zinc, iodine, and selenium are higher in lactation than in pregnancy (Table 11-3). Iron, magnesium, folate, and niacin requirements decrease, and the recommendations for thiamin, calcium, vitamin D, phosphorus, and vitamin K are the same as for pregnant women.

Environmental Contaminants

One observed difference between the milk of vegetarians and omnivores is in the level of environmental contaminants (Figure 11-1). The passage of certain contaminants into breast milk has been noted since 1951.[187] The substances of most concern are those that are soluble in fat and are toxic. These include the pesticides DDT, chlordane, heptachlor, and dieldrin and industrial compounds or byproducts, such as polychlorinated biphenyls (PCBs) and polychlorinated dibenzo-dioxins. Approximately 30% of breast milk contains higher than allowable levels (as determined by the Food and Drug Administration and the WHO) of some of these compounds.[188] Potentially toxic environmental pollutants are commonly found in human milk at levels that would prevent its sale as a commercial food for infants.[189]

Studies of vegetarians show lower levels of these compounds in their breast milk. In an analysis of breast milk of Tennessee vegans, levels of 17 chemicals were markedly lower than in the general population.[190] The highest vegan value was lower than the lowest value seen in breast milk samples from the general population. In most cases, levels were only 1–2% of those in the samples from the general population. Similar results were seen in the breast milk of macrobiotic women.[147] Frequency of consumption of meat, dairy, and fish was directly related to milk contamination.[147] Contaminant levels were much higher in the milk of women with a high consumption of meat and animal fat than in the milk of vegetarians who shopped at health food stores.[191] Finally, levels

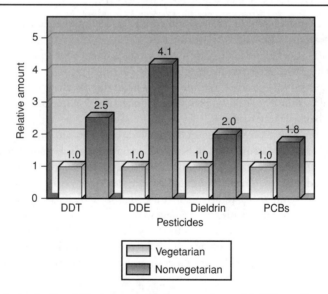

Figure 11-1 Relative levels of pesticides in breast milk from two sisters with different dietary habits. For purposes of the graph, concentrations of pesticides and PCBs in the nonvegetarian sister (32 years of age). Actual values for the nonvegetarian sister for DDT, DDE, dieldrin, and PCBs were 0.50, 1.60, 0.025, and 0.80 mg/kg milk fat, respectively. Values for the vegetarian sister for DDT, DDE, dieldrin, and PCBs were 0.20, 0.39, 0.012, and 0.44 mg/kg milk fat, respectively. *Source:* Data from Noren K. Levels of organochlorine contaminants in human milk in relation to the dietary habits of the mothers. *Acta Paediatr Scand.* 1983;72:811-816.

of DDT, DDE, and PCBs were lowest in the milk of lacto-ovo vegetarians and highest in the milk of women who ate fatty fish from the Baltic Sea. Women on conventional diets fell somewhere in the middle.[192]

Isoflavones

The isoflavone content of breast milk appears to increase as much as 10-fold when the maternal diet includes soy products.[193] Despite this increase, the daily isoflavone intake of breastfed infants remains negligible.[194]

Meal Planning

Breastfeeding vegetarian mothers can follow the same general meal-planning guidelines as pregnant women with slight increases in intake to meet the slightly elevated nutritional requirements of lactation (see Table 11-4). In addition, lactating women should be encouraged to drink plenty of fluids, although women who drink to satisfy the increased thirst that is typical in breastfeeding seem to meet fluid needs. There does not appear to be any advantage to forcing fluids. Small reductions in calories can aid in gradual weight loss without compromising milk output. Severe caloric restriction should be avoided, however, because it can reduce milk volume.

COUNSELING POINTS FOR VEGETARIAN PREGNANCY

- Choose foods that are high in calories and nutrients to support adequate weight gain. Small frequent meals may also help with weight gain.
- Consume 400 µg of folate per day from supplements, fortified foods, or both if you are in a situation where you could become pregnant.
- Pregnant women, ≥19 years of age, need 1000 mg/d day of calcium, at least 11 mg of zinc, and 5 µg of vitamin D. Good sources of calcium are listed in Chapter 5, of zinc in Chapter 6, and of vitamin D in Chapter 7.
- Unless dairy products are consumed regularly, include foods that are fortified with vitamin B_{12} or use B_{12} supplements. Maternal vitamin B_{12} stores do not appear to be transferred to the fetus.
- Iron supplements are commonly used to support the additional iron needs in pregnancy.
- Consume foods high in iron along with foods high in vitamin C to promote iron absorption.
- Promote DHA synthesis by using oils that are high in linolenic acid (canola, flaxseed, and walnut) to maintain DHA stores in pregnancy.
- Simple dietary changes can help to alleviate some of the discomforts of pregnancy. For example, avoiding an empty stomach can help with nausea, high-fiber diets and drinking plenty of liquids can help with constipation, and eating smaller, more frequent meals can help with heartburn.

COUNSELING POINTS FOR VEGETARIAN LACTATION

- Avoid severely limiting calories when breastfeeding, which can lead to decreased milk volume.
- Increase dietary linolenic acid (flaxseed oil, canola oil, ground flaxseeds, and walnuts) and limit linoleic acid (corn, sunflower, and safflower oils) and trans fatty acids to increase the

Case Study

Emily is a 25-year-old woman pregnant for the first time. She follows a lacto-ovo vegetarian diet. She was referred because of concerns about weight gain. Emily was slightly underweight prior to pregnancy with a BMI of 18. She has gained 5 pounds at 20 weeks. Although she had some nausea and vomiting early in pregnancy, that has resolved. All labs are normal. She is taking a prenatal supplement (with iron). She works full time as a first-grade teacher and is very active.

24-hour recall:

Breakfast:
　1 oz fortified ready-to-eat cereal with ½ cup low-fat milk and ½ cup strawberries

Snack at school:
　¼ cup soynuts with ¼ cup raisins

Lunch at school:
　Sandwich with 2 ounces cheese, shredded lettuce, sliced tomato; apple; carton low-fat milk

Dinner:
　Stir-fry with 2 cups bok choy, broccoli, and Chinese cabbage, ½ cup tofu, 1 cup rice
　½ cup sliced pineapple

Snack:
　½ cup milk; crackers with 2 tbsp almond butter
　Approximate nutrient analysis: 2051 kcal; 88 g pro; 1330 mg Ca; 33.3 mg iron; meets recommendations for vitamins

To discuss:

What suggestions can you make to help Emily gain weight?

Emily is very concerned about whether or not her diet is adequate in protein. What will you tell her?

Emily's prenatal supplement contains:

Vitamin A palmitate	2000 IU	Folic acid	800 μg
Vitamin C	100 mg	Vitamin B$_{12}$	10 μg
Vitamin D	400 IU	Biotin	100 μg
Vitamin E	5 IU	Calcium	200 mg
Thiamin	2 mg	Iron	27 mg
Riboflavin	3 mg	Magnesium	60 mg
Niacin	20 mg	Zinc	16 mg
Vitamin B$_6$	3 mg	Copper	2 mg

Evaluate the supplement and whether or not it contains appropriate amounts of vitamin A, vitamin B$_{12}$, calcium, iron, zinc, and iodine considering your client's diet.

After a successful pregnancy and delivery, Emily is exclusively breastfeeding her 6-week-old infant. She wants to move to a vegan diet.

To discuss:

What are key nutrients for someone on a vegan diet that you will review with her?

What suggestions will you make for food choices to replace milk, cheese, and eggs in her diet?

Should she continue to take a prenatal vitamin? Why or why not?

amount of linolenic acid found in milk. Higher levels of linolenic acid may help the breast-fed infant make DHA (an important fatty acid).

- Unless dairy foods are consumed regularly, include foods that are fortified with vitamin B_{12} or use B_{12} supplements because maternal stores of vitamin B_{12} do not appear to be available to the nursing infant.

REFERENCES

1. Craig WJ, Mangels AR. Position of the American Dietetic Association: Vegetarian diets. *J Am Diet Assoc.* 2009; 109:1266–1282.
2. Vegetarian Nutrition in Pregnancy. American Dietetic Association Evidence Analysis Library Web site. http://www .adaevidencelibrary.com/topic.cfm?cat=3125.
3. Stuebe AM, Oken E, Gillman MW. Associations of diet and physical activity during pregnancy with risk for excessive gestational weight gain. *Am J Obstet Gynecol.* 2009;201:58.e1–e8.
4. Butte NF, King JC. Energy requirements during pregnancy and lactation. *Public Health Nutr.* 2005;8(7A):1010–1027.
5. Prentice AM, Goldberg GR. Energy adaptations in human pregnancy: limits and long-term consequences. *Am J Clin Nutr.* 2000;71:1226S–1232S.
6. Food and Nutrition Board, Institute of Medicine. *Dietary Reference Intakes for Energy, Carbohydrate, Fiber, Fat, Fatty Acids, Cholesterol, Protein, and Amino Acids.* Washington, DC: National Academies Press; 2002.
7. Rasmussen KM, Yaktine AL. *Weight Gain During Pregnancy: Reexamining the Guidelines.* Washington, DC: Institute of Medicine, National Research Council; 2009.
8. Carter JP, Furman T, Hutcheson HR. Preeclampsia and reproductive performance in a community of vegans. *South Med J.* 1987;80:692–697.
9. Thomas J, Ellis FR. The health of vegans during pregnancy. *Proc Nutr Soc.* 1977;36:46A.
10. Ward RJ, Abraham R, McFadyen IR, et al. Assessment of trace metal intake and status in a Gujerati pregnant Asian population and their influence on the outcome of pregnancy. *Br J Obstet Gynaecol.* 1988;95:676–682.
11. King JC, Stein T, Doyle M. Effect of vegetarianism on the zinc status of pregnant women. *Am J Clin Nutr.* 1981;34:1049–1055.
12. Abu-Assal MJ, Craig WJ. The zinc status of pregnant women. *Nutr Rep Int.* 1984;29:485–494.
13. Drake R, Reddy S, Davies J. Nutrient intake during pregnancy and pregnancy outcome of lacto-ovo vegetarians, fish-eaters and non-vegetarians. *Veg Nutr.* 1998;2:45–52.
14. Lakin V, Haggarty P, Abramovich DR. Dietary intake and tissue concentrations of fatty acids in omnivore, vegetarian, and diabetic pregnancy. *Prostaglandins Leukot Essent Fatty Acids.* 1998;58:209–220.
15. Dagnelie PC, van Staveren WA, van Klaveren JD, Burema J. Do children on macrobiotic diets show catch-up growth? *Eur J Clin Nutr.* 1988;42:1007–1016.
16. Dagnelie PC, van Staveren WA, Vergote FJVRA, et al. Nutritional status of infants aged 4 to 18 months on macrobiotic diets and matched omnivorous control infants: A population-based mixed-longitudinal study. II. Growth and psychomotor development. *Eur J Clin Nutr.* 1989;43:325–328.
17. Shull MW, Reed RB, Valadian I, et al. Velocities of growth in vegetarian preschool children. *Pediatrics.* 1977;60:410–417.
18. King JC. Physiology of pregnancy and nutrient metabolism. *Am J Clin Nutr.* 2000;71:1218S–1222S.
19. Hornstra G. Essential fatty acids in mothers and their neonates. *Am J Clin Nutr.* 2000;71 (suppl):1262S–1269S.
20. Martinez M. Tissue levels of polyunsaturated fatty acids during early human development. *J Pediatr.* 1992;120: S129–S138.
21. Reddy S, Sanders TA, Obeid O. The influence of maternal vegetarian diet on essential fatty acid status of the newborn. *Eur J Clin Nutr.* 1994;48:358–368.
22. Judge MP, Harel O, Lammi-Keefe CJ. A docosahexaenoic acid-functional food during pregnancy benefits infant visual acuity at four but not six months of age. *Lipids.* 2007; 42:117–122.

23. Szajewska H, Horvath A, Koletzko B. Effect of n-3 long-chain polyunsaturated fatty acid supplementation of women with low-risk pregnancies on pregnancy outcomes and growth measures at birth: a meta-analysis of randomized controlled trials. *Am J Clin Nutr.* 2006;83:1337–1344.

24. Carlson SE. Docosahexaenoic acid supplementation in pregnancy and lactation. *Am J Clin Nutr.* 2009;89(2): 678S–684S.

25. Monique DM, von Houwelingen AC, Hornstra G. Long-chain polyunsaturated fatty acids, pregnancy, and pregnancy outcome. *Am J Clin Nutr.* 2000;71(suppl):285S–291S.

26. Davis B, Kris-Etherton P. Achieving optimal essential fatty acid status in vegetarians: current knowledge and practice implications. *Am J Clin Nutr.* 2003;78 (suppl):640S–646S.

27. Williams CM, Burdge G. Long-chain n-3 PUFA: plant v. marine sources. *Proc Nutr Soc.* 2006;65:42–50.

28. DeGroot RH, Hornstra G, van Houwelingen AC, Roumen F. Effect of alpha-linolenic acid supplementation during pregnancy on maternal and neonatal polyunsaturated fatty acid status and pregnancy outcome. *Am J Clin Nutr.* 2004;79:251–260.

29. Akabas SR, Deckelbaum RJ. Summary of a workshop on n-3 fatty acids: current status of recommendations and future directions. *Am J Clin Nutr.* 2006;93(suppl):1536S–1538S.

30. Conquer JA, Holub BJ. Supplementation with an algae source of docosahexaenoic acid increases (n-3) fatty acid status and alters selected risk factors for heart disease in vegetarian subjects. *J Nutr.* 1996;126:3032–3039.

31. Jensen CL, Voigt RG, Prager TC, et al. Effects of maternal docosahexaenoic acid on visual function and neurodevelopment in breastfed term infants. *Am J Clin Nutr.* 2005;82:125–132.

32. Simopoulos AP, Leaf A, Salem N. Conference report: workshop on the essentiality of and recommended dietary intakes for omega-6 and omega-3 fatty acids. *J Am Coll Nutr.* 1999;18:487–489.

33. Emken EA, Adlof RO, Gulley RM. Dietary linoleic acid influences desaturation and acylation of deuterium-labeled linoleic and ALAs in young adult males. *Biochem Biophys Acta.* 1994;1213:277–228.

34. Decsi T, Burus I, Molnar S, et al. Inverse association between trans isomeric and long-chain polyunsaturated fatty acids in cord blood lipids of full-term infants. *Am J Clin Nutr.* 2001;74:364–368.

35. Institute of Medicine, Food and Nutrition Board. *Dietary Reference Intakes for Vitamin A, Vitamin K, Arsenic, Boron, Chromium, Copper, Iodine, Iron, Manganese, Molybdenum, Nickel, Silicon, Vanadium, and Zinc.* Washington, DC: National Academy Press; 2001.

36. Centers for Disease Control and Prevention. Recommendations to prevent and control iron deficiency in the United States. *MMWR.* 1998;47(No. RR-3):1–29.

37. O'Brien KO, Zavaleta N, Abrams SA, et al. Maternal iron status influences iron transfer to the fetus during the third trimester of pregnancy. *Am J Clin Nutr.* 2003;77:924–930.

38. Allen LH. Anemia and iron deficiency: effects on pregnancy outcome. *Am J Clin Nutr.* 2000;71:1280S–1284S.

39. Brabin BJ, Hakimi M, Pelletier D. An analysis of anemia and pregnancy-related maternal mortality. *J Nutr.* 2001; 131:604S–615S.

40. Barrett JF, Whittaker PG, Williams JG, et al. Absorption of non-haem iron from food during normal pregnancy. *Brit Med J.* 1994;309:79–82.

41. World Health Organization. Iron and folate supplementation. 2007. http://www.who.int/making_pregnancy_safer/publications/Standards1.8N.pdf.

42. Finley DA, Dewey KG, Lonnerdal B, Grivetti LE. Food choices of vegetarians and nonvegetarians during pregnancy and lactation. *J Am Diet Assoc.* 1985;85:678–685.

43. Monsen ER, Balintfy JL. Calculating dietary iron bioavailability: refinement and computerization. *J Am Diet Assoc.* 1982;80:307–311.

44. Whittaker P. Iron and zinc interactions in humans. *Am J Clin Nutr.* 1998;68:442S–446S.

45. Institute of Medicine, Food and Nutrition Board. *Dietary Reference Intakes for Calcium, Phosphorus, Magnesium, Vitamin D, and Fluoride.* Washington, DC: National Academy Press; 1997.

46. Prentice A. Maternal calcium metabolism and bone mineral status. *Am J Clin Nutr.* 2000;71(suppl):1312S–1316S.

47. Olausson H, Laskey MA, Goldberg GR, et al. Changes in bone mineral status and bone size during pregnancy and the influences of body weight and calcium intake. *Am J Clin Nutr.* 2008;88:1032–1039.

48. O'Brien KO, Donangelo CM, Vargas Zapata CL, et al. Bone calcium turnover during pregnancy and lactation in women with low calcium diets is associated with calcium intake and circulating insulin-like growth factor 1 concentrations. *Am J Clin Nutr.* 2006;83:317–323.

49. Koo WW, Walters JC, Esterlitz J, et al. Maternal calcium supplementation and fetal bone mineralization. *Obstet Gynecol.* 1999;94:577–582.

50. Davey GK, Spencer EA, Appleby PN, et al. EPIC—Oxford: lifestyle characteristics and nutrient intakes in a cohort of 33,883 meat-eaters and 31,546 non meat-eaters in the UK. *Public Health Nutr.* 2003;6:259–268.

51. Roberts SA, Cohen MD, Farfar JO. Antenatal factors associated with neonatal hypocalcaemic convulsions. *Lancet.* 1973;2:809–814.

52. Park W, Paust H, Haufmann HJ, Offermann G. Osteomalacia of the mother—rickets of the newborn. *Eur J Pediatr.* 1987;146:292–293.

53. Iq-bal SJ, Garrick DP, Howl A. Evidence of continuing "deprivational" vitamin D deficiency in Asians in the UK. *J Hum Nutr Diet.* 1994;7:47–52.

54. Ford JA, Calhoun EM, McIntosh WB, et al. Biochemical response of late rickets and osteomalacia to a chupatty-free diet. *BMJ.* 1972;3:446–447.

55. Stadler VG, Schmid R, Held U, et al. Serological and radiological improvement of vitamin D-deficiency rickets on treatment with vitamin D in spite of a calcium-free diet. *Ann Pediatr.* 1962;199:215–225.

56. Dent CE, Round JM, Bowe DJF, et al. Effects of chappatia and ultraviolet irradiation on nutritional rickets in an Indian immigrant. *Lancet.* 1973;2:1282–1284.

57. Cooks WT, Asquith P, Ruck N, et al. Rickets, growth and alkaline phosphatase in urban adolescents. *BMJ.* 1974; 2:293–297.

58. Carlson E, Kipps M, Lockie A, Thomson J. A comparative evaluation of vegan, vegetarian and omnivore diets. *J Plant Foods.* 1985;6:89–100.

59. Lamberg-Allardt C, Karkkainen M, Sepanen R, Bistrom H. Low serum 25-hydroxyvitamin D concentrations and secondary hyperparathyroidism in middle-aged white strict vegetarians. *Am J Clin Nutr.* 1993;58:684–689.

60. Lloyd T, Schaeffer JM, Walker MA, Demers LM. Urinary hormonal concentrations and spinal bone densities of premenopausal vegetarian and nonvegetarian women. *Am J Clin Nutr.* 1991;54:1005–1010.

61. Nieman DC, Underwood BC, Sherman KM, et al. Dietary status of Seventh-day Adventist vegetarian and non-vegetarian elderly women. *J Am Diet Assoc.* 1989;89:1763–1769.

62. Alexander D, Ball MJ, Mann J. Nutrient intake and haematological status of vegetarians and age-sex matched omnivores. *Eur J Clin Nutr.* 1994;48:538–546.

63. Preece MA, Tomlinson S, Ribot CA, et al. Studies of vitamin D deficiency in man. *Q J Med.* 1975;44:575–579.

64. Hunt SP, O'Riordon JLH, Windo J, Truswell S. Vitamin D status in different subgroups of British Asians. *BMJ.* 1976;2:1351–1354.

65. Wilmana PF, Brodie MJ, Mucklow JC, et al. Reduction of circulating 25-hydroxyvitamin D by antipyrine. *Br J Clin Pharmacol.* 1979;8:523–528.

66. Dandona P, Mohiuddin J, Weerakoon JW, et al. Persistence of parathyroid hypersecretion after vitamin D treatment in Asian vegetarians. *J Clin Endocrinol Metab.* 1984;59:535–537.

67. Isenberg DA, Newham D, Edwards RHT, et al. Muscle strength and pre-osteomalacia in vegetarian and Asian women. *Lancet.* 1982;1:55.

68. Dent CE, Gupta MM. Plasma 25-hydroxyvitamin-D levels during pregnancy in Caucasians and in vegetarian and non-vegetarian Asians. *Lancet.* 1975;2:1057–1060.

69. Henderson JB, Dunnigan MG, McIntosh WB, et al. The importance of limited exposure to ultraviolet radiation and dietary factors in the aetiology of Asian rickets: a risk-factor model. *Q J Med.* 1987;63:413–425.

70. Kumpusalo E, Karinpää A, Jauhiainen M, et al. Multivitamin supplementation of adult omnivores and lactovegetarians: circulating levels of vitamin A, D, and E, lipids, apolipoproteins and selenium. *Int J Vitam Nutr Res.* 1989;60:58–66.

71. Ellis FR, Montegriffo VME. Veganism, clinical findings and investigations. *Am J Clin Nutr.* 1970;23:249–255.

72. Poskit EME, Cole TJ, Lawson DEM. Diet, sunlight, and 25-hydroxyvitamin D in healthy children and adults. *BMJ.* 1979;1:221–223.

73. Hollis BW, Wagner CL. Vitamin D deficiency during pregnancy: an ongoing epidemic. *Am J Clin Nutr.* 2006; 84:273.

74. Institute of Medicine, Food and Nutrition Board. *Dietary Reference Intakes for Thiamin, Riboflavin, Niacin, Vitamin B_6, Folate, Vitamin B_{12}, Pantothenic Acid, Biotin, and Choline.* Washington, DC: National Academy Press; 1998.

75. Lubby AL, Cooperman JM, Donnfeld AM, et al. Observations on transfer of vitamin B_{12} from mother to fetus and newborn. *Am J Dis Child.* 1958;96:532–533.

76. Allen LH. Vitamin B12 metabolism and status during pregnancy, lactation, and infancy. *Adv Exp Med Biol.* 1994; 352:173–186.

77. Bjorke Monsen AL, Ueland PM, Vollset SE, et al. Determinants of cobalamin status in newborns. *Pediatrics.* 2001;108:624–630.

78. Ronnenberg AG, Goldman MB, Chen D, et al. Preconception homocysteine and B vitamin status and birth outcomes in Chinese women. *Am J Clin Nutr.* 2002;76:1385–1391.

79. Cheng PJ, Chu DC, Chueh HY, et al. Elevated maternal midtrimester serum free beta-human chorionic gonadotropin levels in vegetarian pregnancies that cause increased false- positive Down syndrome screening results. *Am J Obstet Gynecol.* 2004;190:442–447.

80. Koebnick C, Hoffmann I, Dagnelie PC, et al. Long-term ovo-lacto vegetarian diet impairs vitamin B-12 status in pregnant women. *J Nutr.* 2004;134: 3319–3326.

81. Neggers YH, Cutter GR, Action RT, et al. A positive association between maternal serum zinc concentration and birth weight. *Am J Clin Nutr.* 1990;51:678–684.

82. Wells HL, James DK, Luxton R, Rennock CA. Maternal leukocyte zinc deficiency at start of third trimester as a predictor of fetal growth retardation. *BMJ.* 1987;294:1054–1056.

83. Caulfield LE, Zavaleta N, Shankar AH, Merialdi M. Potential contribution of maternal zinc supplementation during pregnancy to maternal and child survival. *Am J Clin Nutr.* 1998;68(suppl):499S–508S.

84. King JC. Determinants of maternal zinc status during pregnancy. *Am J Clin Nutr.* 2000;71(suppl):1334S–1343S.

85. Swanson CA, King JC. Zinc and pregnancy outcome. *Am J Clin Nutr.* 1987;46:763–771.

86. Briefel RR, Bialostosky K, Kennedy-Stephenson J, et al. Zinc intake of the U.S. population: findings from the Third National Health and Nutrition Examination Survey, 1988–1994. *J Nutr.* 2000;130:1367S-1373S.

87. Abraham R, Campbell-Brown M, Haines AP, et al. Diet during pregnancy in an Asian community in Britain—energy, protein, zinc, copper, fibre and calcium. *Hum Nutr Appl Nutr.* 1985;39A:23–35.

88. Campbell-Brown M, Ward RJ, Haines AP, et al. Zinc and copper in Asian pregnancies—is there evidence for a nutritional deficiency? *Br J Obstet Gynaecol.* 1985;92:875–885.

89. Swanson CA, King JC. Reduced serum zinc concentration during pregnancy. *Obstet Gynecol.* 1983;62:313–318.

90. Hambidge KM, Krebs NF, Jacobs MA, et al. Zinc nutritional status during pregnancy. *Am J Clin Nutr.* 1983; 37:429–442.

91. Koebnick C, Heins UA, Hoffmann I, et al. Folate status during pregnancy in women is improved by long-term high vegetable intake compared with the average Western diet. *J Nutr.* 2001;131:733–739.

92. O'Brien KO, Zavaleta N, Caulfield LE, et al. Prenatal iron supplements impair zinc absorption in pregnant Peruvian women. *J Nutr.* 2000;13:2251–2255.

93. Hambidge KM, Krebs NF, Sibley L, English J. Acute effects of iron therapy on zinc status during pregnancy. *Obstet Gynecol.* 1987;4:593–596.

94. Dawson EB, Albers J, McGanity. Serum zinc changes due to iron supplementation in teenage pregnancy. *Am J Clin Nutr.* 1989;50:848–852.

95. Institute of Medicine. *Nutrition During Pregnancy.* Washington, DC: National Academy Press; 1990.

96. Kaiser L, Allen LH; American Dietetic Association. Position of the American Dietetic Association: nutrition and lifestyle for a healthy pregnancy outcome. *J Am Diet Assoc.* 2008;108:553–561.

97. Food and Drug Administration. Food standards: amendment of standards of identity for enriched grain products to require addition of folic acid. *Fed Regist.* 1996;61:8781–8789.

98. Scholl TO, Johnson WG. Folic acid: influence on the outcome of pregnancy. *Am J Clin Nutr.* 2000;71(suppl):1295S–1303S.

99. Suitor CW, Bailey LB. Dietary folate equivalents: interpretation and application. *J Am Diet Assoc.* 2000;100:88–94.

100. Hollowell JG, Haddow JE. The prevalence of iodine deficiency in women of reproductive age in the United States of America. *Public Health Nutr.* 2007;10(12A):1532–1539.

101. Remer T, Neubert A, Manz F. Increased risk of iodine deficiency with vegetarian nutrition *Br J Nutr.* 1999;81:45–49.

102. Lighttowler HJ, Davis GJ. The effect of self-selected dietary supplements on micronutrient intakes in vegans. *Proc Nutr Soc.* 1998;58:35A.

103. Krajcovicova M, Buckova K, Klimes I, Sebokova E. Iodine deficiency in vegetarians and vegans. *Ann Nutr Metab.* 2003;47:183–185.

104. Becker DV, Braverman LE, Delange F, et al. Iodine supplementation for pregnancy and lactation—United States and Canada: recommendations of the American Thyroid Association. *Thyroid.* 2006;16:949–951.

105. Teas J, Pino S, Critchley A, Braverman LE. Variability of iodine content in common commercially available edible seaweeds. *Thyroid.* 2004;14(10):836–841.

106. Nishiyama S, Mikeda T, Okada T, et al. Transient hypothyroidism or persistent hyperthyrotropinemia in neonates born to mothers with excessive iodine intake. *Thyroid.* 2004;14:1077–1083.

107. Guan H, Li C, Li Y, et al. High iodine intake is a risk factor of post-partum thyroiditis: result of a survey from Shenyang, China. *J Endocrinol Invest.* 2005;28:876–881.

108. Nagata C, Iwasa S, Shiraki M, et al. Associations among maternal soy intake, isoflavone levels in urine and blood samples, and maternal and umbilical hormone concentrations (Japan). *Cancer Causes Control.* 2006;17(9):1107–1113.

109. McClain RM, Wolz E, Davidovich A, et al. Reproductive safety studies with genistein in rats. *Food Chem Toxicol.* 2007;45(8):1319–1332.

110. Munro IC, Harwood M, Hlywka JJ, et al. Soy isoflavones: a safety review. *Nutr Rev.* 2003;61:1–33.

111. North K, Golding J, The ALSPAC Study Team. A maternal vegetarian diet in pregnancy is associated with hypospadias. *BJU Int.* 2000;85:107–111.

112. Akre O, Boyd HA, Ahlgren M, et al. Maternal and gestational risk factors for hypospadias. *Environ Health Perspect.* 2008;116:1071–1076.

113. Brouwers MM, Feitz WFJ, Roelofs LAJ, et al. Risk factors for hypospadias. *Eur J Pediatr.* 2007;166:671–678.

114. Pierik FH, Burdorf A, Deddens JA. Maternal and paternal risk factors for cryptorchidism and hypospadias: a case-control study in newborn boys. *Environ Health Perspect.* 2004;112:1570–1576.

115. Mangels R. Vegetarian diets in pregnancy. In Lammi-Keefe CJ, Couch S, Philipson E, eds. *Handbook of Nutrition and Pregnancy.* Totowa, NJ: Humana Press; 2008.

116. Committee on Adolescence, American Academy of Pediatrics. Adolescent pregnancy—current trends and issues, 1998. *Pediatrics.* 1999;103:516–520.

117. Chumlea WC, Schubert CM, Roche AF, et al. Age at menarche and racial comparisons in US girls. *Pediatrics.* 2003;111:110–113.

118. Casanueva E, Rosello-Soberon ME, De-Regil LM, et al. Adolescents with adequate birth weight newborns diminish energy expenditure and cease growth. *J Nutr.* 2006;136:2498–2501.

119. Moran VH. A systematic review of dietary assessments of pregnant adolescents in industrialised countries. *Br J Nutr.* 2007;97:411–425.

120. Baker PN, Wheeler SJ, Sanders TA, et al. A prospective study of micronutrient status in adolescent pregnancy. *Am J Clin Nutr.* 2009;89:1114–1124.

121. Ventura SJ, Abma JC, Mosher WD, et al. Estimated pregnancy rates by outcome for the United States, 1990–2004. *Natl Vital Stat Rep.* 2008;56:1–25, 28.

122. Trumbo PR, Ellwood KC. Supplemental calcium and risk reduction of hypertension, pregnancy-induced hypertension, and preeclampsia: an evidence-based review by the US Food and Drug Administration. *Nutr Rev.* 2007;65(2):78–87.

123. Levine RJ, Hauth JC, Curet LB, et al. Trial of calcium to prevent preeclampsia. *N Engl J Med.* 1997;337:69–76.

124. Hofmeyr GJ, Atallah AN, Duley L. Calcium supplementation during pregnancy for preventing hypertensive disorders and related problems. *Cochrane Database Syst Rev.* 2006;(3):CD001059.

125. Vollset SE, Refsum H, Irgens LM, et al. Plasma total homocysteine, pregnancy complications, and adverse pregnancy outcomes: the Hordaland Homocysteine Study. *Am J Clin Nutr.* 2000;71:962–968.

126. Brantsaeter AL, Haugen M, Samuelsen SO, et al. A dietary pattern characterized by high intake of vegetables, fruits, and vegetable oils is associated with reduced risk of preeclampsia in nulliparous pregnant Norwegian women. *J Nutr.* 2009;139:1162–1168.

127. American Dietetic Association. *Medical Nutrition Therapy Evidence-Based Guides for Practice: Nutrition Practice Guidelines for Gestational Diabetes Mellitus.* Chicago, IL: American Dietetic Association; 2001.

128. Centers for Disease Control. Listeriosis. http://www.cdc.gov/nczved/dfbmd/disease_listing/listeriosis_gi.html.

129. Food Safety and Inspection Service, USDA. Protect your baby and yourself from listeriosis. http://origin-www.fsis.usda.gov/Fact_Sheets/Protect_Your_Baby/index.asp.

130. U.S. Department of Health and Human Services and U.S. Department of Agriculture. *Dietary Guidelines for Americans, 2005.* 6th ed. Washington, DC: U.S. Government Printing Office; January 2005.

131. Young GL, Jewell D. Interventions for leg cramps in pregnancy. *Cochrane Database Syst Rev.* 2002;(1):CD000121.

132. Koebnick C, Leitzmann R, Garcia AL, et al. Long-term effect of a plant-based diet on magnesium status during pregnancy. *Eur J Clin Nutr.* 2005;59:219–225.

133. Institute of Medicine. *Nutrition During Lactation.* Washington, DC: National Academy Press; 1991.

134. Lonnerdal B. Effects of maternal dietary intake on human milk composition. *J Nutr.* 1986;116:499–513.

135. Shearer TR, Hadjimarkos DM. Geographic distribution of selenium in human milk. *Arch Environ Health.* 1975; 30:230–233.

136. Finley DA. Effects of vegetarian diets upon the composition of human milk. In: Hamosh M, Goldman AS, eds. *Human Lactation 2. Maternal and Environmental Factors.* New York: Plenum Press; 1986:83–92.

137. Dagnelie PC, van Staveren WA, Roos AH, et al. Nutrients and contaminants in human milk from mothers on macrobiotic and omnivorous diets. *Eur J Clin Nutr.* 1992;46:355–366.

138. Finley DA, Lonnerdal B, Dewey KG, Grivetti LE. Inorganic constituents of breast milk from vegetarian and non-vegetarian women: relationships with each other and with organic constituents. *J Nutr.* 1985;115:772–781.

139. Brown KH, Akhtar NA, Robertson AD, Ahmed MG. Lactational capacity of marginally nourished mothers: relationships between maternal nutritional status and quantity and proximate composition of milk. *Pediatrics.* 1986; 78:909–919.

140. Prentice A, Jarjou LM, Drury PJ, et al. Breast-milk fatty acids of rural Gambian mothers: effects of diet and maternal parity. *J Pediatr Gastroenterol Nutr.* 1989;8:486–490.

141. Finley DA, Lonnerdal B, Dewey KG, Grivetti LE. Breast milk composition: fat content and fatty acid composition in vegetarians and non-vegetarians. *Am J Clin Nutr.* 1985;41:787–800.

142. Emery WB III, Canolty NL, Atchison JM, Dunkley WL. Effects of sampling and dietary fat on gross and fatty acid composition of human milk. *Nutr Rep Int.* 1978;17:63–70.

143. Kramer M, Szoke K, Lindner K, Tarjan R. The effect of different factors on the composition of human milk and its variations. III. Effect of dietary fats on lipid composition of human milk. *Nutr Diet.* 1965;7:71–79.

144. Mellies MJ, Ishikawa TT, Gartside PS, et al. Effects of varying maternal dietary fatty acids in lactating women and their infants. *Am J Clin Nutr.* 1979;32:299–303.

145. Sanders TAB, Ellis FR, Dickerson JWT. Studies of vegans: the fatty acid composition of plasma choline phosphoglycerides, erythrocytes, adipose tissue, and breast milk, and some indicators of susceptibility to ischemic heart disease in vegans and omnivore controls. *Am J Clin Nutr.* 1978;31:805–813.

146. Specker BL, Wey HE, Miller D. Differences in fatty acid composition of human milk in vegetarian and nonvegetarian women: long term effect of diet. *J Pediatr Gastroenterol Nutr.* 1987;6:764–768.

147. Sanders TAB, Reddy S. The influence of a vegetarian diet on the fatty acid composition of human milk and the essential fatty acid status of the infant. *J Pediatr.* 1992;120:S71–S77.

148. Uauy R, Peirano P, Hoffman D, et al. Role of essential fatty acids in the function of the developing nervous system. *Lipids.* 1996;3:S167–S176.

149. Cunnane SC, Francescutti V, Brenna JT, Crawford MA. Breast-fed infants achieve a higher rate of brain and whole body docosahexaenoate accumulation than formula-fed infants not consuming dietary docosahexaenoate. *Lipids.* 2000;35:105–111.

150. Birch EE, Hoffman DR, Uauy R, et al. Visual acuity and the essentiality of docosahexaenoic acid and arachidonic acid in the diet of term infants. *Pediatr Res.* 1998; 44:201–209.

151. SanGiovanni JP, Berkey CS, Dwyer JT, Colditz GA. Dietary essential fatty acids, long- chain polyunsaturated fatty acids, and visual resolution acuity in healthy full-term infants: a systematic review. *Early Hum Dev.* 2000;57:165–188.

152. Birch EE, Garfield S, Hoffman DR, et al. A randomized controlled trial of early dietary supply of long-chain polyunsaturated fatty acids and mental development in term infants. *Dev Med Child Neurol.* 2000;42:174–181.

153. James DCS, Lessen R. Position of the American Dietetic Association: promoting and supporting breastfeeding. *J Am Diet Assoc.* 2009;109:1926–1942.

154. Salem N Jr, Wegher B, Mena P, Uauy R. Arachidonic and docosahexaenoic acids are biosynthesized from their 19-carbon precursors in human infants. *Proc Natl Acad Sci U S A.* 1996;93:49–54.

155. Carnielli VP, Wattimean DJL, Luijendijk IHT, et al. The very low birthweight premature infant is capable of synthesizing arachidonic and 22:6(n-3) from linoleic and linolenic acids. *Pediatr Res.* 1996;40:169–174.

156. Jensen CL, Prager TC, Fraley JK, et al. Effect of dietary linoleic/alpha-linolenic acid ratio on growth and visual function of term infants. *J Pediatr.* 1997;131:200–209.

157. Francois CA, Connor SL, Bolewicz LC, et al. Supplementing lactating women with flaxseed oil does not increase docosahexaenoic acid in their milk. *Am J Clin Nutr.* 2003;77:226–233.

158. Hollis BW, Wagner CL. Vitamin D requirements during lactation: high-dose maternal supplementation as therapy to prevent hypovitaminosis D for both the mother and the nursing infant. *Am J Clin Nutr.* 2004;80(suppl):1752S–1758S.

159. Saadi HF, Sawodu A, Afandi BO, et al. Efficacy of daily and monthly high-dose calciferol in vitamin D-deficient nulliparous and lactating women. *Am J Clin Nutr.* 2007;85:1565–1571.

160. Wagner CL, Hulsey TC, Fanning D, et al. High-dose vitamin D3 supplementation in a cohort of breastfeeding mothers and their infants: a 6-month follow-up pilot study. *Breastfeed Med.* 2006;1:59–70.

161. Hocy H, Linnell JC, Oberholzer VG, Laurance VM. Vitamin B_{12} deficiency in a mother with pernicious anemia. *J R Soc Med.* 1982;75:656–658.

162. Sklar R. Nutritional vitamin B_{12} deficiency in a breast-fed infant of a vegan-diet mother. *Clin Pediatr.* 1986;25:219–221.

163. Kuhne T, Bubl R, Baumgartner R. Maternal vegan diet causing a serious infantile neurological disorder due to vitamin B_{12} deficiency. *Eur J Pediatr.* 1991;150:205–208.

164. Specker BL, Miller D, Norman EJ, et al. Increased urinary methylmalonic acid excretion in breast-fed infants of vegetarian mothers and identification of an acceptable dietary source of vitamin B_{12}. *Am J Clin Nutr.* 1988;47:89–92.

165. Norman EJ. Detection of cobalamin deficiency using the urinary methylmalonic acid test by gas chromatography mass spectrometry. *J Clin Pathol.* 1992;45:382.

166. Specker BL, Black A, Allen L, Morrow F. Vitamin B_{12}: Low milk concentrations are related to low serum concentrations in vegetarian women and to methylmalonic aciduria in their infants. *Am J Clin Nutr.* 1990;52:1073–1076.

167. Black AK, Allen LH, Pelto GH, et al. Iron, vitamin B_{12} and folate status in men and women and during pregnancy and lactation. *J Nutr.* 1994;124:1179–1188.

168. Johnson PR Jr, Roloff JS. Vitamin B-12 deficiency in an infant strictly breast-fed by a mother with latent pernicious anemia. *J Pediatr.* 1982;100:917–919.

169. Allen LH, Rosado JL, Casterline JE, et al. Vitamin B_{12} deficiency and malabsorption are highly prevalent in rural Mexican communities. *Am J Clin Nutr.* 1995;62:1013–1019.

170. Neurologic impairment in children associated with maternal dietary deficiency of cobalamin—Georgia, 2001. *MMWR Morb Mortal Wkly Rep.* 2003;52:61–64.

171. Rana SK, Sanders TAB. Taurine concentrations in the diet, plasma, and urine and breast milk of vegans compared with omnivores. *Br J Nutr.* 1986;56:17–27.

172. Rebouche CJ. Carnitine. In: Shils ME, Olson JA, Shike M, Ross AC, eds. *Modern Nutrition in Health and Disease.* 9th ed. Baltimore, MD: Williams & Wilkins; 1999:505–512.

173. Mitchell ME, Snyder EA. Dietary carnitine effects on carnitine concentrations in urine and milk in lactating women. *Am J Clin Nutr.* 1991;54:814–820.

174. Debski B, Finley DA, Picciano MF, et al. Selenium content and glutathionine peroxidase activity of milk from vegetarian and nonvegetarian women. *J Nutr.* 1989;119:215–220.

175. McGuire MK, Burgert SL, Milner JA, et al. Selenium status of lactating women is affected by the form of selenium consumed. *Am J Clin Nutr.* 1993;58:649–652.

176. WHO. Trace elements in human nutrition and health. Geneva, Switzerland: World Health Organization; 1996.

177. King JC. Enhanced zinc utilization during lactation may reduce maternal and infant zinc depletion. *Am J Clin Nutr.* 2002;75:2–3.

178. Sian L, Krebs NF, Westcott JE, et al. Zinc homeostasis during lactation in a population with a low zinc intake. *Am J Clin Nutr.* 2002;75:99–103.

179. Atkinson SA, Alston-Mills BP, Lonnerdal B, et al. Major minerals and ionic constituents of human and bovine milk. In: Jensen RJ, ed. *Handbook of Milk Composition*. San Diego, CA: Academic Press; 1995:593–619.

180. Prentice A, Jarjou LM, Cole TJ, et al. Calcium requirements of lactating Gambian mothers: effects of a calcium supplement on breastmilk calcium concentration, maternal bone mineral content, and urinary calcium excretion. *Am J Clin Nutr.* 1995;62:58–67.

181. Kalkwarf HJ, Specker BL, Heubi JE, et al. Intestinal calcium absorption of women during lactation and after weaning. *Am J Clin Nutr.* 1996;63:526–531.

182. Specker BL. Do North American women need supplemental vitamin D during pregnancy or lactation? *Am J Clin Nutr.* 1994;59(suppl):484S–491S.

183. Ritchie LD, Fung EB, Halloran BP, et al. A longitudinal study of calcium homeostasis during human pregnancy and lactation and after resumption of menses. *Am J Clin Nutr.* 1998;67:693–701.

184. Hopkinson JM, Butte NF, Ellis K, et al. Lactation delays postpartum bone mineral accretion and temporarily alters its regional distribution in women. *J Nutr.* 2000;130:777–783.

185. Chan GM, McMurry M, Westover K, et al. Effects of increased dietary calcium intake upon the calcium and bone mineral status of lactating adolescent and adult women. *Am J Clin Nutr.* 1987;46:319–323.

186. Delange F. Iodine requirements during pregnancy, lactation and the neonatal period and indicators of optimal iodine nutrition. *Public Health Nutr.* 2007;10:1571–1580.

187. Laug EP, Kunze FM, Prickett CS. Occurrence of DDT in human fat and milk. *Arch Ind Hyg Occup Med.* 1951;3:245–246.

188. Rogan WJ, Bagniewska A, Damstra T. Pollutants in breast milk. *N Engl J Med.* 1980;302:1450–1453.

189. Rogan WJ, Blanton PJ, Portier CJ, Stallard E. Should the presence of carcinogens in breast milk discourage breast feeding? *Regul Toxicol Pharmacol.* 1991;13:228–240.

190. Hergenrather J, Hlady G, Wallace B, Savage E. Pollutants in breast milk of vegetarians. *N Engl J Med.* 1981;304:792.

191. Centinkaya M, Gabel B, Podbielski A, Thiemann W. Untersuchung uber den Zusammenhang Zwischen Ernahrung und Lebensumstanden stillender Mutter und der Kontamination der Muttermilch mit schwerfluchtigen Organochlorverbindungen. *Akt Ernaehr.* 1984;9:157–162.

192. Noren K. Levels of organochlorine contaminants in human milk in relation to the dietary habits of the mothers. *Acta Paediatr Scand.* 1983;72:811–816.

193. Franke AA, Custer LJ. Daidzein and genistein concentrations in human milk after soy consumption. *Clin Chem.* 1996;42:955–964.

194. Setchell KDR, Zimmer-Nechemias L, Cai J, Heubi J. Exposure of infants to phytoestrogens from soy infant formulas. *Lancet.* 1997;350:23–27.

CHAPTER 12

Vegetarian Diets in Infancy

All infants begin life as vegetarians. Meats are generally not introduced into an infant's diet until 6 to 8 months of age. Until that time, infants consume breast milk, cow's milk formula, or soy formula. First solid foods are preferably infant cereals, vegetables, and fruits. Adapting the diet of older infants (6 to 12 months) to a vegetarian meal plan is a fairly simple matter achieved by substituting vegetable proteins, such as pureed beans or tofu, for strained meats.

GROWTH IN VEGETARIAN INFANTS

The birth weights of infants born to vegetarian mothers are similar to birth weight norms and to weights of infants born to nonvegetarian women.[1–5] In some macrobiotic populations, birth weights have been low and have been attributed to low weight gain in the mother during pregnancy.[6,7]

Vegetarian infants grow normally during the first 6 months after birth.[1,2] This is expected because typically infants in both vegetarian and nonvegetarian families consume similar diets during this time. A slightly slower rate of growth among vegetarian infants that is still within the normal range may be attributed to the fact that vegetarian mothers are more likely to breast-feed.[2,8–10] Breastfed infants grow more slowly than formula-fed infants.[11] Although this difference in growth is taken into consideration to some extent in the growth charts released by the Centers for Disease Control and Prevention (CDC),[12] growth charts released by the World Health Organization (WHO) are based on exclusively or predominantly breastfed infants.[13] These growth charts reflect human growth under the optimal conditions of breastfeeding. Either CDC or WHO growth charts can be used to assess the growth of vegetarian infants.

Satisfactory growth indicates that energy needs are being met. Body weight, recumbent length, and head circumference are all used to evaluate growth in infants. Measurements should be obtained using standard procedures and evaluated by plotting the infant's growth curve on standard growth charts. Additional assessment is needed to determine the cause of the altered growth when an infant's weight, length, or head circumference changes unexpectedly from the established growth channel, either accelerating or faltering.[14] Additional assessment is also required when weight for length is≥95th percentile, length for age is <5th percentile, weight for length is <5th percentile, or head circumference for age is <5th or >95th percentile.[14]

When vegetarian infants receive adequate breast milk or formula and good sources of iron, vitamin B$_{12}$, and vitamin D, they grow well throughout infancy.[15,16] Both milk-based and soy formula support normal growth in infants.[17-19]

Poor growth has been seen in young macrobiotic infants and is attributed to inadequate quantities of milk in the diet.[7] Inadequate energy intakes have been reported in some macrobiotic populations.[1,7,20] There are few data on the growth and development of nonmacrobiotic vegetarian infants. Older studies show, however, that restrictive food patterns among some vegetarian groups, coupled with erroneous ideas about what constitutes an appropriate diet for infancy, have led to nutritional deficiencies in some vegetarian infants, particularly those in macrobiotic families. Observations of rickets, iron-deficiency anemia, and vitamin B$_{12}$ deficiency in some vegan infants have led to concerns about the advisability of such diets for infants.[21,22] It is important to note that these deficiencies are linked to unusually restrictive diets that do not conform to appropriate guidelines for feeding vegan infants. Such diets cannot be used as an argument against the use of well-balanced vegan or lacto-ovo vegetarian diets in infancy. Poorly planned diets are dangerous for infants regardless of the dietary beliefs of the parents.

Although such findings do raise concerns about the appropriateness of macrobiotic diets for infants, they do not necessarily rule out macrobiotics for infants and young children. With some adjustments in the emphasis given to the different food groups in the macrobiotic diet, it is possible to plan appropriate macrobiotic diets for infants. At one point, macrobiotic teachers in the United States liberalized some of their guidelines for children.[22]

When parents are knowledgeable about appropriate infant feeding, both lacto-ovo and vegan feeding patterns are safe and adequate. Dietitians who counsel vegetarian parents of infants need to provide appropriate information to assist parents in planning meals that meet their infants' needs.

VEGETARIAN DIETS DURING THE FIRST 6 MONTHS OF INFANCY
Breastfed Infants

Breastfeeding is a wise option for all infants. Today, about 74% of infants receive some breast milk, although only about 33% are being exclusively breastfed at 3 months and only 43% are receiving any breast milk at 6 months.[23] The number of vegetarian mothers who breastfeed is considerably higher than the average in the general population.[2] The American Academy of Pediatrics (AAP) recommends human milk as the exclusive food for infants for at least the first 4 months after birth but ideally for 6 months.[16] A combination of breastfeeding and supplemental foods should be used after that until at least 12 months of age and thereafter as long as mutually desired by the mother and infant.[16] Breastfeeding's advantages over formula feeding include:[24]

- Superior nutritional composition
- Immunologic components
- Lower cost
- Perceived enhanced maternal–infant bonding

- Fewer respiratory and gastrointestinal infections
- Lower risk of otitis media
- Less likelihood of allergies and asthma
- Reduced risk of developing type 1 and type 2 diabetes, heart disease, and childhood leukemia
- Less likelihood of childhood obesity
- Higher intelligence quotient and school performance through adolescence
- More favorable lipid profile and glucose tolerance in adulthood
- Enhanced maternal weight loss postpartum with lactation duration of at least 6 months
- Reduced risk of maternal type 2 diabetes and breast and ovarian cancer
- Time saved from preparing formulas

Appropriate diets for lactating women are discussed in Chapter 11. Infants of both lacto-ovo vegetarian mothers and vegan mothers thrive, and the breast milk of vegetarian women is adequate in nutrients.[1,3,20,25,26]

Vegan women need to be certain that they are consuming foods fortified with vitamin B_{12} or should use a supplement or their infants should receive a supplement (Tables 12-1 and 12-2). Some evidence indicates that vitamin B_{12} from a woman's stores does not appear in her milk and that only vitamin B_{12} consumed during lactation will be available to her infant.[27] Some data suggest that this may not be the case[28] (see Chapter 11 for more information on vitamin B_{12} and lactation). If there is any question about adequate vitamin B_{12} in a woman's diet, a vitamin B_{12} supplement is recommended for her breastfed infant. A severe vitamin B_{12} deficiency in infancy due to inadequate intake of vitamin B_{12} can lead to neurologic damage that does not resolve with vitamin B_{12} supplementation.[29] Symptoms of vitamin B_{12} deficiency can occur as early as age 2 months, although they appear most commonly between 4 and 10 months.[30] Deficiency symptoms include failure to thrive, apathy, irritability, food refusal, megaloblastic anemia, and developmental regression.[30]

Light-skinned infants can make adequate vitamin D if hands and face are exposed to the sun 2 hours per week or if wearing only a diaper for 30 minutes per week.[31] Supplemental vitamin D is commonly prescribed for all breastfed infants. Breastfeeding without vitamin D supplementation is a significant predictor of vitamin D deficiency.[32,33] The AAP recommends vitamin D supplements of 400 IU/d, beginning soon after birth.[34] Infants who are at particular risk for developing vitamin D deficiency include those who are dark skinned because greater sun exposure is needed in these infants; those who live in northern, smoggy areas; and those who are kept covered because of cultural practices. Sunscreen, commonly recommended for infants, can also interfere with vitamin D synthesis. At this time, in the United States, infant vitamin D supplements contain vitamin D derived from animals (often based on lanolin from sheep's wool); vegan vitamin D supplements for infants are not available.

Breast milk is generally low in iron, regardless of the mother's intake. Nevertheless, the bioavailability of this iron is high; approximately 50% is absorbed.[35] Healthy full-term infants can obtain adequate iron from breast milk and from iron stores for the first 6 to 9 months.[36] Recommendations are for iron supplementation beginning by 4 to 6 months, either in the form of supplementary foods like iron-enriched infant cereals or as iron drops.[16,37] Two servings of iron-enriched infant cereals (½ ounce of dry cereal per serving) are needed to meet iron require-

Table 12-1 Recommended Supplements for Vegetarian Infants from Birth to 6 Months

Nutrient	Breastfed Infants	Formula-Fed Infants
Vitamin K	Single dose at birth:	Single dose at birth:
	0.5–1.0 mg intramuscularly	0.5–1.0 mg intramuscularly
	1.0–2.0 orally	1.0–2.0 mg orally
Vitamin D	200 IU (5 μg) beginning within the first 2 months	Infant formulas contain vitamin D
Iron	1 mg/kg per day beginning at 4–6 months	Use iron-fortified infant formula
Vitamin B$_{12}$	0.4 μg from birth to 6 months unless maternal diet has adequate vitamin B$_{12}$	Infant formulas contain vitamin B$_{12}$

Source: Adapted from Mangels AR, Messina V. Considerations in planning vegan diets. I. Infants. *J Am Diet Assoc*. 2001;101:670–677.

Table 12-2 Recommended Supplements for Vegetarian Infants from 6 to 12 Months

Nutrient	Breastfed Infants	Formula-Fed Infants
Vitamin D	400 IU (10 μg)	Infant formulas contain vitamin D; infants ingesting <500 ml/d of vitamin D–fortified formula or milk should be supplemented with 400 IU/d (10 μg)[34]
Iron	1 mg/kg per day if unable to consume sufficient iron from dietary sources	Use iron-fortified infant formula
Fluoride[39]	0.25 mg/d beginning after 6 mo if water contains <0.3 ppm fluoride	0.25 mg/d beginning after 6 mo if water contains <0.3 ppm fluoride
Vitamin B$_{12}$	0.5 μg/d from 6 to 12 mo unless maternal diet is adequate or infant has a daily, reliable source of vitamin B$_{12}$	Infant formulas contain vitamin B$_{12}$
Zinc	Consider for older infants; see text	Infant formulas contain zinc

Source: Adapted from Mangels AR, Messina V. Considerations in planning vegan diets. I. Infants. *J Am Diet Assoc*. 2001;101:670–677.

ments.[16] Provision of adequate iron throughout infancy and the toddler years could reduce the relatively high incidence of iron deficiency seen in toddlers, age 1 to 2 years.[38]

Breast milk fluoride content is very low; therefore, where water is not fluoridated, infants should receive fluoride supplements after about 6 months.[39]

Formula-Fed Infants

Commercial infant formula is recommended for infants who are not breastfed or who are weaned before 1 year of age. There are several types of formulas available.

Standard Formulas

Standard formulas are the most commonly used. They are based on cow's milk that is modified by removal of the butterfat, addition of vegetable oils and carbohydrate, and reduction of protein content. The addition of whey to some of these standard formulas results in a better approximation of the ratio of whey to casein in breast milk. Approximately 75% of infant formula sales in the United States are for formulas containing added arachidonic acid and docosahexaenoic acid derived from microalgae.[16] The AAP recommends that all formulas fed to infants be fortified with iron.[16] There does not appear to be any increased risk of feeding intolerance with use of iron-fortified formulas.[16]

Soy Formulas

Soy formulas contain methionine-, carnitine-, and taurine-fortified soy protein isolate, vegetable oils, and carbohydrate. They are lactose free. Some are also corn free or sucrose free. All soy formulas are fortified with iron and zinc and have calcium, phosphorus, and protein content higher than standard formulas to compensate for lower bioavailability of these nutrients from soy. Infants who are exclusively fed soy formula grow and develop normally.[18,19] These formulas are a common option when an infant is not breastfed and exhibits an allergy to cow's milk protein, is lactose intolerant, or has galactosemia.[17] Although some brands may contain vitamin D derived from animal sources (often lanolin from sheep's wool), they are the only choice for infants in vegan families who are not breastfed. Use of soy formulas is not recommended for preterm infants,[17] and no commercial formula options are available for preterm vegan infants.

Soy formulas contain significant levels of soy isoflavones ranging from 155.1 to 281.4 μg/g.[40] After adjustment for body weight, this can result in an infant having an isoflavone intake considerably higher than an adult consuming 30 g of soy protein daily.[40] Use of soy formulas has been shown to lead to elevated plasma isoflavone levels.[41] Isoflavones are associated with a number of hormonal and nonhormonal effects.[42] Despite this, soy-based infant formulas have been used for >100 years with no apparent adverse effects.[42,43] A study of close to 250 adults (20 to 34 years of age) who had received soy formula as infants found no effect of soy formula on fertility, miscarriage rate, birth defects in offspring, and maturation.[44]

When parents choose soy formula, they must understand the difference between soy formulas for infants and commercial soy beverages. The latter are not an appropriate food for infants.

Formulas with Extensively Hydrolyzed Protein

Bottle-fed infants who are allergic to both cow's milk protein and soy protein are often placed on formulas that contain extensively hydrolyzed casein. Vegan parents may not be willing to feed these formulas to their infants because they contain cow's milk protein. For vegan infants who show intolerance to soy formulas, there are no commercial vegan formula options. This represents a strong argument in favor of breastfeeding in vegan families.

Supplements for Formula-Fed Infants

Both breastfed and formula-fed infants receive a onetime supplement of vitamin K at birth. Infant formula contains many vitamins and minerals so supplements are seldom needed for formula-fed infants. Although use of iron-fortified formula is recommended, formulas that do not contain iron are available. If an infant is receiving formula that is not fortified with iron, iron drops should be started at age 4 to 6 months and should provide 1 mg/kg of iron daily. Infants who are ingesting <500 ml/d of vitamin D–fortified formula or milk should receive a vitamin D supplement of 400 IU/d.[34]

Follow-Up Formulas

Follow-up and "toddler" formulas are marketed for older infants and toddlers who are eating some solid foods. Both cow's milk-based and soy-based follow-up formulas are available. According to the AAP, there is no advantage to using follow-up formulas instead of standard infant formulas in the first year, although they may be helpful for toddlers who are receiving inadequate amounts of iron and other nutrients in their solid foods.[16]

Other Milk Feedings

Homemade formula based on evaporated milk is sometimes chosen as a lower cost alternative to commercial infant formulas. Although these are a better choice than plain cow's milk, they are not recommended. These formulas contain poorly digested fat, inadequate iron and vitamin C, and excessive amounts of phosphorus and sodium. There are no available recipes for nutritionally adequate homemade infant soy formulas. Infants fed soy formula must use a commercial product. When families cannot afford to purchase commercial infant formula, a referral to the Women, Infants, and Children Supplemental Food Program is appropriate.

Infants should receive breast milk or infant formula for the first 12 months. Introduction of unmodified cow's milk (whole, low fat, or non-fat), goat's milk, commercial soy beverages, or other vegetable milks is not recommended during infancy because these foods are not equivalent to breast milk or commercial infant formula in terms of nutrient levels.[16] Early introduction of cow's milk, particularly before 6 months of age, is associated with a greater risk of milk protein allergy, gastrointestinal blood loss, and poor iron status.[45] Cow's milk is low in iron and has inappropriately high levels of protein, sodium, potassium, and chloride.[16] It also is low in essential fatty acids, vitamin C, vitamin E, and zinc.[16] Cow's milk should definitely not be introduced before 6 months and preferably not before 12 months because even in the second half of the first year, use of cow's milk as a primary beverage has been associated with iron-deficiency anemia.[16] If cow's milk is introduced, in small amounts, during the second half of infancy, only whole cow's milk should be used, not low fat or non-fat.

Commercial soy beverages do not provide adequate nutrition for infants and should not be used, except for small amounts in cooking, during the first year. The bioavailability of iron and zinc from soymilk is relatively low. Commercial soymilk also contains inappropriately high levels of protein, sodium, and potassium for infants. The same is true for other vegetable milks, such as commercial rice and almond milks, or the grain preparations described in some macrobiotic books.

SOLID FOODS FOR VEGETARIAN INFANTS

Parents usually view the introduction of solid foods into an infant's diet as an important milestone. For this reason, there is often a tendency to start infants on solid foods before they are ready. Parents may erroneously believe that breast milk or formula is not adequate nutrition for their infant. It is also commonly, and mistakenly, believed that introducing solids will help an infant sleep through the night.

Either breast milk or commercial formula (based on soy or cow's milk) is adequate nutrition for most infants for the first 4 to 6 months (see Table 12-3) as long as appropriate supplements are offered. Age is a poor indicator of readiness for solid foods. Rather, eating habits and physical preparedness provide better cues to whether solid foods are indicated. One developmental sign of readiness for solid foods is the disappearance of the tongue extrusion reflex. The extrusion reflex allows infants to swallow only liquid foods. As long as this reflex persists, infants will push solids out of the mouth with their tongue, so that feeding such foods will be difficult. Between 4 and 6 months of age, the infant is able to move food from the front to the back of the mouth, where it can be swallowed more easily. Another developmental sign of readiness is the ability to sit independently and maintain balance. This allows the infant to express both hunger and satiety by either leaning forward to receive food or pulling back and turning away.

Although solid foods are generally not necessary before 4 months of age, in most cases there is no advantage to delaying their introduction beyond 6 months of age.[16] Introducing foods at this time allows the infant to develop the skills that accompany solid food consumption.

Solid foods will displace some of the milk or formula in an infant's diet. Because both breast milk and infant formula are nutrient-dense foods, it is important that the solid foods offered are also nutrient dense. Parents must understand that solid foods are added specifically to meet the nutrient needs of the growing infant. The recommended diet for infants provides 40–50% of calories as fat and 7–11% as protein.[16,46] Both breast milk and infant formula meet these recommendations. The addition of solid foods will probably alter the macronutrient intake to some extent. Excessive intake of foods that are high in carbohydrate and low in both protein and fat, such as fruits and juices, can produce diets that are not ideal for infants.

Because the first solid foods for infants are frequently cereals, fruits, and vegetables, recommendations for introducing these foods are exactly the same for vegetarian infants as for those in omnivore households. The first solid food for infants is usually an iron-fortified cereal. Rice cereal is an excellent choice because it is hypoallergenic, and commercially prepared infant cereals are usually recommended. The cereal should be mixed with breast milk or formula to make it dilute for first feedings. Solid foods should always be fed from a spoon, not from a bottle. Infants normally resist the unfamiliar spoon initially. If infants begin to choke, however, this is an indication that they are not ready for solid foods.

Parents should offer one new food every 3 or 4 days, watching for signs of allergic reactions after the introduction of each new food. Breast milk or formula feedings should continue as

Table 12-3 Guidelines for Feeding Vegetarian Infants*

First 4–6 mo	4–6 mo	6–8 mo	9–10 mo	11–12 mo
Breast milk or infant formula	Breast milk or infant formula	Breast milk or infant formula	Breast milk or infant formula	Breast milk or infant formula
	Introduce iron-fortified cereal	Iron-fortified infant cereal, toast, crackers, unsweetened dry cereal	Iron-fortified infant cereal, toast, crackers, unsweetened dry cereal, soft bread	Iron-fortified infant cereal, toast, crackers, unsweetened dry cereal, soft bread, rice, pasta
		Strained fruit, fruit juice	Soft or cooked fruit, fruit juice	Soft, canned or cooked fruit, peeled raw fruit, fruit juice
		Strained vegetable, vegetable juice	Soft, cooked mashed vegetable, juice	Soft, cooked pieces of vegetable, vegetable juice
		Tofu, pureed legumes, yogurt, pureed cottage cheese, egg yolks	Tofu, pureed legumes, yogurt, cheese, egg yolks	Tofu, mashed legumes, yogurt, cheese, egg yolks, tempeh, bite-sized pieces of meat analogs

*Overlap in age groups is due to variation in infant developmental rates.
Source: Adapted from Mangels R. Vegan nutrition. In: Wasserman D, ed. *Simply Vegan*. 4th ed. Baltimore, MD: Vegetarian Resource Group; 2006.

usual. Iron-fortified barley or oat cereal is generally the next food to be introduced after rice cereal. First feedings will comprise just 1 or 2 tsp of cereal. Eventually, the infant can progress to two daily servings of cereal for a total of ⅓ to ½ cup of cereal per day.

Some parents may choose to prepare their own infant cereals. Oats, barley, or rice can be processed in a blender until they are finely ground and then cooked until they are smooth. Because these cereals are low in iron, however, breastfed infants should continue to receive an iron supplement, and bottle-fed infants should receive iron-fortified formula.

When infants are consuming ⅓ to ½ cup of cereal per day, mashed fruits and vegetables can be introduced. Again, it is important that parents introduce only one new food every 3 or 4 days so that any sources of allergies can be identified easily. Good choices for first fruits and vegetables are smooth applesauce, pureed canned peaches or pears (canned in their own juice, not in heavy syrup), strained potatoes, carrots, sweet potatoes, and green beans. Mashed banana and avocado are also good first foods for infants and can be easily prepared because they do not need to be cooked.

Most infants begin to drink from a cup at about 7 to 8 months, and fruit juice can be introduced at that time. Apple juice is a good choice. Infants should not be given unpasteurized juice or cider because of the risk of infection with *Escherichia coli* and *Cryptosporidium parvum*.[47] Excessive juice intake in infants has been linked to diarrhea and failure to thrive, so juice should not be introduced before 6 months and should be limited to 4 to 6 ounces daily for children 1 to 6 years old.[16,48]

At around 7 to 8 months, infants are also ready to begin consuming some higher-protein foods. First protein foods for vegetarian infants can be thoroughly cooked and pureed legumes, well-mashed tofu, or soy yogurt. Infants in lacto-ovo vegetarian families can also have pureed cottage cheese, yogurt mixed with mashed fruit, or cooked egg yolks. At this time, parents can introduce some of the stronger-tasting vegetables, such as kale, collards, or other greens. The flavors of these foods can be tempered by blending them with bland or sweet foods. Vegetables can be pureed with avocado, applesauce, tofu, or cottage cheese.

By 10 months, most infants can enjoy finger foods, such as tofu chunks, crackers, and bread. For infants who are teething, gnawing on frozen bagels can be soothing. By their first birthday, infants can have smooth nut and seed butters, such as almond butter, peanut butter, or tahini.

Many parents prefer to use commercially prepared infant foods. Vegetarian parents should be encouraged to make their own baby foods, however, because commercial lines offer a limited variety of foods for vegetarian infants. Foods that will eventually play a significant role in the diets of vegetarian children (e.g., legumes, tofu, and leafy green vegetables) should be introduced in infancy and are seldom available as commercial baby foods. Exhibit 12-1 offers guidelines for home preparation of infant foods.

Adequate calorie intake can be one concern in vegetarian infants. Parents can be counseled on ways to incorporate foods into infant diets that are particularly rich in calories and nutrients. Some ideas include legume spreads, mashed firm tofu (firm tofu tends to be higher in fat and calories than soft tofu), dried fruits processed in a blender with a few teaspoons of water or fruit juice to make a spread, mashed avocado, and nut and seed butters. To avoid choking, nut and seed butters spread on bread or crackers as well as spoonfuls of these butters should not be given to infants prior to their first birthday. Exhibit 12-2 summarizes some feeding practices to avoid in infancy.

Exhibit 12-1 Home Preparation of Infant Foods

- Wash all fruits and vegetables thoroughly. If preparing beans, rinse dried beans under cold running water. Do not use canned vegetables or beans unless they are canned without added sodium.
- Remove skins, seeds, and stringy portions from fruits and vegetables.
- Cook the foods thoroughly until they are soft enough to puree.
- Puree foods in a blender, adding some cooking liquid to reach a smooth consistency.
- Press cooked legumes through a sieve to remove any skins.
- Home-prepared infant foods can be kept in the refrigerator for up to 2 days. They can also be prepared in large quantities and then frozen for later use. Freeze in ice cube trays and defrost only one serving at a time.

Exhibit 12-2 Some Feeding Practices to Avoid in Infancy

- For the first year, avoid feeding infants whole, low-fat, or nonfat cow's milk; regular commercial soy, rice, grain, or nut milk; or goat's milk.
- Feed only breast milk, infant formula, or water in the infant's bottle. Diluted cereal preparations should not be fed in the bottle. Most infants are ready to drink from a cup when fruit juices are offered.
- Do not feed honey or corn syrup to infants <1 year of age; both can cause infant botulism.[74,75]
- Avoid giving infants <4 months of age home-prepared or canned spinach, turnips, beets, carrots, or collard greens because the nitrate level in these foods can cause methemoglobinemia.[16]

SUPPLEMENTS FOR OLDER INFANTS

Table 12-2 provides information on situations where supplements would be indicated for older infants. A vitamin D supplement is recommended for breastfed infants. Breastfed infants need iron supplements if the infant's iron intake is <1 mg/kg per day. Fluoride supplements are indicated if water fluoride content is low. A vitamin B_{12} supplement is indicated for breastfed infants who do not have a daily, reliable source of vitamin B_{12}. Breast milk can be a reliable source if the maternal diet contains regular, adequate sources of vitamin B_{12}. Although zinc supplements are not routinely recommended for vegetarian infants because zinc deficiency is rarely seen,[16] some experts recommend zinc supplements during the time when complementary foods are being introduced if the infant's diet is low in zinc or mainly consists of foods with low zinc bioavailability.[49,50] Zinc intake should not exceed 5 mg/d for 7- to 12-month-olds.[51] Individual assessment of zinc intake is important for vegetarian infants.

THE SPECIAL SUPPLEMENTAL NUTRITION PROGRAM FOR WOMEN, INFANTS, AND CHILDREN AND VEGETARIAN FAMILIES

The Special Supplemental Nutrition Program for Women, Infants, and Children (WIC) was established in 1974 to safeguard the health of low-income women, infants, and children up to 5 years of age who are at nutritional risk by providing nutritious foods to supplement diets, information on healthy eating, and referrals to health care.[52] Eligibility is limited to pregnant, postpartum (up to 6 months), and breastfeeding women; infants up to 1 year; and children 1 to 5 years with income at or below the standard set by each state and who are determined to be at nutritional risk. Participants receive vouchers to purchase specific foods.

For vegetarian infants, vouchers can be used to purchase infant formula, infant cereal, and baby food fruits and vegetables. Cereal, fruits, and vegetables can be purchased through the WIC program from 6 to 11 months of age.

Table 12-4 provides information about foods acceptable to vegetarians that can be purchased with WIC vouchers for children and adults. Due to limitations on the nutrient content of soymilk, only a few brands have been approved.[53] There are no approved substitutions for eggs or for the cheese provided to fully breastfeeding women. Some states provide additional WIC vouchers to be used to purchase fresh fruits and vegetables at farmers' markets.

Table 12-4 Maximum Monthly Allowance of Foods from the WIC Program Suitable for Vegetarian Women and Children[52]

Food Group	Children 1–4 years	Pregnant and Partially Breastfeeding Women (up to 1 year postpartum)	Postpartum Women (up to 6 mo postpartum)	Fully Breastfeeding Women (up to 1 year postpartum)
Single-strength fruit juice	125 fl oz	144 fl oz	96 fl oz	144 fl oz
Milk, calcium-set tofu, soymilk, cheese*	16 qt	22 qt	16 qt	24 qt
Breakfast cereal	36 oz	36 oz	36 oz	36 oz
Eggs	1 doz	1 doz	1 doz	2 doz
Cash vouchers for fruits and vegetables	$6	$8	$8	$10
Whole grains†	2 lb	1 lb		1 lb
Cheese				1 lb
Dried or canned beans, peanut butter	1 lb dry (64 oz canned) beans OR 18 oz peanut butter	1 lb dry (64 oz canned) beans AND 18 oz peanut butter	1 lb dry (64 oz canned) beans OR 18 oz peanut butter	1 lb dry (64 oz canned) beans AND 18 oz peanut butter

*For children, cheese may be substituted for milk at the rate of 1 lb of cheese per 3 quarts of milk. No more than 1 lb of cheese may be substituted for milk except for fully breastfeeding women who can substitute for no more than 2 lb of cheese. With medical documentation, additional amounts of cheese may be substituted in cases of lactose intolerance or other qualifying conditions, up to the maximum allowance for fluid milk.

For children, soy-based beverage and calcium-set tofu may be substituted for milk only with medical documentation for qualifying conditions. Medical documentation is not required for women.

Soy-based beverage may be substituted for milk on a quart for quart basis up to the total maximum allowance of milk. Tofu may be substituted for milk at the rate of 1 pound of tofu per 1 quart of milk up to the total maximum allowance of milk (for children) or up to 4 quarts of milk for partially or non-breastfeeding women or 6 quarts of milk for fully breastfeeding women.

With medical documentation, additional amounts of cheese or tofu may be substituted, up to the maximum allowances for fluid milk, in cases of lactose intolerance or other qualifying conditions.

Soymilk must be fortified to meet the following nutrient levels: 276 mg calcium per cup, 8 g protein per cup, 500 IU vitamin A per cup, 100 IU vitamin D per cup, 24 mg magnesium per cup, 222 mg phosphorus per cup, 349 mg potassium per cup, 0.44 mg riboflavin per cup, and 1.1 μg vitamin B_{12} per cup.

†Whole grains include whole grain bread, bulgur, oatmeal, whole grain barley, and soft corn or whole wheat tortillas.

Exhibit 12-3 Sample Diets for 9-Month-Old Vegan and Omnivore Infants

Meal	Vegan Infant*	Omnivore Infant†
Breakfast	¼ cup iron-fortified cereal with 2 tbsp wheat germ, 6 oz breast milk or formula	¼ cup iron-fortified cereal, ½ tbsp egg yolk, 6 oz breast milk or formula
Snack	¼ slice whole wheat bread	¼ slice whole wheat bread
Midday	1 oz mashed tofu, 1 tbsp steamed, chopped broccoli, 2 tbsp mashed banana, ¼ slice whole wheat bread, 6 oz breast milk or formula	2 tbsp strained chicken, 1 tbsp steamed, chopped broccoli, 2 tbsp mashed banana, ¼ slice whole wheat bread, 6 oz breast milk or formula
Evening	¼ cup iron-fortified infant cereal with 2 tbsp wheat germ, 2 tbsp mashed kidney beans, 1 tbsp mashed winter squash, 1 tbsp applesauce, 6 oz breast milk or formula	¼ cup iron-fortified infant cereal, 2 tbsp strained beef, 1 tbsp mashed winter squash, 1 tbsp applesauce, 6 oz breast milk or formula
Snack	6 oz breast milk or formula, graham cracker	6 oz breast milk or formula, graham cracker

*Breastfed or soy formula fed.
†Breastfed or cow's milk formula fed.

COMPARISON OF SAMPLE MENU PLANS FOR 9-MONTH-OLD VEGAN AND OMNIVORE INFANTS

Vegan diets that follow the guidelines noted here provide roughly the equivalent nutrient intake of omnivore diets, as the sample meal plans for 9-month-old infants in Exhibit 12-3 indicate. The meal plans are for a vegan breastfed or soy formula-fed infant and a breastfed or cow's milk formula-fed nonvegetarian infant. These menu plans differ mainly in that the plant proteins in the vegan plan have been replaced with animal foods in the nonvegetarian plan. Table 12-5 compares the percentage of the recommended dietary allowances (RDAs) provided by each of these diets. In both cases, when infant formulas (either soymilk or cow's milk based) are used, the nutrient content meets or exceeds the RDAs for infants. For breastfed infants, the nutrient content of the vegan and omnivore diets is adequate for most nutrients with the exception of vitamin D. The omnivore breastfed diet is low in zinc, and the vegan breastfed infant's diet is low in vitamin B_{12}. The levels of vitamins A, B_{12}, D, and C as well as thiamin, riboflavin, and niacin could be expected to vary depending on the mother's diet. In this case, it is assumed that the mother of the vegan infant has a reliable source of vitamin B_{12} in her diet so that milk vitamin B_{12} levels are adequate.

POTENTIAL CONCERNS IN INFANT FEEDING

Cow's Milk Formula and Diabetes

The hypothesis that there is a link between consumption of cow's milk in early infancy and later development of type 1 (insulin-dependent) diabetes remains controversial. Some studies have shown that early consumption of cow's milk, either in untreated form or in commercial

Table 12-5 Percentage RDA or AI met by Vegan and Nonvegetarian Diets for 9-Month-Old Infants on Four Different Diets (Diets Described in Exhibit 12-3)

Nutrient	Vegan, Breastfed	Vegan, Soy Formula Fed	Omnivore, Breastfed	Omnivore Cow's Milk Formula Fed
kcal*	111	108	113	109
Protein*	240	312	219	245
Iron*	136	217	184	108
Calcium	204	296	174	224
Zinc*	233	313	113	233
Vitamin A	99	81	119	114
Thiamin	667	500	450	317
Riboflavin	225	250	208	308
Niacin	250	370	252	342
Pyridoxine (B$_6$)	200	233	100	140
Folate	246	290	113	158
Cobalamin (B$_{12}$)	80[†]	280	260[†]	460
Vitamin C	96	137	100	140
Vitamin D	14	110	26	122

*The percentage RDA for kilocalories and protein are based on a 9-month-old male infant. The percentage RDA for iron and zinc were calculated using the RDA for 7- to 12-month-old infants and were not adjusted for a vegetarian diet. The RDA for iron for infants is based on a bioavailability of 10% rather than the 18% bioavailability used for other age groups.[51] Thus no adjustment needs to be made for infants on vegetarian diets. Although the Institute of Medicine states that vegetarians may need 50% more zinc than nonvegetarians,[51] there is no separate RDA for zinc for vegetarians. The percentage RDA for zinc in Table 12-5 for vegan infants is probably somewhat high because it does not take into account the possible reduced zinc bioavailability from vegan diets.
[†]Vitamin B$_{12}$ level in the breastfed infant's diet will vary depending on maternal diet. Figures in Table 12-5 are based on milk from a woman whose diet contains adequate amounts of vitamin B$_{12}$.

infant formula, increases the risk of developing type 1 diabetes in genetically susceptible infants.[54–58] Not all studies support this finding, however.[59–61] One proposed mechanism for the association between cow's milk exposure and type 1 diabetes is that type 1 diabetes is a T-cell-mediated autoimmune disease in which immunity to insulin leads to islet cell destruction. Early exposure to bovine insulin in cow's milk in genetically susceptible infants may lead to increased production of antibodies to human insulin and to destruction of pancreatic islet cells.[57] Another possibility is that breast milk contains agents that promote maturation of the intestinal mucosa. Infants who do not receive breast milk may have impaired development of mucosa-mediated immunoregulation and, when cow's milk protein is introduced, an immune response may occur leading to destruction of islet cells.[62] If this were the case, genetically susceptible infants would also exhibit an increased immune response to soy formula.[62] However, there are currently no epidemiologic data to support a link between soy and diabetes. Although the issue of early exposure to cow's milk and risk of type 1 diabetes warrants further study, it is an additional reason to recommend breastfeeding for all infants.

Allergies

Approximately 8% of infants develop allergies to one or more foods.[63] Allergies to cow's milk protein are most common; approximately 2.5% of infants are allergic to cow's milk protein.[64] Often, infants with cow's milk allergy are placed on infant soy formulas. Protein hydrolysate formulas should be used for infants intolerant of both cow's milk and soy protein–based formulas and for infants with cow's milk protein-induced enterocolitis or enteropathy.[16]

Vegetarian foods that are most likely to cause allergic reactions include eggs, tree nuts, seeds, peanuts, cow's milk, soy products, and wheat.[16] If solid foods are introduced as single ingredient foods, one at a time, at weekly intervals, it is easier to detect food allergies. For infants at high risk for developing allergies, the AAP recommends[16,65] (1) no maternal dietary avoidance of potential allergens during pregnancy is needed; (2) exclusive breastfeeding for the first 4 to 6 months or use of an extensively hydrolyzed formula if exclusive breastfeeding is not possible or if supplementation is required; and (3) delayed introduction of solid foods until 4 to 6 months of age.

Although breastfed infants appear to be less likely to develop food allergies, they can show adverse reactions to food components in the mother's diet that are passed into her milk. For example, cow's milk protein in the mother's diet can cause an allergic response in her infant.[66] Foods that may cause discomfort include coffee, chocolate, cabbage and other gas-producing vegetables, onions, beans, and chili. Such problems occur in a minority of infants, however. Breastfeeding mothers need not modify their diets unless a specific problem arises.

Colic

Colic, defined as unexplained paroxysms of irritability, fussing, or crying that persists for >3 h/d for >3 days/wk,[67] affects up to 24% of infants in the first months after birth.[68] Numerous causes of and treatments for colic have been proposed including modification of the mother's diet. In one study of breastfed infants, removal of dairy products, soy, wheat, eggs, peanuts, tree nuts, and fish from the mothers' diets resulted in a reduction of symptoms of colic.[69] Another study found that maternal intake of cruciferous vegetables including cabbage, cauliflower, and broccoli, cow's milk, onion, and chocolate was related to colic symptoms.[70] There is also some evidence that colic is related to the infant's diet. In 27 colicky infants who were given a protein-hydrolysate formula in place of cow's milk formula for 5 days, 24 had a marked decrease in crying time.[71] Soy formula used in place of cow's milk formula has also been shown to reduce colic symptoms.[72] Some infants with colic have a significant reduction in symptoms when maternal diet is changed (for breastfed infants) or when changes are made in infant formula.[73] The cause of colic is unknown. Positive results seen with maternal or infant dietary changes may be due to a placebo effect. Dietary interventions may be helpful, however, for some infants.

MACROBIOTIC DIETS IN INFANCY

Several studies of macrobiotics in the United States and the Netherlands have revealed nutritional deficiencies in macrobiotic infants.[21,22] Nutrients of greatest concern are vitamin B_{12}, vitamin D, calcium, and iron. Energy levels have also been found to be too low in some macrobiotic infants.

The percentage of mothers who breastfeed is high among macrobiotics, and they tend to breastfeed for longer periods than the general population.[10] When macrobiotic infants are weaned, it is often onto a homemade grain-based milk that is low in protein, calories, iron, and calcium and devoid of vitamin B_{12} and vitamin D. These water-based cereal porridges can be the major component of the weanling's diet.[7] Tofu, legumes, and vegetables, including sea vegetables, may be added several months after weaning. Although some seeds, particularly sesame seeds, are used in the infant's diet, added fats are strongly discouraged among macrobiotics.

Potential problems with macrobiotic diets for infants center on the following:

- Tofu, legumes, vegetables, and sea vegetables may be the sole sources of calcium for weaned macrobiotic infants. Although these foods can provide adequate calcium for children and adults, they are consumed in amounts that are too small in the infant diet to meet calcium needs.
- A diet based solely on grains, vegetables, and legumes with no added fats appears to be too high in bulk to meet infant calorie needs.
- The use of fortified foods is often prohibited on macrobiotic diets.
- Although the macrobiotic diet is not always vegetarian (some macrobiotics use fish or fish oil), when the weaned infant is consuming only unfortified plant foods the diet contains no vitamin B_{12} or vitamin D.

Dietitians who counsel parents of macrobiotic infants may face some challenges in developing healthy infant diets that conform to macrobiotic guidelines. Many of these parents will be willing to make adjustments to the diets of their infants, however, especially if the nutrition counselor makes every possible effort to work within the guidelines of the macrobiotic principles. Also, proponents of macrobiotics actually follow many versions of the diet, so that it should not be assumed that all macrobiotic infants are being fed deficient diets. Many are well nourished. The following suggestions can help ensure safe macrobiotic diets for infants:

- Practitioners have suggested that macrobiotic infants and children should receive milk in their diet.[21] Because dairy products have never been a part of macrobiotic diets, their adoption would represent a fundamental change in dietary philosophy that may not be acceptable to most macrobiotics. Soy products such as tofu, miso, and soybeans, however, are included in macrobiotic meals; therefore, a fortified soy formula may be more acceptable.
- Sea vegetables should be limited in the diet of macrobiotic infants whose intake of vitamin B_{12} is low. Although these foods may contain some active B_{12}, they can also contain

analogs that may interfere with the absorption of active vitamin B_{12}.[11] The amounts used in infant diets typically provide only negligible amounts of other nutrients, such as calcium.

- A source of dietary fat, such as margarine or vegetable oil added to other foods, should be included in the infant's diet.
- Fiber intake of infants should be reduced by sieving grains before cooking them or by using some refined grains.
- Frequent sun exposure should be encouraged to ensure adequate vitamin D synthesis.
- A vitamin B_{12} supplement should be provided.

CONCLUSION

Although infancy, particularly the period after weaning, can be a time of great nutritional vulnerability, it is relatively easy to provide nutritious vegetarian diets for these youngest family members.

COUNSELING POINTS FOR PARENTS OF VEGETARIAN INFANTS

- Choose breast milk for all milk feedings for the first year if possible. Infants who are not breastfed should receive a commercial iron-fortified infant formula for the first year. Vegan infants who are not breastfed receive soy infant formula.
- Avoid using soy milk, rice milk, homemade formulas, unmodified cow's milk, goat's milk, and vegetable milks to replace breast milk or commercial infant formula during the first year. These foods are not nutritionally adequate for infants.
- Begin vitamin D supplements shortly after birth for breastfed infants and iron supplements (or food fortified with iron) at 4 to 6 months. Breastfed infants whose mothers do not consume dairy products and foods fortified with vitamin B_{12} or B_{12} supplements regularly will need vitamin B_{12} supplements.
- Use fluoride supplements when water is not fluoridated.
- Consider using a zinc supplement if the weaning infant's diet consists mainly of grains and legumes because zinc is not as well absorbed from these foods. Good sources of zinc can be found in Chapter 6.
- Introduce iron-fortified cereal when the infant shows appropriate signs of readiness, usually between 4 and 6 months.
- Gradually offer additional solid foods, including pureed vegetables, fruits, beans, tofu, and cottage cheese.
- Introduce foods that are commonly eaten by vegetarians like legumes, tofu, and leafy green vegetables early by preparing these foods for weaning infants following the guidelines in Exhibit 12-1.
- Use foods that are rich in calories and nutrients like legume spreads, tofu, and mashed avocado when the infant is being weaned.

Case Study

Ethan is a 6-month-old whose family is vegan. Up until now he has been exclusively breastfed. What food would you recommend as a first food? Should he be receiving any supplements?

At age 9 months, Ethan is eating a variety of baby foods and continuing to breastfeed avidly. His weight and height are both at the 75th percentile and he is growing at an appropriate rate. His mother wants to know when she should stop breastfeeding. What do you suggest? She also asks for suggestions for finger foods for Ethan. What will you tell her?

REFERENCES

1. Dwyer JT, Palombo R, Thorne H, et al. Preschoolers on alternate life-style diets. *J Am Diet Assoc.* 1978;72:264–270.
2. O'Connell JM, Dibley MJ, Sierra J, et al. Growth of vegetarian children: The Farm study. *Pediatrics.* 1989;84:475–481.
3. Dwyer JT, Andrew EM, Valadian I, Reed RB. Size, obesity, and leanness in vegetarian preschool children. *J Am Diet Assoc.* 1980;77:434–439.
4. King JC, Stein T, Doyle M. Effect of vegetarianism on the zinc status of pregnant women. *Am J Clin Nutr.* 1981;34:1049–1055.
5. Drake R, Reddy S, Davies J. Nutrient intake during pregnancy and pregnancy outcome of lacto-ovo-vegetarians, fish-eaters and non-vegetarians. *Veg Nutr.* 1998;2:45–52.
6. Dagnelie PC, van Staveren WA, van Klaveren JD, Burema J. Do children on macrobiotic diets show catch-up growth? *Eur J Clin Nutr.* 1988;42:1007–1016.
7. Dagnelie PC, van Staveren WA, Vergot FJVRA, et al. Nutritional status of infants aged 4 to 18 months on macrobiotic diets and matched omnivorous control infants: A population- based mixed-longitudinal study. II. Growth and psychomotor development. *Eur J Clin Nutr.* 1989;43:325–338.
8. van Staveren WA, Dhuybetter JHM, Bons A, et al. Food consumption and height/weight status of Dutch preschool children on alternative diets. *J Am Diet Assoc.* 1985;85:1579–1584.
9. Sanders TAB. Growth and development of British vegan children. *Am J Clin Nutr.* 1988;48:822–825.
10. Dagnelie PC, van Staveren WA, Verschuren SAJM, Hautvast JGAJ. Nutritional status of infants aged 4 to 18 months on macrobiotic diets and matched omnivorous control infants: a population-based mixed-longitudinal study. I. Weaning pattern, energy and nutrient intake. *Eur J Clin Nutr.* 1989;43:311–323.
11. Dewey KG, Heinig MJ, Nommsen LA, et al. Growth of breast-fed and formula-fed infants from 0 to 18 months: the DARLING study. *Pediatrics.* 1992;89:1035–1041.
12. Kuczmarski RJ, Ogden CL, Guo SS, et al. 2000 CDC growth charts for the United States: methods and development. National Center for Health Statistics. *Vital Health Stat.* 2002;11:246.
13. World Health Organization. The WHO Child Growth Standards. 2006. http://www.who.int/childgrowth/standards/en/.
14. Use and interpretation of the CDC growth charts. http://www.cdc.gov/nccdphp/dnpa/growthcharts/00binaries/growthchart.pdf.
15. Craig WJ, Mangels AR. Position of the American Dietetic Association: Vegetarian diets. *J Am Diet Assoc.* 2009; 109:1266–1282.
16. Committee on Nutrition, American Academy of Pediatrics. *Pediatric Nutrition Handbook.* 6th ed. Elk Grove Village, IL: American Academy of Pediatrics; 2009.
17. Bhatia J, Greer F; American Academy of Pediatrics Committee on Nutrition. Use of soy protein-based formulas in infant feeding. *Pediatrics.* 2008;121(5):1062–1068.

18. Lasekan JB, Ostrom KM, Jacobs JR, et al. Growth of newborn, term infants fed soy formulas for 1 year. *Clin Pediatr.* 1999;38:563–571.

19. Mendez MA, Anthony MS, Arab L. Soy-based formulae and infant growth and development: a review. *J Nutr.* 2002;132:2127–2130.

20. Dwyer JT, Andrew EM, Berkey C, et al. Growth in "new" vegetarian preschool children using the Jenss-Bayley curve fitting technique. *Am J Clin Nutr.* 1983;37:815–827.

21. Dagnelie PC, van Staveren WA. Macrobiotic nutrition and child health: results of a population-based, mixed-longitudinal cohort study in the Netherlands. *Am J Clin Nutr.* 1994;59(suppl):1187S–1196S.

22. Dagnelie PC, Vergot F, van Staveren WA, et al. High prevalence of rickets in infants on macrobiotic diets. *Am J Clin Nutr.* 1990;51:202–208.

23. Centers for Disease Control. Breastfeeding Report Card, United States: Outcome Indicators. 2009. http://www.cdc.gov/breastfeeding/data/report_card2.htm.

24. James DCS, Lessen R. Position of the American Dietetic Association: promoting and supporting breastfeeding. *J Am Diet Assoc.* 2009;109:1926–1942.

25. Sanders TAB, Purves R. An anthropometric and dietary assessment of the nutritional status of vegan preschool children. *J Hum Nutr.* 1981;35:349–357.

26. Shull MW, Reed RB, Valadian I, et al. Velocities of growth in vegetarian preschool children. *Pediatrics.* 1977;60:410–417.

27. Lubby AL, Cooperman JM, Donnfeld AM, et al. Observations on transfer of vitamin B_{12} from mother to fetus and newborn. *Am J Dis Child.* 1958;96:532–533.

28. Specker BL, Black A, Allen L, Morrow F. Vitamin B_{12}: low milk concentrations are related to low serum concentrations in vegetarian women and to methylmalonic aciduria in their infants. *Am J Clin Nutr.* 1990;52:1073–1076.

29. von Schenck U, Bender-Gotze C, Koletzko B. Persistence of neurological damage induced by dietary vitamin B-12 deficiency in infancy. *Arch Dis Child.* 1997;72:137–139.

30. Dror DK, Allen LH. Effect of vitamin B12 deficiency on neurodevelopment in infants: current knowledge and possible mechanisms. *Nutr Rev.* 2008;66:250–255.

31. Specker BL, Valanis B, Hertzberg V, et al. Sunshine exposure and serum 25-hydroxyvitamin D concentrations in exclusively breast-fed infants. *J Pediatr.* 1985;107:372–376.

32. Ziegler EE, Hollis BW, Nelson SE, Jeter JM. Vitamin D deficiency in breastfed infants in Iowa. *Pediatrics.* 2006;118(2):603–610.

33. Gordon CM, Feldman HA, Sinclair L, et al. Prevalence of vitamin D deficiency among healthy infants and toddlers. *Arch Pediatr Adolesc Med.* 2008;162(6):505–512.

34. Wagner CL, Greer FR; American Academy of Pediatrics Section on Breastfeeding; American Academy of Pediatrics Committee on Nutrition. Prevention of rickets and vitamin D deficiency in infants, children, and adolescents. *Pediatrics.* 2008;122:1142–1152.

35. Dallman PR. Iron deficiency in the weanling: a nutritional problem on the way to resolution. *Acta Paediatr Scand Suppl.* 1986;323:59–67.

36. Bueche JL, Lessen R. Nutritional requirements during pregnancy and lactation and normal infant nutrition. In: Edelstein S, Sharlin J, eds. *Life Cycle Nutrition A Evidence-Based Approach.* Sudbury, MA: Jones and Bartlett; 2009:39–80.

37. Centers for Disease Control and Prevention. Recommendations to prevent and control iron deficiency in the United States. *MMWR.* 1998;47(No. RR-3):1–29.

38. Centers for Disease Control and Prevention. Iron deficiency-United States, 1999–2000. *MMWR Morb Mortal Wkly Rep.* 2002;51:897–899.

39. American Academy of Pediatric Dentistry, Council on Clinical Affairs. Guidelines on fluoride therapy. *Pediatr Dent.* 2005–2006;27(7 Reference Manual):90–91.

40. Franke AA, Cutler LJ, Tanaka Y. Isoflavones in human breast milk and other biological fluids. *Am J Clin Nutr.* 1998;68(suppl):1466S–1473S.

41. Setchell KDR, Zimmer-Nechemias L, Cai J, Heubi J. Exposure of infants to phytoestrogens from soy infant formulas. *Lancet.* 1997;350:23–27.

42. Setchell KDR. Phytoestrogens: the biochemistry, physiology, and implications for human health of soy isoflavones. *Am J Clin Nutr.* 1998;68(suppl):1333S–1346S.

43. Merritt RJ, Jenks BH. Safety of soy-based infant formulas containing isoflavones: the clinical evidence. *J Nutr.* 2004; 134:1220S–1224S.

44. Strom BL, Schinnar R, Ziegler EE, et al. Exposure to soy-based formula in infancy and endocrinological and reproductive outcomes in young adulthood. *JAMA.* 2001;286:807–814.

45. Ziegler EE. Milk and formulas for older infants. *J Pediatr.* 1990;117:S76–S79.

46. Food and Nutrition Board, Institute of Medicine. *Dietary Reference Intakes for Energy, Carbohydrate, Fiber, Fat, Fatty Acids, Cholesterol, Protein, and Amino Acids.* Washington, DC: National Academies Press; 2002.

47. Outbreaks of *Escherichia coli* O157:H7 infection and Cryptosporidiosis associated with drinking unpasteurized apple cider—Connecticut and New York, October 1996. *MMWR.* 1997;46:4–8.

48. Smith MM, Lifshitz F. Excess fruit juice consumption as a contributing factor in nonorganic failure to thrive. *Pediatrics.* 1994;93:438–443.

49. Allen LH. Zinc and micronutrient supplements for children. *Am J Clin Nutr.* 1998; 68(suppl):495S–498S.

50. Krebs NF. Zinc supplementation during lactation. *Am J Clin Nutr.* 1998;68(suppl):509S–512S.

51. Institute of Medicine, Food and Nutrition Board. *Dietary Reference Intakes for Vitamin A, Vitamin K, Arsenic, Boron, Chromium, Copper, Iodine, Iron, Manganese, Molybdenum, Nickel, Silicon, Vanadium, and Zinc.* Washington, DC: National Academy Press; 2001.

52. Special Supplemental Nutrition Program for Women, Infants and Children (WIC): Revisions in the WIC Food Packages; Interim Rule. Federal Register, Code of Federal Regulations, 7CFR, Part 246, Dec. 6, 2007;72:68966–69032.

53. WIC Food Packages. Frequently Asked Questions. http://www.fns.usda.gov/wic/policyandguidance/wicfaqs-food packages.htm#VI.

54. Gerstein HC. Cow's milk exposure and type I diabetes mellitus. *Diabetes Care.* 1993;17:13–19.

55. Dahl-Jorgensen K, Honer G, Hanssen KF. Relationship between cow's milk consumption and incidence of IDDM in childhood. *Diabetes Care.* 1991;14:1081–1083.

56. Hypponen E, Kenward MG, Virtanen SM, et al. Infant feeding, early weight gain, and risk of type 1 diabetes. Childhood Diabetes in Finland Study Group. *Diabetes Care.* 1999;22:1961–1965.

57. Vaarala O, Knip M, Paronen J, et al. Cow's milk formula feeding induces primary immunization to insulin in infants at genetic risk for type 1 diabetes. *Diabetes.* 1999;48:1389–1394.

58. Paronen J, Knip M, Savilahti M, et al. Effect of cow's milk exposure and maternal type 1 diabetes on cellular and humoral immunization to dietary insulin in infants at genetic risk for type 1 diabetes. Finnish trial to reduce IDDM in the Genetically at Risk Study Group. *Diabetes.* 2000;49:1657–1665.

59. Norris JM, Beaty B, Klingensmith G, et al. Lack of association between early exposure to cow's milk protein and beta-cell autoimmunity. Diabetes Autoimmunity Study in the Young. *JAMA.* 1996;276:609–614.

60. Norris JM, Scott FW. A meta-analysis of infant diet and insulin-dependent diabetes mellitus: do biases play a role? *Epidemiology.* 1996;7:87–92.

61. Couper JJ, Steele C, Beresford S, et al. Lack of association between duration of breast-feeding or introduction of cow's milk and development of islet autoimmunity. *Diabetes.* 1999;48:2145–2149.

62. Harrison LC, Honeyman MC. Cow's milk and type 1 diabetes. The real debate is about mucosal immune function. *Diabetes.* 1999;48:1501–1507.

63. Sicherer SH, Sampson HA. Food allergy. *J Allergy Clin Immunol.* 2006;117(2 suppl):S470–S475.

64. Sampson HA. Update on food allergy. *J Allergy Clin Immunol.* 2004;113:805–819.

65. Greer FR, Sicherer SH, Burks AW; American Academy of Pediatrics Committee on Nutrition; American Academy of Pediatrics Section on Allergy and Immunology. Effects of early nutritional interventions on the development of atopic disease in infants and children: the role of maternal dietary restriction, breastfeeding, timing of introduction of complementary foods, and hydrolyzed formulas. *Pediatrics.* 2008;121(1):183–191.

66. Kilshaw PJ, Cant AJ. Passage of maternal dietary proteins into human breast milk. *Arch Allergy Appl Immunol.* 1984;75:8–15.

67. Hill DJ, Hosking CS. Infantile colic and food hypersensitivity. *J Pediatr Gastroenterol Nutr.* 2000;30:S67–S76.

68. Clifford T, Campbell K, Speechley K, et al. Infant colic: empirical evidence of the absence of an association with source of early infant nutrition. *Arch Pediatr Adol Med.* 2002;156:1123–1128.

69. Hill D, Roy N, Heine R, et al. Effect of a low-allergen maternal diet on colic among breastfed infants: a randomized, controlled trial. *Pediatrics.* 2005;116:e709–e715.

70. Lust KD, Brown JE, Thomas W. Maternal intake of cruciferous vegetables and other foods and colic symptoms in exclusively breast-fed infants. *J Am Diet Assoc.* 1996;96:46–48.

71. Lothe L, Lindberg T. Cow's milk whey protein elicits symptoms of infantile colic in colicky formula-fed infants: a double-blind crossover study. *Pediatrics.* 1989;83: 262–266.

72. Campbell JP. Dietary treatment of infant colic: a double-blind study. *J R Coll Gen Pract.* 1989;39:11–14.

73. Garrison MM, Christakis DA. A systematic review of treatments for infant colic. *Pediatrics.* 2000:106:184–190.

74. Centers for Disease Control and Prevention (CDC). Botulism. http://www.cdc.gov/ncidod/dbmd/diseaseinfo/botulism_g.htm.

75. Kautter DA, Lilly T, Solomon HM, Lynt RK. Clostridium botulinum spores in infant foods: a survey. *J Food Prot.* 1982;45:1028.

CHAPTER 13

Preschool and School-Age Children

Vegetarian diets are appropriate for children of all ages.[1] Approximately 3% of 8- to 18-year-old children follow a vegetarian diet; close to 1% are vegan and 6% avoid red meat (but may eat poultry or fish).[2] Many parents, both vegetarian and omnivore, express concerns about their children's eating behavior and nutritional needs.

There is certainly a basis for concern about children's eating habits. National surveys have shown that a number of nutrients, including iron, zinc, calcium, magnesium, folate, and vitamins A, E, and C, as well as fiber, may be consumed in less than recommended amounts by omnivorous American children.[3,4] Additionally, 80–90% of American children 4 to 13 years of age do not meet recommendations for vegetables and fruits, and only 13% have two or more servings of whole grains daily.[3] More than a third of 6- to 11-year-olds are overweight or at risk for overweight.[5] Ironically, it is vegetarian diets that are frequently pointed out as needing to be "appropriately planned" or "well planned."[1]

GROWTH OF VEGETARIAN CHILDREN

According to both the American Dietetic Association and the American Academy of Pediatrics, growth of vegetarian and vegan children is similar to that of nonvegetarian children if menu planning is adequate.[1,6] Growth of vegetarian children tends to vary depending on the type of vegetarian diet followed. Based on limited available data, it appears that lacto-ovo vegetarian children exhibit growth similar to that of their nonvegetarian peers. Little information about the growth of nonmacrobiotic vegan children is available, although findings suggest that growth may be somewhat slower in younger children but that heights are similar to those of omnivores among older children. Poor growth in vegan children is observed primarily in macrobiotic populations.[7–9]

Studies of Seventh-day Adventist children, who are mostly lacto-ovo vegetarians, show that growth rates equal or exceed those of nonvegetarians.[10–12] This is true even when the control group consists of children from southern California, who are taller and heavier than national standards.[11] When Adventist vegetarian children 7 to 18 years of age were compared with Adventist nonvegetarian children, the vegetarians were slightly taller.[11] One exception is seen in Seventh-day Adventist preadolescent girls, who tend to be slightly shorter than controls, a finding that may be linked to the fact that Adventist girls have a later onset of the adolescent growth spurt.[12] Similarly, school-age vegetarian children in Britain had heights and weights that were not significantly different from nonvegetarians.[13] Lacto-ovo vegetarian children in Taiwan and in China had heights and weights that were comparable to the local population.[14,15]

Growth of British vegan (nonmacrobiotic) children 1 to 18 years of age has also been shown to be normal. In one study, heights and weight of vegan children were within the normal range.[16] Boys tended to be slightly shorter and lighter than British standards; girls tended to be slightly lighter.[17] Similarly, a study of 404 vegan children 4 months to 10 years of age who lived on The Farm, a vegan community in western Tennessee, showed that although they were slightly shorter than controls at ages 1 through 5 years, they were comparable in height by age 10 years.[18] Weights were not significantly different from norms except at age 9 and 10 years when children were lighter than controls.[18] In an earlier study of 48 children from The Farm, however, of 28 boys only 3 met or exceeded the 50th percentile for height, and 7 were below the 5th percentile.[19]

Childhood feeding practices in macrobiotic families can be significantly different from those in other vegan families. Some macrobiotic diets may be too low in calories to support optimal growth because fats are often severely limited in these diets.[20] Smaller size in macrobiotic children has been attributed to inadequate calories,[7,8,17,21–24] calcium,[7,17,24,25] vitamin B_{12},[8,19,26,27] riboflavin,[25] and zinc.[27,28]

Most studies of growth of vegetarian children are dated and based on relatively few cohorts. For example, for the studies of macrobiotic children just noted, the same group of Boston children was examined repeatedly, generating a fairly large body of literature on the growth of macrobiotics but all of it focusing on the same small group of children.

Children with any of the following characteristics require additional assessment:[29] an unexpected change from the established growth channel, either accelerating or faltering; weight for height at or above the 95th percentile; height for age <5th percentile; weight for height <5th percentile.

DIETS OF VEGETARIAN CHILDREN

Several factors make it difficult to generalize about the nutritional status of vegetarian children. First, dietary intake varies considerably depending on the type of vegetarian diet followed. Second, there is limited information about dietary intakes of vegetarian children, and much of the information that exists is derived from studies of macrobiotic children. Macrobiotic diets can be much more restrictive than nonmacrobiotic vegan or vegetarian diets, and therefore nutritional profiles will be different. Third, many of the studies of vegetarian children were conducted before vegetarian products fortified with calcium, vitamin D, and vitamin B_{12} were widely available. In addition, better access to information about vegetarian diets serves to make it increasingly easy to plan healthy diets for vegetarian children.

Much attention has been focused on the question of whether vegetarian children have had healthy diets in the past. The more relevant question, however, is whether healthy diets can be planned for vegetarian children. The answer is that they can, and with ease. A brief review of findings on the intake of vegetarian children can help dietitians highlight appropriate foods in counseling sessions and focus on the particular areas of the diet that may deserve special attention.

Protein

Average protein intake of vegetarian children (lacto-ovo, vegan, and macrobiotic) generally meets or exceeds recommendations,[8,14,15,19,26,27,30–33] although vegetarian children consume less protein than omnivore children.[15,31,32,34] Adequate energy intake is an important consideration in meeting protein needs; when diets are too low in calories, protein is catabolized for energy, raising total protein needs. Therefore, providing adequate calories is an important goal in diet planning for all children.

Recommended intakes of amino acids in childhood vary[35,36] as shown in Table 13-1. This variability is due to the use of different techniques for assessing amino acid needs. Typically, children's diets that meet or exceed protein recommendations and include a variety of protein sources supply adequate amounts of amino acids.

Although protein combining at meals is not necessary for adults, it may be helpful in meeting protein needs of infants and young children. One study in children has shown that the supplementary effect of beans added to a corn-based diet was less when beans were eaten >6 hours after corn was eaten.[37] Because children eat frequently throughout the day, their meals are likely to be timed closely enough to provide the benefits of complementary amino acid profiles without conscious protein combining at each meal. Sample food combinations that will appeal to many vegetarian children are presented in Exhibit 13-1.

Plant proteins differ from animal proteins in amino acid composition and digestibility.[35] These differences may increase protein needs of vegan children. Some have suggested an additional 30–35% protein for vegan children age 1 to 2 years, 20–30% for 2- to 6-year-olds, and 15–20% for children >6 years,[38] although these figures are somewhat arbitrary. This represents 1 to 9 g of protein above the RDA, depending on the child's age (Table 13-2). Protein needs are generally met when vegan children's diets contain adequate energy and a variety of plant foods.

Table 13-1 Amino Acid Recommendations for Children

Amino Acid	Recommended Dietary Allowance[35]* (mg/kg per day)	World Health Organization[36]† (mg/kg per day)
Histidine	16	12
Isoleucine	22	27
Leucine	49	44
Lysine	46	35
Methionine + cysteine	22	18
Phenylalanine + tyrosine	41	30
Threonine	24	18
Tryptophan	6	4.8
Valine	28	29

*These recommendations are for children 4 to 8 years of age.
† These recommendations are for children 3 to 10 years of age.

Exhibit 13-1 Examples of Meals and Snacks That Offer Children Complementary Proteins

- Rice pudding made with soymilk
- Bagel or bread spread with almond butter, sunflower butter, or tahini
- Hummus in pita bread
- Bean burrito with pinto beans in a flour tortilla
- Textured soy protein taco with corn tortilla
- Soup with barley and diced tofu
- Soup with macaroni and beans

Table 13-2 Protein Recommendations for Vegan Children*

Age/Gender	Weight (kg)	Protein Recommendation (g/kg)	Protein Recommendation (g/d)
1–2 years M/F	11	1.4–1.5	15–16
2–3 years M/F	13	1.3–1.4	17–18
4–6 years M/F	18	1.1–1.2	20–22
6–8 years M/F	23	1.1	25
9–13 years M/F	36	1.1	40
14–18 years M	61	1.0	61
14–18 years F	54	1.0	54

*Protein recommendation is based on the *Dietary Reference Intakes for Energy, Carbohydrate, Fiber, Fat, Fatty Acids, Cholesterol, Protein, and Amino Acids*[35] increased as described in the text to adjust for lower amino acid quality and digestibility of foods commonly used by vegan children.

Fat

Fat intake among adult vegans averages about 30% of calories, which is lower than the intake among the general population and comes closer to meeting dietary guidelines than omnivore diets. Vegetarian children may also consume a diet that is lower in fat than that of omnivore children,[14,15,25,39] although one study found no difference in the fat intake of meat-eating and non-meat-eating preschoolers in Britain.[34]

As long as calories are adequate, relatively low-fat diets support growth in children.[40–42] In a study of 7-month to 5-year-old nonvegetarian children, there were no differences in growth between those whose fat intake was between 21% and 38% of calories.[40] Similarly, no differences in growth according to fat intake (<30%, 30.0–34.9%, and >34.9%) were noted among nonvegetarian children in an Australian retrospective study.[43]

A number of expert groups have established recommended fat levels for children. The Pediatric Panel of the National Cholesterol Education Program recommends that all children >2 years of age consume a diet that derives ≤30% of calories from fat and 8–10% of calories from saturated fat.[44] The American Heart Association recommends that children and adolescents limit total fat to 20–30% and saturated fat to <10% of total calories.[45] The American Academy of Pediatrics recommends that after the first 2 years, children's diets should be gradually limited in dietary fat so that 20–30% of calories come from fat.[6] This type of diet should be used throughout childhood and adolescence. The Dietary Guidelines for Americans recommend a total fat intake of 30–35% of calories for 2- to 3-year-olds and 25–35% for 4- to 18-year-olds.[46] Although recommendations vary, it is clear that some limitation of dietary fat and saturated fat is appropriate for children after 2 years of age.

Vegetarian children clearly have the edge here because they consume diets that are lower in total fat[14,15,25,39] and cholesterol[27] and have lower blood cholesterol levels than nonvegetarian children.[15,27,33,47] Vegetarian children >2 years should limit foods that are high in saturated fat and use food high in total fat only in moderate amounts. Children in lacto-ovo vegetarian families should consume low-fat dairy products, and the use of these products should be moderate. In all families, it is wise to limit the use of processed foods, snack foods, and baked goods, all of which can be high in fat and sodium and sometimes offer negligible nutrients. Although calories are an important concern for the young vegetarian child, so is nutrient density.

Very-low-fat diets (10–15% of calories from fat) do not appear to offer significant health benefits for children without specific medical conditions. These diets sometimes eliminate all high-fat foods (e.g., nuts and seeds) and added fats and oils, and they greatly limit or eliminate soy products, which tend to be higher in fat. The inclusion of small amounts of nuts, seeds, and soy products can make it easier for vegan children to meet nutrient needs. Because toddlers and preschoolers can have difficulty meeting calorie needs, especially on vegetarian diets that tend to be higher in bulk, the judicious use of added fats can support adequate energy intake in these children.

Calcium

Limited data indicate the calcium intake of lacto-ovo vegetarian children exceeds recommendations.[39] This is to be expected because, in many cases, dairy products replace meat in lacto-ovo vegetarian diets. Chinese lacto-ovo vegetarian children who consumed small amounts of eggs and dairy products had calcium intakes below recommendations, although their calcium intakes were similar to local nonvegetarian children and bone mineral density was comparable to local children.[14] The calcium content of adult vegan diets is lower than that of both lacto-ovo vegetarian and nonvegetarian diets (Appendix G), and limited data indicate that the calcium content of diets of vegan children is lower than recommended levels (Appendix O).[17,48] Calcium intake of some macrobiotic children has been shown to be quite low.

Adequate calcium is especially important during childhood to promote bone health and to reduce the risk of fractures in childhood and adulthood.[49–52] Children who were on macrobiotic diets that were low in calcium and vitamin D in early childhood (birth to approximately age 6 years) had lower bone mineral content at age 9 to 15 years.[53] The current Adequate Intake (AI) for calcium in children is 500 mg for 1- to 3-year-olds, 800 mg for 4- to 8-year-olds, and 1300 mg for 9- to 13-year-olds.[54]

In many cultures, particularly those with a high incidence of lactose intolerance, dairy products are not commonly used, and calcium intakes are much lower than in Western countries. Studies in these countries may provide insights into calcium needs of vegan children. Higher calcium intakes (342 vs 1056 mg/d) in Gambian children on near-vegan diets have been shown to improve bone mineral status.[55] Chinese children with very low calcium intakes also had improved bone density after 18 months of calcium supplementation.[56] Genetics may be an important factor in determination of bone density, however, and lifestyle differences between Western vegetarian children and children in developing countries may also contribute to different calcium needs. In any case, there is no evidence that vegan children need less calcium than nonvegetarians.

Until more information is available, it is prudent to advise that all children, whether vegan, lacto-ovo vegetarian, or nonvegetarian, consume the recommended level of calcium. As discussed in Chapter 5, many plant foods are rich in calcium. The calcium needs of small children can be met by using plant foods that are naturally high in calcium. For example, a 5-year-old with a good appetite might consume the following amounts of foods in 1 day:

- ¼ cup grains
- 2 slices bread
- ½ cup vegetables
- ½ cup legumes
- 3 cups unfortified soymilk
- 2 tbsp nuts/seeds
- ½ cup fruit
- 1 tbsp blackstrap molasses

When calcium-rich foods in each of these groups are consumed, it is possible to meet the recommendations for calcium even without the use of fortified foods. Table 13-3 illustrates food choices for the groups just listed that would produce a diet that meets or exceeds the calcium AI for ages 1 to 8 years.

Appetite and calorie needs vary greatly among preschoolers, however, and many children may eat less than the amounts noted in Table 13-3. Also, children who are picky eaters may not always be willing to consume many foods that are calcium rich. Therefore, most guidelines for feeding vegan children recommend regular use of a calcium-fortified soymilk.[38,57–60] If children dislike soymilk or are allergic to it, calcium-fortified rice milk is an alternative. It has a sweeter taste that may appeal to many children. Soymilk is more nutrient rich overall, however, and is a better first choice. If rice milk is used as the primary beverage, provision of other foods that supply protein and energy should be stressed. Calcium-fortified juice is also a good choice for children, although juices should be used in moderation in children's diets. Even with the use of fortified foods, it is important to emphasize foods that are naturally rich in calcium in the diets of all children.

The addition of even small amounts of foods that are rich in calcium can significantly increase calcium intake. Although many children may refuse sea vegetables, some may tolerate small amounts of these mineral-rich foods in a broth or wrapped around a child-sized nori roll. Adding blackstrap molasses to recipes can also boost calcium intake considerably.

In addition to dietary factors, regular, weight-bearing physical activity is important for bone health in children.[61] The Dietary Guidelines for Americans recommend that children participate in at least 60 minutes of physical activity on most, preferably all, days of the week.[46]

Table 13-3 Food Choices That Meet or Exceed the Adequate Intake for Calcium for 1- to 8-Year-Old Children

Food	Calcium Content (mg)
¼ cup cooked rice	5
One slice bread	15
½ English muffin	46
¼ cup cooked broccoli	16
¼ cup cooked collards	89
¼ cup calcium-set tofu	217
¼ cup baked beans	22
2 tbsp almond butter	86
3 cups unfortified soymilk	182
1 tbsp blackstrap molasses	200
½ orange	30
Total	908

Source: Data from USDA National Nutrient Database for Standard Reference, Release 22, 2009 and manufacturers' information.

Vitamin D

Children can make adequate vitamin D with sun exposure. For light-skinned children in sunny climates, exposing the hands and face to the sun two or three times a week in the summer for about 20 to 30 minutes each is enough to provide adequate vitamin D.[62] Sunscreen interferes with vitamin D synthesis. As use of sunscreen becomes more common, dietary sources of vitamin D become more important.

A regular source of dietary vitamin D is recommended for children who are otherwise at risk for vitamin D deficiency. This would include dark-skinned children or those who live in northern or very polluted areas. Furthermore, because sun exposure may be erratic and sunscreen use is increasing, consumption of dietary or supplemental sources of vitamin D is prudent for all children.

Although fish oil and egg yolk can provide some natural vitamin D, this nutrient is poorly supplied by foods; fortification is nearly always depended on to provide adequate vitamin D in the diets of children and adults. In the United States, milk is the most commonly recognized fortified food. Lacto-ovo vegetarian children generally have no problem meeting vitamin D needs if they consume cow's milk. By law, vitamin D–fortified cow's milk must provide 400 IU (10 µg) of vitamin D per quart. The AI for vitamin D for children age 1 to 13 years is 5 µg (200 IU)/d.[54] The American Academy of Pediatrics recommends that children consuming <1000 ml/d of vitamin D–fortified formula or milk receive a vitamin D supplement of 400 IU/d.[63]

Rickets due to vitamin D deficiency has been seen in some macrobiotic children illustrating the necessity of reliable sources of vitamin D for children.[64-66] A number of vegan products are vitamin D fortified, including various brands of soymilk or rice milk and many commercial cereals (see Table 7-10 for examples of cereals that are fortified with vitamin D) and orange juice. The vitamin D content of fortified soy and rice milks ranges from 160 to 720 IU per quart.

Vitamin D deficiency in infants and toddlers has been effectively treated with daily low-dose vitamin D_2 or vitamin D_3 (2000 IU/d) as well as with a weekly higher dose of vitamin D_2 (50,000 IU/wk).[67]

Vitamin B$_{12}$

Because dairy products are rich in vitamin B_{12}, lacto-ovo vegetarians generally get enough of this nutrient, although their intake is lower than that of omnivores. Vegan diets are theoretically devoid of this nutrient unless fortified foods are used, however. Some studies of vegan children find that their vitamin B_{12} intakes are below recommendations.[33] Vitamin B_{12} deficiency has been seen in macrobiotic children when fortified foods were not used.[68,69] Fortunately, a variety of B_{12}-fortified products are available, including many brands of soymilk, meat analogs, and breakfast cereals (Table 7-1).

Iron

Iron-deficiency anemia is the most common childhood nutritional problem. Children <24 months, particularly those age 9 to 18 months are at the highest risk for developing iron deficiency.[70] The iron content of adult vegetarian diets is generally higher (Appendix H) than non-vegetarian diets. This also appears to be the case for the iron intake of vegetarian children, particularly vegan children.[17,48] Limited data suggest that iron deficiency is no more likely to occur in vegetarian children than nonvegetarian children,[71] but lower hemoglobin[72] and ferritin[15,34] levels have been reported in vegetarian children.

Excessive consumption (>3 cups daily after age 1 year) of milk and other dairy products can increase the risk for iron deficiency because cow's milk is devoid of iron and, in the diets of young children, can displace iron-rich foods in the diet.[70] It can also inhibit iron absorption[73-75] and cause iron loss through intestinal bleeding.[76] Because young children have fairly high iron needs and eat relatively small quantities of food, the inclusion of iron-dense foods should be stressed.

Many plant foods are high in iron, but because the iron from plant foods is less well absorbed than that from meat, techniques for maximizing iron absorption should be used. Inclusion of some iron-fortified or iron-enriched refined foods in children's meals is often helpful. Fortified cereals and enriched bread, rice, and pasta are good choices. Vitamin C greatly enhances the absorption of nonheme iron in the diet; parents may need help to plan meals for toddlers and older children that include both an iron-rich food and a vitamin C–rich food. Good meal combinations include pasta with tomato sauce, cereal with orange juice, fruit salad with dried fruits added, and soymilk and strawberry shake. Some vegetables, such as spinach, broccoli, and other greens, are rich in both iron and vitamin C. Table 13-4 illustrates an iron-rich menu for a 1- to 3-year-old vegetarian child.

Table 13-4 Iron-Rich Food Choices for a Vegetarian Child 1 to 3 Years of Age*

Meal/Snack	Food	Iron (mg)[†]
Breakfast	Cream of Wheat, instant, fortified, cooked, $1/3$ cup	3.9
	Orange slices (vitamin C source)	
Lunch	Tofu, firm, ¼ cup	1.7
	Whole wheat bread, ½ slice	0.4
	Collard greens, chopped, steamed, ¼ cup	0.5
	Strawberries (vitamin C source)	
Dinner	Lentils, cooked, ¼ cup	1.6
	Green peas, cooked, ¼ cup	0.6
	Enriched pasta, ¼ cup	0.4
	Tomato sauce (vitamin C source)	
Snacks	Hummus, ¼ cup	0.8
	Dried apricots, stewed, ¼ cup	0.6
	Ready-to-eat cereal, enriched, ½ cup	2.2
	Orange juice (Vitamin C source)	
Total		**12.7**

*Additional foods should be added to meet other nutrient needs.
[†] The RDA for iron for 1- to 3-year-old vegetarians is 12.6 mg.
Source: Data from USDA National Nutrient Database for Standard Reference, Release 22, 2009 and manufacturers' information.

Zinc

There is little available information about the zinc content of the diets of vegetarian children. Limited data suggest that the average zinc densities (mg/kcal) of diets of vegetarian and nonvegetarian children are similar.[34,77,78] Although many plant foods are rich in zinc, bioavailability is lower on a vegetarian diet. Both fiber and phytate may inhibit zinc absorption. Serving more refined foods can reduce the zinc content of the diet, however, because much of the zinc is lost from a food when it is processed. Techniques that can enhance zinc absorption in children's diet include emphasizing foods that are good sources of both zinc and protein (nuts and legumes), using yeast-leavened breads and fermented soy products (tempeh and miso), and soaking dried beans and discarding the soaking water prior to cooking.[79] Zinc supplementation should be considered on an individual basis and may be indicated in young children following a vegan diet based on high-phytate cereal and legumes.[80]

NUTRITIONAL ASSESSMENT

Counseling protocol always involves some assessment of the client's initial dietary or nutritional status. Assessment may be limited to a review of the current eating habits but is more likely to involve some additional elements, such as a medical history review, anthropometric measurements, clinical observations, and review of laboratory data. Any or all of these techniques can be used to assess the nutritional status or needs of vegetarian clients. A medical history review is especially important to ascertain special dietary needs. Along with biochemical assessment, it can also be used to identify any long-term problems of malnutrition. In children, ongoing anthropometric measurements are especially useful in this regard. Standard growth charts from the National Center for Health Statistics should be used to assess growth.[81]

GUIDELINES FOR MEAL PLANNING FOR VEGETARIAN CHILDREN

Children can follow the same menu-planning guidelines as adults. Vegetarian children's diets should include a wide variety of grains, legumes, vegetables, fruits, nuts, and seeds. Foods emphasized for children are somewhat different than for adults, however, and serving sizes differ depending on the child's age and appetite. Although not a dietary necessity, vegetarian children meet nutrient needs most easily if some type of milk is consumed. Milk can be a fortified soymilk or other vegetable milk or low-fat cow's milk (or whole cow's milk before the age of 2 years). These milks can provide significant amounts of calcium, vitamin D, and vitamin B$_{12}$ in the diet. This chapter includes a food guide for younger children (1 to 3 years) that features three servings per day of fortified soymilk or cow's milk (Table 13-5). Of course, breast milk is also an option, and some children may consume breast milk well into their second year.

As noted earlier, children can meet vitamin D needs via sun exposure under optimal conditions, and calcium needs can be met using a variety of plant foods that are naturally rich in this nutrient. Even so, children, particularly toddlers and preschoolers, tend to consume small quantities of

Table 13-5 Meal Planning Guidelines for Children, 1 to 3 Years of Age

Food	Servings per Day	Serving Sizes
Grains	6+	½–1 slice bread; ¼–½ cup cooked cereal, grain, or pasta; ½–1 cup ready-to-eat cereal
Legumes, nuts, and other protein-rich foods	2+ (vegan children should include at least 1 serving per day of nuts or seeds or 1 full-fat soy product)	¼–½ cup cooked beans, tofu, tempeh, or textured vegetable protein; 1 oz meat analog; 1–2 tbsp nuts, seeds, or nut or seed butter; 1 egg; ¾ oz cheese; ½ cup yogurt
Vegetables	2+	¼–½ cup cooked; ½–1 cup raw
Fruits	3+	¼–½ cup canned; ½ cup juice; ½ medium piece of fruit
Fats	3–4	1 tsp margarine or oil
Fortified soymilk, cow's milk, or breast milk	3	1 cup

Source: Adapted from Messina V, Mangels AR. Considerations in planning vegan diets. II. Children. *J Am Diet Assoc* 2001;101:661–669.

vegetables and legumes. Also, sun exposure can vary depending on climate. Therefore, it may be somewhat difficult to meet these needs without the use of fortified products.

Nuts and seeds may also play an important role in children's diets. These foods provide an easy way to boost calorie intake and intake of minerals such as zinc and manganese. For this reason, it is advisable that vegetarian children, particularly vegans, include a daily serving of nuts or seeds in their diet.

The use of supplemental foods can also add significantly to a child's nutrient intake. Good choices are nutritional yeast (Vegetarian Support Formula, Red Star brand) that is reliably rich in vitamin B_{12} and blackstrap molasses. Ideas for incorporating these foods in the diets of children include the following:

- Blackstrap molasses
    Add to baked beans
    Use in muffin, cake, or cookie batter
    Mix into milkshakes
    Add to bean or vegetable stews
    Mix with peanut butter or other nut butters and spread thinly on sandwiches
- Nutritional yeast
    Mix into baked beans or other bean dishes
    Mix into white sauce to create a cheese-like sauce to use over vegetables or macaroni
    Sprinkle over popcorn (for older children)
    Add to veggie burgers or loaves
    Add to scrambled tofu
    Sprinkle over pasta dishes like spaghetti or veggie lasagna
    Add to yeast dough to make cheesy breadsticks or rolls
    Add to milk mixture when making French toast or pancakes
    Add to cream soups or mashed potatoes

Parents of vegan children should identify a regular source of vitamin B_{12} to be included in their children's diet. This might be a fortified soymilk, Vegetarian Support Formula nutritional yeast, fortified breakfast cereals, fortified meat analogs, or a vitamin supplement. At least one to two servings of vitamin B_{12}-rich foods (see Chapter 10 for a list of these foods) should be eaten daily by 1- to 3-year-olds; two servings per day for 4- to 13-year-olds. Parents of macrobiotic children in particular should understand that sea vegetables and soy products such as tempeh and miso are not reliable sources of vitamin B_{12}.

Meal-planning guidelines for younger children (1 to 3 years) are shown in Table 13-5. These guidelines use smaller serving sizes to meet the needs of younger children. The meal-planning guidelines for older children (4 to 13 years) presented in Table 13-6 use the food guide presented in Chapter 10 with some adaptations to meet the needs of children.

MILK IN THE DIETS OF VEGETARIAN CHILDREN

Milk can be a favorite food of children, vegetarian or otherwise. As noted earlier, milk can play an important nutritional role in children's diets. The type of milk chosen—breast milk, cow's

Table 13-6 Meal-Planning Guidelines for Children, 4 to 13 Years of Age

	Number of Servings per Day*	
Food Group	4- to 8-year-olds	9- to 13-year-olds
Grains	8	10
Legumes, nuts, and other protein-rich foods	5	6
Vegetables	4	4
Fruits	2	2
Fats	2	3
Calcium-rich foods	6	10

*Suggested minimum number of servings. Depending on energy needs, children may need addi-tional servings from one or more food groups. See Chapter 10 for additional information on foods in each food group and serving sizes.

milk, soymilk, or other vegetable milks such as rice milk, nut milk, or almond milk—depends on the child's diet (vegan children will consume soy or other vegetable milk) and age (breast milk is not commonly consumed in large amounts beyond 2 years of age).

Prior to their first birthday, infants should receive breast milk or an infant formula. After that, either fortified full-fat soymilk or whole cow's milk can be introduced to many infants. Soymilk introduction for vegan infants should be delayed if the infant is not growing well or does not have good sources of iron and zinc in the diet because soymilk is relatively low in calories, fat, iron, and zinc. Use of unflavored milks should be encouraged so that children do not develop a preference for very sweet beverages. Because soymilk has a fat content similar to reduced fat cow's milk, children <2 years of age who use soymilk as a primary beverage should have other fat sources added to their diet so that dietary fat is not overly limited.

Fortified rice milk is low in calories and protein and therefore is not recommended as the pri-mary beverage for young children. Although unfortified vegetable milks (oat, nut, multigrain) can provide dietary variety, they are generally not recommended for use as a primary beverage for vegetarian children unless the diet contains other sources of nutrients like calcium, vitamin D, and vitamin B_{12} that are commonly found in fortified soymilk.

Where consumption of cow's milk is excessive, iron deficiency can be one outcome because cow's milk contains virtually no iron and because calcium and milk both inhibit iron absorption, although the long-term effects of high calcium intakes on iron status are less certain. Therefore, cow's milk should be limited in the diets of young children to no more than 3 cups/d. Although soymilk contains some iron, it is not well absorbed, and overconsumption of this food can displace other nutrient-rich foods in the diet so soymilk consumption may need to be limited if it appears to be excessive.

There have been reports in the literature of an increased risk of diabetes among susceptible chil-dren when cow's milk is consumed. Initial studies linked consumption of cow's milk, either as unmodified milk or as cow's milk infant formula, during the first year of life to an elevated risk for diabetes.[82] Cow's milk consumption throughout childhood is associated with development of type 1 (insulin-dependent) diabetes.[83,84]

Whether these findings justify limiting or even eliminating cow's milk in children's diets remains an issue of debate. It is clear, however, that no one food group should be depended on to provide a particular nutrient. The food guide presented in Chapter 10 illustrates how calcium-rich foods are found in many food groups.

SOY IN THE DIETS OF VEGETARIAN CHILDREN

Although there are no data on average soy consumption of vegetarian children in the United States, children age 8 to 9 years living in Taiwan, where soy is used as a staple food, were estimated to have an isoflavone intake of 36.6 mg/d or about 1.13 mg of isoflavones/kg body weight.[85] This is equivalent to about 1 serving of tofu. Some vegetarian children may have intakes considerably higher than this. Use of soyfoods in childhood is associated with a lower risk of breast cancer in Asian American women.[86]

Soy products are attractive for many reasons. They are convenient, a good source of nutrients, and often resemble foods that are eaten by nonvegetarians. Other foods like bean burgers, seitan, and even peanut butter and jelly still provide convenience and meet the desire to have a food that looks like what peers are eating while simultaneously adding to dietary variety.

COUNSELING PARENTS OF VEGETARIAN CHILDREN

Feeding toddlers and preschoolers is a challenge to most parents, whether or not the family is vegetarian. The food intake of children can seem fairly erratic because their appetite tends to follow their rate of growth. Appetite is generally good in infancy when a child is growing quickly, but by the preschool years both growth and appetite slow, and children begin to form strong food and eating preferences. Disinterest in food is generally evident in most toddlers and preschoolers.

General guidelines for encouraging good eating habits in a young child combine a respect for the child's independence with a healthy dose of parental control. Allowing the child to make food decisions in an environment that includes a wide variety of nutritious foods is believed to eventually lead to a wider acceptance of healthful foods. Parents may be interested to learn that children who frequently eat dinner with their family in their home are more likely to have a healthier diet overall.[87]

Introducing New Foods to Young Children

A number of factors affect the acceptance of new foods by young children. Seeing friends eat foods is one aspect of increasing a food's acceptability.[88] Foods that are emphasized in vegetarian diets may not be typical fare for the average young child, and vegetarian children are unlikely to see these foods in preschool or at friends' homes. Because many of these foods, including dried beans and green leafy vegetables, are foods that make significant contributions to the nutrient intakes of vegetarians, and early exposure may affect later food acceptance,[89] other strategies for promoting consumption of key foods need to be developed.

Familiarity is an important dimension of food preference for toddlers and preschoolers. As many as 15 positive experiences with a food may be needed before a child regularly accepts that food.[88] Therefore, acceptance of a new food may be a multistep process for young children. They may need to see the food on their plate several times before they are willing to try it. Not all parents are aware of the need to repeatedly offer foods to young children. In one study 25% of mothers of toddlers concluded that their child disliked a food after refusing it one or two times.[90]

The attitude with which parents present foods is also important. Children learn which foods are acceptable and which are not in part by observing adult reactions to foods.[91] Therefore, it is imperative that children see parents enjoying a wide range of healthy vegetarian foods.

When parents are introducing new foods to a preschooler, it may help to include one well-liked food in a meal and to offer the new food in a tiny amount. Food preferences can be erratic at this age, however; a food that is a favorite one week may be refused the next week. Similarly, children may suddenly begin to eat a food that they previously disliked.

Preventing Choking

Choking is a concern for toddlers who have not fully developed their chewing and swallowing abilities. Foods that could easily lodge in the esophagus should be avoided. Table 13-7 identifies foods that should be modified for or avoided by toddlers to reduce the risk of choking. A caregiver should supervise mealtimes and distractions such as television should be minimized. Children should sit down to eat and should never run, walk, play, or lie down with food in their mouths.[92]

Getting Children to Eat Vegetables and Legumes

Most children enjoy a varied selection of grains, fruits, juices, and nuts. Many, however, reject a variety of vegetables and legumes. These foods can be important contributors of nutrients in

Table 13-7 Foods to Avoid or Modify to Reduce the Risk of Choking in Toddlers and Young Preschoolers (<4 Years of Age)

Food	Avoid/Modify
Popcorn	Avoid
Chunks of raw carrots, celery	Avoid
Hard, gooey, or sticky candy; chewing gum	Avoid
Apples and other hard fruit	Cut into small pieces no larger than ½ in;[92] avoid giving large chunks
Vegetarian hot dogs	Slice lengthwise and then crosswise
Nut and seed butters	Spread thinly on crackers; avoid eating by the spoonful
Nuts	Grind nuts finely and add to foods
Grapes and cherries	Halve; remove seeds and pits
Cherry tomatoes	Quarter
String cheese, other cheese	Cut into small pieces

the diets of vegetarian children and should be introduced early and regularly. Some tips for introducing more of these foods into the diets of children include the following:

- Make foods as easy to eat as possible. Young children like finger foods, including chunks of braised tofu or strips of steamed vegetables.
- Make mealtimes fun by incorporating raw vegetables into salads in the shapes of animals and other familiar objects. Serve mashed beans with fat-free chips for dipping. Have the child thread steamed vegetables and marinated tofu onto skewers, broil lightly and serve.
- Some children do not care for mixed dishes. Beans may be more acceptable when served as a single food, rather than in a casserole.
- Try different colors and shapes of beans. Red kidney beans, black soybeans, and speckled pinto beans are often well liked.
- Vary the ways in which foods are served. Raw vegetables may be more acceptable than cooked ones. Offer vegetables with dips. A child who rejects chunks of tofu may enjoy it pureed into a cheese sauce with macaroni. Researchers at Southern Illinois University found that tofu incorporated into familiar dishes was well accepted by preschoolers.[93]
- Involve children in food preparation to increase their interest in a new meal. Family gardens can be one way to pique a child's interest in vegetables.
- Dilute the taste of strongly flavored vegetables, such as kale, collards, or other greens, by blending them with bland-tasting foods, such as tofu, avocado, or ricotta cheese.
- Some vegetables can be incorporated in small amounts into well-liked dishes. Greens can be finely shredded and mixed into soups or spaghetti sauce. Finely chopped vegetables can be added to nut or bean loaves or burgers. Shredded carrots and zucchini can be added to muffin or quick bread batters.

Getting Children to Drink Milk

The following suggestions are for any type of milk (soy, nonsoy vegetable milks, or cow's milk):

- Use milk in shakes with frozen or fresh fruit. Soft or silken tofu can be blended in for a thicker shake.
- Cook hot cereals with milk.
- Use milk in cream soups and puddings.
- Add milk to the batter of baked goods.
- Try serving milk at your child's favorite temperature. Some children prefer it warmed a bit; others like it icy cold.

Meeting Calorie Needs

A first step in helping children meet calorie needs is providing an atmosphere that fosters good eating habits at mealtime. Children should be rested, and mealtime should be pleasant with no distractions, such as toys or television.

If appetite is poor in a toddler or preschooler, it can be made worse by a plate that is overloaded with food. Parents should serve small portions and let the child ask for more. Appetite will vary from day to day in the same child and will be different among different children within the same age group. Children need to judge when they are full and should not be forced to finish everything on their plate.

Because children have considerable calorie and nutrient needs and their stomach capacity is small, a pattern of three meals per day is not sufficient for the average child. Snacks are an important means of meeting nutrient needs. Good snack ideas for vegetarian children include the following:

- Muffins
- Fruit-flavored milkshakes or smoothies using cow's or vegetable milk
- Vegetable soup with crackers
- Crackers spread thinly with nut butter
- Trail mix (for older children)
- Popcorn (for older children)
- Pretzels
- Oatmeal cookies or graham crackers with juice
- Frozen bananas
- Frozen juice bars
- Dried fruits
- Fresh fruit
- Yogurt with fruit
- Bagel or English muffin half with fruit spread
- Cold cereal with or without milk
- Vegetables with dip (salsa or blended and flavored tofu, for example)
- Microwaved potato or sweet potato

The high fiber content of vegetarian meals can fill a child up quickly. Where calorie needs are not easily being met, parents may wish to limit the use of high-fiber foods in their child's diet. Good choices for nutritious refined grains are hot cereals such as farina or Cream of Rice, many ready-to-eat cereals, muffins made with half white flour and half whole wheat flour, applesauce, fruit juice, and white rice. Parents can also peel fruits such as apples to make them easier to eat.

High-calorie foods can also play a role in the diets of vegetarian children. Good choices include legume spreads, nut butters, tofu and nut butter spreads, avocado as a sandwich spread or in small chunks, soymilk shakes with fruits, and dried fruit spreads. Small amounts of added fats, such as mayonnaise (eggless mayonnaise is available for vegans) on sandwiches, a small amount of margarine on vegetables or bread, or foods sautéed in oil, can also help boost a child's calorie intake.

Prevention of Overweight and Obesity

Overweight in childhood has also been associated with increased risk of overweight or obesity in adulthood.[94] The most recent estimates of childhood obesity prevalence in the United States come from the National Health and Nutrition Examination Survey, 2003–2004.[5] Among 2- to

5-year-olds, 26.2% were overweight or at risk of overweight (body mass index for age at $\geq$85th percentile) and 37.2% of 6- to 11-year-olds were overweight or at risk of overweight.[5] Although vegetarian children appear to be at a lower risk of having excess body weight than nonvegetarian children,[15] vegetarian children can become overweight. Dietitians may need to offer guidance to families to help them determine if their child is at risk of obesity due to eating habits, family history, or other factors. Some strategies that can reduce the risk of obesity in susceptible children include the following:

- Increased physical activity
- Education about appropriate portion sizes
- Limiting juice consumption to 4 to 6 oz daily for 1- to 6-year-olds and to 8 to 12 oz daily for 7- to 18-year-olds[6]
- Avoiding soft drinks and other calorically dense foods
- Limiting screen time (television, computers) and avoiding eating while watching television
- Not using food as a reward or punishment
- Serving regularly scheduled healthy meals and snacks
- Having parents serve as role models for the child in terms of eating and activity
- Getting adequate amounts of sleep

The Transition to a Vegetarian Diet

Although many children are vegetarian from birth, there will be times when parents of older children decide that their family will change to a vegetarian diet. Some families will do this gradually; others will make a more sudden change. Children often respond well to a clear explanation of the rationale for and the extent of the change in eating habits. Familiar foods like peanut butter sandwiches, pasta, and tacos can help with the transition. New foods should be gradually introduced. If unintentional weight loss occurs or the child's rate of growth slows unexpectedly, it may be necessary to add more concentrated calorie sources and reduce the fiber content of the child's diet.

Vegetarian Diets for School-Age Children

Growth during the school years is slow and steady, and appetite will reflect this to some degree. Food-related problems, such as food jags, have usually played themselves out by this time, although strong food preferences (and dislikes) can persist.

The overall eating behavior of children is bound to change when they enter school. For one thing, snacks will be less frequent, so that well-balanced meals become more important than ever. If children are left to get themselves ready for school in the morning, there may be a tendency to skip breakfast. After-school activities may interfere with after-school snacks and perhaps even with family mealtime. Many children may also participate in the school's lunch program, which may offer few options for vegetarian children.

Some children may exhibit discomfort with their vegetarian diet. Peer pressure is an important influence in this age group. Also, children may be exposed to nutrition education lessons in school that are at variance with the family's eating practices. The child may learn for the first time that vegetarianism is an "alternative" dietary choice. Among older school-age children, however, vegetarian diet is increasingly viewed as attractive, so that many vegetarian children will continue to be comfortable with this choice. Where children are not comfortable with being different, parents can pack lunches that appear more "mainstream" if these are acceptable to the child. For example, sandwiches can be made using soy cheese or meat analogs. Soymilk can be saved for snacks and at-home meals, and juice can be packed in bag lunches.

The decision to let a child experiment with foods that are not a part of the family's chosen diet is strictly a family decision based on philosophical concerns and needs to be assessed in reference to the family's own values. Where children are resistant to the family's vegetarian diet, the outcome will be different among families, and there is no right or wrong resolution to the issue.

MEALS AT SCHOOL

When children enter school, at least one meal per day is eaten away from home. Although some schools have vegetarian choices, offerings may be limited especially for vegan children.[95]

National School Lunch Program

The National School Lunch Program (NSLP) was started in the 1940s to provide low-cost nutritious meals to hungry children. Today, it serves >30.5 million students daily[96] and is a critically important means of ensuring adequate nutrient intake among low-income children. Schools that participate in the NSLP must serve meals that provide a third of the RDA for protein and several other nutrients and that are consistent with the applicable recommendations of the most recent Dietary Guidelines (e.g., ≤30% calories from fat, <10% of calories from saturated fat). In an effort to keep costs low, school lunch programs depend on millions of dollars' worth of donated foods from the U.S. Department of Agriculture (USDA) each year. In some schools, these foods, which include eggs, cheese, butter, ground pork, ground beef, and milk, may represent a significant percentage of the food served in school cafeterias.

The NSLP allows vegetarian protein sources including certain soy products, cheese, eggs, cooked dried beans, yogurt, peanuts, peanut butter, other nut or seed butters, tree nuts, and seeds to be used.[97] There is no requirement that vegetarian meals be served, although schools are permitted to provide substitute foods for children who are medically certified as having a special dietary need.[98] Soymilk can be provided for children if they supply a written statement from a parent or guardian identifying a special dietary need.[99] Soymilks must meet specific nutrient standards, and schools are responsible for costs that exceed federal reimbursement levels.[99]

Schools can choose one of four approaches to meal planning. The Traditional Food-Based Menu Planning Approach requires schools to offer five food items from four food groups (meat/meat alternative, vegetables and/or fruits, grains/breads, and milk). Minimum portion sizes are established by age. The Enhanced Food-Based Menu Planning Approach is similar to the Traditional Menu Planning Approach but has increased amounts of grains/breads and fruits and vegetables. The Nutrient Standard Menu Planning Approach and the Assisted Nutrient Standard Menu Planning Approach are computer-based menu planning systems that allow menu planners to plan meals that meet a specific nutrient standard. These approaches can allow use of more vegetarian menu items than the more traditional approaches. For example, although tofu is not considered a vegetable protein product under the Food-Based Menu Planning Approaches, it could easily be included in the School Lunch Program under the Nutrient Standard Menu Planning Approaches.

Bringing Lunch to School

Lunches brought from home are frequently the best option for many vegetarian children. Parents can plan lunches around a child's food preferences, so there is more likelihood that all the meal will be consumed. Parents have much greater control over the amount of fat in the diet. For children in vegetarian families, there is the opportunity for increased variety in these meals, and for vegan children, lunches brought from home are the only viable option in most school systems.

The following suggestions for bag lunches will appeal to many children:

- Sandwiches:
    Hummus spread with sliced tomatoes and lettuce
    Almond or peanut butter with shredded carrots
    Peanut butter blended with pureed tofu, ricotta cheese, or dried fruits
    "Missing egg salad" (egg salad with chopped tofu in place of the eggs and vegan mayonnaise)
    Avocado blended with chopped or shredded raw vegetables
    Peanut butter mixed with crushed pineapple and raisins
    "No-tuna salad" (chopped chickpeas flavored with kelp powder and lemon in place of tuna)
    Submarine sandwich with cheese (soy or dairy), lettuce, tomatoes, and other sliced vegetables
    Veggie deli slices with sliced tomatoes
    Bean loaves or burgers with ketchup or salsa
    Baked falafel in pita bread
    Tofu burgers with catsup, mustard, pickle relish, lettuce, and tomatoes on a bun
    Cheese with sliced apples
    Mashed kidney beans and salsa in a whole wheat tortilla
- Instead of a sandwich:
    Pasta salad
    Yogurt, dairy or soy
    Baked beans
    Hummus with crackers and vegetable dippers
    Pancakes with veggie sausage
    Peanut butter noodles
    Sushi
    English muffin pizzas
    Hearty soup or chili in an unbreakable thermos
    Leftovers in an unbreakable thermos

- Lunch box stuffers:
    Fresh fruit
    Raw carrots, celery, or zucchini rounds or strips
    Trail mix
    Dried fruit
    Rice cakes
    Muffins, scones
    Pretzels
- Beverages:
    Individual containers of soy, rice, or almond milk
    Juice
    Water
- Treats:
    Oatmeal cookies or other homemade cookies
    Homemade small fruit pies
    Graham crackers
    Granola bars

When perishable items are packed in a lunch box, an ice pack should be used. A small container of frozen juice can also be used and should keep foods cold but defrost by lunchtime.

COUNSELING POINTS FOR PARENTS OF VEGETARIAN CHILDREN

- Ensure adequate energy intake to support growth by using fats in forms like nuts, seeds, and soy products to provide a concentrated source of calories.
- Avoid restricting fat in diets of children <2 years of age. Older children should limit foods high in saturated fat and consume a diet containing moderate amounts of fat.
- Use a variety of foods to meet protein needs. Conscious protein combining at each meal does not appear to be necessary because children eat frequently throughout the day.
- Young children (1 to 3 years) need 500 mg of calcium per day. Older children (4 to 8 years) need 800 mg daily. Good sources of calcium are listed in Chapter 5.
- Use foods fortified with vitamin D like breakfast cereals, cow's milk, orange juice, and soy milk to meet vitamin D needs.
- Unless dairy products are consumed regularly, include foods that are fortified with vitamin B_{12} or use B_{12} supplements. Tempeh and sea vegetables are not reliable sources of vitamin B_{12}.
- Consume foods high in iron along with foods high in vitamin C to enhance iron absorption.
- Young children (1 to 3 years) need at least 3 mg of zinc per day. Older children (4 to 8 years) need at least 5 mg daily. Good sources of zinc are listed in Chapter 6. Techniques like using yeast-leavened breads and fermented soy products can increase the amount of zinc absorbed.
- Provide frequent healthful snacks like crackers and nut butter, cold cereal, fruit or vegetables with dip, and fruit smoothies.

Case Studies

Ashley is a 10-year-old girl who has followed a near-vegan diet for about 8 months. Her family is not vegetarian.

A typical day includes:

Toast with margarine and jelly and juice for breakfast.

Saltines, a granola bar, fruit, and Kool-Aid for lunch.

Pasta or potatoes or rice with vegetables and bread and juice for dinner.

Ashley's weight (70 lb) is appropriate for her age and height.

She has a good appetite.

Her parents are very concerned about her refusal to eat eggs, meat, and milk and wonder if she is getting enough calcium, iron, and protein.

To discuss:

Which nutrients do you think Ashley's diet is lacking?

What do you suggest?

Four-year-old Kevin was doing very well on his vegan diet (near 50th percentile for height and weight) until he stopped nursing about 18 months ago. He is now at the 10th percentile for height and weight.

Kevin's parents are very health-conscious vegans and feed him mainly fresh raw organic fruits and vegetables and juices. They do not use refined grains but do use many whole grains. They also eat a variety of dried beans. They seldom use oils but will eat some nuts.

Kevin drinks 1½ cups of fortified soymilk daily. He eats three meals and two snacks and takes a multivitamin/mineral supplement (containing iron, zinc, vitamin D, and vitamin B_{12}) every day. His diet provides about 1150 calories and is about 17% fat. His estimated energy requirement is 1500 to 1600 calories. His diet also has >35 g of fiber.

Kevin's parents and his pediatrician are concerned about his poor growth.

To discuss:

What suggestions can you make to help increase Kevin's calorie intake and to promote growth?

REFERENCES

1. Craig WJ, Mangels AR. Position of the American Dietetic Association: Vegetarian diets. *J Am Diet Assoc.* 2009;109:1266–1282.
2. Stahler C. How many youth are vegetarian? The Vegetarian Resource Group Web site. http://www.vrg.org/journal/vj2005issue4/vj2005issue4youth.htm. Posted October 7, 2005.
3. Guenther PM, Dodd KW, Reedy J, et al. Most Americans eat much less than recommended amounts of fruits and vegetables. *J Am Diet Assoc.* 2006;106:1371–1379.
4. Ballew C, Kuester S, Serdula M, et al. Nutrient intakes and dietary patterns of young children by dietary fat intakes. *J Pediatr.* 2000;136(2):181–187.
5. Ogden CL, Carroll MD, Curtin LR, et al. Prevalence of overweight and obesity in the United States, 1999–2004. *JAMA.* 2006;295(13):1549–1555.

6. Committee on Nutrition, American Academy of Pediatrics. *Pediatric Nutrition Handbook.* 6th ed. Elk Grove Village, IL: American Academy of Pediatrics; 2009.

7. Dagnelie PC, van Staveren WA, Vergote FJVRA, et al. Nutritional status of infants aged 4 to 18 months on macrobiotic diets and matched omnivorous control infants: a population-based mixed-longitudinal study. II. Growth and psychomotor development. *Eur J Clin Nutr.* 1989;43:325–338.

8. Dwyer JT, Andrew EM, Berkey C, et al. Growth in "new" vegetarian preschool children using the Jenss-Bayley curve fitting technique. *Am J Clin Nutr.* 1983;37:815–827.

9. van Dusseldorp M, Arts ICW, Bergsma JS, et al. Catch-up growth in children fed a macrobiotic diet in early childhood. *J Nutr.* 1996;126:2977–2983.

10. Sabaté J, Linsted KD, Harris RD, Johnston PK. Anthropometric parameters of schoolchildren with different lifestyles. *Am J Dis Child.* 1990;144:1159–1163.

11. Sabaté J, Linsted KD, Harris RD, Sanchez A. Attained height of lacto-ovo vegetarian children and adolescents. *Eur J Clin Nutr.* 1991;45:51–58.

12. Sabaté J, Llorca C, Sanchez A. Lower height of lacto-ovo vegetarian girls at preadolescence: an indicator of physical maturation today? *J Am Diet Assoc.* 1992;92:1263–1264.

13. Nathan I, Hackett AF, Kirby S. A longitudinal study of the growth of matched pairs of vegetarian and omnivorous children, aged 7–11 years, in the north-west of England. *Eur J Clin Nutr.* 1997;51:20–25.

14. Leung SSF, Lee R, Sung R, et al. Growth and nutrition of Chinese vegetarian children in Hong Kong. *J Paediatr Child Health.* 2001;37:247–253.

15. Yen C-E, Yen C-H, Huang M-C, et al. Dietary intake and nutritional status of vegetarian and omnivorous preschool children and their parents in Taiwan. *Nutr Res.* 2008;28:430–436.

16. Sanders TAB. Growth and development of British vegan children. *Am J Clin Nutr.* 1988;48:822–825.

17. Sanders TAB, Purves R. An anthropometric and dietary assessment of the nutritional status of vegan preschool children. *J Hum Nutr.* 1981;35:349–357.

18. O'Connell JM, Dibley MJ, Sierra J, et al. Growth of vegetarian children: The Farm study. *Pediatrics.* 1989;84:475–481.

19. Fulton JR, Hutton CW, Stitt KR. Preschool vegetarian children. *J Am Diet Assoc.* 1980;76:360–365.

20. Kushi M, Kushi A. *Macrobiotic Child Care and Family Health.* Tokyo, Japan: Japan Publications; 1986.

21. Shull MW, Reed RB, Valadian I, et al. Velocities of growth in vegetarian preschool children. *Pediatrics.* 1977;60:410–417.

22. Shull M, Valadian I, Reed RB, et al. Seasonal variations in preschool vegetarian children's growth velocities. *Am J Clin Nutr.* 1978;31:1–11.

23. Dwyer JT, Andrew EM, Valadian I, Reed RB. Size, obesity, and leanness in vegetarian preschool children. *J Am Diet Assoc.* 1980;77:434–439.

24. Brown PT, Bergan JG. The dietary status of "new" vegetarians. *J Am Diet Assoc.* 1975;67:455–459.

25. van Staveren WA, Dhuyvetter JHM, Bons A, et al. Food consumption and height/weight status of Dutch preschool children on alternative diets. *J Am Diet Assoc.* 1985;85:1579– 1584.

26. Dagnelie PC, van Staveren WA, Vergote FJVRA, et al. Increased risk of vitamin B_{12} and iron deficiency in infants on macrobiotic diets. *Am J Clin Nutr.* 1989;50:818–824.

27. Dwyer JT, Dietz WH Jr, Andrews EM, Suskind RM. Nutritional status of vegetarian children. *Am J Clin Nutr.* 1982;35:204–216.

28. Kramer LB, Osis D, Coffey J, Spencer H. Mineral and trace element content of vegetarian diets. *J Am Coll Nutr.* 1984;3:3–11.

29. Use and interpretation of the CDC growth charts. http://www.cdc.gov/nccdphp/dnpa/growthcharts/00binaries/growthchart.pdf.

30. Dwyer JT, Miller LC, Arduino NL, et al. Mental age and IQ of predominantly vegetarian children. *J Am Diet Assoc.* 1980;76:143–147.

31. van Staveren WA, Dhuyvetter JHM, Bons A, et al. Food consumption and height/weight status of Dutch preschool children on alternative diets. *J Am Diet Assoc.* 1985;85:1579–1584.

32. Dagnelie PC, van Staveren WA, Verschuren SAJM, Hautvast JGAJ. Nutritional status of infants aged 4 to 18 months on macrobiotic diets and matched omnivorous control infants: a population-based mixed longitudinal study. I. Weaning pattern, energy and nutrient intake. *Eur J Clin Nutr.* 1989;43:311–323.

33. Ambroszkiewicz J, Klemarczyk W, Chechowska M, et al. Serum homocysteine, folate, vitamin B_{12} and total antioxidant status in vegetarian children. *Adv Med Sci.* 2006;51:265–268.

34. Thane CW, Bates CJ. Dietary intakes and nutrient status of vegetarian preschool children from a British national survey. *J Hum Nutr Diet.* 2000;13:149–162.

35. Food and Nutrition Board, Institute of Medicine. *Dietary Reference Intakes for Energy, Carbohydrate, Fiber, Fat, Fatty Acids, Cholesterol, Protein, and Amino Acids.* Washington, DC: National Academy Press; 2002.

36. WHO/ FAO /UNU Expert Consultation. Protein and Amino Acid Requirements in Human Nutrition. WHO Technical Bulletin #935. Geneva, Switzerland: WHO, 2007.

37. Young VR, Pellett PL. Plant proteins in relation to human protein and amino acid nutrition. *Am J Clin Nutr.* 1994;59(suppl):1203S–1212S.

38. Messina V, Mangels AR. Considerations in planning vegan diets. II. Children. *J Am Diet Assoc.* 2001;101:661–669.

39. Tayter M, Stanek KL. Anthropometric and dietary assessment of omnivore and lacto-ovo-vegetarian children. *J Am Diet Assoc.* 1989;89:1661–1663.

40. Lagstrom H, Seppanen R, Jokinen E, et al. Influence of dietary fat on the nutrient intake and growth of children from 1 to 5 y of age: the Special Turku Coronary Risk Factor Intervention Project. *Am J Clin Nutr.* 1999;69:516–523.

41. Obarzanek E, Hunsberger SA, van Horn L, et al. Safety of a fat-reduced diet: the Dietary Intervention Study in Children (DISC). *Pediatrics.* 1997;100:51–59.

42. Niinikoski H, Lapinleimu H, Viikari J, et al. Growth until 3 years of age in a prospective, randomized trial of a diet with reduced saturated fat and cholesterol. *Pediatrics.* 1997;99:687–694.

43. Boulton TJC, Magarey AM. Effects of differences in dietary fat on growth, energy and nutrient intake from infancy to eight years of age. *Acta Paediatr.* 1995;84:148–150.

44. National Cholesterol Education Program. Introduction to the Heart Healthy Diet. http://www.nhlbisupport.com/cgi-bin/chd1/step1intro.cgi.

45. Williams CL, Hayman LL, Daniels SR, et al. Cardiovascular health in childhood: a statement for health professionals from the Committee on Atherosclerosis, Hypertension, and Obesity in the Young (AHOY) of the Council on Cardiovascular Disease in the Young, American Heart Association. *Circulation.* 2002;106:143–160.

46. U.S. Department of Health and Human Services and U.S. Department of Agriculture. *Dietary Guidelines for Americans, 2005.* 6th ed. Washington, DC: U.S. Government Printing Office, January 2005.

47. Ruys J, Hickie JB. Serum cholesterol and triglyceride levels in Australian adolescent vegetarians. *BMJ.* 1976;2:87.

48. Sanders TAB, Manning J. The growth and development of vegan children. *J Hum Nutr Diet.* 1992;5:11–21.

49. Kalkwarf HJ, Khoury JC, Lanphear BP. Milk intake during childhood and adolescence, adult bone density, and osteoporotic fractures in US women. *Am J Clin Nutr.* 2003;77:257–265.

50. Goulding A, Williams SM, Gold EJ, et al. Bone mineral density in girls with forearm fractures. *J Bone Miner Res.* 1998;13:143–148.

51. Black RE, Williams SM, Jones IE, et al. Children who avoid drinking cow milk have low dietary calcium intakes and poor bone health. *Am J Clin Nutr.* 2002;76:675–680.

52. Goulding A, Rockell JE, Black RE, et al. Children who avoid drinking cow's milk are at increased risk for prepubertal bone fractures. *J Am Diet Assoc.* 2004;104(2):250–253.

53. Parsons TJ, van Dusseldorp M, van der Vliet M, et al. Reduced bone mass in Dutch adolescents fed a macrobiotic diet in early life. *J Bone Miner Res.* 1997;12:1486–1494.

54. Institute of Medicine, Food and Nutrition Board. *Dietary Reference Intakes for Calcium, Phosphorus, Magnesium, Vitamin D, and Fluoride.* Washington, DC: National Academy Press; 1997.

55. Dibba B, Prentice A, Ceesay M. Effect of calcium supplementation on bone mineral accretion in Gambian children accustomed to a low-calcium diet. *Am J Clin Nutr.* 2000;71:544–549.

56. Lee WTK, Leung SSF, Wang S-H, et al. Double-blind, controlled calcium supplementation and bone mineral accretion in children accustomed to a low-calcium diet. *Am J Clin Nutr.* 1994;60:744–750.

57. Haddad EH. Development of a vegetarian food guide. *Am J Clin Nutr.* 1995;59(suppl):1248S–1254S.

58. Mangels R. Nutrition Section. In: Wasserman D, ed. *Simply Vegan.* 4th ed. Baltimore, MD: Vegetarian Resource Group; 2006:187–197.

59. Davis B, Melina V. *Becoming Vegan.* Summertown, TN: Book Publishing Co.; 2000.

60. Stepaniak J, Melina V. *Raising Vegetarian Children.* Chicago, IL: Contemporary Books; 2003.

61. Hind K, Burrows M. Weight-bearing exercise and bone mineral accrual in children and adolescents: a review of controlled trials. *Bone.* 2007;40:14–27.
62. Specker BL, Valanis B, Hertzberg V, et al. Sunshine exposure and serum 25-hydroxyvitamin D concentrations in exclusively breast-fed infants. *J Pediatr.* 1985;107:372–376.
63. Wagner CL, Greer FR; American Academy of Pediatrics Section on Breastfeeding; American Academy of Pediatrics Committee on Nutrition. Prevention of rickets and vitamin D deficiency in infants, children, and adolescents. *Pediatrics.* 2008;122:1142–1152.
64. Dagnelie PC, Vergote FJRVA, van Staveren WA, et al. High prevalence of rickets in infants on macrobiotic diets. *Am J Clin Nutr.* 1990;51:202–208.
65. Salmon P, Rees JRP, Flanagan M, O'Moore R. Hypocalcaemia in a mother and rickets in an infant associated with a Zen macrobiotic diet. *Isr J Med Sci.* 1981;150:192–193.
66. Dwyer JT, Dietz WH Jr, Hass G, Suskind R. Risk of nutritional rickets among vegetarian children. *Am J Dis Child.* 1979;133:134–140.
67. Gordon CM, Williams AL, Feldman HA, et al. Treatment of hypovitaminosis D in infants and toddlers. *J Clin Endocrinol Metab.* 2008;93:2716–2721.
68. Higginbottom MC, Sweetman L, Nyhan WL. A syndrome of methylmalonic aciduria, homocystinuria, megaloblastic anemia and neurologic abnormalities of a vitamin B12-deficient breast-fed infant of a strict vegetarian. *N Engl J Med.* 1978;299:317–323.
69. Specker BL, Black A, Allen L, Morrow F. Vitamin B_{12}: Low milk concentrations are related to low serum concentrations in vegetarian women and to methylmalonic aciduria in their infants. *Am J Clin Nutr.* 1990;52:1073–1076.
70. Centers for Disease Control and Prevention. Recommendations to prevent and control iron deficiency in the United States. *MMWR.* 1998;47(No. RR-3):1–29.
71. Kim Y-C. *The Effect of Vegetarian Diet on the Iron and Zinc Status of School-Age Children* [master's thesis]. Amherst: University of Massachusetts; 1988.
72. Nathan I, Hackett AF, Kirby S. The dietary intake of a group of vegetarian children aged 7-11 years compared with matched omnivores. *Br J Nutr.* 1996;75:533–544.
73. Gleerup A, Rossander-Hultén L, Gramatkovski E, Hallberg L. Iron absorption from the whole diet: comparison of the effect of two different distributions of daily calcium intake. *Am J Clin Nutr.* 1995;61:97–104.
74. Hallberg L, Rossander-Hultén L, Brune M, Gleerup A. Calcium and iron absorption; mechanism of action and nutritional importance. *Eur J Clin Nutr.* 1992;46:317–327.
75. Hallberg L, Brune M, Erlandsson M, et al. Calcium: effect of different amounts on nonheme- and heme-iron absorption in humans. *Am J Clin Nutr.* 1991;53:112–119.
76. Ziegler EE, Foman SJ, Nelson SE, et al. Cow milk feeding in infancy: further observations on blood loss from the gastrointestinal tract. *J Pediatr.* 1990;16:11–18.
77. Gibson RS. Content and bioavailability of trace elements in vegetarian diets. *Am J Clin Nutr.* 1994;59(suppl):1223S–1232S.
78. Sanders TAB. Vegetarian diets and children. *Pediatr Clin N Am.* 1995;42:955–965.
79. Gibson RS, Yeudall F, Drost N, et al. Dietary interventions to prevent zinc deficiency. *Am J Clin Nutr.* 1998;68(suppl):484S–487S.
80. Allen LH. Zinc and micronutrient supplements for children. *Am J Clin Nutr.* 1998;68(suppl):495S–498S.
81. Kuczmarski RJ, Ogden CL, Grummer-Strawn LH, et al. *CDC Growth Charts: United States. Advance Data from Vital and Health Statistics.* No. 314. Hyattsville, MD: National Center for Health Statistics; 2000.
82. Gerstein HC. Cow's milk exposure and type I diabetes mellitus. *Diabetes Care.* 1994;17:13–19.
83. Virtanen SM, Hypponen E, Laara E, et al. Cow's milk consumption, disease-associated autoantibodies and type 1 diabetes mellitus: a follow-up study in siblings of diabetic children. Childhood Diabetes in Finland Study Group. *Diabet Med.* 1998;15:730–738.
84. Marshall AL, Chetwynd A, Morris JA, et al. Type 1 diabetes mellitus in childhood: a matched case control study in Lancashire and Cumbria, UK. *Diabet Med.* 2004;21(9):1035–1040.
85. Hsiao AK-F, Lyons-Wall PM. Soy consumption in Taiwanese children in Taipei. *J Nutr.* 2000;130(suppl):705S.
86. Korde LA, Wu AH, Fears T, et al. Childhood soy intake and breast cancer risk in Asian American women. *Cancer Epidemiol Biomarkers Prev.* 2009;18(4):1050–1059.

87. Gillman MW, Rifas-Shiman SL, Frazier AL, et al. Family dinner and diet quality among older children and adolescents. *Arch Fam Med*. 2000;9(3):235–240.

88. Dovey TM, Staples PA, Gibson EL, et al. Food neophobia and 'picky/fussy' eating in children: a review. *Appetite*. 2008;50(2–3):181–193.

89. Skinner JD, Carruth BR, Bounds W, et al. Do food-related experiences in the first 2 years of life predict dietary variety in school-aged children? *J Nutr Educ Behav*. 2002;34:310–315.

90. Carruth BR, Ziegler PJ, Gordon A, Barr SI. Prevalence of picky eaters among infants and toddlers and their caregivers' decisions about offering a new food. *J Am Diet Assoc*. 2004;104(1 suppl 1):S57–S64.

91. Skinner J, Carruth BR, Moran J, et al. Toddlers' food preferences: concordance with family members' preferences. *J Nutr Educ*. 1998;30:17–22.

92. American Academy of Pediatrics. Healthy Children Web site. Prevention of choking. http://www.healthychildren.org/English/health-issues/injuries- emergencies/Pages/Choking-Prevention.aspx.

93. Ashraf H-R, Schoeppel C, Nelson JA. Use of tofu in preschool meals. *J Am Diet Assoc*. 1990;90:1114–1116.

94. Margarey AM, Daniels LA, Boulton TJ, et al. Predicting obesity in early adulthood from childhood and parental obesity. *Int J Obes Relat Metab Disord*. 2003;27:505–513.

95. Physicians Committee for Responsible Medicine. Healthy School Lunches. 2008 School Lunch Report Card. Physicians Committee for Responsible Medicine Web site. http://www.healthyschoollunches.org/reports/report2008_intro.cfm Posted Autumn 2008.

96. National School Lunch Program. USDA Web site. http://www.fns.usda.gov/cnd/lunch/AboutLunch/NSLPFactSheet.pdf.

97. Modification of the "Vegetable Protein Products" requirements for the National School Lunch Program, School Breakfast Program, Summer Food Service Program and Child and Adult Care Food Program. (7 CFR 210, 215, 220, 225, 226) *Fed Regist*. March 9, 2000;65:12429–12442.

98. US Department of Agriculture, Food and Nutrition Service. Accommodating Children with Special Needs in the School Nutrition Programs. Food and Nutrition Service Web site. http://www.fns.usda.gov/cnd/Guidance/special_dietary_needs.pdf. Posted Fall 2001.

99. Fluid Milk Substitutions in the School Nutrition Programs. (7CFR Parts 210 and 220) Federal Register. September 12, 2008;73:52903–52908.

CHAPTER 14

Vegetarian Diets for Adolescents

Vegetarian adolescents represent a rapidly growing segment of the vegetarian population. A 2005 poll provides insights into how many adolescents in the United States are vegetarian.[1] This poll found that 3% of 8- to 18-year-olds never ate meat, fish, or poultry; approximately 1% were vegan. About 7% of 13- to 18-year-olds reported that they never ate red meat. In this survey, meat avoidance was more common in girls with 8% of girls and 4% of boys avoiding red meat. Red meat avoidance was highest in mid-adolescence in girls with 11% of 13- to 15-year-old girls and 9% of 16- to 18-year-old girls avoiding red meat. Similarly, about 2.5% of ninth graders who were studied in Ontario, Canada, were vegetarian with vegetarianism more commonly seen in girls.[2]

Teens are often attracted to both animal rights and environmental arguments for a meatless diet. Although some teens grow up in vegetarian households, an increasing number who live in omnivore households are choosing a vegetarian diet. As a result, teens' diets may be a subject of great concern to parents, and some adolescents may not have the support of parents in planning vegetarian meals.

ADOLESCENT EATING HABITS

Several studies have focused on the eating habits and nutrient intakes of vegetarian teenagers (Appendixes L, M, N, and O). These studies suggest that, in general, vegetarian teens have better diets than nonvegetarian teens. For example, one study found that female vegetarian adolescents consumed 40% more fiber and 20% more vitamin C than omnivore adolescents.[3] Another study found that vegetarian adolescents were twice as likely to consume fruits or vegetables, a third as likely to consume sweets, and a fourth as likely to eat salty snack foods more than once a day compared to omnivore adolescents.[4] Other studies report that vegetarian adolescents consume more legumes, nuts, and vegetables and have lower intakes of fat and saturated fats than omnivores.[5,6] A Swedish study found that vegan adolescents were much more likely than nonvegetarian adolescents to meet or exceed recommendations for fruits and vegetables; they also had lower intakes of candy and chocolate.[7]

Vegetarian adolescents may also be more interested in where their food comes from and how it is grown and produced. One study of >2500 adolescents found that vegetarian teens were more likely to identify having food that is grown locally, organically produced, not genetically engineered, and not processed as being important to them.[8] Nutrition professionals working with adolescents must be aware of these and other food-related issues.

Omnivore teenagers tend to have diets that are too high in fat and sugar and too low in fiber and complex carbohydrates.[9,10] Obesity is a significant problem among American teenagers. Based on the National Health and Nutrition Examination Survey (NHANES) 2003–2004, 34.3% of adolescents in the United States (age 12 to 19 years) were classified as at risk for overweight or obesity (body mass index [BMI] for age ≥85th percentile).[11] Approximately 1.1 million adolescents in the United States have the metabolic syndrome, characterized by central adiposity, elevated triglycerides, low high-density lipoprotein cholesterol, elevated blood pressure, and elevated fasting blood glucose.[12] Teens' diets also are often too low in zinc, folate, calcium, iron, vitamin A, and magnesium.[13-15] Poor nutrition in adolescence may have long-term health implications. Adult obesity,[16,17] coronary heart disease,[18] hypertension,[19] cancer,[20] and osteoporosis[21] all appear to be affected by diet during the teen years.

In many cases vegetarian teens have diets that are markedly better than those of their nonvegetarian peers.[3-7] Clearly, a vegetarian diet can be a health-promoting alternative to the traditional American diet. This is especially true if use of a vegetarian diet in adolescence leads to health-promoting dietary practices throughout adulthood.

Food habits of adolescents are often driven by their increased desire for independence. Other factors, including busy schedules, peer pressure, skipping meals, increased snacking and use of fast foods, and body image issues, contribute to the poor nutrition seen in many teens. Nutrition is often a low priority for this age group, regardless of dietary practice.[22]

GROWTH OF VEGETARIAN ADOLESCENTS

Growth is faster during the growth spurt of adolescence than at any other time in life, with the exception of infancy. Fifty percent of adult weight and 15–25% of adult height are acquired during puberty.[23,24] During the 2 to 3 years of fastest adolescent growth, a boy can add 10 inches to his height. Nearly half the skeleton is formed during the adolescent years as well.[24] Growth is erratic during this period, however. The actual growth spurt lasts for 2 to 4 years. For girls, it generally occurs between the ages of 9 and 11.5 years with the fastest growth seen in the year preceding menarche. For boys, the growth spurt occurs later, generally between the ages of 11 and 15 years. Boys grow faster and for a longer period of time than girls, and they also gain more muscle tissue, whereas girls deposit more fat. For example, during the peak of their growth spurt, boys increase their body protein content an average of 3.8 g/d, whereas girls increase by 2.2 g/d.[25]

Although nutrient needs can be high during some periods in adolescence, appetite tends to follow growth, so that teens eat more when they are growing fastest. Also, calorie needs are quite high compared with nutrient needs, so that appropriate nutrient density of diets can actually be lower in adolescence than in adulthood.

Limited data are available on the growth of vegetarian adolescents, although studies suggest there is little difference between vegetarians and omnivores.[3,5,26-29] In a study of 1800 lacto-ovo

Table 14-1 Interpretation of BMI-for-Age Percentiles for Adolescents

BMI-for-Age Percentile Value	Nutritional Status Indicator
≥95th	Overweight
≥85th and <95th	At risk of overweight
<5th	Underweight

Source: Data from Centers for Disease Control and Prevention. Use and interpretation of the CDC growth charts. http://www.cdc.gov/nccdphp/dnpa/growthcharts/resources/growthchart.pdf.

vegetarians between the ages of 7 and 18 years, vegetarians were slightly taller than omnivores; among Adventists, vegetarians were taller than nonvegetarians.[30] The exception was 11- and 12-year-old girls, who were slightly shorter than their omnivore peers. Male Swedish vegans (16 to 20 years old) weighed less and had a lower BMI than did omnivore male adolescents; no difference in weight or BMI was seen between vegan and omnivore females.[31]

Although later age of menarche has been observed in some older studies of vegetarian girls,[32,33] more recent studies[34–36] suggest that when nutrient and energy needs are met, age at menarche does not differ between vegetarians and nonvegetarians.

Growth charts that evaluate weight-for-age may be problematic in adolescents because of variability in the age of sexual maturity and peak growth. BMI-for-age charts are recommended to assess weight in relation to stature.[37] Table 14-1 provides guidelines for interpreting BMI-for-age percentiles.

NUTRIENT NEEDS OF VEGETARIAN ADOLESCENTS

Nutrient needs of adolescents vary depending on their growth rate. Some teens may experience their growth spurt at age 10, whereas for others it may not occur until several years later. Therefore, the age divisions in the Dietary Reference Intakes may not reflect the actual growth pattern of the individual adolescent. Calculating energy and protein using the equations shown in the text of the Dietary Reference Intakes rather than relying on a single value can better estimate the needs of an individual adolescent.

Calorie Needs

Teenagers have high calorie needs. On a body weight basis, they require more calories than adults. Energy needs actually vary considerably among teenagers, however, and in the same teen over time depending on the growth rate at any given age and the level of physical activity. Some teens who are involved in athletics can have exceptionally high calorie needs. This represents an advantage because it encourages greater food consumption among teenagers and increases the likelihood of meeting nutrient needs. For proper growth and development, teenagers should meet those calorie needs. Exhibit 14-1 provides information on the calculation of calorie needs for adolescents. Limited data suggest little difference in caloric intake between vegetarian and omnivore adolescents (Appendix L).

A significant portion of American adolescents more than meet their calorie needs and frequently have diets that are too high in both fat and total calories. The result of this overconsumption is

Exhibit 14-1 Calculation of the Estimated Energy Requirement for Adolescents (9 through 18 years)[38]

- Determine adolescent's:

  Age in years (A)

  Weight in kilograms (W)

  Height in meters (H)

  Physical activity level (PA)

  - If adolescent is sedentary, PA = 1
  - If adolescent is low active, PA = 1.13 for males, 1.16 for females
  - If adolescent is active, PA = 1.26 for males, 1.31 for females
  - If adolescent is very active, PA = 1.42 for males, 1.56 for females

- Calculate estimated energy requirement (EER) using the following equations:

$$\text{Male EER} = 88.5 - (61.9 \times A) + PA \times (26.7 \times W + 903 \times H) + 25 \text{ kcal}$$

$$\text{Female EER} = 135.3 - (30.8 \times A) + PA \times (10 \times W + 934 \times H) + 25 \text{ kcal}$$

Example:

14 year-old female, 50 kg, 1.6 m, active

$$\text{EER} = 135.3 - (30.8 \times 14) + 1.31 \times (10 \times 50 + 934 \times 1.6) + 25 \text{ kcal}$$
$$= 135.3 - 431.2 + 2612.7 + 25 \text{ kcal}$$
$$= 2342 \text{ kcal}$$

---

reflected in high rates of overweight. At the other end of the spectrum, some adolescents markedly restrict energy intakes and may follow very low-fat diets. These practices can compromise growth. Adolescents with weight issues, whether overweight or underweight, can benefit from nutrition counseling.

Protein

Protein should provide about 6–8% of calories in a physically active teenager's diet.[38] Because of lower energy needs, sedentary teens need to get a higher percentage of energy from protein, around 8–11%.[38] Recommendations for adults call for at least 10% of calories from protein,[38] so the amount of protein recommended for adolescents is often a slightly smaller percentage of calories than is the case for adults. Vegan adolescents may need slightly more protein than other adolescents to allow for amino acid composition and digestibility (Exhibit 14-2).[39] This is equivalent to between 7% and 10% of calories from protein for active teens and 10–13% for sedentary teens. Vegetarian adults easily meet protein needs with vegans, who typically have somewhat lower protein intakes than other vegetarians consuming between 10% and 12% of their calories in the form of protein. Consequently, it is likely that vegetarian or vegan teens will meet their protein needs because often, relatively speaking, they actually need less protein than adults. Of course vegetarian teens who avoid or excessively limit protein-rich foods such as soy products,

Exhibit 14-2 Calculation of Protein Recommendations for Adolescents[38]

- If the adolescent follows a primarily lacto-ovo or lacto vegetarian diet, use the unadjusted RDA for protein to calculate needs.
  - For ages 9 to 13 years, the protein RDA is 0.95 g/kg per day
  - For ages 14–18 years the protein RDA is 0.85 g/kg per day
- If the adolescent follows a primarily vegan diet, use the adjusted RDA for protein to calculate needs. (Adjustments are based on Messina and Mangels,[39] increased as described in the text to allow for lower amino acid quality and digestibility of foods commonly eaten by vegan adolescents.)
  - For ages 9 to 13 years, the adjusted protein RDA is 1.1 g/kg per day
  - For ages 14 to 18 years, the adjusted protein RDA is 1.0 g/kg per day

Examples:

14-year-old girl, lacto-ovo vegetarian, 50 kg
- 50 kg × 0.85 g/kg per day = 42.5 g/d

13-year-old boy, vegan, 47 kg
- 47 kg × 1.1 g/kg per day = 51.7 g/d

---

beans, nuts, nut butters, and dairy products and eggs (if lacto-ovo vegetarian) can fall short of protein needs.[40]

Limited data suggest protein intakes of vegetarian adolescents tend to be above requirements and similar to nonvegetarians (Appendix L). One study of Swedish vegan adolescents found that 53% of their protein intake was from bread, cereals, pasta, and rice; 24% from legumes; and 14% from vegetables and potatoes.[7] These results illustrate the roles that several food groups play in supplying protein to vegan diets. There is no need to emphasize dietary protein when counseling vegetarian adolescents unless the diet is inadequate in energy or contains few good sources of protein (dried beans, grains, soy products, dairy products, or eggs).

Calcium and Vitamin D

The recommendation for calcium for teenagers is 1300 mg/d,[41] although some experts recommend intakes as high as ≥1500 mg/d.[42] Calcium needs probably vary considerably throughout the teenage years according to the rate of growth. Typically, between age 10 and 20 years, boys accumulate 210 mg of calcium daily, girls 110 mg/d. During the peak growth spurt, these amounts increase to 400 and 260 mg, respectively.[25,43]

Adolescence represents an important time for development of bone mass, with half of adult bone calcium accumulating during this period.[44] During peak skeletal growth, which occurs at a mean age of 12.5 years for girls and 14.0 years for boys, close to a quarter of adult bone calcium is deposited.[45,46] Calcium absorption and bone calcium deposition increase significantly at the beginning of the physical changes associated with puberty, which take place around 10 years of age in the average girl.[47] The adequate intake for calcium increases at age 9 years from 800 mg/d to 1300 mg/d to support the increased calcium needed to support maximal bone calcium deposition.[41] Calcium absorption decreases in later puberty beginning 2 to 3 years after menarche.[47,48]

In the short term, high calcium intakes by pubertal children appear to lead to optimal bone mineralization. However, in healthy adolescents and young adults, calcium intakes that are below recommendations but close to the average calcium intake in the United States (about 800 to 900 mg/d in adolescent girls and 950 to 1050 mg/d in adolescent boys[49]) when combined with weight-bearing exercise appear to support long-term rates of bone mineralization that are comparable to those of adolescents who had higher calcium intakes during puberty.[42] Very low calcium intakes (especially those <500–600 mg/d) can compromise long-term bone health. Although calcium absorption increases with very low intakes, the increased absorption is not able to compensate for lower intake overall, and a markedly reduced amount of calcium absorbed results.[50]

Although some evidence links higher calcium intakes in childhood and adolescence with greater bone mass in adulthood,[51–53] other studies find that exercise is a more important determinant of bone health than calcium intake provided calcium intake is in the range of 600 to 1400 mg/d.[54,55] Physical activity appears to make a significant contribution to bone development and should be promoted.[56,57] Adequate vitamin D status also appears to be necessary for bone development in adolescence.[58] The American Academy of Pediatrics recommends a vitamin D intake of at least 400 IU/d for adolescents.[59]

Calcium intakes of some vegetarian adolescents are considerably below recommendations (Appendix O). Because of uncertainty about the exact amount of calcium needed to promote maximal bone density, it is prudent for vegetarian teenagers to strive to meet the calcium recommendation. Calcium-rich foods that are likely to appeal to teenagers include calcium-fortified orange juice, almond butter, tahini, figs, calcium-fortified soymilk, calcium-set tofu, textured soy protein, soy nuts, English muffins, and corn tortillas. Beans and dark leafy green vegetables can also boost calcium intake considerably but may not be well liked by all teens. The use of some type of calcium-rich milk seems advisable for most teenagers. This can include fortified soymilk, fortified rice milk, or cow's milk. Nondairy fortified vegetable milks can be good choices because they also often supply vitamin D and vitamin B_{12}. Regardless of the type of milk chosen, it is wise to encourage all teenagers to explore a variety of calcium-rich foods rather than depend on one food group to provide this nutrient. Vitamin D sources include sunlight exposure and fortified foods including some brands of soymilk, cow's milk, some cheeses, some cereals, and some juices (Chapter 7). Calcium and vitamin D supplements represent another option to aid in achieving adequate intakes of these nutrients.

Teens should also be encouraged to avoid full-fat dairy products. When cow's milk is chosen, skim or 1% should be used. Cheese and ice cream can provide calcium, but they do so at the risk of an increased intake of saturated fat and cholesterol and should be used on a limited basis unless they are reduced-fat versions.

Iron

Iron-deficiency anemia is the most common nutritional deficiency in the world and in American female adolescents.[60,61] Teenage girls in particular, because of their lower calorie intake and their greater iron needs, require a particularly iron-dense diet. The recommended dietary allowance (RDA) for iron for vegetarian adolescent girls is 26 mg/d.[62] Girls need an additional 1.1 mg/d of iron during the growth spurt, and boys need an additional 2.9 mg/d.[62] Vegetarian diets, particularly vegan diets, are often higher in iron than omnivore diets, although nonheme iron has a lower absorption rate. In a study of U.S. adolescents, lacto-ovo vegetarians consumed more iron than omnivores (11.4 mg vs 9.5 mg), although neither group appeared to meet the RDA for adolescent girls.[28] In contrast, studies of Canadian female adolescents found iron intake was similar or lower between lacto-ovo vegetarians and omnivores, and twice as many vegetarians as omnivores had ferritin levels indicative of depleted iron stores.[3-5] Fewer vegetarians, however, had two or more abnormal indexes of iron status.[3] These results suggest that adolescent women, regardless of vegetarian status, may need counseling on dietary choices to improve their iron status.

Excessive use of dairy products can be a disadvantage because dairy foods are devoid of iron, and both calcium and milk are potent inhibitors of iron absorption.[63] Long-term supplementation with calcium, however, when calcium supplements are not taken with meals, does not appear to have a detrimental effect on the iron status of adolescent girls.[64] Adolescents should be counseled to use milk in moderation and to avoid dairy products with high-iron meals and iron supplements. Including a vitamin C source with high-iron meals promotes iron absorption. Vegetarian sources of iron that appeal to many teenagers include bran flakes, instant oatmeal, bread, nuts, nut butters, potatoes, and dried fruits.

Vitamin B$_{12}$

The RDA for vitamin B$_{12}$ is twice as high for 14- to 18-year-olds compared to 4- to 8-year-old children.[65] These recommendations can easily be met by lacto-ovo vegetarians who consume 3 cups of cow's milk or the equivalent. Vegans need to use fortified foods or supplements. At least three servings of vitamin B$_{12}$-rich foods (see Chapter 10 for a list of these foods) should be eaten daily by 14- to 18-year-olds.

One study has shown that although vegetarian teens had lower vitamin B$_{12}$ intakes than nonvegetarian teens, the average vitamin B$_{12}$ intake of both groups was above the current RDA.[6] There is some evidence that adolescents who had low dietary vitamin B$_{12}$ intakes as infants and children (due to an unsupplemented macrobiotic diet) may need more vitamin B$_{12}$ than current recommendations to achieve normal blood vitamin B$_{12}$ levels.[66] Marginal vitamin B$_{12}$ status in adolescents has been associated with impaired cognitive function.[67] This reinforces the importance of ensuring the intakes of optimal amounts of vitamin B$_{12}$ for children and adolescents.

A cobalamin deficiency may mimic the symptoms of other diseases including Lyme disease and Guillain-Barré syndrome. One case report found normal serum vitamin B$_{12}$ levels in a vegan adolescent who had a variety of symptoms including gait disturbance, mental status changes, and fatigue.[68] Cobalamin deficiency was diagnosed based on elevated serum methylmalonate and homocysteine levels.

Zinc

Zinc is needed for growth and sexual maturation in adolescence. Zinc is absorbed somewhat less well from vegetarian diets than from omnivore diets, so it is important that all teenagers get enough of this nutrient.[62,69] In Canadian female adolescents, zinc intake was about 15% lower among vegetarians than omnivores[3] and averaged 11 mg/d.[5] However, in a small study of British adolescents, vegetarian zinc intake was higher (9.3 mg vs 7.6 mg) than that of omnivores.[70] Simple modifications of existing vegetarian diets can lead to increased zinc intakes.[71] Dairy products can significantly contribute to the zinc intake of lacto-ovo vegetarians. Good plant sources of zinc for teenagers include whole grains, legumes, and nuts. The RDA for zinc is 11 mg/d for 14- to 18-year-old boys, 9 mg/d for 14- to 18-year-old girls, and 8 mg/d for 9- to 13-year-old boys and girls.[62] Vegetarians may need up to 50% more zinc, depending on the composition of their diet.[62]

MEAL-PLANNING GUIDELINES FOR VEGETARIAN ADOLESCENTS

Adolescents can follow meal-planning guidelines that are similar to those for adults and can use the same serving sizes, but they often require more servings from some of the food groups (Table 14-2). As is true for adults, many different food patterns can offer adequate nutrition. In many cases, adolescents in Western countries may find it easiest to meet nutrient needs if nutrient-rich milk, either vegetable milk or cow's milk, is used daily.

As for adults, the number of servings in each of the food groups represents the minimum. Boys in general and both boys and girls who are at a period of rapid growth or who are physically active may require more than the number of servings represented in Table 14-2.

Dietitians may be called on to counsel vegetarian teenagers or families with vegetarian teenagers in planning appropriate menus. Special care may be required in discussing food habits with teenagers because these clients can interpret criticism of food habits as personal criticism. Also, food choices can be a point of intense conflict in families, especially where teenagers choose a diet that is different from that of the rest of the family. It is important to elicit support for, and interest in, the teen's diet from the parents. Many nonvegetarian parents agree to allow a teenager to choose vegetarianism but may be reluctant to participate actively in menu planning and food preparation to support this dietary choice. Wherever possible, dietitians should encourage parents to become active participants in the teen's efforts to consume a vegetarian diet.

Some adolescents may experience difficulty in planning appropriate vegetarian diets if parents do not willingly cooperate by purchasing "special" foods such as soymilk, beans, vegetarian burgers,

Table 14-2 Food Guide for Vegetarian Adolescents

Food Group	Number of Servings* per Day
Grains	10
Legumes, nuts, and other protein-rich foods	6
Vegetables	4
Fruit	3
Fats	3
Calcium-rich foods	10

*Suggested minimum number of servings. Many adolescents need additional servings from one or more food groups, depending on energy needs. See Chapter 10 for additional information on foods in each food group and serving sizes.

Table 14-3 Strategies for Counseling Vegetarian Adolescents

Concern	Counseling Strategies
Adolescent's diet is very high in carbohydrate (pasta, bread, bagels, etc.) and very low in other foods.	Determine and address reasons for limited diet (lack of food preparation knowledge, convenience, taste preference, etc.). Recommend addition of beans, nuts, and soy as spreads (hummus, peanut butter) and additions to dishes. Recommend increased use of fruits and vegetables.
Possible overreliance on convenience foods.	Determine and address reasons for limited diet.
Adolescent's diet consists mainly of veggie burgers and tofu hot dogs.	Suggest other foods that are easy to prepare including bean burritos and heat-and-eat Indian foods. Recommend fresh fruits and vegetables as convenient snacks or part of a meal.
Overconsumption of junk food. Adolescent believes personal health is of little concern and that any food that is vegetarian is healthy.	Address health concerns with a high-fat, high-sugar diet. Recommend healthier snacks and work with teen to develop a healthier eating plan.
Adolescent is trying to lose weight by limiting intake to mainly salads (lettuce and cucumbers) and diet sodas.	Assess teen's weight status and determine if referral for eating disorder evaluation is indicated. If teen does not have an eating disorder and would benefit from weight control, develop an eating plan that will promote gradual weight loss while providing adequate nutrition.
Adolescent is trying to gain weight to improve sports performance.	Assess teen's weight status and determine if weight gain is needed. If it is, suggest several meals and snacks with emphasis on convenient, nutritious, energy-dense foods. Suggest snack ideas including nuts and nut butters, dried fruits, granola, soy products, and whole grain crackers. Assess adolescent's intake of energy and nutrients and make recommendations as needed to increase intake of nutrients that are low.

and so forth. Good nutrition is not a high priority with most teenagers, so that they may need some supervision from parents in planning menus. Sincere interest in, and acceptance of the vegetarian eating plan, will encourage teens to accept some menu-planning guidance from parents. Table 14-3 provides information about some concerns that may be encountered when working with adolescent vegetarians and counseling strategies for these situations.

Introducing more vegetarian meals that the whole family enjoys, such as spaghetti with tomato sauce or bean burritos, can be a unifying approach to mealtime, especially in a family where the teen's dietary change has disrupted family mealtimes. So can using more meals that can be served with and without meat. Spaghetti can be served meatless to the vegetarian teen and with meat to the rest of the family. Mealtime can include a variety of ingredients for tacos or burritos, and individuals can make their own according to their preferences. Stir-fries can be made with meat added at the last minute after a portion for the vegetarian teen has been removed.

Exhibit 14-3 Ideas for Quick and Portable Snacks and Meals for Teenagers

- Dried fruits
- Trail mix
- Popcorn
- Rice cakes
- Yogurt
- Leftover pizza or frozen pizza slices
- Milkshakes
- Hummus in pita bread
- Muffin and juice
- Bagel with peanut butter
- Peanut butter and banana sandwich
- Almond butter on crackers
- Instant soup

If parents are especially resistant to the idea of serving more vegetarian options at mealtimes, the dietitian may need to work with the teenager to plan meals that the teenager can prepare himself or herself. Also, vegetarian teens who have been raised in omnivore households may not be familiar with many foods that can be important staples in vegetarian diets, such as whole grains, leafy green vegetables, soymilk, nut butters, legumes, and tofu. The dietitian may need to work with both the teenager and the parents to identify stores in the community that sell these foods and to explore ways to introduce these foods into the teen's diet.

Teens are likely to have different eating styles than those of adults and children. Convenience and time considerations are important factors in food choices by adolescents.[72] Teenagers consume many of their calories as snacks and consume many meals away from home. Some teenagers may begin to skip breakfast because of lack of time or because they are not hungry in the morning. Often meals will be purchased out, but portable meals and snacks can make it easier for vegetarian adolescents to have constant access to nutritious food choices. Parents can improve the chances that teenagers will make appropriate meal choices by stocking the kitchen with healthful foods that can serve as quick snacks, portable meals, and even breakfasts that can be consumed en route to school. Exhibit 14-3 lists some ideas for portable snacks and meals.

NUTRITION-RELATED CONCERNS IN ADOLESCENTS

Acne

Acne is a common concern among adolescents. It is characterized by plugged pores, pimples, and nodules. Hormonal changes, as seen in adolescence, appear to play a role in acne. Diet's role is controversial. For most adolescents, chocolate and greasy foods do not appear to affect acne. In some adolescents, specific foods appear to trigger an acne outbreak so the keeping of a food and symptom diary may be helpful in identifying problematic foods. Positive associations have been found between the intake of skim milk and acne in adolescent boys,[73] between cow's milk of all types and acne in adolescent girls,[74] and between a high glycemic index diet and acne,[75] although additional research is needed. These findings have led some to suggest that a dairy-free low-glycemic index diet be a treatment option for acne, either alone or as an adjunct to topical or oral medications.[76]

Adolescent Pregnancy

See Chapter 11, "Pregnancy and Lactation," for information about adolescent pregnancy.

Sports Nutrition for Adolescents

Many adolescents participate in sports whether as part of an organized team or as individuals. Vegetarian diets can meet the needs of athletes.[77,78] As is true for all athletes, regardless of age or dietary choice, appropriate nutrition is required for peak performance. To ensure adequate nutrition, adolescent athletes may need to be reminded of the importance of three meals (including breakfast) and several snacks.

For most sports activities, carbohydrates, whether from dietary intake or from stored glycogen, provide the most energy. Generally, athletes should get at least 50% of their calories from carbohydrates to provide energy and to prevent the catabolism of muscle protein. The amount of carbohydrates required depends on the sport, the athlete's gender, and energy expenditure. A general recommendation for athletes is from 6 to 10 g/kg body weight per day.[79]

Protein needs for adolescents participating in endurance sports (sustained activity over a long period of time) and in resistance training may be somewhat higher than the current RDA. The recommendations for adults are as follows:[79]

- Endurance athletes: 1.2 to 1.4 g/kg per day
- Resistance-trained athletes: 1.2 to 1.7 g/kg per day

These recommendations are for elite highly trained athletes and are not necessarily applicable to recreational and nonelite athletes.[80] Limited information is available on the protein needs of the adolescent athlete participating in endurance sports or resistance training while still requiring additional protein to support growth. It is likely that protein intakes in the range just indicated will meet or exceed adolescent protein needs. These higher protein needs are frequently met simply through the increased energy intake seen in many athletes. An inadequate intake of total protein is not likely to be a concern for most vegetarian athletes except for those who are following a low protein diet and trying to limit energy intake.[81] In some cases it may be necessary to emphasize concentrated sources of protein such as soyfoods. Some energy bars can provide significant amounts of protein and calories and are often vegan.

Hydration is an important consideration for athletic performance. Athletes should be encouraged to monitor their fluid intake and output and to strive for light yellow or clear urine. Fluid intake before, during, and after exercise should be:[45]

- 1 to 2 hours before exercise: 6 to 12 ounces fluid
- During exercise (especially if >1 hour): 8 ounces fluid every 20 minutes (more if weight is > 60 kg)
- After exercise: Replace losses with 15 to 23 ounces/0.5 kg weight loss

---

Exhibit 14-4 Food Guide for Young Female Athletes (2000 Calories, 20% Protein, 30% Fat, 50% Carbohydrate, 1500 mg Calcium

- 11 servings grains
- 9 servings legumes, nuts, and other protein-rich foods
- 4 servings vegetables
- 4 servings fruit
- 4–5 servings fat
- 12 servings calcium-rich foods

Note: See Chapter 10 for additional information on foods in each food group and serving sizes.

Because even marginal iron status can inhibit optimal athletic performance, athletes should be encouraged to have an adequate iron intake and to monitor iron status as needed. Similar to iron, inadequate calcium intake is common in adolescents, both athletes and nonathletes. Although physical activity does promote an increased bone mass, adequate intake of key nutrients like calcium, protein, and vitamin D is necessary for this to occur. Exhibit 14-4 offers guidelines for menu planning to achieve adequate intakes of macronutrients and calcium. This plan needs to be adapted to meet energy needs >2000 kcal/d.

Amenorrhea in Athletes

Secondary amenorrhea, typically defined as the absence of three or more consecutive menstrual periods after menarche, occurs in some female athletes. The prevalence of secondary amenorrhea was reported to be as high as 65% among long-distance runners age 15 to 21 years with lower prevalence rates seen in other athletes.[81] Although amenorrhea can be linked to disordered eating behavior, this is not always the cause. In athletes, amenorrhea may be related to an energy deficit due to increased needs secondary to intense training. Stress and hormone changes associated with exercise have also been proposed as explanations for athletic amenorrhea.[82] An athlete with amenorrhea should be evaluated for the other components of the female athlete triad, namely bone density loss and disordered eating. In addition, other causes of secondary amenorrhea should be ruled out by a physician.

Secondary amenorrhea in athletes appears to be related to a dysfunction of the hypothalamus due to an energy deficit. This leads to a marked reduction in bone formation and, to a lesser extent, a reduction in bone resorption.[83] The potential consequences of the lower bone mineral density (BMD) resulting from athletic amenorrhea include an increased risk of stress fractures[84–85] as well as increased risk for osteoporosis later in life. Alterations in bone metabolism with athletic amenorrhea differ from the reduction in bone formation and increased bone resorption seen in women with primary ovarian failure. Although weightbearing exercise is commonly recommended as a means of increasing BMD, exercise does not appear to compensate adequately for the reduced bone formation seen in amenorrheic athletes.[86,87]

Hormone replacement therapy is often used to treat hypothalamic amenorrhea. This treatment has had mixed results in terms of BMD.[88] A more satisfactory treatment appears to be achievement of a normal BMI, decreased exercise, and increased caloric intake. The increases in BMD that occur with weight gain are greater than those seen when amenorrhea is treated with hormone replacement alone.[88] Weight gain leading to a BMI of 19 to 20.5 kg/m² in amenorrheic athletes is associated with a resumption of menses and improved BMD.[83] Treatment strategies include at least 1 rest day per week, increasing caloric intake by 200 to 300 kcal/d, and meeting recommendations for calcium, vitamin D, B vitamins, iron, and zinc.[89,90]

Eating Disorders

Eating disorders occur in approximately 0.5–5% of adolescent females.[91] They are much less common in males, with only about 5–10% of all cases occurring in males.[91] The most common eating disorders include anorexia nervosa, characterized by self-starvation, which occurs in about 0.5% of adolescent girls, and bulimia nervosa, a bingeing and purging syndrome that affects 1–5% of adolescent girls.[91] In addition, there are a number of individuals with milder behavior that does not meet strict diagnostic criteria but who still experience the effects of an eating disorder. Table 14-4 provides some characteristics of the two most common types of eating disorders.

The association between vegetarian diets and eating disorders is controversial and not completely understood. Eating disorders have a complex etiology, and the use of a vegetarian diet does not appear to increase the risk of developing an eating disorder.[92,93] Limited data suggest that vegetarian diets are sometimes selected as a way to hide a preexisting eating disorder[94] with vegetarianism chosen before the onset of anorexia nervosa in only 6% of cases examined in one study.[95] Some adolescents may choose a vegetarian or partially vegetarian diet as a socially acceptable way to limit their food and possibly fat intake and in this way make it less likely that parents and peers will realize they have an eating disorder.

A number of studies have reported that self-described vegetarians were at higher risk of disordered eating.[4,96–100] Other studies do not find this and report either no significant difference between self-described vegetarians and nonvegetarians in measures including eating restraint score and perception of weight status[101,102] or that vegetarians have lower restraint scores than nonvegetarians.[92] A problem with many of these studies is that they do not differentiate between true

Table 14-4 Characteristics of Anorexia Nervosa and Bulimia Nervosa

Anorexia Nervosa	Bulimia Nervosa
Low body weight for age and height with refusal to maintain a minimally normal weight for age and height	Episodes of binge eating with sense of lack of control of behavior
Intense fear of gaining weight	Recurrent use of self-induced vomiting; laxatives, diuretics, or other medications; fasting; or excess exercise to prevent weight gain
Disturbed perception of body weight and shape	Self-image greatly influenced by body shape and weight
Amenorrhea (in postmenarchal females)	

vegetarians who avoid meat, fish, and poultry and those self-described "vegetarians" who eat chicken, fish, and possibly red meat. This failure to differentiate may lead to false conclusions. Several studies suggest that if vegetarians are properly classified, eating disorders are not more prevalent in vegetarians.[102,103] In addition, some assessment tools may give vegetarians higher dietary restraint scores simply because they are vegetarian.[102] Some studies suggest that adolescents who describe themselves as lapsed vegetarians are more likely to use extreme weight control methods, like vomiting and laxatives, than current vegetarians or nonvegetarians.[100] Apparently some adolescents try a variety of diets, including vegetarian diets, in an attempt to lose weight. When weight loss does not occur on a vegetarian diet, they move on to other methods. Self-described vegetarians whose main motivation for their dietary choice is weight loss appear to be at a higher risk for developing eating disorders than vegetarians with other motivations such as animal welfare or personal health.[92,103]

The clinician's task is to distinguish between individuals who are vegetarian but not eating disordered and those who have an eating disorder and follow a vegetarian or near-vegetarian diet. In doing this, the following should be considered:

- Did parents or peers express concern about eating disordered behaviors before the adoption of a vegetarian diet?
- Does the food record show abstention from high-fat or high-calorie foods?
- Is a primary motivation for the vegetarian diet weight loss?
- Has the adolescent followed other diets for short periods of time?
- Has the adolescent been vegetarian for <2 years?
- Does the adolescent display symptoms of an eating disorder?
- Is the adolescent still eating poultry, fish, and/or red meat but self-identifying as a vegetarian? Answers of "yes" to one or more questions require further investigation and possible referral to an eating disorders specialist.

Eating disorders are multifaceted and complex. In some cases, vegetarianism is prohibited for patients recovering from eating disorders. The efficacy of this has not been studied. The American Psychiatric Association's guidelines for treatment of anorexia nervosa call for a meal plan that "ensures nutritional adequacy and that none of the major food groups are avoided."[104] It is not necessary to give up vegetarianism to meet these guidelines. What is important for the treatment process is to understand the motivation for a vegetarian diet.[105] If the primary motivation for choosing a vegetarian diet is based on ethics and a commitment to it as a healthy lifestyle, use of a nutritionally adequate, varied vegetarian diet should not conflict with treatment goals. If the main motivation is weight loss, however, continuing with a vegetarian diet may be counterproductive to treatment goals.

COUNSELING POINTS FOR VEGETARIAN ADOLESCENTS AND THEIR PARENTS

- Ensure adequate energy intake to support the rapid growth adolescent years.
- Protein needs are usually met easily unless energy intakes are inadequate or diets contain few good sources of protein like beans, grains, and soyfoods.

- Adolescents need 1300 mg of calcium per day. Good sources of calcium are listed in Chapter 5.
- Daily physical activity is important for bone health.
- Consume foods high in iron along with foods high in vitamin C to enhance iron absorption.
- Unless dairy products are consumed regularly, include foods that are fortified with vitamin B_{12} or use B_{12} supplements.
- Vegetarian meals can be incorporated into family eating styles by planning meatless meals that the whole family enjoys or by offering entrees that can be served with or without meat.
- Some simple and convenience items such as instant soups or prepared sandwich spreads can be quick meals that require little or no preparation. Having these foods on hand can make it possible for the teen vegetarian to prepare some of his or her own meals and snacks.
- Most vegetarians do not have eating disorders but vegetarian diets may be used to mask an eating disorder. Investigate further if other signs of eating disorders are present.
- Female vegetarian athletes may benefit from diets that include additional energy, higher levels of fat, and generous amounts of calcium.

Case Studies

Sandra is a 15-year-old lifelong lacto-ovo vegetarian. Her father has recently discovered that he has type 2 diabetes. Sandra has elevated cholesterol and is about 30 pounds above ideal weight.

A typical day includes:

A 3 egg omelet, 2 slices of toast with butter for breakfast
A grilled cheese sandwich, French fries, and a milkshake for lunch
Fried tofu with black bean sauce and a couple of slices of carrot, a cup of white rice, whole milk, and a bowl of ice cream for dinner.
Snacks include potato chips, diet soft drinks, and an energy bar.

To discuss:

What are your concerns with Sandra's diet?
What modifications can you suggest?

Julie is a 15-year-old on the cross-country team. During the season (now), she runs 50 to 60 miles weekly. She has recently decided to become vegan because of concerns about animals and because many of her teammates are vegan.

Julie's parents are concerned because she has lost 5 lb in the past month. Julie is 5′2″ tall and weighs 98 lb (BMI: 18.3).

Julie has noticed that her racing times are not as good as they used to be. She and her coach are troubled but not certain what to do about this. Julie does not display any symptoms of an eating disorder other than weight loss.

(continued)

A typical day includes:

Peanut butter crackers and a glass of juice for breakfast
A veggie burger and fries for lunch
A couple of bean burritos and iced tea for dinner
Snacks include rice cakes, peanut butter crackers, and lemonade
Her estimated calorie requirement is 2000 kcal; estimated intake is 1500 kcal.

To discuss:

What can Julie do to improve her diet?
What foods can she add knowing that she has limited time to prepare foods?
What role should her parents take?

REFERENCES

1. Stahler C. How many youth are vegetarian? *Vegetarian J.* 2005;24(4).
2. Greene-Finestone LS, Campbell MK, Gutmanis IA, et al. Dietary intake among young adolescents in Ontario: associations with vegetarian status and attitude toward health. *Prev Med.* 2005; 40:105–111.
3. Donovan UM, Gibson RS. Iron and zinc status of young women aged 14–19 years consuming vegetarian and omnivorous diets. *J Am Coll Nutr.* 1995;14:463–472.
4. Neumark-Sztainer D, Story M, Resnick MD, Blum RW. Adolescent vegetarians: a behavioural profile of a school-based population in Minnesota. *Arch Pediatr Adolesc Med.* 1997;151:833–838.
5. Donovan UM, Gibson RS. Dietary intakes of adolescent females consuming vegetarian, semi-vegetarian, and omnivorous diets. *J Adolesc Health.* 1996;18:292–300.
6. Perry CL, McGuire MT, Neumark-Sztainer D, et al. Adolescent vegetarians: how well do their dietary patterns meet the healthy people 2010 objectives? *Arch Pediatr Adolesc Med.* 2002;156:431–437.
7. Larsson CL, Johansson GK. Young Swedish vegans have different sources of nutrients than young omnivores. *J Am Diet Assoc.* 2005;105:1438–1441.
8. Robinson-O'Brien R, Larson N, Neumark-Sztainer D, et al. Characteristics and dietary patterns of adolescents who value eating locally grown, organic, nongenetically engineered, and nonprocessed food. *J Nutr Educ Behav.* 2009; 41:11–18.
9. Troiano RP, Briefel RR, Carroll MD, Bialostosky K. Energy and fat intakes of children and adolescents in the United States: data from the National Health and Nutrition Examination Surveys. *Am J Clin Nutr.* 2000;72(suppl):1343S–1353S.
10. Briefel RR, Johnson CL. Secular trends in dietary intake in the United States. *Annu Rev Nutr.* 2004;24:401–431.
11. Ogden CL, Carroll MD, Curtin LR, et al. Prevalence of overweight and obesity in the United States, 1999–2004. *JAMA.* 2006;295(13):1549–1555.
12. Ford ES, Li C, Zhao G, et al. Prevalence of the metabolic syndrome among U.S. adolescents using the definition from the International Diabetes Federation. *Diabetes Care.* 2008;31:587–589.
13. Cavadini C, Siega-Riz AM, Popkin BM. U.S. adolescent food intake trends from 1965 to 1996. *Arch Dis Child.* 2000;83:18–24.
14. Ogden CL, Flegal KM, Carroll MD, Johnson CL. Prevalence and trends in overweight among US children and adolescents, 1999–2000. *JAMA.* 2002; 288:1728–1732.
15. ARS/USDA. Continuing Survey of Food Intakes of Individuals, 1994–96, 1998, Table Set 17: Food and Nutrient Intakes by Children, 1994–96, 1998. http://www.barc.usda.gov/bhnrc/foodsurvey/pdf/scs_all.pdf.
16. Guo SS, Chumlea WC. Tracking of body mass index in children in relation to overweight in adulthood. *Am J Clin Nutr.* 1999;70(suppl):145S–148S.

17. Guo SS, Wu W, Chumlea WC, et al. Predicting overweight and obesity in adulthood from body mass index values in childhood and adolescence. *Am J Clin Nutr.* 2002;76:653–658.

18. McGill HC Jr, McMahan CA, Herderick EE, et al. Origin of atherosclerosis in childhood and adolescence. *Am J Clin Nutr.* 2000;72(suppl):1307S–1315S.

19. Falkner B, Sherif K, Michel S, et al. Dietary nutrients and blood pressure in urban minority adolescents at risk for hypertension. *Arch Pediatr Adolesc Med.* 2000;154:918–922.

20. Law M. Dietary fat and adult diseases and the implications for childhood nutrition: an epidemiologic approach. *Am J Clin Nutr.* 2000;72(suppl):1291S–1296S.

21. Misra M. Long-term skeletal effects of eating disorders with onset in adolescence. *Ann N Y Acad Sci.* 2008;1135:212–218.

22. Story M, Resnick M. Adolescents' views on food and nutrition. *J Nutr Educ.* 1986;18:188–192.

23. Tanner JM. *Fetus into Man: Physical Growth from Conception to Maturity.* Cambridge, MA: Harvard University Press; 1978.

24. Jaffe A. Why adolescent medicine? *Med Clin N Am.* 2000;84:769–785.

25. Forbes GB. Nutritional requirements in adolescence. In: Suskind RM, ed. *Textbook of Pediatric Nutrition.* New York, NY: Raven Press; 1981:381–392.

26. Hardinge MG, Stare FJ. Nutritional studies in vegetarians. 1. Nutritional, physical, and laboratory studies. *J Clin Nutr.* 1954;2:73–82.

27. Cooper R, Allen A, Goldberg R, et al. Seventh-day Adventist adolescents-life-style patterns and cardiovascular risk factors. *West J Med.* 1984;140:471–477.

28. Persky VW, Chatterton RT, Van Horn LV, et al. Hormone levels in vegetarian and nonvegetarian teenage girls: potential implications for breast cancer risk. *Cancer Res.* 1992;50:578–583.

29. Hebbelinck M, Clarys P, De Malsche A. Growth, development, and physical fitness of Flemish vegetarian children, adolescents, and young adults. *Am J Clin Nutr.* 1999;70(suppl):579S–585S.

30. Sabate J, Linsted KD, Harris RD, Sanchez A. Attained height of lacto-ovo vegetarian children and adolescents. *Eur J Clin Nutr.* 1991;45:51–58.

31. Larsson CL, Johansson GK. Dietary intake and nutritional status of young vegans and omnivores in Sweden. *Am J Clin Nutr.* 2002;76:100–106.

32. Sanchez A, Kissinger DG, Phillips RL. A hypothesis on the etiological role of diet on age of menarche. *Med Hypothesis.* 1981;7:1339–1345.

33. Kissinger DG, Sanchez A. The association of dietary factors with the age of menarche. *Nutr Res.* 1987;7:471–479.

34. Hebbelinck M, Clarys P, De Malsche A. Growth, development, and physical fitness of Flemish vegetarian children, adolescents, and young adults. *Am J Clin Nutr.* 1999;70(suppl):579S–585S.

35. Barr SI. Women's reproductive function. In: Sabate J, ed. *Vegetarian Nutrition.* Boca Raton, FL: CRC Press; 2001:221–249.

36. Rosell M, Appleby P, Key T. Height, age at menarche, body weight and body mass index in life-long vegetarians. *Public Health Nutr.* 2005;8:870–875.

37. Kuczmarski RJ, Ogden CL, Grummer-Strawn LH, et al. CDC Growth Charts: United States. Advance data from vital and health statistics; No. 314. Hyattsville, MD: National Center for Health Statistics; 2000.

38. Food and Nutrition Board, Institute of Medicine. *Dietary Reference Intakes for Energy, Carbohydrate, Fiber, Fat, Fatty Acids, Cholesterol, Protein, and Amino Acids.* Washington, DC: National Academies Press; 2002.

39. Messina V, Mangels AR. Considerations in planning vegan diets. II. Children. *J Am Diet Assoc.* 2001;101:661–669.

40. Borrione P, Spaccamiglio A, Salvo RA, et al. Rhabdomyolysis in a young vegetarian athlete. *Am J Phys Med Rehabil.* 2009;88(11):951–954.

41. Institute of Medicine, Food and Nutrition Board. *Dietary Reference Intakes for Calcium, Phosphorus, Magnesium, Vitamin D, and Fluoride.* Washington, DC: National Academy Press; 1997.

42. Abrams SA. Calcium supplementation during childhood: long-term effects on bone mineralization. *Nutr Rev.* 2005;63:251–255.

43. McKay HA, Bailey DA, Mirwald RL, et al. Peak bone mineral accrual and age at menarche in adolescent girls: a 6-year longitudinal study. *J Pediatr.* 1998;133:682–687.

44. Theintz G, Buchs B, Rizzoli R, et al. Longitudinal monitoring of bone mass accumulation in healthy adolescents: evidence for a marked reduction after 16 years of age at the levels of lumbar spine and femoral neck in female subjects. *J Clin Endocrinol Metab.* 1992;75:1060–1065.

45. Kleinman RE, ed. *Pediatric Nutrition Handbook.* Elk Village, IL: American Academy of Pediatrics; 2009.

46. Bailey DA, Martin AD, McKay HA, et al. Calcium accretion in girls and boys during puberty: a longitudinal analysis. *J Bone Miner Res.* 2000;15:2245–2250.

47. Abrams SA, Copeland KC, Gunn SK, et al. Calcium absorption, bone mass accumulation, and kinetics increase during early pubertal development in girls. *J Clin Endocrinol Metab.* 2000;85:1805–1809.

48. Bonjour J-P, Theintz G, Buchs B, et al. Critical years and stages of puberty for spinal and femoral bone mass accumulation during adolescence. *J Clin Endocrinol Metab.* 1991;73:555–563.

49. Ervin RB, Wang CY, Wright JD, et al. Dietary intake of selected minerals for the United States population: 1999–2000. *Adv Data.* 2004;27:1–5.

50. Abrams SA, Griffin IJ, Hicks PD, et al. Pubertal girls only partially adapt to low dietary calcium intakes. *J Bone Mineral Res.* 2004;19:759–763.

51. Nieves JW, Golden AL, Siris E, et al. Teenage and current calcium intake are related to bone mineral density of the hip and forearm in women aged 30–39 years. *Am J Epidemiol.* 1995;141:342–351.

52. Halioua L, Anderson JJ. Lifetime calcium intake and physical activity habits: independent and combined effects on the radial bone of healthy premenopausal Caucasian women. *Am J Clin Nutr.* 1989;49:534–541.

53. Teegarden D, Lyle RM, Prouix WR, et al. Previous milk consumption is associated with greater bone density in young women. *Am J Clin Nutr.* 1999;69:1014–1017.

54. Lloyd T, Petit MA, Lin HM, et al. Lifestyle factors and the development of bone mass and bone strength in young women. *J Pediatr.* 2004;144:776–782.

55. Lloyd T, Beck TJ, Lin HM, et al. Modifiable determinants of bone status in young women. *Bone.* 2002;30:416–421.

56. Lloyd T, Chinchilli VM, Johnson-Rollings N, et al. Adult female hip bone density reflects teenage sports-exercise patterns but not teenage calcium intake. *Pediatrics.* 2000;106:40–44.

57. Bailey DA, McKay HA, Mirwald RL, et al. A six-year longitudinal study of the relationship of physical activity to bone mineral accrual in growing children: the university of Saskatchewan bone mineral accrual study. *J Bone Miner Res.* 1999;14:1672–1679.

58. Lehtonen-Veromaa MKM, Mottonen TT, Nuotio IO, et al. Vitamin D and attainment of peak bone mass among peripubertal Finnish girls: a 3-y prospective study. *Am J Clin Nutr.* 2002;76:1446–1453.

59. Wagner CL, Greer FR. American Academy of Pediatrics Section on Breastfeeding; American Academy of Pediatrics Committee on Nutrition. Prevention of rickets and vitamin D deficiency in infants, children, and adolescents. *Pediatrics.* 2008;122:1142–1152.

60. DeMaeyer EM, Adiels-Tegman M. The prevalence of anemia in the world. *World Health Stat Q.* 1985;38:302–316.

61. Centers for Disease Control and Prevention. Recommendations to prevent and control iron deficiency in the United States. *MMWR.* 1998;47(No. RR-3):1–29.

62. Institute of Medicine, Food and Nutrition Board. *Dietary Reference Intakes for Vitamin A, Vitamin K, Arsenic, Boron, Chromium, Copper, Iodine, Iron, Manganese, Molybdenum, Nickel, Silicon, Vanadium, and Zinc.* Washington, DC: National Academy Press; 2001.

63. Hallberg L, Rossander-Hultén, Brune M, Gleerup A. Calcium and iron absorption: mechanism of action and nutritional importance. *Eur J Clin Nutr.* 1991;46:317–327.

64. Ilich-Ernst JZ, McKenna AA, Badenhop NE, et al. Iron status, menarche, and calcium supplementation in adolescent girls. *Am J Clin Nutr.* 1998;68:880–887.

65. Institute of Medicine, Food and Nutrition Board. *Dietary Reference Intakes for Thiamin, Riboflavin, Niacin, Vitamin B_6, Folate, Vitamin B_{12}, Pantothenic Acid, Biotin, and Choline.* Washington, DC: National Academy Press; 1998.

66. van Dusseldorp M, Schneede J, Refsum H, et al. Risk of persistent cobalamin deficiency in adolescents fed macrobiotic diet in early life. *Am J Clin Nutr.* 1999;69:664–671.

67. Louwman MWJ, van Dusseldorp M, van de Vijver FJR, et al. Signs of impaired cognitive function in adolescents with marginal cobalamin status. *Am J Clin Nutr.* 2000;72:762–769.

68. Licht DJ, Berry GT, Brooks DG, et al. Reversible subacute combined degeneration of the spinal cord in a 14-year-old due to a strict vegan diet. *Clin Pediatr.* 2001;40:413–415.

69. Hunt JR, Matthys LA, Lykken GI. Reduced zinc absorption from a lacto-ovo vegetarian diet. *Am J Clin Nutr.* 1995;61:908.

70. Treuherz J. Possible inter-relationship between zinc and dietary fibre in a group of lacto-ovo vegetarian adolescents. *J Plant Foods.* 1982;4:89–95.

71. Gibson RS, Donovan UM, Heath AL. Dietary strategies to improve the iron and zinc nutriture of young women following a vegetarian diet. *Plant Foods Hum Nutr.* 1997;51:1–16.

72. Neumark-Sztainer D, Story M, Perry C, Casey MA. Factors influencing food choices of adolescents: findings from focus-group discussions with adolescents. *J Am Diet Assoc.* 1999;99:929–934, 937.

73. Adebamowo CA, Spiegelman D, Berkey CS, et al. Milk consumption and acne in teenaged boys. *J Am Acad Dermatol.* 2008;58(5):787–793.

74. Adebamowo CA, Spiegelman D, Berkey CS, et al. Milk consumption and acne in adolescent girls. *Derm Online J.* 2006;12(4):1.

75. Smith RN, Mann NJ, Braue A, et al. A low-glycemic-load diet improves symptoms in acne vulgaris patients: a randomized controlled trial. *Am J Clin Nutr.* 2007;86:107–115.

76. Danby FW. Diet and acne. *Clin Dermatol.* 2008;26(1):93–96.

77. Barr SI, Rideout CA. Nutritional concerns for vegetarian athletes. *Nutrition.* 2004;20:696–700.

78. Craig WJ, Mangels AR. Position of the American Dietetic Association: vegetarian diets. *J Am Diet Assoc.* 2009;109:1266–1282.

79. Rodriguez NR, DiMarco NM, Langley S, et al. Position of the American Dietetic Association, Dietitians of Canada, and the American College of Sports Medicine: nutrition and athletic performance. *J Am Diet Assoc.* 2009;109:509–527.

80. Venderley AM, Campbell WW. Vegetarian diets. Nutritional considerations for athletes. *Sports Med.* 2006;36:293–305.

81. Dusek T. Influence of high intensity training on menstrual cycle disorders in athletes. *Croat Med J.* 2001;42:79–82.

82. American College of Sports Medicine. The female athlete triad. Position stand. *Med Sci Sport Exerc.* 1997;29:i–ix.

83. Zanker CL, Cooke CB. Energy balance, bone turnover, and skeletal health in physically active individuals. *Med Sci Sports Exerc.* 2004;36:1372–1381.

84. Kadel NJ, Teitz CC, Kronmal RA. Stress fractures in ballet dancers. *Am J Sports Med.* 1992;20:445–449.

85. Bennett KL, Malcolm SA, Thomas SA, et al. Risk factors for stress fractures in track and field athletes. *Am J Sports Med.* 1996;24:810–818.

86. Nichols JF, Rauh MJ, Barrack MT, et al. Bone mineral density in female high school athletes: interactions of menstrual function and type of mechanical loading. *Bone.* 2007;41:371–377.

87. Kahn KM, Warren MP, Stiehl A, et al. Bone mineral density in active and retired ballet dancers. *J Dance Med Sci.* 1999;3:15–23.

88. Warren MP, Chua AT. Exercise-induced amenorrhea and bone health in the adolescent athlete. *Ann NY Acad Sci.* 2008;1135:244–252.

89. Gamboa S, Gaskie S, Atlas M. What's the best way to manage athletes with amenorrhea? *J Family Prac.* 2008;57:740–750.

90. Manore MM. Dietary recommendations and athletic menstrual dysfunction. *Sports Med.* 2002;32:887–901.

91. American Academy of Pediatrics, Committee on Adolescence. Identifying and treating eating disorders. *Pediatrics.* 2003;111:204–211.

92. Janelle KC, Barr SI. Nutrient intakes and eating behavior scores of vegetarian and nonvegetarian women. *J Am Diet Assoc.* 1995;95:180–186, 189.

93. Barr SI. Vegetarianism and menstrual cycle disturbances: is there an association? *Am J Clin Nutr.* 1999;70(suppl):549S–554S.

94. Martins Y, Pliner P, O'Connor R. Restrained eating among vegetarians: does a vegetarian eating style mask concerns about weight? *Appetite.* 1999;32:145–154.

95. O'Connor AM, Touyz WS, Dunn SM, Beumont PJ. Vegetarianism in anorexia nervosa? A review of 116 consecutive cases. *Med J Aust.* 1987;147:540–542.

96. Bas M, Karabudak E, Kiziltan G. Vegetarianism and eating disorders: association between eating attitudes and other psychological factors among Turkish adolescents. *Appetite.* 2005;44:309–315.

97. Gilbody SM, Kirk SFL, Hill AJ. Vegetarianism in young women: another means of weight control? *Int J Eat Disord.* 1999;26:87–90.

98. Klopp SA, Heiss CJ, Smith HS. Self-reported vegetarianism may be a marker for college women at risk for disordered eating. *J Am Diet Assoc.* 2003;103:745–747.

99. McClean JA, Barr SI. Cognitive dietary restraint is associated with eating behaviors, lifestyle practices, personality characteristics and menstrual irregularity in college women. *Appetite.* 2003;40:185–192.

100. Robinson-O'Brien R, Perry CL, Wall MM, et al. Adolescent and young adult vegetarianism: better dietary intake and weight outcomes but increased risk of disordered eating behaviors. *J Am Diet Assoc.* 2009;109:648–655.

101. Barr SI, Broughton TM. Relative weight, weight loss efforts and nutrient intakes among health-conscious vegetarian, past vegetarian and nonvegetarian women ages 18 to 50. *J Am Coll Nutr.* 2000;19:781–788.

102. Fisak B, Peterson RD, Tantleff-Dunn S, et al. Challenging previous conceptions of vegetarianism and eating disorders. *Eating Weight Disord.* 2006;11:195–200.

103. Perry CL, McGuire MT, Neumark-Sztainer D, et al. Characteristics of vegetarian adolescents in a multiethnic urban population. *J Adolesc Health.* 2001;29:406–416.

104. American Psychiatric Association. Treatment of patients with eating disorders, 3rd ed. *Am J Psych.* 2006; 163(7 suppl): 4–54.

105. Finnigan B. Vegetarianism and disordered eating. National Eating Disorders Information Centre. 2004. http://www.nedic.ca/knowthefacts/documents/Vegetarianismanddisorderedeating.pdf

CHAPTER 15

Vegetarian Diets for Older People

A 2009 poll found that 2% of Americans, ≥65 years of age never ate meat, fish, or poultry and 1% did not use any animal products.[1] These percentages are similar to those for all adults, suggesting that vegetarianism is not limited to younger adults. The number of older vegetarians may be on the rise. First, in the United States the older segment of the population is growing more rapidly than any other age group.[2] Second, some evidence suggests that the number of vegetarians is growing, and those who choose a meatless diet appear to make this a long-term choice.[3] Third, life expectancy is higher for vegetarians than for nonvegetarians.[4] As a result, dietitians need to be prepared to address the concerns of older vegetarians. Diet is an issue of importance for all older Americans. Calorie needs decrease with aging, but needs for calcium, vitamin D, and vitamin B_6 increase (Table 15-1). There is also evidence that protein needs increase and that vitamin B_{12} supplements are important for all older people. All of these nutrients are of particular interest in the diets of older vegetarians.

DIETARY STATUS OF OLDER VEGETARIANS

There are few recent studies of older vegetarians worldwide and a very limited number of studies of older vegetarians in the United States. The available data indicate, however, that nutrient intake of older vegetarians is similar to or better than that of older nonvegetarians (Appendices P, Q, and R). In a study of Dutch vegetarians, for example, age 65 to 99 years, intakes of fiber, carbohydrate, fat, and protein were closer to recommendations than intakes of nonvegetarians.[5] Intake of zinc was somewhat low, however, and although iron intake was adequate, there was a higher incidence of poor iron status among the vegetarians[5] (these minerals are discussed in Chapter 6). In another study, elderly Canadian Seventh-day Adventist women had lower protein and energy intakes but higher copper, selenium, and magnesium intakes than nonvegetarians.[6] Adventist women with an average age of 71 years consumed less cholesterol and saturated fat and more carbohydrate, fiber, magnesium, vitamin A, vitamin E, thiamin, pantothenic acid, copper, folate, and manganese than nonvegetarian women of a similar age. The nonvegetarians also had diets that were low in vitamins B_6 and E. Both groups had low intakes of vitamin D and zinc,

Table 15-1 Nutrients for Which Recommendations Change with Aging (Based on Institute of Medicine Recommendations)

	Age 31–50		Age 51–70		Age 70+	
	M	F	M	F	M	F
Calcium AI (mg)	1000	1000	1200	1200	1200	1200
Vitamin D AI (μg)	5	5	10	10	15	15
Chromium AI (μg)	35	25	30	20	30	20
Iron RDA (mg)	8	18	8	8	8	8
Iron RDA (mg) vegetarians	14	33	14	14	14	14
Vitamin B_6 RDA (mg)	1.3	1.3	1.7	1.5	1.7	1.5
Vitamin B_{12} RDA (μg)	2.4	2.4	2.4*	2.4*	2.4*	2.4*

*The Food and Nutrition Board recommends that vitamin B_{12} needs be met after the age of 51 years with supplements or fortified foods.
Source: Based on Institute of Medicine Recommendations.

however.[7] Two other studies of older Adventist vegetarian women also indicate intake to be equal to or superior to that of nonvegetarians.[8,9]

Although studies indicate that most older vegetarians have dietary intakes that are comparable to those of omnivores, dietary adequacy of all older people is an issue of concern because caloric intake often decreases, requiring diets to become more nutrient dense.

NUTRIENT NEEDS OF OLDER VEGETARIANS

Calories

As people age, muscle mass decreases and percentage body fat increases in response to both hormonal changes and decreased physical activity. These changes can be significant. At age 60 years, on average men and women have 7 lb (3.2 kg) and 3.5 lb (1.6 kg) fewer pounds of muscle tissue, respectively, than they did at 20 years of age.[10] After age 70, men lose 1.6 kg and women lose 0.6 kg of lean tissue per decade, on average.[11] Reduced lean body mass, along with decreased physical activity in some adults, results in decreased calorie needs. Equations have been developed that predict energy requirements for adults ages ≥19 years.[12] Age is a parameter in these equations. An age-related decline in energy expenditure is predicted to be approximately 10 kcal/year for men and 7 kcal/year for women beginning at age 19.[12] Most of the reduction is due to reduced metabolic rate, although a small amount is also due to decreased physical activity and possibly to a reduced thermic effect of food.

The estimated energy requirement (EER) varies considerably for different age individuals. For example, a 30-year-old man weighing 165 lb, 6 feet tall (body mass index [BMI]: 22.5 kg/m²), with a low physical activity level, has an EER of approximately 2800 kcal/d. Assuming no change in weight, height, or activity level, his EER at age 60 would be 2500 kcal/d and at age 80 it would be 2300 kcal/d. Similarly, a 30-year-old woman weighing 134 lb, 5 feet 6 inches tall (BMI:

21.5 kg/m^2), with a low physical activity level, has an EER of about 2100 kcal/d. Again, assuming no change in weight, height, or physical activity level, her EER at age 60 would be 1900 kcal/d and at age 80 it would be 1800 kcal/d.

Even with lower energy requirements, however, there is some concern that older people do not meet those needs. According to the National Health and Nutrition Examination Survey (NHANES) III, men and women age 70 to 79 years consumed an average of only 1880 and 1600 kcal/d, respectively; intakes of those ≥80 years were even lower.[13] Inadequate energy intake can lead to unintentional weight loss. The extent of this problem is illustrated by the report that more than a quarter of women 55 to 69 years of age have had at least one unintentional weight loss episode of ≥20 lb[14] and that more than a quarter of women 65 to 74 years of age have lost at least 15% of their body weight.[15] Unintentional weight loss is associated with a higher mortality rate.[16] Underweight in older people is a marker for chronic disease, frailty, and dementia.[17] Older people with a BMI <22 kg/m^2 had a higher mortality than those with higher BMIs even when results were adjusted for smoking status, chronic disease, and other factors likely to affect both BMI and mortality.[18] Low BMI is also associated with increased fracture risk.[19]

Decreased calorie intake with aging is not a problem as long as ideal body weight is maintained, but it does make it more difficult to meet nutrient needs. Some older people may have energy intakes so low that appropriate nutrient densities are difficult to achieve.[20] Caloric intake of elderly vegetarians appears to be slightly lower than that of nonvegetarians, but the data vary considerably (Appendix P).

Protein

The current recommended dietary allowances (RDAs) for protein for adults ages ≥51 years are not different from those of younger adults (0.8 g/kg body weight [bw]).[12] These recommendations were based on a meta-analysis of nitrogen balance studies that concluded there was not enough evidence to recommend a higher protein intake for older adults.[21] This analysis included only one study relevant to older adults, however.[22] Some researchers have called for higher protein recommendations for older people, citing factors such as less efficient protein use with aging.[23–26] Gersovitz et al found that at caloric intake usual for older people, protein intakes at the RDA level (0.8 g/kg bw) did not maintain nitrogen balance in more than half of the subjects.[23] Similar results were obtained by Campbell et al.[24] Protein recommendations of 1 to 1.25 g/kg bw for elderly adults have been proposed.[27,28] Other studies and reviews do not support higher protein needs for the elderly.[29,30] More research in this area is clearly needed.

Sarcopenia, the loss of muscle mass and strength that occurs with aging, affects all elderly adults to some extent and contributes to a decline in functional ability. Both resistance exercise and protein intakes above the RDA have been shown to be helpful in reducing or reversing sarcopenia.[31] Vegetarian diets providing 133–145% of the RDA for protein (with 0.6 g/kg of protein from soy) in conjunction with resistance training in older men led to similar increases in muscle mass compared to nonvegetarian diets and resistance training.[32,33]

Given their possible increased protein needs, older Americans may be consuming too little protein. The median dietary intake of protein for men and women >71 years was 72.5 g/d and 56.4 g/d, respectively.[12] Some research shows that protein supplements improve bone mineral density but do not affect hip fracture risk.[34] Other research suggests that protein has favorable effects on bone health in the elderly only if they are consuming adequate amounts of calcium.[35,36]

Vegetarians, including older vegetarians, consume diets that are lower in protein than omnivore diets (Appendix P). This may be advantageous for some. Excess protein, especially nondairy animal protein,[37] may exacerbate the decline in kidney function that is often seen in aging. Replacing animal protein with plant protein may help preserve kidney function, especially in those with mild renal insufficiency.[37] However, it is important that all older vegetarians consume a variety of protein-rich foods and select protein-dense foods, such as soy products and legumes. Older vegetarians should strive for protein intakes that meet or slightly exceed the RDA.

Calcium

Bone loss begins prior to menopause in women and is highest within the first 1 to 5 years after menopause; bone loss slows after that, although higher rates of loss have been seen in women ≥85 years of age.[38] Men also lose bone mass at rates that are lower than those seen in women,[39] but older men, like older women, have an increased risk of osteoporosis and fracture.[40]

Calcium supplementation at a level of ≥1200 mg/d has been associated with reduced bone loss and reduced fracture risk in men and women age ≥50 years with the greatest effect seen in those with low dietary calcium intakes.[41] The calcium adequate intake (AI) for men and women >51 years of age is 1200 mg.[42] Despite evidence that calcium absorption decreases with age,[43,44] the Food and Nutrition Board (FNB) concluded there were not enough data to increase the calcium AI for those >70 years.[42]

Calcium intakes of older adults are frequently below recommendations. Results from NHANES III showed that 60% of men and 66% of women age ≥60 years had calcium intakes that were below the Healthy People 2010[45] calcium objective of 924 mg/d.[46] As indicated in Appendix R, older vegetarians commonly have calcium intakes below the current AI of 1200 mg/d and frequently have intakes lower than the Healthy People 2010 objectives.

About 25% of adults in the United States have lactose intolerance;[47] consequently, many older people are unable to drink milk without experiencing some discomfort, although modest quantities of milk can be tolerated.[48] However, some older people may no longer be able to tolerate milk. If milk has represented an important part of the diet in the past, it may be difficult for the older person to identify alternative sources of calcium. Lactase-fortified milk can be one option. Many older people may also enjoy calcium-fortified soymilk and other nondairy milks. Other sources of well-absorbed calcium include calcium-fortified orange juice and calcium supplements.[49] Dietitians can help older clients identify a wide variety of calcium-rich foods, including calcium-rich vegetables, beans, and nuts. However, it is difficult to achieve the calcium AI for older people even with the inclusion of dairy foods in the diet. Many older vegetarians, particularly vegans, benefit from the use of supplements and/or fortified foods.

Vitamin D

NHANES III found that as many as 30% of older people (≥60 years) had serum 25(OH)D levels indicative of insufficiency.[50] These lower levels are associated with decreased calcium absorption,[51] an increased risk of falls,[52] lower bone mass,[53,54] and an increased risk of fracture in the elderly.[52] Those living in northern regions are more likely to experience vitamin D deficiency.[55]

Compared to younger people, older people may be at increased risk for vitamin D deficiency for the following reasons:

- Less sun exposure due to decreased mobility and concerns about skin cancer
- Decreased vitamin D synthesis; young adults make as much as four times more vitamin D in their skin than older adults[56,57]
- Impaired renal synthesis of 1,25-dihydroxyvitamin D, possibly due to a decreased renal mass and/or an impaired response to parathyroid hormone[58]
- Increased vitamin D requirements due to medications commonly used by the elderly[42]
- Intakes below recommendations[59]

The AI for vitamin D is 10 μg (400 IU) for those 51 to 70 years and 15 μg (600 IU) for those >70 years.[42] Higher intakes of vitamin D appear to promote bone health. Supplements containing at least 800 IU of vitamin D and 1200 mg of calcium were effective in reducing fracture risk and bone loss in a meta-analysis of supplementation studies conducted in people age ≥50 years.[41] In lieu of adequate sun exposure, fortified foods or vitamin D supplements are the only reliable means of ensuring adequate vitamin D status. The only foods that naturally provide this vitamin are eggs and some fatty fish. In the United States, fortified milk is an important source of vitamin D. As noted earlier, however, many older people do not drink cow's milk. Other good sources of this nutrient include fortified soymilk and rice milks and fortified breakfast cereals (Table 7-2).

Iron

Anemia is relatively common in older people with 26% of men and 20% of women age ≥85 years having anemia.[60] About a sixth of anemias in older people in the United States are due to iron deficiency.[60] Older people with anemia, even mild anemia (hemoglobin <11 g/dL) are at higher risk for mortality and for declining physical ability.[61,62] Poor iron status can also lead to impaired immunity.[63]

Iron intakes of older adults in the United States are usually close to recommendations.[46] Limited information on iron intakes of older vegetarians suggest that they are similar to those of nonvegetarians (Appendix R). Intakes of vegetarians are typically lower than the iron RDA for vegetarians, however. Good sources of iron for older vegetarians include iron-fortified breakfast cereals and vegetarian "meats," dried beans, soyfoods, and whole grains (Table 6-3).

Vitamin B₁₂

Older people, regardless of dietary habits, may be at risk for vitamin B_{12} deficiency. Epidemiologic studies suggest, based on serum values, that vitamin B_{12} deficiency among older people is more common than once thought.[64-66] For example, >20% of Americans age ≥60 years are considered to have marginal vitamin B_{12} depletion based on serum levels.[64,65] Several instances of either extremely low serum levels of vitamin B_{12} or outright B_{12} deficiency have been seen in older vegans and vegetarians.[67-76]

In older people, the main cause of vitamin B_{12} deficiency is impaired absorption of cobalamin from food.[77] This is due to atrophic gastritis, which leads to a reduced ability to release the vitamin from food. Atrophic gastritis may occur in as much as 30% of the population >50 years[78] and in as much as 37% of those ≥ 80 years.[79] This condition also leads to increases in levels of bacteria in the intestines that may compete for vitamin B_{12},[80,81] although these bacteria may also synthesize vitamin B_{12}.[82] Other factors contributing to the poor vitamin B_{12} status of the elderly may include a compromised functioning of the vitamin B_{12} binding proteins and depleted B_{12} stores.[83]

There is evidence that some of the physical, psychological, and emotional changes often attributed to aging might actually be caused by marginal vitamin B_{12} deficiency. These include depression, restlessness, irritability, mood swings, panic disorders, phobic disorders, impotence, confusion, disorientation, memory loss, concentration difficulties, hearing loss, dementia, chronic fatigue, apathy, insomnia, and even psychotic episodes.[84-86] Not all research supports this, however; a 2007 systematic review found no association between blood concentrations of vitamin B_{12} and cognition or the risk of Alzheimer's disease.[87] Marginal or deficient vitamin B_{12} status has been associated with poorer bone health in elderly women[88] and in vegetarians.[89]

In addition, lower vitamin B_{12} levels have been associated with increased serum homocysteine, which may be a risk factor for vascular disease among both the young and the elderly.[90,91] Some studies,[92-95] but not all,[96,97] have demonstrated higher levels of homocysteine among vegetarian subjects. De Jong and coworkers reported a 25% reduction in blood homocysteine concentrations when elderly subjects consumed 0.25 mg of folic acid and 2.5 µg of vitamin B_{12} per day from fortified foods.[98]

The current RDA for vitamin B_{12} for older people is 2.4 µg, the same as for younger adults.[78] Because of malabsorption problems, it is not clear that simply increasing dietary vitamin B_{12} intake among older people will actually increase blood levels.[99-102] However, although absorption of vitamin B_{12} from food decreases with age, absorption of crystalline vitamin B_{12} does not. Therefore, the FNB advises that all older people use fortified foods or supplements to meet most of their vitamin B_{12} needs.[78] So older vegetarians who get most of their vitamin B_{12} from fortified foods and supplements may actually have better vitamin B_{12} status than older nonvegetarians who rely on meat or poultry for their vitamin B_{12}. Older people, including vegetarians, are encouraged to maintain a good, rather than just an adequate, vitamin B_{12} status.[86]

Calls to fortify flour with vitamin B_{12} in the United States and other industrialized countries have been mainly due to a desire to improve the vitamin B_{12} status of the elderly.[77] Due to the cost of the fortificant, the Flour Fortification Initiative recommended a level of 2 µg/100 g of flour, which would result in an average intake (based on typical flour consumption in the United States) of 3 µg/d.[77] Not all experts support this fortification program until further studies on issues including risk of toxicity and evidence of benefits of low-dose vitamin B_{12} supplementation on cognitive decline are conducted.[86,103,104]

Vitamin B$_6$

A limited number of studies suggest that vitamin B$_6$ requirements increase with age.[78] Both plasma vitamin B$_6$ levels and parameters of vitamin B$_6$ status have been shown to be low in older people.[105–108] The RDA for vitamin B$_6$ for older people is 1.7 mg and 1.5 mg for men and women, respectively,[78] and is higher than for younger adults, but some research suggests that requirements for older people may actually be as high as 2.0 mg.[109] Selhub et al found that serum homocysteine levels were higher in older people when B$_6$ intakes were <2.0 mg.[110] Serum homocysteine is affected by vitamin B$_6$, vitamin B$_{12}$, and folate status and possibly by riboflavin status. Because hyperhomocysteinemia has been associated with cognitive decline,[87] the role of vitamin B$_6$ in cognitive deficit in the elderly has been studied. Overall, there does not appear to be an association between serum vitamin B$_6$ and cognition.[87]

Riboflavin

In the past, riboflavin recommendations have been lower for older people because of their reduced calorie intakes. However, research shows that the riboflavin needs of older people are similar to those of younger people,[111] and the most recent RDAs of 1.3 mg/d for men and 1.1 mg/d for women >70 years[78] reflect this. Older vegetarians consuming a high-carbohydrate, low-fat diet, however, might require somewhat less riboflavin (about 5–10% less) than older omnivores consuming less carbohydrate because, in a metabolic feeding study, subjects consuming a high-carbohydrate, low-fat (20% fat) diet required less dietary riboflavin to achieve normal riboflavin status than subjects consuming a high-fat diet (30% fat).[84] This may be because a high-carbohydrate diet leads to greater riboflavin synthesis by the intestinal bacteria, some of which is absorbed.[84]

NUTRITIONAL FACTORS AFFECTING COGNITIVE FUNCTION

Close to 4.6 million older people worldwide become cognitively impaired each year.[112] Nutritional factors can play a role in cognitive function. The deterioration of cognitive processes may be due, in part, to oxygen free radicals.[113] Thus diets that are high in antioxidants such as vitamin E and possibly vitamin C may play a protective role.[113] Elevated serum homocysteine levels increase the risk of Alzheimer's disease,[87,114] although an association with blood levels or dietary intakes of folate or vitamins B$_6$ and B$_{12}$ has not been seen consistently.[87,115] Due to a limited number of good quality studies, additional research is recommended.[87] Omega-3 fatty acids may also play a role in prevention and treatment of Alzheimer's disease, although results are inconsistent.[116] (Chapter 4 provides more information on this topic.)

MEAL PLANNING FOR OLDER PEOPLE

It is increasingly evident that nutritional needs of older people demand the attention of dietitians.[117] This is a stage where energy needs begin to decrease while nutrient needs remain the same or may even increase. It is clear that changes in dietary habits are warranted and that special attention should be given to nutrient-dense foods. In addition, there are certain challenges to meeting the dietary needs of older people. A variety of physical, social, and psychological conditions that may accompany aging can affect food choices; also, lifelong dietary habits can be difficult to change. Food habits of people in their 70s and 80s may require special attention because some research indicates that those 60 to 70 years of age make more healthful food choices than those 75 to 85 years.[118]

Dietitians need to work closely with older clients to develop strategies for meeting dietary requirements in the face of many complicating factors whether the client is vegetarian or not. Older vegetarians can follow the same meal-planning guidelines for younger vegetarian adults outlined in Chapter 10. By avoiding the use of low nutrient dense foods, it should be possible to achieve adequate nutrient intake within an appropriate caloric allowance. It is especially important to include daily servings of foods that are fortified with vitamins D and B_{12}. Older people should also be encouraged to include plenty of fluids in their diets to help prevent constipation and dehydration.

FACTORS THAT AFFECT FOOD CHOICES

In helping older people make food choices, it is important to evaluate a variety of factors that may affect those choices (Exhibit 15-1).

Decreased Appetite

Taste acuity diminishes with aging. This may be due more to a decline in the sense of smell than to the reduced number of taste buds seen with aging.[119] Loss of the ability to smell and taste food frequently leads to a poor appetite and can result in weight loss and malnutrition.[17,119] Loss of smell can make it more difficult to distinguish weak tastes. There may be a tendency to over-salt foods to make them more flavorful and because of a decline in the ability to taste salt.[120] Dietitians can help clients choose flavorful foods that are low in sodium. A number of salt-free herb blends are available. Lemon juice, herb-flavored vinegars, and other condiments can help perk up food flavors. Spicy dishes may also appeal to some older people. In formulating recommendations, however, it is necessary to realize that many older Seventh-day Adventists avoid black pepper and sometimes vinegar as well.

Many older people may show an increased desire for sweets. In younger people, intensely sweet foods are perceived as unpleasant, but with aging this response to sweet foods diminishes, and sweet flavors are more acceptable.[121,122] Dietitians can take advantage of this by encouraging consumption of sweet foods that offer good nutrition. Some examples are chopped dried fruits mixed into hot cereals, fruit smoothies or fruit-flavored milkshakes, blackstrap molasses added to bean dishes, baked fruits, and fruit-oat crisps.

Anorexia can also be a side effect of drugs. Poor appetite can be exacerbated by loneliness and isolation. Feelings of loneliness have been found to be inversely related to caloric intake.[123] In addition, depression and dementia have both been associated with decreased appetite and weight loss in older people.[124]

Exhibit 15-1 Recommendations for Healthful Food Choices for Older Vegetarians

Considerations in food choices for older people to make good food choices include convenience of preparation, ease of chewing, and cost.

Convenient foods include:
Pasta with prepared sauce
Canned soup with crackers (choose low-sodium soups where possible)
Textured vegetable protein with canned meatless sloppy joe sauce
Frozen vegetarian burgers
Vegetarian baked beans
Peanut butter sandwich
Instant soup (many are lower in sodium than canned soups)
Bagel with fruit spread or nut butter
Cereal with milk
Instant hot cereal with fresh, canned, or dried fruit
Frozen pizza
Cottage cheese and fruit
Prepared bean tacos
Homemade bean tacos using canned refried beans or reconstituted dried refried beans
Instant flavored rice mixes tossed with cooked frozen vegetables
Three-bean salad
Baked potatoes
Tofu marinated in barbecue sauce and baked in the oven
Instant mashed potatoes
Canned low-sodium vegetables
Frozen vegetables
Canned and instant soups

Easy-to-chew foods:
White bread
Couscous
Potatoes
Sweet potatoes
Cooked cereals
Cooked and canned vegetables with high water content (winter and summer squash; eggplant)
Stewed fruit
Tofu
Textured vegetable protein
Creamed soups
Beans, particularly canned
Nut butters

Affordable foods:
Macaroni and cheese mix from a box
Canned beans
Baked potatoes
Peanut butter
Quick (not instant) oatmeal
Textured soy protein
Frozen greens

Decreased Mobility and Dexterity

For many older people, cooking may present some difficulties. In one study, approximately 4% and 17% of noninstitutionalized Americans >65 and 85 years of age, respectively, reported that they could not prepare their own meals because of a health or physical problem.[125] Many homebound older persons report difficulties in preparing meals. Assistance with meal preparation is the most frequent form of help received by elderly users of home health care services.[117]

Using some convenience foods such as canned soups and frozen entrees can help older people with limited cooking ability choose healthy meals. Although many of these are high in fat and sodium, they can be used occasionally provided that most of the dietary choices are whole foods that are low in fat and sodium. Frozen entrees with reduced fat and sodium are also available, although these tend to be expensive. Also, many packaged items, particularly those wrapped tightly in cellophane, can be difficult to open for older people with poor hand strength and coordination. All these factors need to be considered in helping older people make food choices that include easy-to-prepare items.

Appliances that make preparation easier include microwave ovens, food processors, and slow cookers. Many older people may need to be taught to use these, however. Also, older people with poor eyesight may not be able to read preparation directions on packages, so that unfamiliar cooking techniques may require some help.

Finally, the dietitian may be able to help clients identify community resources for seniors. Meals on Wheels (a national network of programs that provide congregate and home-delivered meals to the elderly, funded by the federal Elderly Nutrition Program) has a 4-week set of vegetarian menus.[126] Exhibit 15-2 offers suggestions for menu substitutions provided by federal guidelines. These could meet the needs of vegetarians and also could result in meals that are more likely to appeal to minority populations. It may also be possible to arrange for special meals where resources allow. In more populated areas, some Seventh-day Adventist churches may be involved

---

Exhibit 15-2 Possible Substitutions in the USDA Food Guide Meal Plan That Produce Meals Suitable for Vegetarians

---

Substitutions for 1 oz cooked meat:[127]

> 1 egg
> 1 oz cheese
> ½ cup cooked dried beans, peas, lentils, or tofu
> 2 tbsp peanut butter
> ⅓ cup nuts
> ¼ cup cottage cheese

Source: National Resource Center on Nutrition, Physical Activity & Aging. Older Americans Act Nutrition Programs Toolkit. 2005. http://nutritionandaging.fiu.edu/OANP_Toolkit/toolkit%20update%202.7.06.pdf. Accessed February 8, 2010.

in providing low-cost vegetarian meals to seniors. Cafeterias in Seventh-day Adventist hospitals also offer inexpensive vegetarian meals.

Problems with Chewing

Many older people have problems chewing tough or hard foods. A dental referral may be advised to make sure that dentures are properly fitted. A healthy diet can also easily be planned around foods that are soft and easy to chew. Refined grains, such as white bread and rolls, couscous, and white rice, can be easier to chew than their whole grain counterparts. Although adequate fiber is an important concern in the diets of older people, vegetarians are likely to be consuming much more fiber than their nonvegetarian peers. As long as some whole fiber-rich foods are emphasized in the diet, the moderate use of refined foods is certainly acceptable in the diets of vegetarians.

Many fiber-rich foods can be easy to eat. These include baked potatoes (rich in fiber even without the skin), sweet potatoes, oatmeal, multigrain hot cereals, cooked vegetables (especially softer vegetables such as zucchini, winter squash, and eggplant), stewed or baked fruits, and well-cooked beans.

Tofu is easy to chew and can be used in a variety of ways, including cubes of tofu in soups, creamed tofu pureed with vegetables and served as a cream soup or sauce over rice, and crumbled tofu mixed with mayonnaise as a sandwich filling. Textured soy protein, particularly the granular form, has a texture similar to that of ground beef and makes an easy-to-prepare meat substitute. Cream of vegetable soups or soups with pasta and well-cooked vegetables are popular with many older people. Beans can be cooked to a tender stage to make them easy to chew and digest. Nut butters on soft bread provide a nutrient- and calorie-rich meal or snack.

Cost Constraints

Limited income is a common constraint for seniors and may affect food purchases. Dietitians can help them plan low-cost meals that are nutritious. This can be particularly difficult in view of some of the other potential restrictions just discussed. For example, seniors who are cooking for themselves only and/or have trouble preparing meals are likely to gravitate toward convenience foods, which tend to be expensive. Some convenience foods are inexpensive, however, and some low-cost foods are relatively easy to prepare.

Where seniors are unable to meet their living expenses, the dietitian needs to be able to make referrals to the appropriate social agencies to arrange for financial help. Local food banks and charitable institutions can also offer assistance.

SAMPLE MENUS FOR OLDER VEGETARIANS

When planning meals for seniors, there may be many factors to take into consideration. Important goals include helping clients choose foods that are nutrient rich and are enjoyed, that fit well within the senior's budget, and that consider any constraints in meal preparation ability and eating ability. The menus shown in Exhibit 15-3 follow the meal-planning guide in Chapter 10 and use foods that are likely to meet the needs of seniors.

Exhibit 15-3 Two-Day Menu for Older Vegetarians*

Meal	Day 1	Day 2
Breakfast	¾ cup quick oatmeal with ½ cup fortified soymilk and ½ sliced banana, 1 cup calcium-fortified orange juice	1 cup bran flakes with ½ cup fortified soymilk; one slice toast; coffee, tea, or herbal tea
Snack	½ cup canned peaches, 1 oat bran muffin, 1 cup herbal tea	Fruit smoothie with ½ cup calcium-fortified orange juice, ½ banana, ¼ cup strawberries, ½ cup calcium-set tofu
Lunch	Sloppy joes (½ cup textured soy protein with ½ cup Manwich sauce), one whole wheat hamburger bun, 1 cup cooked collards, 1 cup water	1 cup spaghetti with 1 cup spaghetti sauce and ½ cup chickpeas, 1 cup steamed broccoli, 1 cup juice
Snack	One slice toast with 2 tbsp almond butter; 1 cup calcium-fortified soymilk	Four saltines with 2 tbsp almond butter; 1 cup calcium-fortified soymilk
Dinner	One small baked potato, ½ cup vegetarian baked beans, 1 cup steamed fresh or frozen kale, one slice bread, ½ stewed figs, 1 cup decaffeinated coffee	1 cup canned or instant or homemade lentil soup, four crackers, 1 cup steamed frozen or fresh asparagus, sliced tomatoes, 1 whole wheat roll with margarine, ½ cup canned fruit cocktail, 1 cup water

*Additional foods may be needed to meet energy needs. Foods supplying omega-3 fats should be used daily (see Chapter 10). If fortified foods, such as soymilk and breakfast cereals do not provide enough vitamin B_{12} and vitamin D to meet needs, supplements of these vitamins should be used.

COUNSELING POINTS FOR OLDER VEGETARIANS

- Most older people require supplements or fortified foods that provide vitamin D and calcium.
- As calorie needs decrease with aging, it is important to reduce food intake to avoid unwanted weight gain. However, inadequate caloric intake and underweight are also unhealthful.
- Emphasize nutrient-dense foods in the diet. As calorie needs decrease, requirements for most nutrients stay the same. For some nutrients, like calcium, vitamin D, and vitamin B_6, recommendations increase with age.
- Although this is not reflected in the RDAs, protein needs may increase with aging. Emphasize foods that are good sources of protein such as soyfoods and legumes, and, for lacto-ovo vegetarians, lower fat dairy foods.
- Keep sodium intake moderate. Other ways to intensify the flavor of foods include adding herb-flavored vinegar, fresh lemon juice, salsa and other condiments using hot peppers, and sodium-free herb mixes.
- Identify foods that provide fiber but are soft for those who have problems chewing.
- Identify foods that are easily prepared and affordable.

Case Studies

Bill is a 75-year-old man whose wife has recently died. He has followed a lacto-ovo vegetarian diet for most of his life and is doing his best to prepare meals. Bill has limited knowledge of food preparation because this was mainly his wife's responsibility. He has little interest in food or eating and has lost 10 lb in the past 3 months. He has no family support because his only child died about 6 years ago. In addition, Bill is on a fixed income and has lost several teeth due to gum disease. He plans to see a dentist in a few months when he has saved some money but is currently having difficulty chewing foods like raw fruits and vegetables and nuts.

What are Bill's main nutritionally related problems?

What suggestions do you have for Bill?

The congregate meals program in your community has received many requests from participants for vegetarian meals and has contacted you for menu planning. Use the Administration on Aging Guidelines (http://www.aoa.gov/AoARoot/AoA_Programs/OAA/oaa_full.asp#_Toc153957696) to plan three lunch menus that will be appropriate for vegetarians and meet the guidelines. Menus should include options that would allow them to be used by vegan participants.

REFERENCES

1. Personal communication. Charles Stahler, The Vegetarian Resource Group, February 2010.
2. Goulding MR, Rogers ME, Smith SM. Public health and aging: trends in aging—United States and worldwide. *MMWR.* 2003;52:101–106.
3. Yankelovich, Skelly, White/Clancy, Shulman, Inc. The American vegetarian: coming of age in the 90s (a study of the vegetarian marketplace conducted by Vegetarian Times, Inc.). Oak Park, IL, 1992.
4. Fraser GB, Shavlik DJ. Ten years of life. Is it a matter of choice? *Arch Intern Med.* 2001;161:1645–1652.
5. Brants HA, Lowik MR, Westenbrink S, et al. Adequacy of a vegetarian diet at old age (Dutch Nutrition Surveillance System). *J Am Coll Nutr.* 1990; 9:292–302.
6. Gibson RS, Anderson BM, Sabry JH. The trace metal status of a group of post-menopausal vegetarians. *J Am Diet Assoc.* 1983; 82:246–250.
7. Nieman DC, Underwood BC, Sherman KM, et al. Dietary status of Seventh-day Adventist vegetarian and non-vegetarian elderly women. *J Am Diet Assoc.* 1989; 89:1763–1769.
8. Hunt IF, Murphy NJ, Henderson C. Food and nutrient intake of Seventh-day Adventist women. *Am J Clin Nutr.* 1988; 48:850–851.
9. Marsh AG, Christiansen DK, Sanchez TV, et al. Nutrient similarities and differences of older lacto-ovo vegetarian and omnivorous women. *Nutr Rep Int.* 1989;39:19–24.
10. Gallagher D, Visser M, DeMeersman RE, et al. Appendicular skeletal muscle mass: effects of age, gender, and ethnicity. *J Appl Physiol.* 1997;83:229–239.
11. Gallagher D, Ruts E, Visser M, et al. Weight stability masks sarcopenia in elderly men and women. *Am J Physiol Endocrinol Metab.* 2000;279:E366–E375.
12. Food and Nutrition Board, Institute of Medicine. *Dietary Reference Intakes for Energy, Carbohydrate, Fiber, Fat, Fatty Acids, Cholesterol, Protein, and Amino Acids.* Washington, DC: National Academy Press; 2002.
13. Briefel RR, McDowell MA, Alaimo K, et al. Total energy intake of the US population: the third National Health and Nutrition Examination Survey, 1988–1991. *Am J Clin Nutr.* 1995;62(5 suppl):1072S–1080S.

14. French SA, Jeffery RW, Folsom AR, et al. History of intentional and unintentional weight loss in a population-based sample of women aged 55 to 69 years. *Obes Res.* 1995;3(2):163–170.

15. Williamson DF. Descriptive epidemiology of body weight and weight change in U.S. adults. *Ann Intern Med.* 1993; 119:646–649.

16. French SA, Folsom AR, Jeffery RW, Williamson DF. Prospective study of intentionality of weight loss and mortality in older women: the Iowa Women's Health Study. *Am J Epidemiol.* 1999;149(6):504–514.

17. Bales CW, Ritchie CS. Sarcopenia, weight loss, and nutritional frailty in the elderly. *Annu Rev Nutr.* 2002. 22:309–323.

18. Gulsvik AK, Thelle DS, Mowé M, Wyller TB. Increased mortality in the slim elderly: a 42 years follow-up study in a general population. *Eur J Epidemiol.* 2009;24(11):683–690.

19. Miller MD, Thomas JM, Cameron ID, et al. BMI: a simple, rapid and clinically meaningful index of under-nutrition in the oldest old? *Br J Nutr.* 2009;101(9):1300–1305.

20. Roberts SB, Hajduk CL, Howarth NC, et al. Dietary variety predicts low body mass index and inadequate macro-nutrient and micronutrient intakes in community-dwelling older adults. *J Gerontol A Biol Sci Med Sci.* 2005;6A:613–621.

21. Rand WM, Pellett PL, Young VR. Meta-analysis of nitrogen balance studies for estimating protein requirements in healthy adults. *Am J Clin Nutr.* 2003;77:109–127.

22. Millward DJ. Sufficient protein for our elders? *Am J Clin Nutr.* 2008;88:1187–1188.

23. Gersovitz M, Motil K, Munro HN, et al. Human protein requirements: assessment of the adequacy of the current recommended dietary allowance for dietary protein in elderly men and women. *Am J Clin Nutr.* 1982;35:6–14.

24. Campbell WW, Crim MC, Dallal GE, et al. Increased protein requirements in elderly people: new data and retro-spective reassessments. *Am J Clin Nutr.* 1994;60:501–509.

25. Castaneda C, Charnley JM, Evans WJ, Crim MC. Elderly women accommodate to a low-protein diet with losses of body cell mass, muscle function, and immune response. *Am J Clin Nutr.* 1995;62(1):30–39.

26. Kurpad AV, Vaz M. Protein and amino acid requirements in the elderly. *Eur J Clin Nutr.* 2000;54(suppl 3): S131–S142.

27. Campbell WW. Dietary protein requirements of older people: is the RDA adequate? *Nutrition Today.* 1996; 31:192–197.

28. Chernoff R. Protein and older adults. *J Am Coll Nutr.* 2004;23(6 suppl):627S–630S.

29. Campbell WW, Johnson CA, McCabe GP, Carnell NS. Dietary protein requirements of younger and older adults. *Am J Clin Nutr.* 2008;88:1322–1329.

30. Millward DJ, Roberts SB. Protein requirements of older individuals. *Nutr Res Rev.* 1996;9:67–87.

31. Campbell WW. Synergistic use of higher-protein diets or nutritional supplements with resistance training to counter sarcopenia. *Nutr Rev.* 2007;65:416–422.

32. Haub MD, Wells AM, Campbell WW. Beef and soy-based food supplements differentially affect serum lipoprotein-lipid profiles because of changes in carbohydrate intake and novel nutrient intake ratios in older men who resistive-train. *Metabolism.* 2005;54:769–774.

33. Haub MD, Wells AM, Tarnopolsky MA, Campbell WW. Effect of protein source on resistive-training-induced changes in body composition and muscle size in older men. *Am J Clin Nutr.* 2002;76:511–517.

34. Darling AL, Millward DJ, Torgerson DJ, Hewitt CE, Lanham-New SA. Dietary protein and bone health: a system-atic review and meta-analysis. *Am J Clin Nutr.* 2009;90:1674–1692.

35. Rapuri PB, Gallagher JC, Gatbatzja V. Protein intake: effects on bone mineral density and the rate of bone loss in elderly women. *Am J Clin Nutr.* 2003;77:1517–1525.

36. Dawson-Hughes B, Harris SS. Calcium intake influences the association of protein intake with rates of bone loss in elderly men and women. *Am J Clin Nutr.* 2002;75(4):773–779.

37. Knight EL, Stampfer MJ, Hankinson SE, et al. The impact of protein intake on renal function decline in women with normal renal function or mild renal insufficiency. *Ann Intern Med.* 2003;138:460–467.

38. Ensrud KE, Palermo L, Black DM, et al. Hip and calcaneal bone loss increase with advancing age: longitudinal results from the study of osteoporotic fractures. *J Bone Miner Res.* 1995;10:1778–1787.

39. Hannan MT, Felson DT, Dawson-Hughes B, et al. Risk factors for longitudinal bone loss in elderly men and women: the Framingham Osteoporosis Study. *J Bone Miner Res.* 2000;15(4):710–720.

40. Khosla S. Update in male osteoporosis. *J Clin Endocrinol Metab.* 2010;95:3–10.
41. Tang BMP, Eslick GD, Nowson C, et al. Use of calcium or calcium in combination with vitamin D supplementation to prevent fractures and bone loss in people aged 50 years and older: a meta-analysis. *Lancet.* 2007;370:657–666.
42. Institute of Medicine, Food and Nutrition Board. *Dietary Reference Intakes for Calcium, Phosphorus, Magnesium, Vitamin D, and Fluoride.* Washington, DC: National Academy Press; 1997.
43. Heaney RP, Gallagher JC, Johnston CC, et al. Calcium nutrition and bone health in the elderly. *Am J Clin Nutr.* 1982;36:986–1013.
44. Weaver CM. Age related calcium requirements due to changes in absorption and utilization. *J Nutr.* 1994;124:1418S–1425S.
45. U.S. Department of Health and Human Services. *Objectives for Improving Health.* Washington, DC: US Government Printing Office; 2000. *Healthy People 2010,* vol 2, 2nd ed.
46. Ervin RB, Kennedy-Stephenson J. Mineral intakes of elderly adult supplement and non-supplement users in the Third National Health and Nutrition Examination Study. *J Nutr.* 2002;132:3422–3427.
47. Coffin B, Azpiroz F, Guarner F, et al. Selective gastric hypersensitivity and reflex hyporeactivity in functional dyspepsia. *Gastroenterology.* 1994;107:1345–1351.
48. Johnson AO, Semenya JG, Buchowski MS, et al. Adaptation of lactose maldigesters to continued milk intakes. *Am J Clin Nutr.* 1993;58:879–881.
49. Martini L, Wood RJ. Relative bioavailability of calcium-rich dietary sources in the elderly. *Am J Clin Nutr.* 2002;76:1345–1350.
50. Looker AC, Dawson-Hughes B, Calvo MS, et al. Serum 25-hydroxyvitamin D status of adolescents and adults in two seasonal subpopulations from NHANES III. *Bone.* 2002;30:771–777.
51. Heaney RP. Vitamin D and calcium interactions: functional outcomes. *J Clin Nutr.* 2008;88(suppl):541S–544S.
52. Dawson-Hughes B. Serum 25-hydroxyvitamin D and functional outcomes in the elderly. *J Clin Nutr.* 2008;88(suppl):537S–540S.
53. Bischoff-Ferrari HA, Dietrich T, Orav EJ, Dawson-Hughes B. Positive association between 25-hydroxy vitamin D levels and bone mineral density: a population-based study of younger and older adults. *Am J Med.* 2004;116:634–639.
54. Cranney A, Weiler HA, O'Donnell S, Puil L. Summary of evidence-based review on vitamin D efficacy and safety in relation to bone health. *Am J Clin Nutr.* 2008;88(suppl):513S–519S.
55. Rosen CJ, Morrison A, Zhou H, et al. Elderly women in northern New England exhibit seasonal changes in bone mineral density and calciotropic hormones. *Bone Miner.* 1994;25:83–92.
56. Holick MF, Matsuoka LY, Wortsman J. Age, vitamin D, and solar ultraviolet. *Lancet.* 1989; 2:1104–1105.
57. Need AG, Morris HA, Horowitz M, Nordin C. Effects of skin thickness, age, body fat, and sunlight on serum 25-hydroxyvitamin D. *Am J Clin Nutr.* 1993;58:882–885.
58. Tsai KS, Heath H 3rd, Kumar R, Riggs BL. Impaired vitamin D metabolism with aging in women. Possible role in pathogenesis of senile osteoporosis. *J Clin Invest.* 1984;73:1668–1672.
59. Moore C, Murphy MM, Keast DR, Holick MF. Vitamin D intake in the United States. *J Am Diet Assoc.* 2004;104(6):980–983.
60. Guralnik JM, Eisenstaedt RS, Ferrucci L, et al. Prevalence of anemia in persons 65 years and older in the United States: evidence for a high rate of unexpected anemia. *Blood.* 2004;104:2263–2268.
61. Kikuchi M, Inagaki T, Shinagawa N. Five-year survival of older people with anemia: variation with hemoglobin concentration. *J Am Geriatr Soc.* 2001;49:1226–1228.
62. Penninx BWJH, Guralnik JM, Onder G, et al. Anemia and decline in physical performance among older persons. *Am J Med.* 2003;115:104–110.
63. Heuberger R. Special topics in nutrition and the older adult: diet, life-style, disease, and pharmacologic considerations. In: Edelstein S, Sharlin J, eds. *Life Cycle Nutrition: A Evidence-Based Approach.* Sudbury, MA: Jones & Bartlett; 2009:377–408.
64. Pfeiffer CM, Caudill SP, Gunter EW, et al. Biochemical indicators of B vitamin status in the US population after folic acid fortification: results from the National Health and Nutrition Examination Survey 1999–2000. *Am J Clin Nutr.* 2005;82:442–450.

65. Pfeiffer CM, Johnson CL, Jain RB, et al. Trends in blood folate and vitamin B-12 concentrations in the United States, 1988–2004. *Am J Clin Nutr.* 2007;86:718–727.

66. Campbell AK, Miller JW, Green R, et al. Plasma vitamin B-12 concentrations in an elderly Latino population are predicted by serum gastrin concentrations and crystalline vitamin B-12 intake. *J Nutr.* 2003;133:2770–2776.

67. Murphy MF. Vitamin B12 deficiency due to a low-cholesterol diet in a vegetarian. *Ann Intern Med.* 1981;94:57–58.

68. Wokes F, Badenoch J, Sinclair HM. Human dietary deficiency of vitamin B12. *Am J Clin Nutr.* 1955;16:590–602.

69. Wokes F. Anaemia and vitamin B12 dietary deficiency. *Proc Nutr Soc.* 1956;15:134–141.

70. Harrison RJ, Booth CC, Mollin DL. Vitamin-B12 deficiency due to defective diet. *Lancet.* 1956;1:727–728.

71. Connor PM, Pirola RC. Nutritional vitamin B12 deficiency. *Med J Aust.* 1963;2:451–453.

72. Winawer SJ, Strieiff RR, Zamcheck N. Gastric and hematological abnormalities in a vegan with nutritional vitamin B12 deficiency: effect of oral vitamin B12. *Gastroenterology.* 1967;3:130–135.

73. Carmel R. Nutritional vitamin B12 deficiency. Possible contributory role of subtle vitamin B12 malabsorption. *Ann Intern Med.* 1978;88:647–649.

74. Kwok T, Cheng G, Woo J, et al. Independent effect of vitamin B12 deficiency on hematological status in older Chinese vegetarian women. *Am J Hematol.* 2002;70(3):186–190.

75. Su TC, Jeng JS, Wang JD, et al. Homocysteine, circulating vascular cell adhesion molecule and carotid atherosclerosis in postmenopausal vegetarian women and omnivores. *Atherosclerosis.* 2006;184(2):356–362.

76. Waldmann A, Koschizke JW, Leitzmann C, Hahn A. Homocysteine and cobalamin status in German vegans. *Public Health Nutr.* 2004;7(3):467–472.

77. Allen LH. How common is vitamin B-12 deficiency? *Am J Clin Nutr.* 2009;89(suppl):693S–696S.

78. Institute of Medicine, Food and Nutrition Board. *Dietary Reference Intakes for Thiamin, Riboflavin, Niacin, Vitamin B6, Folate, Vitamin B12, Pantothenic Acid, Biotin, and Choline.* Washington, DC: National Academy Press; 1998.

79. Krasinski SD, Russell RM, Samloff IM, et al. Fundic atrophic gastritis in an elderly population. Effect on hemoglobin and several serum nutritional indicators. *J Am Geriatr Soc.* 1986;34:800–806.

80. Suter PM, Golner BB, Goldin BR, et al. Reversal of protein-bound vitamin B12 malabsorption with antibiotics in atrophic gastritis. *Gastroenterology.* 1991;101:1039–1045.

81. Nilsson-Ehle H, Landahl S, Lindstedt G, et al. Low serum cobalamin levels in a population study of 70- and 75-year-old subjects. Gastrointestinal causes and hematological effects. *Dig Dis Sci.* 1989;34:716–723.

82. Herbert V. Vitamin B-12: plant sources, requirements, and assay. *Am J Clin Nutr.* 1988;48:852–858.

83. Van Asselt DZ, van den Broek WJ, Corstens CBL, et al. Free and protein-bound cobalamin absorption in healthy middle-aged and older subjects. *J Am Geriatr Soc.* 1996;44:949–953.

84. Houston DK, Johnson MA, Nozza RJ, et al. Age-related hearing loss, vitamin B-12, and folate in elderly women. *Am J Clin Nutr.* 1999;69:564–571.

85. Baik HW, Russell RM. Vitamin B12 deficiency in the elderly. *Annu Rev Nutr.* 1999;19:357–377.

86. Smith AD, Refsum H. Vitamin B-12 and cognition in the elderly. *Am J Clin Nutr.* 2009;89(suppl):707S–711S.

87. Raman G, Tatsioni A, Chung M, et al. Heterogeneity and lack of good quality studies limit association between folate, vitamins B-6 and B-12, and cognitive function. *J Nutr.* 2007;137:1789–1794.

88. Dhonukshe-Rutten RAM, Lips M, de Jong N, et al. Vitamin B-12 status is associated with bone mineral content and bone mineral density in frail elderly women but not in men. *J Nutr.* 2003;133:801–807.

89. Herrmann W, Obeid R, Schorr H, et al. Enhanced bone metabolism in vegetarians—the role of vitamin B12 deficiency. *Clin Chem Lab Med.* 2009;47(11):1381–1387.

90. McCully KS. Homocysteine, vitamins, and vascular disease prevention. *Am J Clin Nutr.* 2007;86(5):1563S–1568S.

91. Ford ES, Smith SJ, Stroup DF, et al. Homocysteine and cardiovascular disease: a systematic review of the evidence with special emphasis on case-control studies and nested case- control studies. *Int J Epidemiol.* 2002;31:59–70.

92. DeRose DJ, Charles-Marcel ZL, Jamison JM, et al. Vegan diet-based lifestyle program rapidly lowers homocysteine levels. *Prev Med.* 2000;30:225–233.

93. Mann NJ, Li D, Sinclair AJ, et al. The effect of diet on plasma homocysteine concentrations in healthy male subjects. *Eur J Clin Nutr.* 1999;53:895–899.

94. Mezzano D, Munoz X, Martinez C, et al. Vegetarians and cardiovascular risk factors: hemostasis, inflammatory markers and plasma homocysteine. *Thromb Haemost.* 1999;81:913–917.

95. Krajcovicova-Kudlackova M, Blazicek P, Kopcova J, et al. Homocysteine levels in vegetarians versus omnivores. *Ann Nutr Metab.* 2000;44:135–138.
96. Houghton LA, Green TJ, Donovan UM, et al. Association between dietary fiber intake and the folate status of a group of female adolescents. *Am J Clin Nutr.* 1997;66:1414–1421.
97. Haddad EH, Berk LS, Kettering JD, et al. Dietary intake and biochemical, hematologic, and immune status of vegans compared with nonvegetarians. *Am J Clin Nutr.* 1999;70:586S– 593S.
98. De Jong N, Chin A Paw MJM, de Groot L, et al. Nutrient dense foods and exercise in frail elderly: effects on B vitamins, homocysteine, methylmalonic acid, and neuropsychological functioning. *Am J Clin Nutr.* 2001;73:338–346.
99. Allen LH, Casterline J. Vitamin B-12 deficiency in elderly individuals: diagnosis and requirements. *Am J Clin Nutr.* 1994;60:12–14.
100. Herbert V. Vitamin B-12 and elderly people. *Am J Clin Nutr.* 1994;59:1093–1095.
101. Russell RM. Vitamin B12 and elderly people. Reply to V Herbert. *Am J Clin Nutr.* 1994;59:1094–1095.
102. Hurwitz A, Brady DA, Schaal SE, et al. Gastric acidity in older adults. *JAMA.* 1997;278:659–662.
103. Green R. Is it time for vitamin B-12 fortification? What are the questions? *Am J Clin Nutr.* 2009;89(suppl):712S–716S.
104. Refsum H, Smith AD. Are we ready for mandatory fortification with vitamin B-12? *Am J Clin Nutr.* 2008;88(2):253–254.
105. Rose CS, Gyorgy P, Butler M, et al. Age differences in vitamin B6 status of 617 men. *Am J Clin Nutr.* 1976;29:847–853.
106. Suter PM, Russell RM. Vitamin requirements of the elderly. *Am J Clin Nutr.* 1987;45:501–512.
107. Munro HN, Suter PM, Russell RM. Nutritional requirements of the elderly. *Annu Rev Nutr.* 1987;7:23–49.
108. Madigan SM, Tracey F, McNulty, et al. Riboflavin and vitamin B-6 intakes and status and biochemical response to riboflavin supplementation in free-living elderly people. *Am J Clin Nutr.* 1998;68:389–395.
109. Ribaya-Mercado JD, Russell RM, Sahyoun N, et al. Vitamin B-6 requirements of elderly men and women. *J Nutr.* 1991;121:1062–1074.
110. Selhub J, Jacques PF, Wilson PW, et al. Vitamin status and intake as primary determinants of homocysteinemia in an elderly population. *JAMA.* 1993;270:2693–2698.
111. Boisvert WA, Mendoza I, Castaneda C, et al. Riboflavin requirement of healthy elderly humans and its relationship to macronutrient composition of the diet. *J Nutr.* 1993;123:915–925.
112. Ferri CP, Prince M, Brayne C, et al. Global prevalence of dementia: a Delphi consensus study. *Lancet.* 2005;366:2112–2117.
113. Grodstein F, Chen J, Willett WC. High-dose antioxidant supplements and cognitive function in community-dwelling elderly women. *Am J Clin Nutr.* 2003;77:975–984.
114. Seshadri S, Beiser A, Selhub J, et al. Plasma homocysteine as a risk factor for dementia and Alzheimer's disease. *N Engl J Med.* 2002;346:476–483.
115. Balk EM, Raman G, Tatsioni A, et al. Vitamin B6, B12, and folic acid supplementation and cognitive function. A systematic review of randomized trials. *Arch Intern Med.* 2007;167:21–30.
116. Cole GM, Ma QL, Frautschy SA. Omega-3 fatty acids and dementia. *Prostaglandins Leukot Essent Fatty Acids.* 2009;81(2–3):213–221.
117. Kuczmarski MF, Weddle DO. Position paper of the American Dietetic Association. Nutrition across the spectrum of aging. *J Am Diet Assoc.* 2005;105:616–633.
118. Fischer CA, Crockett SJ, Heller KE, Skauge LH. Nutrition knowledge, attitudes, and practices of older and younger elderly in rural areas. *J Am Diet Assoc.* 1991;91:1398–1401.
119. Boyce JM, Shone GR. Effects of aging on smell and taste. *Postgrad Med.* 2006;82:239–241.
120. Morley JE. Decreased food intake with aging. *J Gerontol.* 2001;56A:81–88.
121. Mojet J, Heidema J, Christ-Hazelhof E. Taste perception with age: generic or specific losses in supra-threshold intensities of five taste qualities? *Chem Senses.* 2003;28(5):397–413.
122. Kamath SK. Taste acuity and aging. *Am J Clin Nutr.* 1982;36:766–775.
123. Walker D, Beauchene RE. The relationship of loneliness, social isolation, and physical health to dietary adequacy of independently living elderly. *J Am Diet Assoc.* 1991;91:300–304.

124. Morley JE. Anorexia of aging: physiologic and pathologic. *Am J Clin Nutr.* 1997;66:760–773.

125. US Department of Health and Human Services (DHHS) PHS, Centers for Disease Control and Prevention. *Physical Functioning of the Aged—United States, 1984.* Hyattsville, MD: US Department of Health and Human Services; 1989. DHHS publication (PHS) 89–1595.

126. Havala S, Abate T. The National Meals on Wheels Foundation Vegetarian Initiative: a unique collaboration. *J Nutr Elderly.* 1997;17:45–50.

127. National Resource Center on Nutrition, Physical Activity & Aging. Older Americans Act Nutrition Programs Toolkit. 2005. http://nutritionandaging.fiu.edu/OANP_Toolkit/toolkit%20update%202.7.06.pdf.

PART IV

Practical Implications

16

Carbohydrates, Fat, and Chronic Disease

Vegetarian diets may be especially effective in reducing the risk for diabetes and cardiovascular disease (CVD) and also for the management of these diseases. Vegetarians typically have lower intakes of total and saturated fat, and they consume more fiber and complex carbohydrates than omnivores. They are also less likely to be obese. However, there are unresolved issues regarding the roles of carbohydrate and fat in the prevention and treatment of chronic diseases. These questions may be particularly relevant to vegetarians because of their typically higher carbohydrate intake. This chapter provides a brief overview of issues related to macronutrient content of diets as they impact management of chronic disease and offers some guidelines for counseling vegetarians.

GLYCEMIC INDEX

The glycemic index (GI) ranks foods according to their effect on postprandial glycemia and is determined by ingesting 50 g of carbohydrate and comparing the area under the resultant serum glucose response curve to that generated by 50 g of pure glucose in the same individual (some earlier studies used white bread as the reference). By setting the response to glucose at 100, the relative values of other foods can be ascertained. The ingestion of individual carbohydrate-containing foods elicits a widely varied postprandial serum glucose response even when the quantity of carbohydrate is held constant.[1] Although there is considerable variability within and between subjects, individual carbohydrate-containing foods have characteristic GIs.[2,3] The glycemic load (GL) of a food or meal is the product of its GI and the amount of carbohydrate in the food or meal, and it is calculated as follows: GL= (GI × carbohydrate content per serving)/100.

Foods with a low GI include oats, barley, bulgur, legumes, pasta, pumpernickel bread, apples, oranges, milk, and yogurt. Variation in the rate of the absorption of carbohydrates from different foods is almost certainly the primary explanation for why foods have different GIs.[4] Factors that appear to slow carbohydrate absorption include a higher amylose-to-amylopectin ratio, acid, protein, fat, lactose, fructose, decreased ripeness of fruits, and rawness or undercooking. Fiber, which increases the viscosity of the intestinal contents and slows the interaction between starch and

417

enzymes, also results in a lower GI.[5] However, although the fiber content—particularly viscous fiber—of food does impact the GI, the predominant factor affecting absorption appears to be the physical state of the carbohydrate rather than fiber content.[6]

Particle size explains why the GI of 1-inch cubes of boiled potato is increased by 25% when the potatoes are mashed[7] and why ground brown rice produces a greater blood glucose and insulin response than unground brown rice.[8] However, some types of brown rice have a similar GI to some types of white rice. Corn flakes, which are fully gelatinized and thus likely to be rapidly absorbed and digested, have a high GI, and pasta because of its dense food matrix has a low GI.[9] For this reason, the GI of a food cannot be intuitively determined, and distinctions between simple and complex carbohydrates have little relevance to this concept. For example, a baked potato has a GI of 93, much higher than the GI of 65 for sucrose, which is relatively low because half of the molecule is composed of fructose, which does not contribute to serum glucose levels.

The Glycemic Index and Chronic Disease

Prospective studies have found that high-GI diets in combination with low fiber intakes increase the risk of type 2 diabetes more than twofold,[10,11] and clinical studies of persons with diabetes have found improved glycemic control with low-GI diets.[12–16] For example, in a 6-month parallel trial of 210 patients with type 2 diabetes, subjects following a low-GI diet had a greater decrease in glycosylated hemoglobin (HbA_{1c}) compared to those following a high cereal fiber diet (-0.5% vs -0.18%).[16] In agreement, in people with type 1 diabetes, low-GI diets were correlated with lower HbA_{1c}.[17]

Although some studies have not found support for the importance of GI in glucose control[18] or insulin sensitivity,[19] a recent Cochrane review of randomized controlled trials (RCTs) found that in people with diabetes, a low-GI diet led to improved glycemic control and a 0.5% decrease in HbA_{1c} in comparison to subjects on higher GI diets or measured carbohydrate exchange diets.[20]

Beyond diabetes, there is interest in the impact of the GI and GL on overall chronic disease risk.[21] A meta-analysis of 37 prospective observational studies involving predominantly female subjects concluded that diets with a high GI or GL were associated with increased risk of type 2 diabetes, heart disease, gallbladder disease, breast cancer, and all diseases combined.[22] Similarly, in the Nurses' Health Study, after 10 years of follow-up, the dietary GL was found to be directly associated with the risk of coronary heart disease (CHD) even after adjustment for age, smoking status, total energy intake, and other CHD risk factors. The relative CHD risk of women with the highest GL was twice that of women with the lowest GL. Risk was even more pronounced in overweight and obese women.[23]

The GI has also been studied in regard to weight control. For example, in a longitudinal study of 572 healthy adults, Ma et al[24] found a positive association between GI and body mass index (BMI). However, in an analysis of 8195 adults, GI was associated with BMI in women but not men, and the association was no longer significant after adjusting for fiber and energy intake.[25] Finally, some studies[26–28] but not all[29,30] have found low-GI diets to be beneficial for weight loss.

Critics have suggested that the usefulness of the GI is limited by within-person and between-person variability[31] and that it adds unnecessary complexity to nutrition education messages.

However, the GI is commonly used by practitioners in Canada, Australia, New Zealand, France, and the United Kingdom. Use of the GI may not be any more difficult a concept for some clients than the effects of different types of fatty acids on health. For those who are able to translate information about the GI into dietary practice, and for whom a lower GI diet may impact health, incorporating this message into dietary counseling may be useful. Although the American Diabetes Association concluded there is insufficient evidence to conclude that low-GL diets reduce the risk for diabetes, they suggest that low-GI foods that are rich in fiber are to be encouraged and may provide a modest additional benefit to the monitoring of total carbohydrate intake.[32]

The Glycemic Index in Vegetarian Diets

Vegetarian diets are typically higher in carbohydrates than omnivore eating patterns, but they may also have a lower GI[33] and be associated with improved insulin sensitivity. For example, Hua et al[34] found that in a comparison of 30 lacto-ovo vegetarians and 30 meat eaters, the vegetarians were more insulin sensitive. Insulin sensitivity was also better in Taiwanese lacto-ovo vegetarian women[35] and Chinese vegetarians[36] compared to omnivores. Among the Chinese vegetarians, insulin sensitivity correlated with years on a vegetarian diet.

Vegetarian diets are also typically lower in protein and somewhat lower in total fat compared to omnivore eating patterns. Research suggests that, although foods high in protein and fat have a lower GI, they actually raise insulin levels and thus may lead to hyperinsulinemia.[37–40] In one study, consumption of a meal containing cottage cheese produced an insulin response that was 3.6 times greater than that following ingestion of glucose.[41] Increases in insulin response to a protein load may increase disease risk.[42,43] However, one study showed that protein levels not exceeding 9 g per 50 g of carbohydrate had no effect on insulin response.[39] Therefore, vegetarian diets, which are typically more moderate in protein than omnivore diets, may improve glucose tolerance and insulin response. This is especially likely if these diets are based on plant foods with a lower GI.

DIABETES

In 2005, an estimated 20.8 million Americans had diabetes, and the number is estimated to triple by 2050.[44] The prevalence of impaired fasting glucose among the U.S. population may be as high as 6.9%.[45] And, according to some experts, as much as 25% of the population may be insulin resistant.[46] Insulin resistance or insensitivity can lead to hyperinsulinemia, which may increase risk for heart disease, diabetes, and possibly cancer. Based on data from the National Health and Nutrition Examination Survey (NHANES) III, nearly 12 million overweight people in the United States have prediabetes.[47] Diabetes is also increasingly a problem in developing countries where the prevalence of this disease is expected to increase 48% between 1995 and 2025, about twice the increase expected for developed countries.[48] Particularly striking is the increase in type 2 diabetes among young people.

Diet has played in important role in the treatment of diabetes since the early part of the 20th century, although recommendations have changed in accordance with a better understanding of this disease. Because it was recognized several centuries ago that people with diabetes excreted sugar in their urine, early recommendations were to restrict carbohydrates, especially simple sugars. However, dietary recommendations for carbohydrate intake when expressed as a percentage of total calories increased from 20% in 1921 to ≤60% in 1986. The current recommendation is for both dietary fat and carbohydrate intake to be determined on an individual basis and to be dictated by the achievement of treatment goals.

Lifestyle appears to play a significant role in the risk of developing type 2 diabetes. For example, within a given ethnic population, rural dwellers are far less likely to have diabetes than urban dwellers,[48] and the rate of diabetes is higher among Japanese who move to Hawaii or California than among those who live in Japan, and is higher among Yemenites who move to Israel than among those who live in Yemen.[49]

The first person to describe diabetes was a Hindu physician who noted 3000 years ago that the disease occurred in people who were "gluttonous and obese."[50] In 1927, Elliot Joslin wrote, "With an excess of fat diabetes begins."[51] Today, it is well recognized that obesity dramatically elevates the risk for type 2 diabetes. According to an analysis of the U.S. population, among nonobese persons age 45 to 54 years with a BMI of 22.5, the risk of type 2 diabetes was 3.0% for men and 3.2% for women. The risk increased with increasing BMIs.[52] Duration of obesity also correlates with risk. The younger the age of obesity onset, the greater the risk for diabetes.[53] Research suggests that BMI cut points for risk may be lower among Asians compared to other groups.[32]

Abdominal fat is much more closely related to diabetes risk than are hip and thigh fat.[54-56] In the Nurses' Health Study, after controlling for BMI and most other commonly accepted risk factors for diabetes, the relative risk of diabetes for women in the 90th percentile of waist-to-hip ratio was 3.1-fold greater than for women in the 10th percentile.[55]

Moderate weight loss (5% of body weight) has been associated with decreased insulin resistance and improved glycemic control.[57] Weight loss also lowers risk for developing type 2 diabetes.[58,59] Exercise is also related to a reduced risk for diabetes. According to one systematic review, people who engage in even moderate physical activity are as much as 30% less likely to develop diabetes than sedentary individuals.[60]

People with diabetes are at a marked increased risk of CHD.[61] Although CHD rates have declined among the general population, this has not been the case for diabetic patients.[62] The most common pattern of dyslipidemia in people with type 2 diabetes is elevated triglyceride and decreased high-density lipoprotein cholesterol (HDL-C) levels.[63] Also, people with type 2 diabetes often have a preponderance of smaller, dense low-density lipoprotein (LDL) particles, which may increase atherogenicity even if the absolute concentration of LDL-cholesterol (LDL-C) is not elevated.[64] Therefore, the American Diabetic Association recommends that LDL-C reduction be given a higher priority than elevating HDL-C or lowering triglyceride levels.[63]

It is also very important to prevent or control hypertension in people with diabetes to prevent damage to the organs[65,66] and to reduce the risk of renal damage because diabetic nephropathy is a major cause of renal failure, accounting for 20% of patients starting dialysis.[67,68]

Vegetarian Diets and Diabetes

The evidence suggests that vegetarians are less likely to develop type 2 diabetes compared to the general population. In an analysis of the Adventist Health Study-1, the age-adjusted risk of developing type 2 diabetes for vegetarian, semi-vegetarian, and nonvegetarian men was 1.00, 1.35, and

1.97, and for women was 1.00, 1.08, and 1.93, respectively.[69] And analyses based on cross-sectional data obtained at baseline from participants in the Adventist Health Study-2 suggests that risk for type 2 diabetes is lower by nearly half for vegetarians compared to nonvegetarians after adjusting for lifestyle factors and BMI.[70] In this study, even occasional meat or fish consumption increased risk. Red meat intake was also associated with increased risk of diabetes in the Women's Health Study.[71]

The higher fiber and perhaps lower saturated fat content of vegetarian diets suggests that these diets come closer to the eating pattern that reduces risk for developing diabetes than meat-containing diets. Whole grains, cereal fibers, and magnesium have also been independently associated with a reduced risk for diabetes.[72,73] Furthermore, the lower rates of hypertension among vegetarians may help to control some of the complications of this disease. Also, the amount and type of protein in vegetarian diets may have some impact on complications of diabetes. The American Diabetes Association recommends that people with diabetes consume diets that are 10–20% protein. A prevailing hypothesis has been that high-protein diets can adversely affect kidney function, and that therefore diabetic patients should limit protein intake.[74] Although some data have questioned the validity of this approach other findings are supportive.[75–77] Furthermore, protein type may impact renal function. In this regard, there is evidence that soy protein may favorably affect renal function and provide important benefits for people with diabetes (see Chapter 9).

High-Carbohydrate versus High Monounsaturated Fat Diets in the Management of Diabetes

According to the dietary recommendations of the American Diabetes Association, the distribution of calories between fat and carbohydrate can vary and should be individualized according to nutrition assessment and treatment goals. There has been considerable success in the management of diabetic patients with low-fat, high-fiber, high-carbohydrate vegetarian diets including reductions in insulin requirements and serum glucose levels.[78–83] For example, in a study of 99 free-living adults with type 2 diabetes, although both a low-fat vegan diet (10% of energy from fat, 15% protein, 75% carbohydrate) and a conventional diabetes diet (15–20% protein, 60–70% carbohydrate and monounsaturated fat) were associated with significant weight loss and reductions in HbA_{1c}, the benefits were greater in response to the vegan diet.[84]

Anderson et al[85,86] have shown that in type 1 diabetics, a high-carbohydrate, high-fiber diet enhances peripheral glucose disposal and decreases basal insulin requirements without affecting triglyceride levels. Despite fiber intakes as high as 70 g/d, Anderson has found good compliance with these types of diets,[87] and among subjects studied by Barnard et al[88] a low-fat vegan diet had an acceptability similar to a conventional diabetes diet.

In addition, studies using amounts of fiber that are closer to that typically consumed by vegetarians have been shown to be effective in managing diabetes. For example, in a randomized crossover study, Chandalia et al[89] fed 13 patients with type 2 diabetes identical diets for 6 weeks, differing only in fiber content; one contained 24 g of total fiber (including 8 g soluble fiber), the amount recommended by the American Diabetes Association, and the other, 50 g (including 25 g soluble fiber). No fiber supplements were used in the study. The high-fiber diet improved glycemic control and decreased hyperinsulinemia and significantly lowered both serum cholesterol and triglyceride levels. Similarly, Giacco et al[15] found that in comparison to type 1 diabetic patients consuming a low-fiber diet (15 g/d) for 24 weeks, patients fed the high-fiber (39 g/d) diet had significantly lower daily blood glucose concentrations, experienced fewer hypoglycemic events, and had lower HbA_{1c} levels. Both the low- and high-fiber diets were composed of natural foodstuffs, and both triglyceride and LDL-C levels decreased on the high-fiber diet.

These data suggest that fiber has a favorable impact on the management of diabetes. Even though the American Diabetes Association considers the evidence on the role of soluble fiber in blood glucose control to be inconclusive, the position of the Nutrition Study Group of the European Association for the Study of Diabetes is that it is effective.[90]

Replacing some of the carbohydrate in a diet with monounsaturated fats has also been shown to improve diabetic control. In a meta-analysis that included nine studies comparing the effects of diets high in total fat (37–50%) and monounsaturated fat (22–33%) with those high in carbohydrate (about 60%), Garg found that the higher-fat diets improved lipoprotein profiles by decreasing triglyceride levels and causing modest increases in HDL-C levels, and that they improved glycemic control relative to the high-carbohydrate diets.[91] Substituting unsaturated fats for saturated fats has also been found to improve insulin sensitivity.[92,93] In contrast, Gerhard et al[94] found no differences in HbA_{1c} levels between people with diabetes following a low-fat or high monounsaturated fatty acid (MUFA) diet.

CARDIOVASCULAR DISEASE

Results from recent analyses have challenged the long-held notion that saturated fat intake increases CHD risk. For example, a systematic review of prospective cohort studies and RCTs by Mente et al[95] found only very weak support for the association between saturated fat, total fat, meat, milk or eggs and CHD. Dietary factors that reduced risk were vegetables, nuts, monounsaturated fats, and Mediterranean and prudent dietary patterns. Factors positively associated with CHD were trans fats, high-GI foods, and a Western dietary pattern. In agreement, a meta-analysis of 21 prospective studies by Siri-Tarino et al[96] found no significant evidence for concluding that saturated fat intake was associated with an increased risk of CHD or CVD. This analysis has garnered considerable attention, and not unexpectedly, some have raised questions about the validity of the findings on methodological grounds.[97]

The presumed benefits of diets low in saturated fat may actually be due to higher polyunsaturated fatty acid (PUFA) intake or a higher dietary ratio of PUFA to saturated fat. Importantly, although very-low-fat vegan or semi-vegan diets deriving no more than 10% of calories from fat have been found to be effective for weight loss and management of CVD, findings from prospective studies and RCTs indicate that replacing saturated and trans fat with unsaturated fats is more effective than simply lowering total fat for reducing the risk of CHD.[98] A meta-analysis of controlled feeding studies found that moderate-fat and low-fat diets similarly decreased LDL-C, but the moderate fat diets lowered HDL-C to a lesser extent.[99] Furthermore, some data suggest there may be disadvantages to consuming very-low-fat diets.[100–105]

Effects of Low-Fat Diets on Risk Factors for Heart Disease

Diets low in fat and high in carbohydrate can produce what has been termed atherogenic lipoprotein phenotype[106] or atherogenic dyslipidemia in sedentary overweight people. This pattern is characterized by high triglycerides, decreased HDL-C, and small LDL-C particles.

The protective effect of HDL-C on CHD risk is well established in both men and women but appears to be particularly pronounced in women. Data suggest that every 1 mg increase in HDL-C decreases CHD risk by 2% in men and 3% in women.[107] Consequently, the total cholesterol-to-HDL-C ratio is often viewed as a better predictor of CHD risk than LDL-C alone. When expressed as percentage change from baseline, diets in which saturated fat is replaced by carbohydrate usually lower LDL-C and HDL-C to a similar extent such that the total cholesterol-to-HDL-C ratio is unchanged.[108] However, if levels of HDL-C are already low, low-fat diets do not produce further reductions.[109] In women, because a 1% decrease in HDL-C raises risk of CHD to a greater extent than a 1% reduction in LDL-C lowers risk, it could be argued that very-low-fat diets actually increase CHD risk.

However, the relevance to CHD risk of dietary-induced reductions in HDL remain unknown, and populations consuming low-fat diets have low risks of CHD despite low HDL-C levels.[110–112] One explanation may be that the decrease in HDL-C that occurs in response to a low-fat diet results from a decrease in the synthesis of apolipoprotein A-1, the main protein that carries HDL-C in the bloodstream. In contrast, low HDL-C levels in people on typical Western diets occur as a result of an increase in apo A-1 clearance,[113–115] although there is some disagreement on this point.[116] Therefore, in assessing CHD risk, it may be inappropriate to conclude that diet-induced decreases in HDL-C are equivalent to low HDL-C levels within a population. It has also been suggested that higher HDL-C levels in people consuming higher fat diets occur as an adaptive response, which is only necessary to reverse cholesterol transport, to deal with the greater metabolic load imposed by high-fat diets.[117]

Nevertheless, population data indicate that low HDL-C levels represent an increased risk of CHD even when total cholesterol levels are <200 mg/dl.[118] An analysis of 21,448 subjects enrolled in the EPIC-Norfolk study found that among healthy men and women, the ratio of total cholesterol to HDL-C and levels of triglycerides were both more strongly linked to risk for CHD than LDL-C levels alone.[119] And populations with very low cholesterol levels often have in common a number of lifestyle factors, such as a low incidence of obesity, which may mitigate any undesirable effects resulting from low HDL-C levels.[120] These other factors may not be present in Westerners who adopt low-fat diets.

Because studies suggest that replacing dietary carbohydrate with unsaturated fat is as effective in reducing LDL-C as replacing saturated fat with carbohydrate, but without the corresponding reduction in HDL-C,[121–123] very-low-fat diets are not necessarily the right approach for all individuals. Also, certain higher fat foods like tree nuts have been shown to reduce serum cholesterol levels with decreases greater than predicted from their fatty acid content.[124–126]

Although a meta-analysis concluded that elevated triglycerides are an independent risk factor for heart disease,[127] there is considerable disagreement over the role of triglycerides in the etiology of CHD.[128–131] However, elevated triglyceride levels are recognized as a target for intervention according to the American Diabetes Association consensus panel.[63] Furthermore, in an analysis of seven clinical trials, hypertriglyceridemia was identified as an important predictor of plaque progression among patients with the metabolic syndrome.[132]

That carbohydrate feeding can lead to an increase in triglyceride levels was first observed during the late 1950s.[133] Based on observations of populations, some argue that the carbohydrate-induced hypertriglyceridemia is a transient phenomenon. But studies have found that elevations in triglycerides persist in subjects who have been studied for as long as 2 years.[102]

Another issue is the extent to which carbohydrate type or form influences triglyceride levels. More recent analyses suggest that hypertriglyceridemia is due to higher amounts of simple carbohydrates and a higher GL.[134,135] In a recent intervention by Barnard et al,[84] triglyceride levels were lowered among the subjects following a high (66.6% of kcal) carbohydrate diet versus no change in the group following conventional guidelines from the American Diabetes Association. But in contrast, Parks et al[136] found that after feeding a low-fat, high-carbohydrate diet that was based on whole foods high in fiber and low in simple carbohydrates, triglyceride levels still increased by 60%. Overall, however, the evidence suggests that diets higher in starch and fiber are less likely to cause hypertriglyceridemia than isocaloric diets that are high in monosaccharides and disaccharides.[131,137] In addition, exercise and weight loss can greatly diminish or prevent the carbohydrate-induced hypertriglyceridemia.

Studies suggest that low-fat diets also decrease LDL particle size.[138,139] As noted previously, small, dense LDLs are associated with increased risk of CHD[140] and are thought to be the most atherogenic because they enter the artery wall more easily. Research from the University of California at Berkeley has shown that approximately a third of men who manifested LDL subclass phenotype A (large buoyant LDL) while consuming a high-fat diet (40–46% of calories) converted to phenotype B (small, dense LDL) with a reduction in fat to 20–24% of energy.[141] This group of investigators found that upon a further reduction in fat intake to 10% of calories, approximately a third of men who were stable phenotype A during the 20–24% fat diet converted to phenotype B.[103] Although these studies have potentially important implications, they have been criticized on several grounds including the fact that the high-fat diets were higher in fiber than the low-fat diets. However, other research has found that diets high in monounsaturated fats or a Mediterranean diet pattern are associated with increased LDL particle size in comparison to high-carbohydrate diets.[142,143]

Despite the positive effects on blood lipids associated with diets higher in unsaturated fat, consumption of high-fat meals may have disadvantages. High-fat meals can contribute to exaggerated postprandial lipemia, which may adversely affect endothelial function, and increase activated factor VII levels, which may increase platelet aggregation.[144,145] In a review of findings on fat and postprandial lipids, Sanders suggested limiting fat to no more than 30 g per meal.[146] However, lipids are cleared more rapidly in people who are physically active,[147] and effects on endothelial function have been shown to be blocked by pretreatment with antioxidant vitamins C and E, suggesting an oxidative mechanism. Cortes et al also found that adding walnuts to a high-fat meal improved endothelial function.[148]

In conclusion, diets low in total fat or moderate in unsaturated fat both have potential advantages for managing CVD and can offer options in nutrition therapy for vegetarians and vegans.

METABOLIC SYNDROME

Metabolic syndrome refers to a cluster of abnormalities including but not limited to glucose intolerance, increased blood pressure, high plasma triglyceride concentrations and low-HDL-C concentrations, all thought to be brought about by insulin insensitivity/resistance.[46] Individuals who are insulin insensitive are resistant to insulin-stimulated glucose uptake. According to some estimates, as much as 25% of the nonobese, nondiabetic population are insulin resistant despite having a normal oral glucose tolerance test. Factors that increase plasma glucose and insulin may modulate the effects of insulin resistance, which in turn increases risk of type 2 diabetes. Interestingly, Facchini et al proposed that hyperinsulinemia is the missing link between oxidative stress and age-related diseases.[149]

Insulin resistance results from an interaction between genetic makeup and the environment and is associated with obesity, lack of exercise, aging, smoking, and certain drugs that antagonize the action of insulin.[150] The first approach to improving insulin sensitivity is weight loss, which is effective in approximately 50% of the insulin-resistant cases.[139,151,152] Physical activity increases insulin sensitivity independently of weight loss. Saturated fat may decrease insulin sensitivity, as may a high-carbohydrate diet, especially when composed of high-GI foods.[153]

Overall, the evidence supports a role for insulin resistance as a risk factor in CVD[154–157] and diabetes, although not all studies support insulin resistance's role in CVD.[158,159] An analysis of NHANES III data showed that people with metabolic syndrome had a higher risk for CVD than individuals with diabetes who did not have metabolic syndrome.[160] In fact, elevated insulin levels are thought by some to increase risk even when the other risk factors associated with metabolic syndrome are controlled.[161–163]

In contrast, some findings suggest that the metabolic syndrome has no greater predictive value for CHD compared to the Framingham algorithm that is based on age, sex, smoking, blood pressure, total cholesterol, HDL-C, and diabetes.[164,165] In the Gubbio population study, a prospective study of 2650 adults, the only factors contributing to the predictive power of the metabolic syndrome were HDL-C levels and systolic blood pressure.[166] A joint statement from the American Diabetes Association and the European Association for the Study of Diabetes suggested that more research is needed before the metabolic syndrome can actually be designated a "syndrome" and that its clinical utility has yet to be determined.[167]

WEIGHT CONTROL

For adults, overweight is defined as a BMI of 25.0 to 29.9, and obesity is defined as a BMI of ≥30.0.[168] Based on NHANES data, the prevalence of obesity in 2007–2008 was 32.2% among men and 35.5% among women.[169] Although the prevalence of obesity is increasing, the increases appear to be smaller than in previous years.[169] Vegetarians tend to be thinner than nonvegetarians (Appendix D), but whether dietary differences contribute to this difference is unclear.

Among adults trying to maintain weight loss, approximately 40% reduce fat intake without specifically restricting caloric intake.[170] In the general population, fat intake as a percentage of calories has decreased from 36% in the 1980s to 34% in the 1990s, although because caloric intake has increased, absolute fat intake has actually increased.[171] Low-fat foods will likely not contribute to a reduction in caloric intake unless these foods have a reduced energy density.[172]

In a review on the role of dietary fat in obesity, Golay and Bobbioni concluded that dietary fat induces overconsumption and weight gain through its high caloric density.[173] Flatt maintains that because fat stores are not tightly regulated, dietary fat, much more so than dietary carbohydrate, leads to obesity.[174] However, some nutrition researchers have questioned the efficacy of low-fat diets for weight loss.[175,176] Willett and Leibel have stated that fat consumption within the range of 18–40% of total caloric intake has little relationship with body fatness.[177]

Although many agree that low-fat diets lead to weight loss in the short term, questions remain about their long-term effectiveness. In a meta-analysis of the efficacy of low-fat diets in reducing body weight in nondiabetic individuals that involved 16 trials and nearly 2000 individuals, Astrup et al found that subjects on the ad libitum low-fat diets lost on average 3.2 kg more than control subjects. However, weight loss plateaued after 3 to 6 months.

One randomized intervention study demonstrated that 2 years after a major weight loss, a group of obese subjects who consumed an ad libitum low-fat diet regained on average 5.9 kg less than a group who cut down on all calories equally.[178] Some data suggest that the efficacy of low-fat diets can be enhanced by substituting protein for some of the carbohydrate in the diet,[179] and a comprehensive analysis reported not unexpectedly that exercise plus dietary changes is more effective at long-term weight loss than diet alone.[180]

Several short-term clinical studies have shown low-fat vegetarian diets lead to weight loss, but caloric intake was also reduced in these trials.[82,181] One of the longest studies of a low-fat vegetarian diet was the Lifestyle Heart Trial, which involved comprehensive lifestyle changes that included a vegetarian low-fat diet (<10%) diet, stress reduction, exercise, and counseling. The intervention group lost approximately 11 kg after 1 year; however, at 5 years approximately half of that weight loss was regained despite good adherence to the low-fat diet.[182] Subjects who began with an average weight of 201 pounds (91.4 kg) ended up weighing 188 pounds. This degree of weight loss can have important physiologic benefits but it is often viewed unsatisfactorily by obese subjects.[183]

In contrast, calorie-controlled diets that are moderate in fat content may increase satiety and improve compliance.[184] Diets high in monounsaturated fats in particular increase adipose tissue metabolism and may facilitate weight loss. Monounsaturated fats have a higher oxidation rate in comparison with saturated fat.[185] In the Nurses' Health Study, nut consumption—a high-fat food—was related to improved weight control.[186] Higher protein intakes may also improve satiety on calorie-controlled diets[187] and may promote loss of fat tissue while sparing lean body mass.[179,188] However, as noted, high-protein foods may lead to hyperinsulinemia despite their lack of effect on blood glucose levels. The American Diabetes Association does not recommend high-protein diets for weight loss.[32] Diets using plant proteins, however, may avoid some of the disadvantages associated with usual high-protein weight loss plans. In a randomized parallel study of 47 subjects, Jenkins et al found that a low-carbohydrate, high-protein plant-based diet (26% carbohydrate, 31% protein, 43% fat) deriving protein from gluten, soy, nuts, vegetables, and cereals had more beneficial effects on lipids compared to a low-fat, high-carbohydrate plan, and there was no difference in insulin resistance between the groups.[189]

As noted previously, findings about the effects of low-GI diets on weight loss are conflicting. And in a comparison of four different types of diets providing varying levels of carbohydrate, fat, and protein over 2 years, there was no difference in weight loss, satiety, hunger, and satisfaction among the different groups, suggesting that macronutrient content is of minor importance in achieving weight control.[190] Finally, a growing body of research suggests that dietary monotony may help to control calorie intake.[191] The recent popularity and self-reported success of very-low-carbohydrate diets may be due to severe restrictions on variety that result in a reduced caloric intake.

COUNSELING VEGETARIANS WITH CHRONIC DISEASE

Diets high in complex carbohydrates or moderately high in unsaturated fats, particularly monounsaturated fats, may be beneficial in control of diabetes and in reducing risk for heart disease and obesity. Some research suggests that incorporating some higher fat foods into menus confers benefits over very-low-fat eating plans. The World Health Organization suggests that minimal fat intakes should be 15% of energy for adults or 20% for women of reproductive age or those with BMI <18.5. Maximum recommended total fat intake is 30–35% of calories.[192] Based on findings about high-fat meals and postprandial lipids, some have recommended that fat intake should be no more than 30 g per eating occasion. Findings regarding benefits of the glycemic index for preventing or managing chronic disease and as a part of weight control programs are conflicting, but low-GI foods are likely to confer some benefits to healthy eating plans.

Vegetarian diets can be effective in the management of chronic disease and weight loss. Vegetarians are less likely to be obese than omnivores. They have lower intakes of saturated fat and cholesterol, and higher intakes of fiber and antioxidants. Some may consume foods that have been linked specifically to reduced disease incidence.

General principles for counseling vegetarian clients with chronic disease are the same as for omnivores. The following points can be useful in working with vegetarian clients.

- *Replace saturated fat* with unsaturated fats, particularly monounsaturated. Good sources of monounsaturated fats include many nuts and some seeds, olives, avocado, olive oil, and canola oil. Exhibit 16-1 lists some vegetarian foods that are high in saturated fat.
- *Reduction in total fat* may be helpful for those who need to lose weight. Exhibit 16-2 offers suggested low-fat vegetarian snacks. However, avoidance of all high-fat foods may not be advantageous, and some clients may have more success with moderate fat intakes.
- *Higher protein intake* may improve satiety and help in retention of muscle mass during weight loss. Including more plant sources of protein in meals can help to produce weight-loss

---

Exhibit 16-1 Vegetarian Foods High in Saturated Fat

Whole milk

Cheese

Dairy fats, including sour cream, ice cream, cream, butter

Crackers

Commercial baked products

Home-baked products made with butter

Processed snack foods such as microwave popcorn, some snack chips

Dishes prepared with coconut milk

Exhibit 16-2 Low-Fat Vegetarian Snacks

Baked potato	Bagels
Steamed vegetable	Reduced fat crackers
Salad with low-fat dressing	Rice cakes
Fruit salad	Air-popped popcorn
Ready-to-eat cereals with low-fat milk	Soft pretzels with mustard
Whole grain breads	Baked fruit

diets that are low in saturated fat and cholesterol. Exhibit 16-3 lists vegetarian foods that are good sources of protein.

- *Weight loss* is an important goal in the management of chronic disease. It can reduce risk for diabetes and improve diabetic control by reducing insulin insensitivity. It also helps to raise HDL-C, reduces triglyceride levels, and lowers total cholesterol.
- *Foods with a low glycemic* index may be helpful in the control and prevention of diabetes, heart disease, metabolic syndrome, and obesity, although these relationships are not conclusive. Whether or not the GI is useful in a counseling setting depends on the needs and motivation of the client. For some clients with diabetes, carbohydrate counting may be more practical. However, vegetarian diets can easily be based on foods with a low GI when whole plant foods form the basis of the diet and foods like legumes are included often in meals. It is important for clients to understand that it is not necessary to choose only low-GI foods but to choose these foods often. Exhibit 16-4 presents guidelines for choosing low-GI meals.

Exhibit 16-3 Protein-Rich Vegetarian Foods

	Protein (g)	Kcal
3 oz seitan (wheat gluten)	18	90
1 burger made from soy protein	13	70
½ cup cottage cheese (1% fat)	14	81
½ cup beans	7.6	120
2 tbsp peanut butter	8	188
½ cup cooked quinoa	4.1	111
2 tbsp chopped walnuts	2.2	95.6

Source: Data from USDA National Nutrient Database for Standard Reference, Release 22, 2009 and manufacturers' information.

Exhibit 16-4 Meal-Planning Tips for Reducing Glycemic Load

Reduce the glycemic load of meals by choosing:

"Grainy" breads made from intact, sprouted, or coarsely chopped grains rather than flour

Sourdough and pumpernickel bread

Cereals made from whole oat groats or rolled oats (rather than ready-to-eat cereals)

Whole raw fruits rather than juices and dried or canned fruit

Raw and lightly cooked vegetables

Regular full-fat soymilk instead of reduced-fat milk

Foods flavored with acidic ingredients, such as lemon juice, lime juice, vinegar, and tomatoes

Beans cooked from scratch rather than canned

Meals that include protein and fat

- *Exercise* is important in the management of chronic disease because of its role in weight loss or maintenance and its positive effects on insulin sensitivity, HDL-C levels, triglycerides, and blood pressure.
- *Replacing animal protein with plant protein* may be helpful in preventing renal insufficiency in people with diabetes. The extent to which this may help vegetarians, whose diets are already generally low in animal protein, is not known.
- *Reducing sodium intake* is important for many people in the management of hypertension.
- *Increasing antioxidant intake* may help to reduce risk for heart disease. Although vegetarian diets tend to be high in antioxidants, this may not be true for those who depend to a great extent on refined foods and dairy products and whose intake of fruits and vegetables is low. More consumption of fruit and vegetables and of whole plant foods increases antioxidant intake. Vegetable oils, nuts, and avocado can be important sources of vitamin E and are sometimes avoided by those vegetarians following very-low-fat diets.
- *An adequate intake of essential fatty acids* is important in the prevention of chronic disease (Chapter 4).
- *Reduced intake of trans-fatty acids* may reduce risk for heart disease and enhance conversion of essential fatty acids to long-chain omega-3 fatty acids (Chapter 4).
- *Specific foods like nuts and soyfoods* have been shown to play roles in reducing blood cholesterol and preventing heart disease. (See Chapter 9 for more information about soyfoods and chronic disease.)
- *The Exchange Lists for Meal Planning* are useful for clients who desire more structured guidelines, particularly for weight control or management of diabetes. Exhibit 16-5 provides exchanges for common vegetarian foods. Vegan clients can choose fortified soymilk from the milk exchange or, if desired, they can omit the milk exchanges. It is important to identify other sources of calcium, vitamin B_{12}, and perhaps vitamin D, in this case.

Exhibit 16-5 Exchanges for Vegetarian Foods

Food	Exchanges
1 tofu hot dog	1 lean meat or meat substitute
1 Boca Burger	1 lean meat or meat substitute + ½ starch
1 Boca Burger (vegan)	1 very lean meat or meat substitute + ½ starch
1 Gardenburger	1 lean meat or meat substitute + 1 starch
1 Garden Vegan Burger	1 very lean meat or meat substitute + 1 starch
2 oz seitan	1 lean meat or meat substitute + 1 starch
3 tbsp soynuts	1 high-fat meat or meat substitute + 1 starch
1 oz meatless deli slices	1 lean meat or meat substitute
3 strips soy bacon	1 lean meat or meat substitute
¼ cup prepared TVP	1 lean meat or meat substitute
2 tbsp tahini	1 high-fat meat or meat substitute
⅓ cup cooked quinoa	1 starch
¾ cup mung bean (cellophane) noodles	1 starch
½ cup cooked polenta	1 starch
½ cup cooked soba noodles	1 starch
½ cup vegetarian baked beans	2 starch
1.5 oz soy cheese (no casein)	1 starch + 1 fat
1 cup soymilk	1 low-fat milk
1 cup light soymilk	½ low-fat milk
1 cup rice milk	1 starch + 1 fruit
1 cup almond milk	½ starch
1 cup oat milk	1 skim milk + 1 starch
6 oz soy yogurt, fruited	1 starch + ½ fruit
1½ tbsp tofu mayonnaise (Nayonaise)	1 fat
2 tsp tofu cream cheese	1 fat

Case Study

Alexa is a 62-year-old woman who has been trying to lose weight and reduce her cholesterol levels for the past 6 months. She has attempted to eliminate as much fat from her diet as possible and is trying to increase her exercise by walking a mile every morning. She lost 14 pounds during the first

(continued)

4 months but has not been able to lose any more weight since then. She would like to lose an additional 20 pounds. Her recent blood work shows a modest decline in total cholesterol but also a drop in HDL-C so that the ratio of total cholesterol to HDL-C has not changed. She has also experienced an increase in triglycerides, which are moderately high. She feels that her diet is boring and finds that she is incorporating more nonfat sweets into meals.

Here is her 24-hour recall:

Breakfast
    ¼ cup egg replacer cooked in 1 tbsp reduced-fat margarine
    1 slice of whole wheat toast with 1 tbsp raspberry jam
    1 cup orange juice

Midmorning snack
    ½ cup nonfat strawberry yogurt with 2 tbsp nonfat granola

Lunch
    1 cup canned vegetable soup
    2 nonfat rice cakes
    Banana
    ½ cup nonfat chocolate ice cream

Afternoon snack
    Baked tortilla chips with salsa

Dinner
    1 cup brown rice
    ½ cup black beans flavored with salsa
    Tossed green salad with nonfat dressing
    ½ cup steamed green beans

Evening snack
    2 nonfat oatmeal cookies

Alexa's concerns:

Her weight loss has stopped, HDL levels have decreased, and triglycerides are modestly increased. She is bored with her food choices and finds them unsatisfying. What changes would you suggest to help make her meals more interesting while addressing concerns about weight control and blood lipids?

REFERENCES

1. Crapo PA, Reaven G, Olefsky J. Postprandial plasma glucose and insulin response to different complex carbohydrates. *Diabetes Care.* 1977;26:1178–1183.
2. Foster-Powell K, Miller JB. International tables of glycemic index. *Am J Clin Nutr.* 1995;62:871S–890S.
3. Wolever TM, Jenkins DJ, Jenkins AL, Josse RG. The glycemic index: methodology and clinical implications. *Am J Clin Nutr.* 1991;54(5):846–854.
4. Wolever TM. Metabolic effects of continuous feeding. *Metabolism.* 1990;39:947–951.
5. Wolever TM. Relationship between dietary fiber content and composition in foods and the glycemic index. *Am J Clin Nutr.* 1990;51:72–75.

6. Trout DL, Behall KM, Osilesi O. Prediction of glycemic index for starchy foods. *Am J Clin Nutr.* 1993;58:873–878.

7. Wolever TMS, Katzman-Relle L, Jenkins AL, Vuksan V, Josse RG, Jenkins DJA. Glycemic index of 102 complex carbohydrate foods in patients with diabetes. *Nutr Res.* 1994;14:651–669.

8. Jenkins DJA, Jenkins AL, Wolever TM, Rao AV. Simple and complex carbohydrates. *Nutr Rev.* 1986;44:44–49.

9. Englyst KN, Englyst HN, Hudson GJ, Cole TJ, Cummings JH. Rapidly available glucose in foods: an in vitro measurement that reflects the glycemic response. *Am J Clin Nutr.* 1999;69(3):448–454.

10. Salmeron J, Ascherio A, Rimm EB, et al. Dietary fiber, glycemic load, and risk of NIDDM in men. *Diabetes Care.* 1997;20(4):545–550.

11. Salmeron J, Manson JE, Stampfer MJ, Colditz GA, Wing AL, Willett WC. Dietary fiber, glycemic load, and risk of non-insulin-dependent diabetes mellitus in women. *JAMA.* 1997;277(6):472–477.

12. Brand JC, Colagiuri S, Crossman S, Allen A, Roberts DC, Truswell AS. Low-glycemic index foods improve long-term glycemic control in NIDDM. *Diabetes Care.* 1991;14(2):95–101.

13. Wolever TM, Jenkins DJ, Vuksan V, et al. Beneficial effect of a low glycaemic index diet in type 2 diabetes. *Diabet Med.* 1992;9(5):451–458.

14. Frost G, Wilding J, Beecham J. Dietary advice based on the glycaemic index improves dietary profile and metabolic control in type 2 diabetic patients. *Diabet Med.* 1994;11(4):397–401.

15. Giacco R, Parillo M, Rivellese AA, et al. Long-term dietary treatment with increased amounts of fiber-rich low-glycemic index natural foods improves blood glucose control and reduces the number of hypoglycemic events in type 1 diabetic patients. *Diabetes Care.* 2000;23(10):1461–1466.

16. Jenkins DJ, Kendall CW, McKeown-Eyssen G, et al. Effect of a low-glycemic index or a high-cereal fiber diet on type 2 diabetes: a randomized trial. *JAMA.* 2008;300(23):2742–2753.

17. Wolever TM, Hamad S, Chiasson JL, et al. Day-to-day consistency in amount and source of carbohydrate associated with improved blood glucose control in type 1 diabetes. *J Am Coll Nutr.* 1999;18(3):242–247.

18. Mayer-Davis EJ, Dhawan A, Liese AD, Teff K, Schulz M. Towards understanding of glycaemic index and glycaemic load in habitual diet: associations with measures of glycaemia in the Insulin Resistance Atherosclerosis Study. *Br J Nutr.* 2006;95(2):397–405.

19. Liese AD, Schulz M, Fang F, et al. Dietary glycemic index and glycemic load, carbohydrate and fiber intake, and measures of insulin sensitivity, secretion, and adiposity in the Insulin Resistance Atherosclerosis Study. *Diabetes Care.* 2005;28(12):2832–2838.

20. Thomas D, Elliott EJ. Low glycaemic index, or low glycaemic load, diets for diabetes mellitus. *Cochrane Database Syst Rev.* 2009;(1):CD006296.

21. Joint Food and Agricultural Organization/World Health Organization Expert Consultation, 1997. *Carbohydrates in Human Nutrition.* Rome, Italy: Food and Agricultural Organization; 1998.

22. Barclay AW, Petocz P, McMillan-Price J, et al. Glycemic index, glycemic load, and chronic disease risk—a meta-analysis of observational studies. *Am J Clin Nutr.* 2008;87(3):627–637.

23. Liu S, Willett WC, Stampfer MJ, et al. A prospective study of dietary glycemic load, carbohydrate intake, and risk of coronary heart disease in US women. *Am J Clin Nutr.* 2000;71(6):1455–1461.

24. Ma Y, Olendzki B, Chiriboga D, et al. Association between dietary carbohydrates and body weight. *Am J Epidemiol.* 2005;161(4):359–367.

25. Mendez MA, Covas MI, Marrugat J, Vila J, Schroder H. Glycemic load, glycemic index, and body mass index in Spanish adults. *Am J Clin Nutr.* 2009;89(1):316–322.

26. de Rougemont A, Normand S, Nazare JA, et al. Beneficial effects of a 5-week low- glycaemic index regimen on weight control and cardiovascular risk factors in overweight non-diabetic subjects. *Br J Nutr.* 2007;98(6):1288–1298.

27. Abete I, Parra D, Martinez JA. Energy-restricted diets based on a distinct food selection affecting the glycemic index induce different weight loss and oxidative response. *Clin Nutr.* 2008;27(4):545–551.

28. Maki KC, Rains TM, Kaden VN, Raneri KR, Davidson MH. Effects of a reduced-glycemic-load diet on body weight, body composition, and cardiovascular disease risk markers in overweight and obese adults. *Am J Clin Nutr.* 2007;85(3):724–734.

29. Philippou E, McGowan BM, Brynes AE, Dornhorst A, Leeds AR, Frost GS. The effect of a 12-week low glycaemic index diet on heart disease risk factors and 24 h glycaemic response in healthy middle-aged volunteers at risk of heart disease: a pilot study. *Eur J Clin Nutr.* 2008;62(1):145–149.

30. Das SK, Gilhooly CH, Golden JK, et al. Long-term effects of 2 energy-restricted diets differing in glycemic load on dietary adherence, body composition, and metabolism in CALERIE: a 1-y randomized controlled trial. *Am J Clin Nutr.* 2007;85(4):1023–1030.

31. Williams SM, Venn BJ, Perry T, et al. Another approach to estimating the reliability of glycaemic index. *Br J Nutr.* 2008;100(2):364–372.

32. Bantle JP, Wylie-Rosett J, Albright AL, et al. Nutrition recommendations and interventions for diabetes: a position statement of the American Diabetes Association. *Diabetes Care.* 2008;31(suppl 1):S61–S78.

33. Waldmann A, Strohle A, Koschizke JW, Leitzmann C, Hahn A. Overall glycemic index and glycemic load of vegan diets in relation to plasma lipoproteins and triacylglycerols. *Ann Nutr Metab.* 2007;51(4):335–344.

34. Hua NW, Stoohs RA, Facchini FS. Low iron status and enhanced insulin sensitivity in lacto-ovo vegetarians. *Br J Nutr.* 2001;86(4):515–519.

35. Hung CJ, Huang PC, Li YH, Lu SC, Ho LT, Chou HF. Taiwanese vegetarians have higher insulin sensitivity than omnivores. *Br J Nutr.* 2006;95(1):129–135.

36. Kuo CS, Lai NS, Ho LT, Lin CL. Insulin sensitivity in Chinese ovo-lactovegetarians compared with omnivores. *Eur J Clin Nutr.* 2004;58(2):312–316.

37. Holt SH, Miller JC, Petocz P. An insulin index of foods: the insulin demand generated by 1000-kJ portions of common foods. *Am J Clin Nutr.* 1997;66(5):1264–1276.

38. Gannon MC, Ercan N, Westphal SA, Nuttall FQ. Effect of added fat on plasma glucose and insulin response to ingested potato in individuals with NIDDM. *Diabetes Care.* 1993;16(6):874–880.

39. Westphal SA, Gannon MC, Nuttall FQ. Metabolic response to glucose ingested with various amounts of protein. *Am J Clin Nutr.* 1990;52(2):267–272.

40. Saeed A, Jones SA, Nuttall FQ, Gannon MC. A fasting-induced decrease in plasma glucose concentration does not affect the insulin response to ingested protein in people with type 2 diabetes. *Metabolism.* 2002;51(8):1027–1033.

41. Gannon MC, Nuttall FQ, Neil BJ, Westphal SA. The insulin and glucose responses to meals of glucose plus various proteins in type II diabetic subjects. *Metabolism.* 1988;37(11):1081–1088.

42. Haffner SM. Epidemiology of insulin resistance and its relation to coronary artery disease. *Am J Cardiol.* 1999; 84(1A):11J–14J.

43. Tsuchihashi K, Hikita N, Hase M, et al. Role of hyperinsulinemia in atherosclerotic coronary arterial disease: studies of semi-quantitative coronary angiography. *Intern Med.* 1999;38(9):691–697.

44. Deshpande AD, Harris-Hayes M, Schootman M. Epidemiology of diabetes and diabetes-related complications. *Phys Ther.* 2008;88(11):1254–1264.

45. Harris MI, Flegal KM, Cowie CC, et al. Prevalence of diabetes, impaired fasting glucose, and impaired glucose tolerance in U.S. adults. The Third National Health and Nutrition Examination Survey, 1988–1994. *Diabetes Care.* 1998;21(4):518–524.

46. Reaven GM. Banting lecture 1988. Role of insulin resistance in human disease. *Diabetes.* 1988;37(12):1595–1607.

47. Benjamin SM, Valdez R, Geiss LS, Rolka DB, Narayan KM. Estimated number of adults with prediabetes in the US in 2000: opportunities for prevention. *Diabetes Care.* 2003;26(3):645–649.

48. King H, Aubert RE, Herman WH. Global burden of diabetes, 1995–2025: prevalence, numerical estimates, and projections. *Diabetes Care.* 1998;21(9):1414–1431.

49. West KM. Epidemiology of diabetes and its vascular lesions. New York: Elsevier/North-Holland; 1978.

50. Hazlett BE. Historical perspective: the discovery of insulin. In: Davidson JK, ed. *Clinical Diabetes Mellitus, a Problem Oriented Approach.* New York, NY: Thieme Medical; 1991:2–10.

51. Steiner G. From and excess of fat, diabetics die. *JAMA.* 1989;262:398–399.

52. Thompson D, Edelsberg J, Colditz GA, Bird AP, Oster G. Lifetime health and economic consequences of obesity. *Arch Intern Med.* 1999;159(18):2177–2183.

53. Everhart JE, Pettitt DJ, Bennett PH, Knowler WC. Duration of obesity increases the incidence of NIDDM. *Diabetes.* 1992;41(2):235–240.

54. Bjorntorp P. Abdominal obesity and the development of noninsulin-dependent diabetes mellitus. *Diabetes Metab Rev.* 1988;4(6):615–622.

55. Carey VJ, Walters EE, Colditz GA, et al. Body fat distribution and risk of noninsulin-dependent diabetes mellitus in women. The Nurses' Health Study. *Am J Epidemiol.* 1997;145(7):614–619.

56. Rush EC, Plank LD, Mitchelson E, Laulu MS. Central obesity and risk for type 2 diabetes in Maori, Pacific, and European young men in New Zealand. *Food Nutr Bull*. 2002;23(3 suppl):82–86.

57. Klein S, Sheard NF, Pi-Sunyer X, et al. Weight management through lifestyle modification for the prevention and management of type 2 diabetes: rationale and strategies: a statement of the American Diabetes Association, the North American Association for the Study of Obesity, and the American Society for Clinical Nutrition. *Diabetes Care*. 2004;27(8):2067–2073.

58. Tuomilehto J, Lindstrom J, Eriksson JG, et al. Prevention of type 2 diabetes mellitus by changes in lifestyle among subjects with impaired glucose tolerance. *N Engl J Med*. 2001;344(18):1343–1350.

59. Knowler WC, Barrett-Connor E, Fowler SE, et al. Reduction in the incidence of type 2 diabetes with lifestyle intervention or metformin. *N Engl J Med*. 2002;346(6):393–403.

60. Jeon CY, Lokken RP, Hu FB, van Dam RM. Physical activity of moderate intensity and risk of type 2 diabetes: a systematic review. *Diabetes Care*. 2007;30(3):744–752.

61. Gu K, Cowie CC, Harris MI. Mortality in adults with and without diabetes in a national cohort of the U.S. population, 1971–1993. *Diabetes Care*. 1998;21(7):1138–1145.

62. Vidt DG. Good news for the older patient with diabetes: added cardiovascular risk reduction. *Curr Hypertens Rep*. 1999;1(5):379–380.

63. Haffner SM. Dyslipidemia management in adults with diabetes. *Diabetes Care*. 2004;27 (suppl 1):S68–S71.

64. Haffner SM. Management of dyslipidemia in adults with diabetes [Technical review]. *Diabetes Care*. 1998;21:160–178.

65. de La Sierra A, Ruilope LM. Treatment of hypertension in diabetes mellitus. *Curr Hypertens Rep*. 2000;2(3):335–342.

66. White WB, Prisant LM, Wright JT Jr. Management of patients with hypertension and diabetes mellitus: advances in the evidence for intensive treatment. *Am J Med*. 2000;108(3):238–245.

67. Zeller K, Whittaker E, Sullivan L, Raskin P, Jacobson HR. Effect of restricting dietary protein on the progression of renal failure in patients with insulin-dependent diabetes mellitus [see comments]. *N Engl J Med*. 1991;324(2):78–84.

68. Liew BS, Perry C, Boulton-Jones JM, Simpson K, Paterson K. Diabetic nephropathy: an observational study on patients attending a joint diabetes renal clinic. *QJM*. 1997;90(5):353–358.

69. Fraser GE. Diet as primordial prevention in Seventh-day Adventists. *Prev Med*. 1999;29(6 Pt 2):S18–S23.

70. Tonstad S, Butler T, Yan R, Fraser GE. Type of vegetarian diet, body weight, and prevalence of type 2 diabetes. *Diabetes Care*. 2009;32(5):791–796.

71. Song Y, Manson JE, Buring JE, Liu S. A prospective study of red meat consumption and type 2 diabetes in middle-aged and elderly women: the women's health study. *Diabetes Care*. 2004;27(9):2108–2115.

72. Fung TT, Hu FB, Pereira MA, et al. Whole-grain intake and the risk of type 2 diabetes: a prospective study in men. *Am J Clin Nutr*. 2002;76(3):535–540.

73. Meyer KA, Kushi LH, Jacobs DR Jr, Slavin J, Sellers TA, Folsom AR. Carbohydrates, dietary fiber, and incident type 2 diabetes in older women. *Am J Clin Nutr*. 2000;71(4):921–930.

74. Brenner BM, Meyer TW, Hostetter TH. Dietary protein intake and the progressive nature of kidney disease: the role of hemodynamically mediated glomerular injury in the pathogenesis of progressive glomerular sclerosis in aging, renal ablation, and intrinsic renal disease. *N Engl J Med*. 1982;307(11):652–659.

75. Levey AS, Adler S, Caggiula AW, et al. Effects of dietary protein restriction on the progression of advanced renal disease in the Modification of Diet in Renal Disease Study. *Am J Kidney Dis*. 1996;27(5):652–663.

76. Toeller M, Buyken AE. Protein intake—new evidence for its role in diabetic nephropathy [editorial]. *Nephrol Dial Transplant*. 1998;13(8):1926–1927.

77. Knight EL, Stampfer MJ, Hankinson SE, Spiegelman D, Curhan GC. The impact of protein intake on renal function decline in women with normal renal function or mild renal insufficiency. *Ann Intern Med*. 2003;138(6):460–467.

78. Barnard RJ, Massey MR, Cherny S, O'Brien LT, Pritikin N. Long-term use of a high- complex-carbohydrate, high-fiber, low-fat diet and exercise in the treatment of NIDDM patients. *Diabetes Care*. 1983;6(3):268–273.

79. Barnard RJ, Lattimore L, Holly RG, Cherny S, Pritikin N. Response of non-insulin- dependent diabetic patients to an intensive program of diet and exercise. *Diabetes Care*. 1982;5(4):370–374.

80. Garg A, Bantle JP, Henry RR, et al. Effects of varying carbohydrate content of diet in patients with non-insulin-dependent diabetes mellitus [see comments]. *JAMA*. 1994;271(18):1421–1428.

81. Simpson HC, Simpson RW, Lousley S, et al. A high carbohydrate leguminous fibre diet improves all aspects of diabetic control. *Lancet*. 1981;1(8210):1–5.

82. Nicholson AS, Sklar M, Barnard ND, Gore S, Sullivan R, Browning S. Toward improved management of NIDDM: a randomized, controlled, pilot intervention using a lowfat, vegetarian diet. *Prev Med.* 1999;29(2):87–91.

83. Perez-Jimenez F, Lopez-Miranda J, Pinillos MD, et al. A Mediterranean and a high-carbohydrate diet improve glucose metabolism in healthy young persons. *Diabetologia.* 2001;44(11):2038–2043.

84. Barnard ND, Cohen J, Jenkins DJ, et al. A low-fat vegan diet and a conventional diabetes diet in the treatment of type 2 diabetes: a randomized, controlled, 74-wk clinical trial. *Am J Clin Nutr.* 2009;89(5):1588S–1596S.

85. Anderson JW, Zeigler JA, Deakins DA, et al. Metabolic effects of high-carbohydrate, high-fiber diets for insulin-dependent diabetic individuals. *Am J Clin Nutr.* 1991;54(5):936–943.

86. Anderson JW, Ward K. High-carbohydrate, high-fiber diets for insulin-treated men with diabetes mellitus. *Am J Clin Nutr.* 1979;32(11):2312–2321.

87. Anderson JW, Gustafson NJ. Adherence to high-carbohydrate, high-fiber diets. *Diabetes Educ.* 1989;15(5):429–434.

88. Barnard ND, Gloede L, Cohen J, et al. A low-fat vegan diet elicits greater macronutrient changes, but is comparable in adherence and acceptability, compared with a more conventional diabetes diet among individuals with type 2 diabetes. *J Am Diet Assoc.* 2009;109(2):263–272.

89. Chandalia M, Garg A, Lutjohann D, von Bergmann K, Grundy SM, Brinkley LJ. Beneficial effects of high dietary fiber intake in patients with type 2 diabetes mellitus [see comments]. *N Engl J Med.* 2000;342(19):1392–1398.

90. Diabetes and Nutrition Study Group of the EASD. Recommendations for the nutritional management of patients with diabetes melitus. *Diabetes Nutr Metab.* 1995;8:1–4.

91. Garg A. High-monounsaturated-fat diets for patients with diabetes mellitus: a meta-analysis. *Am J Clin Nutr.* 1998;67(3 suppl):577S–582S.

92. Lovejoy JC, Smith SR, Champagne CM, et al. Effects of diets enriched in saturated (palmitic), monounsaturated (oleic), or trans (elaidic) fatty acids on insulin sensitivity and substrate oxidation in healthy adults. *Diabetes Care.* 2002;25(8):1283–1288.

93. Summers LK, Fielding BA, Bradshaw HA, et al. Substituting dietary saturated fat with polyunsaturated fat changes abdominal fat distribution and improves insulin sensitivity. *Diabetologia.* 2002;45(3):369–377.

94. Gerhard GT, Ahmann A, Meeuws K, McMurry MP, Duell PB, Connor WE. Effects of a low-fat diet compared with those of a high-monounsaturated fat diet on body weight, plasma lipids and lipoproteins, and glycemic control in type 2 diabetes. *Am J Clin Nutr.* 2004;80(3):668–673.

95. Mente A, de Koning L, Shannon HS, Anand SS. A systematic review of the evidence supporting a causal link between dietary factors and coronary heart disease. *Arch Intern Med.* 2009;169(7):659–669.

96. Siri-Tarino PW, Sun Q, Hu FB, Krauss RM. Meta-analysis of prospective cohort studies evaluating the association of saturated fat with cardiovascular disease. *Am J Clin Nutr.* 2010;91(3):535–546.

97. Stamler J. Diet-heart: a problematic revisit. *Am J Clin Nutr.* 2010;91(3):497–499.

98. Hu FB. Diet and lifestyle influences on risk of coronary heart disease. *Curr Atheroscler Rep.* 2009;11(4):257–263.

99. Cao Y MD, Pelkman CL, Zhao G, Townsend SM, Kris-Etherton PM Effects of moderate (MF) versus lower fat (LF) diets on lipids and lipoproteins: a meta-analysis of clinical trials in subjects with and without diabetes. *J Clin Lipidol.* 2008;3:19–32.

100. Connor WE, Connor SL. Should a low-fat, high-carbohydrate diet be recommended for everyone? The case for a low-fat, high-carbohydrate diet. *N Engl J Med.* 1997;337(8):562–563; discussion 566–567.

101. Willett WC. Will high-carbohydrate/low-fat diets reduce the risk of coronary heart disease? *Proc Soc Exp Biol Med.* 2000;225(3):187–190.

102. Retzlaff BM, Walden CE, Dowdy AA, McCann BS, Anderson KV, Knopp RH. Changes in plasma triacylglycerol concentrations among free-living hyperlipidemic men adopting different carbohydrate intakes over 2 y: the Dietary Alternatives Study. *Am J Clin Nutr.* 1995;62(5):988–995.

103. Dreon DM, Fernstrom HA, Williams PT, Krauss RM. A very-low-fat diet is not associated with improved lipoprotein profiles in men with a predominance of large, low-density lipoproteins. *Am J Clin Nutr.* 1999;69(3):411–418.

104. Dreon DM, Fernstrom HA, Williams PT, Krauss RM. Reduced LDL particle size in children consuming a very-low-fat diet is related to parental LDL-subclass patterns. *Am J Clin Nutr.* 2000;71(6):1611–1616.

105. Krauss RM, Dreon DM. Low-density-lipoprotein subclasses and response to a low-fat diet in healthy men. *Am J Clin Nutr.* 1995;62(2):478S–487S.

106. Krauss RM. Atherogenic lipoprotein phenotype and diet-gene interactions. *J Nutr.* 2001;131(2):340S–343S.

107. Gordon DJ, Probstfield JL, Garrison RJ, et al. High-density lipoprotein cholesterol and cardiovascular disease. Four prospective American studies. *Circulation.* 1989;79(1):8–15.

108. Mensink RP, Zock PL, Kester AD, Katan MB. Effects of dietary fatty acids and carbohydrates on the ratio of serum total to HDL cholesterol and on serum lipids and apolipoproteins: a meta-analysis of 60 controlled trials. *Am J Clin Nutr.* 2003;77(5):1146–1155.

109. Asztalos B, Lefevre M, Wong L, et al. Differential response to low-fat diet between low and normal HDL-cholesterol subjects. *J Lipid Res.* 2000;41(3):321–328.

110. Knuiman JT, West CE. The concentration of cholesterol in serum and in various serum lipoproteins in macrobiotic, vegetarian and non-vegetarian men and boys. *Atherosclerosis.* 1982;43(1):71–82.

111. Ornish D. Serum lipids after a low-fat diet [letter; comment]. *JAMA.* 1998;279(17):1345–1346.

112. Connor WE, Cerqueira MT, Connor RW, Wallace RB, Malinow MR, Casdorph HR. The plasma lipids, lipoproteins, and diet of the Tarahumara indians of Mexico. *Am J Clin Nutr.* 1978;31(7):1131–1142.

113. Wolf G. High-fat, high-cholesterol diet raises plasma HDL cholesterol: studies on the mechanism of this effect. *Nutr Rev.* 1996;54(1 Pt 1):34–35.

114. Brinton EA, Eisenberg S, Breslow JL. A low-fat diet decreases high density lipoprotein (HDL) cholesterol levels by decreasing HDL apolipoprotein transport rates. *J Clin Invest.* 1990;85(1):144–151.

115. Azrolan N, Odaka H, Breslow JL, Fisher EA. Dietary fat elevates hepatic apoA-I production by increasing the fraction of apolipoprotein A-I mRNA in the translating pool. *J Biol Chem.* 1995;270(34):19833–19838.

116. Ginsberg HN, Kris-Etherton P, Dennis B, et al. Effects of reducing dietary saturated fatty acids on plasma lipids and lipoproteins in healthy subjects: the DELTA Study, protocol 1. *Arterioscler Thromb Vasc Biol.* 1998;18(3):441–449.

117. Hayek T, Ito Y, Azrolan N, et al. Dietary fat increases high density lipoprotein (HDL) levels both by increasing the transport rates and decreasing the fractional catabolic rates of HDL cholesterol ester and apolipoprotein (Apo) A-I. Presentation of a new animal model and mechanistic studies in human Apo A-I transgenic and control mice. *J Clin Invest.* 1993;91(4):1665–1671.

118. Sacks FM. Desirable serum total cholesterol with low HDL cholesterol levels. An undesirable situation in coronary heart disease [editorial; comment]. *Circulation.* 1992;86(4):1341–1344.

119. Arsenault BJ, Rana JS, Stroes ES, et al. Beyond low-density lipoprotein cholesterol: respective contributions of non-high-density lipoprotein cholesterol levels, triglycerides, and the total cholesterol/high-density lipoprotein cholesterol ratio to coronary heart disease risk in apparently healthy men and women. *J Am Coll Cardiol.* 2009;55(1):35–41.

120. Ginsberg GS, Safran C, Pasternak RC. Frequency of low serum high-density lipoprotein cholesterol levels in hospitalized patients with "desirable" total cholesterol levels. *Am J Cardiol.* 1991;68:187–192.

121. Kris-Etherton PM. AHA science advisory: monounsaturated fatty acids and risk of cardiovascular disease. *J Nutr.* 1999;129(12):2280–2284.

122. Katan MB. Effect of low-fat diets on plasma high-density lipoprotein concentrations. *Am J Clin Nutr.* 1998;67(suppl 3):573S–576S.

123. Sanders TA. High- versus low-fat diets in human diseases. *Curr Opin Clin Nutr Metab Care.* 2003;6(2):151–155.

124. Spiller GA, Miller A, Olivera K, et al. Effects of plant-based diets high in raw or roasted almonds, or roasted almond butter on serum lipoproteins in humans. *J Am Coll Nutr.* 2003;22(3):195–200.

125. Sabate J. Nut consumption, vegetarian diets, ischemic heart disease risk, and all-cause mortality: evidence from epidemiologic studies. *Am J Clin Nutr.* 1999;70(3 suppl):500S– 503S.

126. Kelly JH Jr, Sabate J. Nuts and coronary heart disease: an epidemiological perspective. *Br J Nutr.* 2006;96(suppl 2):S61–S67.

127. Austin MA, Hokanson JE, Edwards KL. Hypertriglyceridemia as a cardiovascular risk factor. *Am J Cardiol.* 1998;81(4A):7B–12B.

128. Rubins HB. Triglycerides and coronary heart disease: implications of recent clinical trials. *J Cardiovasc Risk.* 2000;7(5):339–345.

129. Bloomfield Rubins H. The trouble with triglycerides [editorial; comment]. *Arch Intern Med.* 2000;160(13):1903–1904.

130. Havel RJ. Plasma triglycerides and the clinician: time for reassessment. *J Am Coll Cardiol.* 1998;31(6):1258–1259.

131. Parks EJ, Hellerstein MK. Carbohydrate-induced hypertriacylglycerolemia: historical perspective and review of biological mechanisms. *Am J Clin Nutr.* 2000;71(2):412–433.

132. Bayturan O, Tuzcu EM, Lavoie A, et al. The metabolic syndrome, its component risk factors, and progression of coronary atherosclerosis. *Arch Intern Med.* 2010;170(5):478– 484.

133. Ahrens E, Hirsch J, Oette K, Farquhar J, Stein Y. Carbohydrate-induced and fat-induced lipemia. *Trans Assoc Am Physicians* 1961;74:134–146.

134. Liu S, Manson JE, Hu FB, Willett WC. Reply to BO Schneeman. *Am J Clin Nutr.* 2001;73(1):130–131.

135. Howard BV, Van Horn L, Hsia J, et al. Low-fat dietary pattern and risk of cardiovascular disease: the Women's Health Initiative Randomized Controlled Dietary Modification Trial. *JAMA.* 2006;295(6):655–666.

136. Parks EJ, Krauss RM, Christiansen MP, Neese RA, Hellerstein MK. Effects of a low-fat, high-carbohydrate diet on VLDL-triglyceride assembly, production, and clearance. *J Clin Invest.* 1999;104(8):1087–1096.

137. Kasim-Karakas SE, Almario RU, Mueller WM, Peerson J. Changes in plasma lipoproteins during low-fat, high-carbohydrate diets: effects of energy intake. *Am J Clin Nutr.* 2000;71(6):1439–1447.

138. Kasim-Karakas SE, Lane E, Almario R, Mueller W, Walzem R. Effects of dietary fat restriction on particle size of plasma lipoproteins in postmenopausal women. *Metabolism.* 1997;46(4):431–436.

139. Lamarche B, Lemieux I, Despres JP. The small, dense LDL phenotype and the risk of coronary heart disease: epidemiology, patho-physiology and therapeutic aspects. *Diabetes Metab,* 1999;25(3):199–211.

140. Koba S, Hirano T, Kondo T, et al. Significance of small dense low-density lipoproteins and other risk factors in patients with various types of coronary heart disease. *Am Heart J.* 2002;144(6):1026–1035.

141. Dreon DM, Fernstrom HA, Miller B, Krauss RM. Low-density lipoprotein subclass patterns and lipoprotein response to a reduced-fat diet in men. *Faseb J.* 1994;8(1):121–126.

142. Zambon A, Sartore G, Passera D, et al. Effects of hypocaloric dietary treatment enriched in oleic acid on LDL and HDL subclass distribution in mildly obese women. *J Intern Med.* 1999;246(2):191–201.

143. Moreno JA, Perez-Jimenez F, Marin C, et al. The effect of dietary fat on LDL size is influenced by apolipoprotein E genotype in healthy subjects. *J Nutr.* 2004;134(10):2517–2522.

144. Mennen L, de Maat M, Meijer G, et al. Factor VIIa response to a fat-rich meal does not depend on fatty acid composition: a randomized controlled trial. *Arterioscler Thromb Vasc Biol.* 1998;18(4):599–603.

145. Larsen LF, Bladbjerg EM, Jespersen J, Marckmann P. Effects of dietary fat quality and quantity on postprandial activation of blood coagulation factor VII. *Arterioscler Thromb Vasc Biol.* 1997;17(11):2904–2909.

146. Sanders TA. Dietary fat and postprandial lipids. *Curr Atheroscler Rep.* 2003;5(6):445–451.

147. Petitt DS, Cureton KJ. Effects of prior exercise on postprandial lipemia: a quantitative review. *Metabolism.* 2003;52(4):418–424.

148. Cortes B, Nunez I, Cofan M, et al. Acute effects of high-fat meals enriched with walnuts or olive oil on postprandial endothelial function. *J Am Coll Cardiol.* 2006;48(8):1666–1671.

149. Facchini FS, Hua NW, Reaven GM, Stoohs RA. Hyperinsulinemia: the missing link among oxidative stress and age-related diseases? *Free Radic Biol Med.* 2000;29:1302–1306.

150. Smith U. Carbohydrates, fat, and insulin action. *Am J Clin Nutr.* 1994;59(3 suppl):686S– 689S.

151. Riccardi G, Rivellese AA. Dietary treatment of the metabolic syndrome—the optimal diet. *Br J Nutr.* 2000;83(suppl 1): S143–S148.

152. Grundy SM. Hypertriglyceridemia, insulin resistance, and the metabolic syndrome. *Am J Cardiol.* 1999;83(9B):25F–29F.

153. Frost G, Leeds A, Trew G, Margara R, Dornhorst A. Insulin sensitivity in women at risk of coronary heart disease and the effect of a low glycemic diet. *Metabolism.* 1998;47(10):1245–1251.

154. Moller LF, Jespersen J. Fasting serum insulin levels and coronary heart disease in a Danish cohort: 17-year follow-up. *J Cardiovasc Risk.* 1995;2(3):235–240.

155. Pyorala M, Miettinen H, Laakso M, Pyorala K. Hyperinsulinemia predicts coronary heart disease risk in healthy middle-aged men: the 22-year follow-up results of the Helsinki Policemen Study. *Circulation.* 1998;98(5):398–404.

156. Folsom AR, Szklo M, Stevens J, Liao F, Smith R, Eckfeldt JH. A prospective study of coronary heart disease in relation to fasting insulin, glucose, and diabetes. The Atherosclerosis Risk in Communities (ARIC) Study. *Diabetes Care.* 1997;20(6):935–942.

157. Hu G, Qiao Q, Tuomilehto J, Eliasson M, Feskens EJ, Pyorala K. Plasma insulin and cardiovascular mortality in non-diabetic European men and women: a meta-analysis of data from eleven prospective studies. *Diabetologia.* 2004;47(7):1245–1256.

158. Orchard TJ, Eichner J, Kuller LH, Becker DJ, McCallum LM, Grandits GA. Insulin as a predictor of coronary heart disease: interaction with apolipoprotein E phenotype. A report from the Multiple Risk Factor Intervention Trial. *Ann Epidemiol.* 1994;4(1):40–45.

159. Ferrara A, Barrett-Connor EL, Edelstein SL. Hyperinsulinemia does not increase the risk of fatal cardiovascular disease in elderly men or women without diabetes: the Rancho Bernardo Study, 1984–1991. *Am J Epidemiol.* 1994; 140(10):857–869.

160. Alexander CM, Landsman PB, Teutsch SM, Haffner SM. NCEP-defined metabolic syndrome, diabetes, and prevalence of coronary heart disease among NHANES III participants age 50 years and older. *Diabetes.* 2003;52(5):1210–1214.

161. Stout RW. Hyperinsulinemia and atherosclerosis. *Diabetes.* 1996;45(suppl 3):S45–S46.

162. Reaven GM. Diet and syndrome X. *Curr Atheroscler Rep.* 2000;2(6):503–507.

163. Zimmet PZ. Hyperinsulinemia—how innocent a bystander? *Diabetes Care.* 1993;16 (suppl 3):56–70.

164. Wilson PW, D'Agostino RB, Levy D, Belanger AM, Silbershatz H, Kannel WB. Prediction of coronary heart disease using risk factor categories. *Circulation.* 1998;97(18):1837–1847.

165. Stern MP, Williams K, Gonzalez-Villalpando C, Hunt KJ, Haffner SM. Does the metabolic syndrome improve identification of individuals at risk of type 2 diabetes and/or cardiovascular disease? *Diabetes Care.* 2004;27(11): 2676–2681.

166. Menotti A, Lanti M, Zanchetti A, et al. The role of HDL cholesterol in metabolic syndrome predicting cardiovascular events. The Gubbio population study. *Nutr Metab Cardiovasc Dis.* 2010; February 17 (Epub ahead of print).

167. Kahn R, Buse J, Ferrannini E, Stern M. The metabolic syndrome: time for a critical appraisal: joint statement from the American Diabetes Association and the European Association for the Study of Diabetes. *Diabetes Care.* 2005;28(9):2289–2304.

168. Clinical guidelines on the identification, evaluation, and treatment of overweight and obesity in adults: executive summary. Expert Panel on the Identification, Evaluation, and Treatment of Overweight in Adults. *Am J Clin Nutr.* 1998;68(4):899–917.

169. Flegal KM, Carroll MD, Ogden CL, Curtin LR. Prevalence and trends in obesity among US adults, 1999–2008. *JAMA.* 2010;303(3):235–241.

170. Serdula MK, Mokdad AH, Williamson DF, Galuska DA, Mendlein JM, Heath GW. Prevalence of attempting weight loss and strategies for controlling weight. *JAMA.* 1999;282(14):1353–1358.

171. Kennedy ET, Bowman SA, Powell R. Dietary-fat intake in the US population. *J Am Coll Nutr.* 1999;18(3):207–212.

172. Rolls BJ, Miller DL. Is the low-fat message giving people a license to eat more? *J Am Coll Nutr.* 1997;16(6):535–543.

173. Golay A, Bobbioni E. The role of dietary fat in obesity. *Int J Obes Relat Metab Disord.* 1997;21(suppl 3):S2–S11.

174. Flatt JP. McCollum Award Lecture, 1995: diet, lifestyle, and weight maintenance. *Am J Clin Nutr.* 1995;62(4):820–836.

175. Katan MB, Grundy SM, Willett WC. Should a low-fat, high-carbohydrate diet be recommended for everyone? Beyond low-fat diets. *N Engl J Med.* 1997;337(8):563–566; discussion 566–567.

176. Willett WC. Is dietary fat a major determinant of body fat? [published correction appears in *Am J Clin Nutr.* 1999; 70(2):304]. *Am J Clin Nutr.* 1998;67(3 suppl):556S–562S.

177. Willett WC, Leibel RL. Dietary fat is not a major determinant of body fat. *Am J Med.* 2002;113(suppl 9B):47S–59S.

178. Toubro S, Astrup A. Randomised comparison of diets for maintaining obese subjects' weight after major weight loss: ad lib, low fat, high carbohydrate diet v fixed energy intake. *BMJ.* 1997;314(7073):29–34.

179. Skov AR, Toubro S, Ronn B, Holm L, Astrup A. Randomized trial on protein vs carbohydrate in ad libitum fat reduced diet for the treatment of obesity. *Int J Obes Relat Metab Disord.* 1999;23(5):528–536.

180. Miller WC, Koceja DM, Hamilton EJ. A meta-analysis of the past 25 years of weight loss research using diet, exercise or diet plus exercise intervention [see comments]. *Int J Obes Relat Metab Disord.* 1997;21(10):941–947.

181. McDougall J, Litzau K, Haver E, Saunders V, Spiller GA. Rapid reduction of serum cholesterol and blood pressure by a twelve-day, very low fat, strictly vegetarian diet. *J Am Coll Nutr.* 1995;14(5):491–496.

182. Ornish D, Scherwitz LW, Billings JH, et al. Intensive lifestyle changes for reversal of coronary heart disease. *JAMA*. 1998;280(23):2001–2007.

183. Pi-Sunyer FX. Short-term medical benefits and adverse effects of weight loss. *Ann Intern Med*. 1993;119(7 Pt 2): 722–726.

184. McManus K, Antinoro L, Sacks F. A randomized controlled trial of a moderate-fat, low-energy diet compared with a low fat, low-energy diet for weight loss in overweight adults. *Int J Obes Relat Metab Disord*. 2001;25(10):1503–1511.

185. Brunerova L, Smejkalova V, Potockova J, Andel M. A comparison of the influence of a high-fat diet enriched in monounsaturated fatty acids and conventional diet on weight loss and metabolic parameters in obese non-diabetic and type 2 diabetic patients. *Diabet Med*. 2007;24(5):533–540.

186. Bes-Rastrollo M, Wedick NM, Martinez-Gonzalez MA, Li TY, Sampson L, Hu FB. Prospective study of nut consumption, long-term weight change, and obesity risk in women. *Am J Clin Nutr*. 2009;89(6):1913–1919.

187. Layman DK, Boileau RA, Erickson DJ, et al. A reduced ratio of dietary carbohydrate to protein improves body composition and blood lipid profiles during weight loss in adult women. *J Nutr*. 2003;133(2):411–417.

188. Piatti PM, Monti F, Fermo I, et al. Hypocaloric high-protein diet improves glucose oxidation and spares lean body mass: comparison to hypocaloric high-carbohydrate diet. *Metabolism*. 1994;43(12):1481–1487.

189. Jenkins DJ, Wong JM, Kendall CW, et al. The effect of a plant-based low-carbohydrate ("Eco-Atkins") diet on body weight and blood lipid concentrations in hyperlipidemic subjects. *Arch Intern Med*. 2009;169(11):1046–1054.

190. Sacks FM, Bray GA, Carey VJ, et al. Comparison of weight-loss diets with different compositions of fat, protein, and carbohydrates. *N Engl J Med*. 2009;360(9):859–873.

191. Raynor HA, Epstein LH. Dietary variety, energy regulation, and obesity. *Psychol Bull*. 2001;127(3):325–341.

192. Joint FAO/WHO Expert Consultation of Fats and Fatty Acids in Human Nutrition. Interim summary of conclusions and recommendations on total fat and fatty acids. Geneva: November 10–14, 2008.

CHAPTER 17

Vegetarian Food Preparation

Vegetarian diets often include foods that are unfamiliar to many Americans. Clients may have questions about the preparation and use of these products. There are many excellent cookbooks (see Resources section at the end of the book) that can be recommended to vegetarian clients who request recipe suggestions or who wish to hone their cooking skills. In counseling vegetarians, however, it is helpful for the dietitian to have a basic understanding of food preparation. This is especially true for dietitians who offer community presentations on vegetarian diets.

PREPARING GRAINS

The technique for cooking grains is generally the same for most grains, although the amounts of water used and the cooking times vary (Tables 17-1 and 17-2).

1. Rinse the grain thoroughly.
2. Pretoast the grain. This step is optional, although in many cases it helps grains cook more evenly and enhances flavor. To toast grains, heat a large heavy skillet, add the rinsed grain, and stir until the water has evaporated. Continue stirring until the grain begins to pop.
3. Measure liquid into a heavy pot with a tight-fitting lid, and bring the water to a boil. Grains can be cooked in water, vegetable broth, or, for a sweeter flavor, in a mixture of water and apple juice. Grains will not cook well in tomato sauce, so add any tomato products after cooking is completed.
4. Add the grain, return to a boil, then lower heat to simmer. Cover and cook until all the water is absorbed.
5. Most grains will cook best if salt is added after cooking is completed.

PREPARING BEANS

Soaking Methods

The first step in preparing dried beans is to rinse them thoroughly. Then, to reduce cooking time greatly, most beans (except lentils and split peas) should be soaked for several hours. Small

Table 17-1 Cooking Times for Grains*

Grain	Cups Liquid	Cooking Time (minutes)	Yield (cups)
Amaranth	2½	20–25	3
Barley (hulled)	3	90	3½–4
Barley (pearl)	3	50	3½
Bulgur	2	20	3
Couscous	2	5	3
Kamut	3	120	2¾
Millet	2	25	3
Quinoa	2	15	3
Spelt	3	120	3
Wheat berries	3	120	3

*Amounts are for 1 cup dry uncooked grain.

Table 17-2 Grain Cooking Times for Pressure Cookers*

Grain	Cups Liquid	Cooking Time (minutes at high pressure)	Yield (cups)
Amaranth	1¾	4	2
Barley (hulled)	3	40	3½
Barley (pearl)	3	18	3½
Buckwheat	1¾	3	2
Bulgur	1½	6	3
Kamut	3	40	2½
Millet	2–2½	12	3½
Wheat berries	3	40	2

*Instructions are for 1 cup dry uncooked grain.

beans require only about 4 hours of soaking time; large beans should be soaked for 8 hours or overnight. Use any of the following soaking methods.

Soaking Method 1

1. Place the beans in a large bowl or pot, and add 2 cups of fresh cold water for each cup of dried beans.
2. Place in the refrigerator, and allow to soak for 4 to 8 hours.
3. Drain the beans thoroughly.

Soaking Method 2

Clients who experience gas when consuming beans may wish to try this soaking technique:

1. Place the rinsed beans in a large pot with 3 cups of water for each cup of dried beans. Bring to a boil, and boil for 2 minutes. Drain the beans.
2. Add fresh water, again using 3 cups of water for each cup of beans. Let soak for ≥6 hours in the refrigerator.
3. Drain the beans thoroughly.

Soaking Method 3: The Quick-Soak Method

1. Cover the beans with water, and bring to a boil.
2. Remove from heat, cover, and let stand at room temperature for 1 hour.

Cooking Dried Beans

Soaked beans should be drained and then cooked in fresh water. Place the beans in a large heavy pot with 3 cups of water for each cup of soaked beans or 4 cups of water for each cup of unsoaked beans. Bring the water to a boil. Reduce the heat, cover, and simmer until the beans are tender. Table 17-3 gives approximate cooking times for different varieties of beans.

Table 17-3 Cooking Times in Hours for Beans*

Beans	Soaked	Unsoaked	Yield (cups)
Anasazi	2	2½–3	2
Adzuki	1–1½	2–3	2
Black	1½–2	2–3	2
Black-eyed peas	½	1	2
Cannellini	1–1½	2	2
Chickpeas	2	3½–4	2½
Cranberry	2	2–3	2½
Great northern	1–1½	2–3	2¼
Kidney	1½–2	2–3	2
Lentils†		½–¾	2
Lima	¾–1	1½	2
Navy	1½–2	2½–3	2
Pinto	1½–2	2–3	2
Soybeans	2–3	3–4	2½
Split peas†		¾	2

*Yields are for 1 cup of dried uncooked beans.
†No need to soak before cooking.

Table 17-4 Cooking Times for Beans in a Pressure Cooker*

Beans	Soaked	Unsoaked	Yield (cups)
Adzuki	5–9	14–20	2
Anasazi	4–7	20–22	2
Black	9–11	20–25	2
Black-eyed peas†		9–11	2
Cannellini	9–12	22–25	2
Chickpeas	10–12	30–40	2½
Cranberry	9–12	30–35	2¼
Great northern	8–12	25–30	2¼
Kidney	10–12	20–25	2
Lentils†		7–10	2
Lima	5–7	12–15	2½
Navy	6–8	15–25	2
Pinto	4–6	22–25	2¼
Soybeans	9–12	25–35	2¼
Split peas†		8–10	2

*Instructions are for 1 cup of dried uncooked beans. Cooking time is in minutes under high pressure.
†No need to soak before cooking.

Because beans take such a long time to cook, a pressure cooker is an excellent way to prepare them. Follow these steps for pressure-cooking beans.

1. Use 3 cups of water for each cup of soaked beans or 4 cups of water for each cup of unsoaked beans.
2. If using a jiggle-top pressure cooker, add 1 tbsp of oil for each cup of dried beans.
3. Lock the lid into place, and bring to high pressure.
4. Cook at high pressure for the time indicated in Table 17-4.
5. Release the pressure quickly, according to the directions for the cooker.
6. Test the beans, and return to high pressure for a few minutes if they are not quite done.

USING TOFU

Tofu is still an unfamiliar food to many Westerners. Its versatility and ease of use make it a staple in many vegetarian kitchens, however. Tofu has been a staple in Chinese cooking since around 200 BC and is still used every day in most households throughout much of Asia. It is made fresh daily in small tofu shops and sold by street vendors.

Two distinctive features make tofu an especially versatile food. First, because it is relatively bland, it does not compete with other flavors and contributes no strong flavors of its own to a dish. Second, it is a spongy, porous food that absorbs flavors and sauces well. Therefore, tofu works well in a wide variety of dishes, from spicy chili to banana cream pie.

A variety of types of tofu are on the market. Firm tofu works well for stir-fried dishes, for grilling, in salads, or for scrambled tofu. Soft tofu is a much more delicate product with a higher water content. It can be blended to produce sauces, dressings, fruit shakes, cream pies, dips, cheese type fillings for pasta, and salad dressings. Silken tofu is a soft, custardy product. It is more delicate than the other two kinds of tofu and is especially appropriate for shakes and desserts. In addition to regular firm, soft, and silken tofu, a number of baked and flavored tofu products are available.

Tofu can be frozen for up to 5 months. Once defrosted, it has a spongy, chewy texture that is pleasant grilled and in stews or baked in a sauce.

Tofu is available in water tubs, vacuum packs, or aseptic brick packages. It is usually found in the produce section of the supermarket, although it can also be found in the dairy case. Bulk tofu is often available in food cooperatives or in Asian markets. Unless it is aseptically packaged, tofu should be kept refrigerated.

The following ideas can help vegetarian clients introduce tofu into their meals:

- Marinate tofu chunks in tamari or any sauce, and add them to soups and stews.
- Mash tofu with cottage cheese and fresh herbs to make a dip or a sandwich spread.
- Make tofu burgers by mashing tofu with bread crumbs, chopped onions, celery, and seasonings. Form into patties and fry or bake.
- Defrost frozen tofu, marinate in barbecue sauce, and cook on the grill. Serve in rolls with sliced tomatoes and onions.
- Sauté crumbled firm tofu with chopped onion, and add a package of taco seasoning and tomato sauce to create a filling for tacos.
- Blend dried onion soup mix into soft or silken tofu to make onion dip.
- Blend soft tofu with fresh lemon juice, salt, and fresh herbs for a baked potato topping.
- Blend soft tofu with melted chocolate chips to make a pie filling or a pudding-type dessert.
- Replace all or part of the cream in creamed soups with blended silken tofu.
- Replace all or part of the cooked egg in egg salad with diced tofu.
- Use blended firm tofu instead of ricotta cheese in stuffed shells or lasagna.
- Use blended soft tofu in creamy ranch or Thousand Island dressing in place of mayonnaise.

USING TEXTURED VEGETABLE PROTEIN

TVP, which stands for Textured Vegetable Protein, is actually a brand name; the generic name for this product is textured soy protein, or TSP. TVP is the commonly used term, however, and it is often sold in bulk in natural food stores under this name. TVP is made from soy flour and is low in fat and rich in protein, fiber, calcium, iron, and zinc.

TVP is available as a dried granular product. When boiling water is added to it, it takes on a tender, chewy consistency similar to that of ground beef. TVP is also sold in chunks and is sometimes available as a product flavored to taste like beef or chicken. Flavored TVP chunks can be used in stir-fried dishes, soups, stews, and curries. Most TVP sold in grocery stores or natural foods stores is the unflavored granular variety, however. Both unflavored and flavored TVP is also sold by mail.

To use TVP, pour ⅞ cup of boiling water over 1 cup of dry TVP. Let it sit for a few minutes. Chunk-style TVP requires 1 full cup of water for each cup of TVP and may need to be simmered or cooked in a microwave oven to rehydrate fully.

Studies show that unflavored TVP tastes best in tomato sauce-based dishes. It works well as a replacement for the ground beef in chili, tacos, spaghetti sauce, stuffed peppers, stuffed cabbage, and sloppy joes. Rehydrate the TVP, and use it to replace an equal amount of ground beef in those dishes.

USING EGG SUBSTITUTES

Eggs have two important functions in recipes. First, because the protein in eggs coagulates upon heating, eggs help thicken mixtures and hold them together. For example, most meatloaf recipes contain eggs to bind the rest of the ingredients together. Second, eggs help leaven baked goods, making them lighter and fuller. Eggs also add some moisture to these baked goods.

For vegans or others who prefer to cook without eggs, a number of ingredients can take on these roles in most dishes.

Baked Goods

In baked goods, eggs leaven and add some moisture. The following can be used in place of eggs in baking.

- **Flax seed**. Grind 3 level tbsp of flax seed in a blender for several minutes to produce a fine powder. Then add ½ cup of cold water, and blend until the mixture is frothy and viscous and has a texture similar to that of well-beaten whole eggs. This mixture is the equivalent of about two large eggs and can be added to batter whenever eggs are called for. It can also be refrigerated for several days.
- **Soy flour**. Soy flour has properties not found in other flours that help it serve some egg-like functions in baked goods. For each egg in a recipe, substitute 1 heaping tbsp of soy flour and 1 tbsp of water.
- **Mashed fruits**. The addition of mashed banana, applesauce, or pureed prunes can replace the moisture of an egg and make a product somewhat tender. Use ¼ cup of mashed banana, applesauce, or pureed prunes to replace one egg. This will change the flavor of the product and result in a slightly heavier baked good. When using fruit to replace the egg in baked goods, try adding an extra ½ tsp of baking powder for each egg omitted from the recipe.
- The following mixture can replace one egg in the batter of baked goods: 2 tbsp white flour, ½ tbsp vegetable oil, 2 tbsp water, and ½ tsp baking powder.
- Commercial egg replacer is also available. This is a powdered mixture of potato starch, tapioca flour, and leavening agents.

In some products that do not require a great deal of leavening and call for only one egg (e.g., pancakes), it is usually acceptable to leave the egg out. Two or three additional tablespoons of liquid should be added to the batter.

Binding

The following substitutions can be used to bind ingredients in loaves or burgers:

- Tomato paste (thin just a bit with water, but not too much or it will lose its capacity to hold the recipe together)
- Tahini mixed with tomato paste
- Blended tofu (blended with or without white flour)
- Thickened white cream sauce made from flour, margarine, and soymilk
- Mashed potatoes
- Mashed banana
- Flour, matzo meal, or quick oats (use these sparingly because they can give burgers or loaves a heavy, dense quality)
- Moistened bread crumbs

COOKING WITH SWEETENERS

Many vegans choose to avoid white sugar because animal products are involved in its processing; most also avoid honey. Many other sweeteners can be substituted for sugar in recipes, but substituting sweeteners can sometimes change the end result of the product. Also, when sugar is replaced with a liquid sweetener, other liquids in the recipe must be reduced. The following can substitute for 1 cup of refined white sugar:

- 1 cup Sucanat
- 1 cup maple syrup (reduce the liquid in the recipe by 3 to 4 tbsp)
- 1¼ cup molasses (reduce the liquid in the recipe by 6 tbsp; use molasses for only half the sugar in a recipe)
- 1 cup barley malt (reduce the liquid in the recipe by ½ cup)
- 1 cup brown rice syrup (reduce the liquid in the recipe by ½ cup)

Glossary of Vegetarian Foods

Many foods frequently consumed by vegetarians may not be common in mainstream American diets. The growing market for vegetarian products has also resulted in a large selection of vegetarian convenience foods. Some foods commonly found in vegetarian and vegan pantries are listed here.

SOYFOODS

Edamame: Green immature soybeans consumed as a vegetable.

Soybeans: High-protein beans used to make a variety of products that are of importance in the cuisine of Asian cooking.

Soy flour: Flour made from soybeans; can be full fat or defatted.

Soymilk: The rich liquid expressed from soaked soybeans.

Soy nuts: Roasted, soaked soybeans used for snacks or in salads.

Tempeh: A traditional Indonesian product made from fermented soybeans pressed into a solid cake. It can be marinated and grilled, baked in sauces, or used to make sandwich spreads.

Textured Vegetable Protein (TVP): A brand name for textured soy protein, made from soy flour. Available as either granules or chunks and sometimes flavored to taste like meat. Used in place of ground beef in dishes such as chili and tacos or in stews and soups.

Tofu: A mild-tasting porous product made by curdling soymilk and pressing the curds into a solid block.

MEAT ANALOGS

Commercial meat substitutes: Made from soy, gluten (wheat protein), vegetables, nuts, and other plant foods. Soy protein is a common ingredient. Many products are vegan, although some contain cheese, milk products, or eggs. Meat analogs are available as products that mimic burgers, hotdogs, deli slices, chicken nuggets, roasts, turkey breast, chicken, sausages, and ground beef.

Seitan: Sometimes called wheat meat and made from gluten (wheat protein). It is baked and can be used alone as a meat substitute or combined with other ingredients.

MILKS AND DAIRY ANALOGS

Nondairy cheese: Made from almonds, hempseed, rice, and soy. Newer cheese analogs are derived from nuts or from a combination of oils and thickeners. Vegan cream cheese made from soy is also available. Some of these cheeses may contain the milk derivative casein and are not suitable for vegans.

Nondairy frozen desserts: Made from coconut, rice, or soymilk.

Nondairy milks: Made from almonds, coconut, hempseed, oats, rice, and soy. Soymilk is the only variety that has an appreciable protein content. Most of these milks are fortified with calcium, vitamin D, and vitamin B_{12}.

Sour cream substitute: Made from soy; usually vegan.

Yogurt: Made from soy, rice, or coconut milk. Some soy yogurt has added milk and is not vegan.

BEANS

Adzuki beans: A small brownish bean used frequently in Japan and often served mixed in with brown rice or other grains. Popular in macrobiotic cooking.

Anasazi beans: Maroon-and-white speckled beans that are native to the American Southwest and are used in Mexican and southwestern dishes. Can be used interchangeably with pinto beans. Considered an heirloom bean.

Black-eyed peas (cowpeas): Used in salads and often flavored with hot peppers. Because they are quick cooking, they do not require presoaking.

Black turtle beans: Natives of the Caribbean and Central and South America, these beans are important to the cuisine of those areas.

Brown beans: Also called Swedish brown beans, they are used in baked beans.

Cannellini beans: Small white beans used frequently in Italian cooking. When thoroughly cooked, they have a creamy consistency and can be blended with lemon, garlic, and herbs to produce paté or sandwich spreads.

Chickpeas: Called garbanzo beans in Mexican cooking. Popular in vegetarian cooking, especially to produce the Middle Eastern sandwich spread hummus.

Cowpeas: See black-eyed peas.

Cranberry beans: Brownish beans with red spots. These are traditional in New England-style baked beans.

Fava beans: Large brown beans that are a staple in Middle Eastern and Mediterranean cooking. The tough skins must be removed before eating.

Garbanzo beans: *See* chickpeas.

Great northern beans: Large white beans with a mild flavor, used in baked beans or bean soups.

Kidney beans: Available as either a red or white bean. The red variety is traditional in chili.

Lentils: One of the oldest foods known, lentils are used frequently in the cuisines of India and Middle Eastern and Mediterranean countries. Brown lentils are most commonly available, but yellow and orange types are also sold.

Lima beans: Used as a fresh green bean or a dried tan bean. Dried, they are sometimes called butter beans. Available as large or baby limas; used in soups and stews.

Mung beans: Tiny green beans used in soups and purees.

Navy beans (pea beans): Small, roundish tan beans frequently used in soups or baked beans. Most commercial canned baked beans use navy beans.

Pea beans: *See* navy beans.

Pinto beans: Pale beige or pinkish beans with dark brown speckles. A southwestern staple used in chili and spicy bean stews or to make refried beans.

Split peas: Available as green or yellow beans. When well cooked, they develop a creamy consistency and are used to make soup or sauces to use over grains. A staple in Indian cooking.

GRAINS

Amaranth: An ancient grain used by the Aztecs. The seeds are yellowish brown and tiny; cooked amaranth tends to be soupy rather than fluffy, and it is often mixed with other grains.

Barley: An ancient grain with a chewy quality and mild taste. Barley is available as either hulled barley (the whole grain; also called Scotch barley) or pearled barley (which has the bran removed). It is frequently used in soups and stews or sauteed with onions and mushrooms.

Buckwheat: Toasted buckwheat is a Russian grain called kasha; it has a decidedly strong, earthy flavor that works best when mixed with other, mellower grains. Untoasted buckwheat is milder in flavor. All types of buckwheat cook quickly.

Bulgur (bulghur): Whole wheat that has been precooked and dried. It is common in Middle Eastern cuisine and is used to make the popular salad tabouli.

Couscous: A quick-cooking grain made from steamed, dried wheat and used extensively in North Africa. Available as both refined and whole wheat products.

Job's tears: An Asian grain resembling barley that can be added to soups or stews.

Kamut: An ancient Egyptian wheat berry with a chewy consistency and a rich taste.

Kasha: *See* buckwheat.

Millet: A tiny, round, yellowish grain widely used in Asia and Africa. It is often served as a simple grain dish tossed with chopped onions and herbs.

Quinoa: Called the Mother Grain by the Incas, this grain was a staple in the diet of that civilization. Quinoa is coated with saponin and must be thoroughly rinsed before it is cooked.

Rice: Comes in three basic varieties. Long grain rice is fluffy when cooked and ideal for pilaf. Medium grain rice is moist and tender right after cooking but becomes sticky as it cools. Short grain rice is higher in starch and tends to stick together when cooked; it is the traditional rice used in Chinese and Japanese cooking.

Wheat berries: The whole kernel of wheat. Ground wheat berries produce whole wheat flour. Whole wheat berries have a chewy quality and are often mixed with other grains.

Wheat germ: The nutrient-rich germ of the wheat kernel, often added to baked goods or cereals.

SEA VEGETABLES

Alaria: Similar to Japanese wakame; it is harvested off the coast of Maine. Used frequently in soups.

Arame: Precooked, mildly flavored. The large leaves are usually sliced and dried into thin black strands that can be crumbled into soups and stews. Requires little cooking time.

Dulse: A red-colored sea vegetable that does not require cooking and is added to soups and stews.

Hijiki: A black-colored sea vegetable that looks like strands of angel hair pasta. Should be soaked for several minutes before cooking to reduce saltiness. Often added to soups, stews, and vegetables.

Kelp: Usually sold in powdered form to add a salty, briny taste to vegetables or grains.

Kombu: Grows as long flat strips. Often added to beans while they are cooking to improve digestibility.

Nori: Sold in flat dried sheets and often used to make sushi or nori rolls.

Wakame: Often sliced into soups, especially miso soup.

SWEETENERS

Agave nectar: Syrup made from the agave plant and used to replace sugar and honey in vegan recipes.

Barley malt syrup: A liquid sweetener extracted from sprouted roasted barley. It is only about 50% as sweet as sugar.

Stevia: Sweetener derived from leaves of an herb and used in small amounts.

Sucanat: Made from evaporated and granulated sugar cane juice. Can be used to replace sugar in equal amounts.

PRODUCTS USED IN BAKING

Agar: Sometimes called agar-agar; a sea vegetable that can be used in place of gelatin. Sold in flakes or bars and is taste free. Add 2 tbsp agar flakes to 2 cups of simmering water. Continue to simmer until the flakes are dissolved, then allow to gel for 35 minutes in the refrigerator or for 1 hour at room temperature.

Egg replacer: Commercial egg-free powdered egg replacer for use in baked products.

Flax seeds: Tiny brown seeds that are sometimes added to cereals. Ground flax seeds can be used as an egg replacer. They are prone to rancidity and must be stored in the freezer.

CONDIMENTS

Bragg liquid amino acids: A salty, unfermented condiment similar to soy sauce and used the same way.

Brewer's yeast: A by-product of beer making, it is rich in many vitamins and minerals; usually used in supplement form. Not a source of vitamin B_{12}.

Mayonnaise: Eggless varieties made from tofu or oil are available.

Miso: Fermented soybean paste with a salty, earthy flavor. An essential condiment in Japanese cooking, it is used to make miso soup and to flavor sauces, stews, grains, and bean dishes.

Nutritional yeast: An inactive yeast grown on a nutrient-rich culture to produce a condiment that is rich in vitamins and minerals. Red Star brand Vegetarian Support Formula is reliably rich in vitamin B_{12}.

Tahini: Made from pureed sesame seeds to produce a product that is slightly more liquid than peanut butter. A popular ingredient in Middle Eastern cooking.

Tamari: Soy sauce made in the traditional Asian way, which requires long periods of fermentation and aging. It has a much richer taste than commercial American soy sauce.

Vegetarian Worcestershire sauce: Worcestershire sauce made without anchovies; many commercial low-sodium brands are vegetarian.

Resources on Vegetarian Diet

VEGETARIAN RESOURCES FOR DIETITIANS

Organizations

Vegetarian Nutrition Dietetic Practice Group of the American Dietetic Association
  120 South Riverside Plaza, Suite 2000
  Chicago, IL 60606-6995
  (800) 877-1600
  http://www.vegetariannutrition.net

Seventh-day Adventist Dietetic Association
  Department of Nutrition & Dietetics, School of Allied Health Professions
  Loma Linda University, NH 1103
  Loma Linda, CA 92350
  http://www.sdada.org

Vegetarian Resource Group
  PO Box 1463
  Baltimore, MD 21203
  (410) 366-8343
  http://www.vrg.org

Printed Materials

Diet Manual: A Handbook Supporting Vegetarian Nutrition, http://www.llu.edu/pages/nutrition/dietmanualform.pdf

Joan Sabaté, ed. *Vegetarian Nutrition* (Boca Raton, FL: CRC Press, 2001.

Vegetarian Journal's Foodservice Update Quarterly. A newsletter for dietitians and food service directors. Available from the Vegetarian Resource Group, PO Box 1463, Baltimore, MD 21203, (410) 366-8343.

Chef Nancy Berkoff, *Vegan in Volume*. Features 125 quantity vegan recipes for all occasions. Available from the Vegetarian Resource Group, PO Box 1463, Baltimore, MD 21203, (410) 366-8343.

Gary Fraser, *Diet, Life Expectancy and Chronic Disease: Studies of Seventh-day Adventists and Other Vegetarians* (New York, NY: Oxford University Press, 2003).

RESOURCES FOR VEGETARIAN CLIENTS

National Organizations

The Vegetarian Resource Group
    PO Box 1463
    Baltimore, MD 21203
    (410) 366-8343

Physicians Committee for Responsible Medicine
    PO Box 6322
    Washington, DC 20015
    (202) 686-2210

Vegetarian Nutrition Dietetic Practice Group c/o The American Dietetic Association
    120 South Riverside Plaza, Suite 2000
    Chicago, IL 60606-6995
    (800) 877-1600
    http://www.vegetariannutrition.net

Books

Vesanto Melina, MS, RD, and Brenda Davis, RD, *The New Becoming Vegetarian* (Summertown, TN: Book Publishing, 2003).

Suzanne Havala Hobbs, DrPH, *Living Vegetarian for Dummies* (Indianapolis, IN: Wiley, 2010).

Debra Wasserman and Reed Mangels, *Simply Vegan*, 4th ed. (Baltimore, MD: The Vegetarian Resource Group, 2006).

Enette Larson-Meyer, *Vegetarian Sports Nutrition* (Champaign, IL: Human Kinetics, 2006).

Materials Especially for Young People

- Judy Krizmanic, *Teen's Vegetarian Cookbook* (New York, NY: Viking Children's Books, 1999). Filled with very easy recipes in a format that should be attractive to teens.
- Stephanie Pierson, *Vegetables Rock!* (New York, NY: Bantam Books, 1999). Nutrition information, tips, and mostly vegan recipes.
- Dorothy Bates, Bobbie Hinman, and Robert Oser, *Vegetarian Meals for Teens.* (Summertown, TN: Book Publishing Company, 2003). Quick and easy recipes with information on the health benefits of vegetarian diets. Teens.

- Carole Raymond, *Student's Go Vegan Cookbook* (New York, NY: Three Rivers Press, 2006). Vegan recipes. Teens.
- Carole Raymond, *Student's Vegetarian Cookbook* (New York, NY: Prima Publishing, 2003). Vegetarian recipes. Teens.
- Jules Bass and Debbie Harter, *Cooking with Herb, the Vegetarian Dragon: A Cookbook for Kids* (Cambridge, MA: Barefoot Books, 1999). Easy-to-follow directions and tips. Ages 8–12.

Vegetarian Magazines

Vegetarian Journal
PO Box 1463
Baltimore, MD 21203
Bimonthly

Vegetarian Times
PO Box 446
Mount Morris, IL 61054
Monthly

Websites

- The Vegetarian Resource Group: http://www.vrg.org
- Vegan Outreach: http://www.veganhealth.org
- Vegetarian Nutrition: http://www.vegetarian-nutrition.info
- Vegetarian Recipes: http://vegweb.com

MAIL-ORDER VEGETARIAN FOODS

Vegan Essentials: http://www.veganessentials.com
The Vegan Store: http://www.veganstore.com

Appendixes

Appendix A Fiber, Cholesterol, and Macronutrient Intakes of Adult Vegetarians and Nonvegetarians

(Ref)/year	Group[1]/Gender(N)	Country	Age (years)	SDA/NSDA[2]	Kcal[3]	Protein[4] (%)	Fat[4] (%)	CHO[4] (%)	Sat fat[5] (g or %)	PUFA or LA[6]	PUFA: Sat fat[7]	Chol[8] (mg)	Fiber[9]
(1) 1954	LOV M (15)	United States	55	NSDA	3020	13.0	32.1		33.4 g	14.8 g	0.44	333	16.3
	VEG M (14)		51		3260	10.2	35.9		21.3 g	19.0 g	0.89		23.9
	NV M (15)		57		3720	13.4	42.5		67.4 g	16.3 g	0.24	914	10.7
	LOV F (15)		58		2451	13.4	33.9		32.4 g	10.5 g	0.33	350	12.6
	VEG F (11)		49		2400	10.2	36.3		28.3 g	22.2 g	0.78		20.7
	NV F (15)		57		2690	14.0	41.6		46.8 g	11.2 g	0.24	612	8.4
(2) 1963	LOV F (26)	Australia	19	NSDA	1980	10.7	31.8						6.4
	NV F (25)		20		2115	12.2	40.8						4.0
(3) 1968	LOV M/F (206)	United States	15–74	SDA		14.6	32.8		11.1%	5.5%		193	5.7
	NV M/F (106)		15–74	SDA		16.3	37.4		14.1%	5.5%		361	3.8
(4) 1978	VEG M/F (23)	United States	27	NSDA	2233	17.0	32.0	51.0			1.9		
	NV M/F (39)		27		2264	16.0	42.0	41.0			0.44	424	
(5) 1978	LOV F (42)	United States	57	SDA	1600	16.3	32.2	54.8	13.7 g			185	5.9
	NV F (36)		59	NSDA	1579	17.0	35.7	48.9	21.5 g			307	3.9
(6) 1980	LOV M/F (57)	United States	18–40	NSDA	2270	12.2	34.5	51.5					8.9
	LV M/F (14)		18–40		1830	12.2	30.5	59.0					10.8
	VEG M/F (8)		18–40		1665	8.2	28.6	69.9					16.1
	NV F (41)		18–40		2072	16.2	40.0	41.7					4.5
(7) 1980	LOV M (7)	Netherlands	20–26	NI	2833	13.1	34.0	49.7		25.8	0.30	272	48.1
	NV M (7)		18–25		2619	14.2	38.5	44.6		16.6	0.18	279	33.1
(8) 1980	LOV M (15)	United States	28	NSDA	2624	13.7	34.0	54.7				298	
	NV M (25)		27		2684	16.7	40.2	41.1				453	
	LOV F (13)		26		2174	14.5	38.5	51.0				241	
	NV F (24)		26		1859	16.4	38.7	40.5				287	
(9) 1980	LOV F (49)	Canada	53	SDA	1630	14.2							30.9

(Appendix A continued)

Appendix A Fiber, Cholesterol, and Macronutrient Intakes of Adult Vegetarians and Nonvegetarians

(Ref)/ year	Group[1]/ Gender(N)	Country	Age (years)	SDA/ NSDA[2]	Kcal[3]	Protein[4] (%)	Fat[4] (%)	CHO[4] (%)	Sat fat[5] (g or %)	PUFA or LA[6]	PUFA: Sat fat[7]	Chol[8] (mg)	Fiber[9]
(10) 1981	LOV M (11)	Great Britain	28–80	NSDA	2015	13.1	39.3	49.4					36.7
	NV M (18)	Britain	28–80		2300	14.3	40.1	46.5					24.5
	LOV F (14)		28–80		1737	12.9	42.4	48.5					30.1
	NV F (28)		28–80		1656	15.4	41.1	44.3					19.5
(11) 1981	LOV F (5)	United States	22	NI	1329	15.3	34.5	51.8	17.0 g			340	6.2
(12) 1982	LOV F (101)	United States	57	NI	1565	15.2	32.3	56.8	13.2 g			157	6.3
	NV F (107)	States	62		1573	17.4	36.5	47.6	22.1 g			319	4.0
(13) 1982	LOV F (10)	United States	27	NI	1649	13.3	30.6		17.0 g				28.0
	NV F (10)		25		1572	15.8	40.1		27.0 g				12.0
(14) 1982	VEG M (8)	United States	30	NSDA	2910	16.0	43.0	42.0			2.5		
	VEG F (8)	States	29		2451	14.0	41.0	46.0			2.7		
(15) 1983	LOV M (36)	United States	31	NSDA	2532	13.0	36.6	47.7	37.0 g	23.0 g	0.66	340	7.1
	NV M (18)	States	31		2836	14.0	39.4	42.3	46.0 g	20.0 g	0.45	482	4.6
(16) 1983	LOV M/F (75)	United States	NI	SDA		13.5	36.1						
(17) 1983	LOV M (47)	Australia	33	SDA	2610	14.1	34.4	54.1	33.7 g	25.1 g	0.83	191	44.3
	NV M (59)		34	NSDA	2767	14.9	41.3	46.4	50.3 g	18.4 g	0.41	398	24.3
	LOV F (51)		34	SDA	2036	14.2	36.8	51.3	29.2 g	19.0 g	0.77	208	32.6
	NV F (54)		33	NSDA	2007	15.8	41.3	44.6	35.4 g	14.2 g	0.46	308	19.7
(18) 1983	LOV F (14)	United States	33	SDA	1865	13.5	30.9	58.6	16.0 g	12.8 g	0.80	136	
	NV F (9)	States	36	NSDA	1711	14.7	41.0	44.7	22.6 g	10.6 g	0.47	322	
(19) 1983	LOV M (20)	United States	36	SDA	2324	12.7	28.7	60.9	18.8 g	15.4 g	0.81	186	
	NV M (17)	States	44	NSDA	2652	14.6	39.4	46.8	37.2 g	15.0 g	0.40	404	
	LOV F (31)		46	SDA	1776	13.5	30.4	58.6	14.8 g	11.8 g	0.80	168	
	NV F (36)		44	NSDA	1754	14.1	40.0	44.7	22.9 g	11.2 g	0.49	284	

	Group	Country	Age	SDA						g	g	n	ratio	
(20) 1983	LOV F (36)	Canada	69	SDA	1615	14.5								33.2
	NV F (30)		60	NSDA	1727	15.6								20.2
(21) 1984	LOV M (25)	United	39–65	SDA	2128	13.2	27.5	62.4						48.0
	VEG M (9)	States	39–65	SDA	2259	11.7	25.9	67.1						22.0
	NV M (25)		39–65	NSDA	2335	17.5	37.8	42.3						38.0
	LOV F (25)		39–65	SDA	1615	12.9	34.6	55.2						18.0
	VEG F (9)		39–65	SDA	1497	12.9	22.8	68.7						
	NV F (25)		39–65	NSDA	1821	14.7	40.0	43.1						
(22) 1984	VEG M (10)	Great	NI	NSDA	2548	11.0	35.3	53.8						48.0
	NV M (12)	Britain			2524	13.3	40.3	43.3						22.0
	VEG F (12)				2214	12.5	33.7	55.8						38.0
	NV F (12)				1976	14.6	38.3	45.7						18.0
(23) 1985	LOV M/F (17)	Great	34	NSDA	2290	11.5	38.5	48.6						37.0
	VEG M/F (17)	Britain	31		2381	10.2	33.6	56.3						47.0
	NV M/F (17)		35		2313	14.5	40.9	44.3						23.0
(24) 1985	LOV M (12)	United	57	SDA	2667	14.1	34.1	54.0	31.0 g	17.0 g	197			37.0
	NV M (8)	States	56	NSDA	2617	12.7	39.9	38.7	32.0 g	17.0 g	438			20.0
(25) 1985	LV M/F (9)	Great	37	NSDA	NI	14.1	38.5	45.1			296			49.0
	VEG M/F (10)	Britain	35		NI	11.4	32.6	54.5						40.0
	NV M/F (10)		39		NI	14.0	41.0	38.5			375			22.0
(26) 1986	LOV M (14)	South	29	SDA/	2717	11.4	36.6	49.7	13.4	7.7	292	0.72		38.6
	NV M (10)	Africa	29	NSDA	3167	14.1	37.5	41.7	13.1	7.9	467	0.63		22.4
	LOV F (19)		27	SDA/	1916	12.1	38.0	48.5	14.9	8.0	191	0.58		25.6
	NV F (12)		27	NSDA	1890	14.6	38.3	41.0	13.8	8.1	272	0.60		17.3
(27) 1986	LOV M (60)	Israel	55	NSDA	3290	12.1	30.3	57.2						74.4
	NV M (53)		50		2896	16.7	31.0	50.8						42.4
	LOV F (32)		51		2544	11.6	29.6	58.6						58.5
	NV F (60)		52		2389	18.8	32.8	47.4						33.6
(28) 1986	LOV M (14)	Canada	28	NSDA	2401	11.8	37.1	53.5	31.0		245			35
	NV M (14)		21		2809	14.1	38.4	46.7	30.0		368			21
	LOV F (22)		26		1760	14.5	37.3	54.8	21.0		206			25
	NV F (18)		22		2097	15.3	37.8	46.5	29.0		249			19

(Appendix A continued)

Appendix A Fiber, Cholesterol, and Macronutrient Intakes of Adult Vegetarians and Nonvegetarians

(Ref)/ year	Group[1]/ Gender(N)	Country	Age (years)	SDA/ NSDA[2]	Kcal[3]	Protein[4] (%)	Fat[4] (%)	CHO[4] (%)	Sat fat[5] (g or %)	PUFA or LA[6]	PUFA: Sat fat[7]	Chol[8] (mg)	Fiber[9]
(29) 1986	VEG M (8)	Great Britain	18–40	NSDA	2429	11.1	40.7	47.0					46
	NV M (8)		18–40		2381	13.3	39.6	41.4					21
	VEG F (10)		18–40		2071	11.2	34.3	52.4					25
	NV F (10)		18–40		2333	14.9	37.8	43.1					19
(30) 1987	VEG M (11)	Great Britain	32	NSDA	2643	11.0	40.7	47.0			1.18		50
	NV M (11)		31		2381	15.4	39.6	41.4			0.35		22-+
	VEG F (11)		28		1881	11.6	34.3	52.4			1.15		39
	NV F (11)		24		1833	15.1	37.8	43.1			0.45		27
(31) 1988	LOV F (88)	United States	73	SDA	1533	14.2	32.9	56.4				167	5.6
	NV F (278)		79	NSDA	1633	17.1	48.5	46.1				305	4.2
(32) 1988	LOV F (20)	United States	31	NSDA	1814	14.2	31.8	54.9					
	NV F (16)		29		1788	17.0	39.3	44.1					
(33) 1988	LOV M (14)	United States	34	SDA/	2444	12.8	33.6	54.6					7.0
	NV M (13)	States	35	NSDA	2329	13.9	35.6	48.2					3.9
	LOV F (15)		34	SDA/	1742	12.4	33.1	54.4					5.9
	NV F (16)		34	NSDA	1656	14.3	37.2	47.2					3.5
(34) 1989	LV/LOV F (11)	Finland	36	NSDA	1820	12.8	33.5	52.3	33.4	10.3			22.9
	NV F (12)		32		1910	15.0	38.4	43.8	43.2	9.3			17.4
(35) 1989	LOV (9)	United States	58	SDA	1452	13.3	29.3	59.0	16.5 g	12.4 g		142	27.0
	NV (10)	States	56	NSDA	1799	16.6	36.9	45.4	28.0 g	14.3 g		350	16.8
(36) 1989	LOV M (15)	Canada	29	NI	2700	12.6	29.7	58.4	27.0	19.0		296	38.0
	NV M (14)		27		2620	16.6	36.8	48.4	43.0	12.0		524	14.0
(37) 1989	LOV F (144)	United States	67	SDA	1474	14.1	30.8	58.6	15.0 g			155	20.0
	NV F (146)		66	NSDA	1563	16.2	34.9	49.1	20.6 g			243	16.0
(38) 1989	LOV F (10)	United States	67	NI	1612	13.9	36.0				0.75	194	5.2
	NV F (10)		65		1641	16.6	42.0				0.48	294	4.7

Group (n)	Year	Country	Age	Diet	Energy								
(39) B-LOV M/F (51)	1989	United States	55	SDA	2406	11.1	28.0	50.0					10.8
B-NV M/F (49)		States	56	SDA	2504	15.5	36.9	51.4					10.2
W LOV M/F (163)			52	SDA	2340	13.7	31.7	60.0					13.2
W-NV M/F (89)			53	SDA	2225	14.5	36.0	53.6					9.6
(40) LOV M (11)	1989	France	37	NSDA	2100	12.0	33.9	53.1			1.00	296	
NV M (33)			40		2600	14.8	37.7	39.2			0.40	497	
LOV F (26)			35		1700	12.0	36.0	51.8			0.90	188	
NV F (36)			49		1800	16.2	41.5	39.8			0.40	373	
(41) LOV F (23)	1990	United States	72	SDA	1452	12.9	31.7	60.0	12.1%	9.2%	0.845	89	21.5
NV F (14)		States	71	SDA	1363	16.2	35.9	50.2	16.5%	7.9%	0.506	183	13.0
(42) LOV F (12)	1990	United States	76	SDA	1425	13.2	31.6	60.6	10.0 g	7.0 g		72	24.0
NV F (12)		States	72	SDA	1334	16.2	36.4	49.8	17.0 g	7.0 g		181	13.0
(43) LOV M (18)	1990	Netherlands	83	NSDA	1960	12.2	37.2	50.8	15.0 g	8.5 g	0.57	200	33.7
NV M			elderly		2412	13.6	40.8	41.8	17.3 g	6.8 g	0.39	356	27.4
LOV F (26)			81		1667	13.1	37.3	49.8	15.8 g	8.3 g	0.53	216	28.7
NV F			elderly		1879	14.9	40.1	43.2	17.2 g	6.5 g	0.38	294	23.7
(44) LOV M (15)	1990	Netherlands	82	NSDA	2014	11.7	39.3	49.5					33.0
NV M (225)			72		2414	13.6	41.0	41.6					27.0
LOV F (17)			82		1681	12.8	39.1	48.1					28.0
NV F (216)			72		1874	14.9	40.3	42.7					23.0
(45) LOV F (8)	1990	United States	27	NSDA	1814	14.7	27.9	62.8			0.60		11.6
NV F (8)		States	23		2542	14.3	35.4	49.9			0.50		4.7
(46) LOV M (20)	1990	United States	26	SDA	2489	12.7	33.3	56.4	23 g	10 g		184	34.0
VEG M (15)		States	30	SDA	2915	10.7	30.6	65.2	15 g	22 g			50.0
NV M (18)			26	SDA	2061	14.8	34.9	51.6	23 g	7 g		195	16.0
(47) LOV F (18)	1990	Great Britain	30	NSDA	1826	11.9	35.1	48.0				104	29.3
NV F (22)			34		1779	15.8	40.3	40.3				199	16.6
(48) LOV M (26)	1990	Great Britain	41	NSDA	2619	12.2	36.4	47.7	35.2%		0.73	267	41.8
VEG M (26)			41		2571	11.3	33.5	52.5	17.7%		1.85		55.3
NV M (26)			41		2548	14.6	38.1	43.0	37.4%		0.56		35.0
LOV F (26)			45		1952	12.4	39.6	46.4	31.0%		0.63	306	31.3
VEG F (26)			44		1905	12.2	36.2	51.4	15.7%		1.77	201	42.7
NV F (26)			44		1952	15.5	38.7	43.2	30.8%		0.49	266	26.8

(Appendix A continued)

Appendix A Fiber, Cholesterol, and Macronutrient Intakes of Adult Vegetarians and Nonvegetarians

(Ref)/ year	Group[1]/ Gender/(N)	Country	Age (years)	SDA/ NSDA[2]	Kcal[3]	Protein[4] (%)	Fat[4] (%)	CHO[4] (%)	Sat fat[5] (g or %)	PUFA or LA[6]	PUFA: Sat fat[7]	Chol[8] (mg)	Fiber[9]
(49) 1991	LOV F (23)	United States	35	NSDA	1939	12.8	33.9	56.5	21.0 g	15.0 g		106	24.0
	NV F (36)		36		1835	16.6	35.8	48.6	24.0 g	11.0 g		261	14.0
(50) 1991	LOV F (34)	United States	36	SDA	1819	13.9	33.2	58.1	16.0 g	13.0 g		133	26.0
	NV F (41)		29	SDA	1700	17.6	32.3	51.3	19.0 g	9.0 g		198	15.0
(51) 1991	LOV M/F (79)	United States	18–30	NSDA	2800	13.7	34.0	53.8			0.66		10.7
	NV M/F (4821)		18–30		2980	14.9	37.6	45.9			0.50		6.0
(52) 1992	LOV F (28)	United States	63	SDA	1652	15.2	30.5	58.7	16.5 g	10.1 g		98	10.3
	NV F (28)		63	SDA	1657	18.5	33.6	48.1	19.1 g	10.9 g		214	7.6
(53) 1992	LOV F (20)	Scotland	NI	NI	1690	13.0	34.8	53.9					
	NV F (13)				2143	13.0	37.1	52.0					
(54) 1993	LOV M (16)	Great Britain	21–40	NSDA	2238	11.8	37.4	50.0	32.6 g	19.2 g	0.71	275	34.0
	VEG M (18)		21–40		2190	11.9	34.9	52.8	18.0 g	28.6 g	1.79		44.0
	NV M (386)		NI		2452	14.2	38.2	44.4	42.5 g	14.5 g	0.36	396	26.0
	LOV F (36)		21–40		1826	12.3	38.0	48.4	25.1 g	18.5 g	0.94	155	33.0
	VEG F (20)		21–40		1750	10.7	34.5	55.5	15.7 g	22.4 g	1.47		36.0
	NV F (377)		NI		1733	15.2	39.5	45.5	31.9 g	10.4 g	2.96	296	20.0
(55) 1993	LV M/F (14)	Finland	44	NSDA	2029								31.0
	VEG M/F (10)		42		1927								41.0
	NV M/F (12)		33		1778								16.0
(56) 1993	B-LOV M (23)	United States	69	SDA	1900	14.0	30.8	59.8	13.5 g	15.0 g	0.90	84.0	
	B-NV M (29)		65	SDA	2487	14.5	37.1	52.3	25.5 g	24.7 g	0.97	303	
	W-LOV M (83)		67	SDA	2336	13.6	30.8	61.1	17.8 g	19.4 g	1.09	137	
	W-NV M (43)		65	SDA	2078	14.1	33.8	56.8	20.1 g	18.3 g	0.91	183	
(57) 1993	LV M (23)	Taiwan	23	NSDA	2071	11.8	25.1	62.8	9.0 g	30.0 g	3.40	9.0	5.6
	NV M (20)		21		2119	14.7	33.2	52.9	18.5 g	25.9 g	1.30	434	5.8
	LV F (32)		25		1881	12.4	29.5	57.5	10.0 g	31.8 g	3.30	14.0	4.9
	NV F (39)		20		1500	16.0	37.2	47.5	14.9 g	19.2 g	1.30	408	6.5

(58) 1994	LOV M/F (50)	New	26–30	NSDA	2272	12.3	35.4		32.3 g	19.2 g			34.4
	VEG F (5)	Zealand	26–30		1842	12.0	29.6		14.0 g	19.7 g			36.0
	NV M/F (50)		26–30		2608	12.8	34.4		41.5 g	14.8 g			28.2
(59) 1994	LV/VEG M (17)	United	25	NI	3005	13.3	26.1	59.8					
	NV M (40)	States	24		2906	14.6	34.4	52.4					
(60) 1994	LOV (8 M, 4 F)	Finland	36	NI	2298	12.1	31.8	56.5	34.8 g	18.0 g	0.69	303	
	NV M (14)		50		2507	15.9	40.8	40.8	54.7 g	15.6 g	0.28	803	
(61) 1994	LOV M/F (64)	United	47	SDA	2272	12.8	30.0	59.7	16.3 g	19.5 g	1.20	110	36.0
	NV M/F (44)	States	47	SDA	2603	14.7	31.6	56.6	24.9 g	20.7 g	0.83	248	33.8
(62) 1995	LV F (15)	Canada	26	NI	2024	11.3	33.6	57.0	23.8 g	16.1 g	0.70	152	24.7
	VEG F (8)		29		1923	10.8	30.1	62.3	15.1 g	17.3 g	1.36		35.0
	NV F (22)		28		2086	14.8	32.4	54.5	25.2 g	14.6 g	0.64	231	22.4
(63) 1995	VEG (25)	United	36	NI		12	26	62					42.5
	NV (20)	States	33			16	33	50					17.6
(64) 1996	LOV M/F (11)	Great	34	NI	NI		38.4	NDR	16.0%	7.8%			
	VEG M/F (38)	Britain	35				39.5		8.8%	15.0%			
	NV M/F (39)		44				38.2	NDR	16.1%	7.8%			
(65) 1997	LOV F (13)	Scotland	24	NI	1728	12.8	34.1	49.5					
	NV F (20)		23		2184	12.9	36.6	48.2					
(66) 1998	LOV M (12)	New	49	SDA	2280	12.1	25.3	63.3	11.3%	9.1%		163	44.8
	NV M (11)	Zealand	40		2688	13.5	33.9	52.9	16.1%	6.7%		325	33.8
	LOV F (12)		43		1872	12.2	27.8	60.6	9.4%	6.8%		103	40.6
	NV F (12)		39		2016	14.3	33.0	53.1	14.7%	7.6%		232	26.9
(67) 1998	LOV M (939)	United	39	NI									34.3
	NV M (975)	Kingdom	38										25.2
	LOV F (1908)		38										29.2
	NV F (1470)		38										22.8
(68) 1998	LOV F (4)	Scotland	27	NI	2323	14.4	34.0	51.6	42.9 g	12.0 g	0.28		
	NV F (10)		28		2417	16.7	34.3	48.6	43.8 g	11.6 g	0.26		
(69) 1998	LOV F (18)	Great	30	NSDA	1841	11.9	35.1	53.0	11.4%	7.8%		104	29.3
	NV F (22)	Britain	34		1793	15.8	40.3	43.9	15.7%	6.4%		199	16.6

(Appendix A continued)

Appendix A Fiber, Cholesterol, and Macronutrient Intakes of Adult Vegetarians and Nonvegetarians

(Ref)/year	Group[1]/Gender/(N)	Country	Age (years)	SDA/NSDA[2]	Kcal[3]	Protein[4] (%)	Fat[4] (%)	CHO[4] (%)	Sat fat[5] (g or %)	PUFA or LA[6]	PUFA: Sat fat[7]	Chol[8] (mg)	Fiber[9]
(70) 1998	B-LOV M (49)	United States	50	SDA	2356	12.1	30.0	57.7	16.4 g	23.2 g	1.41	112	37.5
	B-VEG M (14)		46		1869	12.0	24.4	63.3	10.3 g	17.4 g	1.69		41.4
	B-LOV F (94)		52		1922	11.7	29.1	58.7	14.0 g	17.3 g	1.24	94	32.1
	B-VEG F (31)		51		1865	11.3	28.2	60.5	10.2 g	19.6 g	1.92		41.1
(71) 1999	LOV F (50)	Australia	25	NSDA	1652	14.1	34.1	51.8	23.0 g	11.5 g	0.50	122	24.4
	NV F (24)		25		1655	17.5	37.2	45.3	28.2 g	9.2 g	0.33	218	17.3
(72) 1999	LOV M (13)	Belgium	18-30	NI	1971								
	LOV F (31)		16-30		1616								
(73) 1999	VEG M (10)	United States	20-60	NI	2230	13	26	61	13 g	21 g	1.62		48
	NV M (10)		20-60		2170	16	32	52	25 g	16 g	0.64	260	20
	VEG F (15)		20-60		1702	12	25	63	12 g	14 g	1.17		38
	NV F (10)		20-60		1978	15	34	51	27 g	15 g	0.56	235	15
(74) 1999	LOV M (10)	Australia	20-50	NI	2143	14.1	29.8	54.3	9.9%	8.3%	0.8	99	37.4
	LOV M (10)		20-50		2877	12.4	32.6	54.8	8.3%	10.7%	1.3	68.8	59.8
(75) 1999	LOV M (46)	Australia	35	NI	NI10	14.7	32.7	50.9	11.9%	7.9%		197	
	VEG M (18)		33			14.1	28.2	57.4	6.6%	9.8%			
	NV M (65)		38			17.9	32.8	45.7	14.3%	5.6%		332	
(76) 2000	LOV M (237)	United Kingdom	46	NI	2131	13.2	31.0	55.8	8.71%	6.12%	0.78	112	
	VEG M (233)		43		1939	12.7	29.9	57.4	4.87%	8.17%	1.71	327	
	NV M (226)		53		2472	16.6	34.0	49.4	11.8%	5.39%	0.49		
(77) 2000	LOV M (37)	France	50	NSDA	1951	11.5	36.6	51.8					
	VEG M (6)		31		2051	15.0		63.4				22	
	LOV F (57)		53		1675	12.8	34.6	52.6					
	VEG F (11)		46		1302	14.8		61.2				24	
(78) 2000	LOV M (39)	Australia	18-50	NI	2520	12.7	29.3	56.7					
	VEG M (10)		18-50		2784	11.6		59.4				29.0	
	NV M (25)		18-50		2640	16.4	33.4	44.1					
	LOV F (50)		25.2		1656	13.0	32.6	51.0					
	NV F (24)		25.3		1656	16.2	35.3	44.2					

Ref	Year	Group (n)	Country		NSDA										
(79)	2000	LV F (28)	Taiwan	38.2	NSDA	1333	14.1	27.0	58.9			2.34		
		NV F (25)		40.4		1619	16.1	30.6	53.3			1.47		
		LV M (21)		37.7		2000	12.6	23.8	63.6			2.31		
		NV M (21)		38.3		2000	15.2	29.2	55.6			1.25		
		LV F (51)		36.6		1524	12.3	23.0	64.7			2.47		
		NV F (53)		36.9		1738	15.0	25.9	59.1			1.15		
(80)	2001	VEG M (54)	United States	57	NSDA	1830	10.3	25.2	71.9	9.4 g	16.4 g	1.74	28.0	47.0
		VEG F (87)		53		1460	10.2	26.9	71.5	8.2 g	13.6 g	1.66	22.0	38.0
(81)	2002	LV F (45)	Taiwan	31–45	NSDA	1524	12	22	66					
		NV F (45)		31–45		1738	15	26	59					
(82)	2002	LOV F (101)	Great Britain	44	NSDA	1855	13.7	31.1	52.4	8.92%	5.73%	0.64	109	23.4
		VEG F (94)		44		1767	13.5	30.6	53.8	5.37%	8.10%	1.51	0	27.9
		NV F (99)		45		1974	17.6	30.6	49.2	9.74%	4.91%	0.50	211	20.9
(83)	2002	LOV M (786)	Great Britain	45	NSDA	2121	13.1	30.9	51.7	9.1%	5.8%	0.71		24.0
		VEG M (272)		40		1919	12.8	28.7	54.7	4.9%	7.8%	1.65		28.2
		NV M (996)		54		2171	16.1	31.5	47.6	10.4%	5.2%	0.56		19.9
		LOV F (3014)		41		1835	13.9	30.4	53.0	9.2%	5.4%	0.66		22.9
		VEG F (467)		37		1696	13.4	28.7	55.5	5.2%	7.6%	1.53		26.5
		NV F (3741)		51		1906	17.4	31.1	49.0	10.0%	5.2%	0.57		20.2
(84)	2002	LOV M/F (14)	Italy	48.5	NSDA	2002	12.2	33.8	54.0					44.8
		VEG M/F (31)		45.8		1930	12.3	23.5	64.2					52.7
(85)	2003	LOV M (3748)	United Kingdom	39	NSDA	2090	13.1	31.1	51.2	9.37%	5.67%	0.68		22.7
		VEG M (770)		35		1907	12.9	28.2	54.9	7.53%	4.99%	1.57		27.7
		NV M (6951)		51		2186	16.0	31.9	46.9	10.7%	5.21%	0.54		18.7
		LOV F (12347)		35		1810	13.8	30.4	52.9	9.33%	5.29%	0.63		21.8
		VEG F (1342)		32		1660	13.5	27.8	56.1	5.11%	7.20%	1.49		26.4
		NV F (22962)		48		1910	17.3	31.5	48.3	5.19%	10.4%	0.54		18.9
(86)	2003	LOV M (2888)	United Kingdom	38	NSDA	2112	13.0	31.2	51.1	9.4%	5.7%	0.61		22.7
		VEG M (570)		35		1960	12.9	28.5	54.3	5.1%	7.7%	1.51		28.1
		NV M (4318)		48		2225	15.8	32.4	46.7	10.9%	5.2%	0.48		18.7
		LOV F (9419)		34		1817	13.8	30.4	52.8	9.4%	5.3%	1.77		21.8
		VEG F (983)		32		1675	13.4	27.9	56.1	5.1%	7.2%	0.71		26.5
		NV F (13506)		45		1914	17.1	31.6	48.3	10.4%	5.1%	0.49		19.0

(Appendix A continued)

Appendix A Fiber, Cholesterol, and Macronutrient Intakes of Adult Vegetarians and Nonvegetarians

(Ref)/ year	Group[1]/ Gender(N)	Country	Age (years)	SDA/ NSDA[2]	Kcal[3]	Protein[4] (%)	Fat[4] (%)	CHO[4] (%)	Sat fat[5] (g or %)	PUFA or LA[6]	PUFA: Sat fat[7]	Chol[8] (mg)	Fiber[9]
(87) 2003	VEG M (48)	Germany	42.4	NI	2381	11.4	31.4	55.8					66.2
	VEG M (19)		45.2		2186	11.4	28.7	57.9					60.1
	VEG F (50)		42.4		1721	12.4	29.2	56.9					41.3
	VEG F (37)		44.5		1617	10.8	28.8	58.4					50.1
(88) 2003	LOV M/F (37)	Taiwan	28.9	NI	2125	11.5	31.5	57.7					19.2
	NV M/F (32)		22.9		1873	13.6	34.2	52.7					10.5
(89) 2004	VEG F (50)	Germany	35.4	NI	1721	11.9							52.3
	VEG F (25)		62.0		1697	11.6							51.0
(90) 2004	VEG M/F (86)	Germany	43.8	NI	2055								
	VEG M/F (45)		44.6		1757								
(91) 2004	LOV M/F (33)	United Kingdom	18–42	NI	1936	12.9	34.2	47.5	11.3%				
	NV M/F (33)		18–42		2127	13.7	35.9	44.2	12.9%				
(92) 2004	LV F (30)	India	49.5	NSDA	1618	9.1	32.3	57.0	10.4 g	30.3 g	2.91		23.5
	LV F htn (26)		48.7		1737	8.9	31.4	57.3	10.0 g	30.1 g	3.01		24.7
	LV M (85)		46.1		2166	9.3	31.4	57.6	14.4 g	38.4 g	2.74		35.0
	LV M htn (83)		47.1		2260	9.1	30.2	57.5	11.0 g	32.8 g	2.98		34.8
(93) 2004	LOV F (6478)	United Kingdom	49	NI	2303	13.1	32.0	55.7	27 g	18 g	0.67		29
	NV F (24738)		54		2370	15.7	32.6	51.5	31 g	16 g	0.52		24
(94) 2005	VEG M/F (21)	United Kingdom	35	NSDA	2342	11.9	32.2	54.7	4.9%	8.0%			
	NV M/F (25)		36		2486	15.1	35.8	44.0	10.9%	5.2%			
(95) 2005	VEG M/F (18)	United States	54.2	NSDA	1285–2432	9.1	43.2	47.7					
	NV M/F (18)		NI		1976–3537	17.9	32.1	50.0					
(96) 2005	LOV M (31)	United States	19–84[11]	NI	2605	13.0	30.6	56.1	29.6 g	17.0 g	0.57	236	29.4
	NV M (869)				2605	16.5	31.9	50.2	30.3 g	16.6 g	0.55	355	19.9
	LOV F (75)				1840	15.3	27.7	56.9	15.2 g	12.4 g	0.82	209	20.9
	NV F (842)				1793	16.0	32.5	51.4	22.6 g	10.9 g	0.48	236	15.5

(97) 2005	LV F (159)	Sweden	51.1	NI	1206	13.5	25.2	59.8	11.1%	3.7%			22.4
	VEG F (83)		54.8		1140	12.4	23.0	62.7	9.0%	4.1%			23.0
	NV F (54257)		52.5		1373	16.3	30.7	50.9	13.0%	4.4%			17.0
(98) 2005	LOV M/F (55)	Germany	18–43[11]	NI	2177	13.4	28.7	54.2		4.4%	167		32.1
	LOV M/F (53)				1928	13.0	31.4	51.6		5.8%	148		34.8
(99) 2005	VEG M/F (98)	Germany	43.4	NI	2053	11.9	30.3	56.4	5.9%	9.1%	18		58.6
	VEG M/F (56)		45.7		1816	11.0	28.8	58.6	6.2%	7.8%	27.8		53.5
(100) 2005	LOV M/F (43)	Germany	25–64[11]	NI	1792	8.4	28.6	53.1	10.3 g	32.5 g	9.2	3.16	59.5
	VEG M/F (43)				1888	8.2	27.5	58.9	7.3 g	36.2 g	0	4.96	59.0
	NV M/F (115)				2055	8.8	28.5	56.2	11.9 g	34.1 g	61.1	2.87	58.1
(101) 2006	LOV M/F (95)	Slovak Republic	37.8	NI	2345	9.3	24.6	64.3					36.2
	NV M/F (107)		38.7		2445	9.2	24.7	64.9					26.7
(102) 2006	LV F (49)	Taiwan	36.6	NSDA	1530	12.2	22.8	66.1	8.3 g				6.6
	NV F (49)		36.9		1696	15.2	26.5	58.4	16.2 g				4.3
(103) 2006	LOV M/F (90)	Slovak Republic	37.7	NI	1945	14.9	32.4	56.8	20.0 g		130		34.8
	NV M/F (46)		37.1		2438	16.8	34.0	49.0	29.3 g		300		29.4
(104) 2007	LOV M (11)	Ireland	37.8	NI	2486	12.7	33.3	55.5			28		
	NV M (17)		42.2		2366	15.9	34.6	51.1			27		
	LOV F (20)		33.8		1888	13.3	32.4	55.5			22		
	NV F (41)		36.6		1936	15.5	34.9	49.4			17		
(105) 2007	LOV M/F (67)	Brazil	47	NI	1748	13	20	68					
	NV M/F (134)		47		1762	17	30	52					
(106) 2008	LO/LSV F (26)	Turkey	29.0	NI	1832	13.4	35.8	49.7	23.1 g	17.2 g	140.2	1.34	25.6
	NV F (26)		27.4		1849	15.7	35.6	48.1	26.0 g	18.1 g	227.1	1.44	21.8
(107) 2008	LOV M/F (21)	Taiwan	34.8	NI	1884	11.3	31.6	58					6.1
	NV M/F (28)		35.9		1944	12.6	36.3	51.3					3.7
(108) 2008	LOV M/F (25)	Austria	36.4	NI			36.9		16.4%	6.6%			
	VEG M/F (37)		29.5				33.2		12.4%	8.6%			
	NV M/F (23)		38.5				36.8		18.2%	4.5%			

(Appendix A continued)

Appendix A Fiber, Cholesterol, and Macronutrient Intakes of Adult Vegetarians and Nonvegetarians

(Ref)/ year	Group[1]/ Gender(N)	Country	Age (years)	SDA/ NSDA[2]	Kcal[3]	Protein[4] (%)	Fat[4] (%)	CHO[4] (%)	Sat fat[5] (g or %)	PUFA or LA[6]	PUFA: Sat fat[7]	Chol[8] (mg)	Fiber[9]
(109) 2008	LO/SV M (20)	Japan	45.2	NI	1983	13.2	24.9	61.6	12.4 g	14.4 g	1.39	193	19.5
	NV M (32)		44.2		1843	15.1	25.1	57.7	13.9 g	12.5 g	0.97	338	11.4
	LO/SVF (50)		45.9		1675	14.6	28.2	58.5	13.3 g	12.0 g	1.14	253	16.3
(110) 2009	VEG F (105)	Vietnam	62	NI	1130	12.5	18.4	69.1					
	NV F (105)		62		1486	16.9	23.4	59.7					
(111) 2009	LO/LV F (19)	Finland	48	NI	1821	12.7	34.6	52.9	36 g	11 g	0.31		
	NV F (21)		43		1817	14.3	37.1	47.6	39 g	9 g	0.23		
(112) 2010	LOV M/F (30)	Belgium	23	NI	2110	13.8	28.6	56.3					
	NV M/F (30)		24		2215	16.5	30.9	50.6					

Notes: [1]Abbreviations: LV, lacto vegetarian; LOV, lacto-ovo vegetarian; VEG, vegan; NV, nonvegetarian; SV, eats chicken and/or fish; NI, not indicated; CHO, carbohydrates; Sat fat, saturated fat; PUFA, polyunsaturated fat; LA, linoleic acid; Chol, cholesterol; B, black; W, white; htn, subjects identified as having hypertension; NDR, no difference reported between vegetarians and nonvegetarians, although no data were reported.

[2]SDA indicates the vegetarians were specifically identified as Seventh-day Adventists, whereas NSDA indicates the vegetarians were not exclusively SDAs, although some SDAs may have been included in the vegetarian group. NI indicates the process by which subjects were recruited for the study was not indicated or the extent to which SDAs composed the vegetarian groups was not possible to determine by the information provided.

[3]A factor of 4.2 was used to convert kilojoules into kilocalories; a factor of 239 was used to convert megajoules into kilocalories.

[4]Values for protein, fat, and carbohydrate are the percentage of calories contributed by each nutrient. The percentage of calories contributed by protein, fat, and carbohydrate was determined by multiplying the number of grams consumed per day, by 4, 9, and 4 calories per gram, respectively, and then dividing the calories provided by each macronutrient by the total number of calories listed in the reference. In some cases, this led to differences between the calculated percentage of calories contributed by each nutrient and the percentage listed in the reference and often resulted in the total percent not equaling 100. In cases where only the percentage of calories for each nutrient was listed and not grams, those percentages were used.

[5]Values for saturated fat are in grams unless indicated by (%), which represents the percentage of total calories provided by saturated fat.

[6]Values for PUFA and LA are in grams unless indicated by (%), which represents the percentage of total calories provided by PUFA or LA.

[7]PUFA-to-saturated fat ratios represent values as listed in the reference or were determined by dividing the number of grams of PUFA or linoleic acid by the number of grams of saturated fat.

[8]No cholesterol values were listed for vegans because theoretically vegans do not consume cholesterol, although in some studies small amounts of cholesterol were reportedly consumed.

[9]Values for fiber are listed as either dietary fiber (g) or crude fiber (g) (references 2, 3, 5, 6, 11, 12, 15, 31, 33, 38, 39, 42, 45, 51, 52, 57). Typically, 1 g of crude fiber represents between 3 and 4 g of dietary fiber.

[10]Energy intake as reported appears impossibly low.

[11]Age range of all study subjects.

ANNOTATED REFERENCES APPENDIX A

1. Hardinge MG, Stare FJ. Nutritional studies of vegetarians. 1. Nutritional, physical, and laboratory studies. *J Clin Nutr.* 1954;2:73–82. Hardinge MG, Stare FJ. Nutritional studies of vegetarians. Dietary and serum levels of cholesterol. *J Clin Nutr.* 1954;2:83–88.
2. Hitchcock NE, English RM. A comparison of food consumption in lacto-ovo vegetarians and non-vegetarians. *Food Nutr Notes Rev.* 1963;20:141–146.
3. West RO, Hayes OB. Diet and serum cholesterol levels. *Am J Clin Nutr.* 1968;21:853–862. *Note:* 3NV consisted of individuals considered to be moderate meat consumers.
4. Burslem J, Schonfeld G, Howald MA, Weidman SW, Miller JP. Plasma apoprotein and lipoprotein lipid levels in vegetarians. *Metabolism.* 1978;27:711–719.
5. Mason RL, Kunkel ME, Ann Davis T, Beauchene RE. Nutrient intakes of vegetarian and nonvegetarian women. *Tenn Farm Home Science.* 1978;1:18–20.
6. Freeland-Graves JH, Bodzy PW, Eppright MA. Zinc status of vegetarians. *J Am Diet Assoc.* 1980;77:655–661.
7. Huijbregtys AWM, Van Schaik A, Van Berge-Henegouwen GP, Van Der Werf SDJ. Serum lipids, biliary composition, and bile acid metabolism in vegetarians as compared to normal controls. *Eur J Clin Invest.* 1980;10:443–449.
8. Taber LAL, Cook RA. Dietary and anthropometric assessment of adult omnivores, fish-eaters, and lacto-ovo vegetarians. *J Am Diet Assoc.* 1980;76:21–29.
9. Anderson BM, Gibson RS, Sabry JH. The iron and zinc status of long-term vegetarian women. *Am J Clin Nutr.* 1981;34:1042–1048.
10. Burr ML, Bates CJ, Fehily AM, Leger AS. Plasma cholesterol and blood pressure in vegetarians. *J Human Nutr.* 1981;35:437–441.
11. King JC, Stein JC, Doyle M. Effect of vegetarianism on the zinc status of pregnant women. *Am J Clin Nutr.* 1981;34:1049–1055.
12. Beauchene RE, Kunkel ME, Bredderman SH, Mason RL. Nutrient intake and physical measurements of aging vegetarian and nonvegetarian women. *J Am Coll Nutr.* 1982;1:131.
13. Goldin BR, Adlercreutz H, Gorbach SL, et al. Estrogen excretion patterns and plasma levels in vegetarian and omnivorous women. *N Engl J Med.* 1982;307:1542–1547.
14. Lock DR, Varhol A, Grimes S, Patsch W, Schonfeld G. Apolipoprotein E levels in vegetarians, *Metabol.* 1982;31:917–921.
15. Liebman M, Bazzarre TL. Plasma lipids of vegetarian and nonvegetarian males: effects of egg consumption. *Am J Clin Nutr.* 1983;38:612–619.
16. Phillips RL, Snowdon DA, Brin BN. Cancer in Vegetarians. In: Wynder EL, Leveille GA, Weisburger GA, Livingston GE, eds. *Environmental Aspects of Cancer. The Role of Macro and Micro Components of Foods.* Food and Nutrition Press, Trumbull, CT; 1983.
17. Rouse IL, Armstrong BK, Beilin LJ. The relationship of blood pressure to diet and lifestyle in two religious populations. *J Hypertension.* 1983;1:65–71.
18. Shultz TD, Leklem JE. Nutrient intake and hormonal status of premenopausal vegetarian Seventh-Day Adventists and premenopausal nonvegetarians. *Nutr Cancer.* 1983;4:247–259.
19. Shultz TD, Leklem JE. Dietary status of Seventh-Day Adventists and nonvegetarians. *J Am Diet Assoc.* 1983;83:27–33.
20. Gibson RS, Anderson BM, Sabry JH. The trace metal status of a group of post-menopausal vegetarians. *J Am Diet Assoc.* 1983;82:246–250. *Note:* Eight of the 36 LOV were vegans.
21. Calkins BM, Whittaker DJ, Nair PP, Rider AA, Turjman N. Diet, nutrition intake, and metabolism in populations at high and low risk for colon cancer. *Am J Clin Nutr.* 1984;40:896–905.
22. Roshanai F, Sanders TAB. Assessment of fatty acid intakes in vegans and omnivores. *Human Nutr: Applied Nutr.* 1984;38A:345–354. *Note:* The intake (g) of saturated fat, linoleic acid and linolenic acid for 10 vegetarians and their controls was 18, 26, and 1.5 for vegetarians and 31, 10, and 1.0 for the nonvegetarian controls. Subject ages were not provided, but vegetarians were age and sex matched with omnivores.
23. Davies GJ, Crowder M, Dickerson JWT. Dietary fibre intakes of individuals with different eating patterns. *Human Nutr: Appl Nutr.* 1985;39A:139–148.

24. Howie BJ, Schultz TD. Dietary and hormonal interrelationships among vegetarian Seventh-day Adventists and non-vegetarian men. *Am J Clin Nutr.* 1985;42:127–134.

25. Lockie AH, Carlson E, Kipps M, Thomson J. Comparison of four types of diet using clinical, laboratory, and psychological studies. *J Royal Coll Gen Prac.* 1985;35:333–336.

26. Faber M, Gouws E, Benadé AJS, Labadarios D. Anthropometric measurements, dietary intake and biochemical data of South African lacto-ovo vegetarians. *S Afr Med J.* 1986;69:733–738.

27. Levin N, Rattan J, Gilat T. Energy intake and body weight in ovo-lacto vegetarians. *J Clin Gastroenterol.* 1986; 8:451–453.

28. Locong A. Nutritional status and dietary intake of a selected sample of young adult vegetarians. *Can Diet Assoc J.* 1986;47:101–106.

29. Rana SK, Sanders TAB. Taurine concentrations in the diet, plasma, urine and breast milk of vegans compared with omnivores. *Br J Nutr.* 1986;56:17–27.

30. Sanders TAB, Key TJA. Blood pressure, plasma renin activity and aldosterone concentrations in vegans and omnivores. *Human Nutr: Appl Nutr.* 1987;41A:204–211.

31. Tylavsky FA, Anderson JJB. Dietary factors in bone health of elderly lacto-ovo vegetarian and omnivorous women. *Am J Clin Nutr.* 1988;48:842–849.

32. Worthington-Roberts BS, Breskin MW, Monsen ER. Iron status of premenopausal women in a university community and its relationship to habitual dietary sources of protein. *Am J Clin Nutr.* 1988; 47:275–279.

33. Kelsay JL, Frazier CW, Prather E, Canary JJ, Clark WM, Powell AS. Impact of variation in carbohydrate intake on mineral utilization by vegetarians. *Am J. Clin Nutr.* 1988;48:875–879.

34. Adlercreutz H, Fotsis T, Hockerstedt K, et al. Diet and urinary estrogen profile in premenopausal omnivorous and vegetarian women and in premenopausal women with breast cancer. *J Steroid Biochem.* 1989;34:527–530.

35. Adlercreutz H, Hamalainen E, Gorbach SL, Goldin BR, Woods MN, Dwyer JT. Diet and plasma androgens in postmenopausal vegetarian and omnivorous women and postmenopausal women with breast cancer. *Am J Clin Nutr.* 1989;49:433–442.

36. Bélanger A, Locong A, Noel C, et al. Influence of diet on plasma steroid and sex plasma binding blobulin levels in adult men. *J Steriod Biochem.* 1989;32:829–833.

37. Hunt IF, Murphy NJ, Henderson C, et al. Bone mineral content in postmenopausal women: comparison of omnivores and vegetarians. *Am J Clin Nutr.* 1989;50:517–523.

38. Marsh AG, Christensen DK, Sanchez TV, Mickelsen O, Chaffee FL. Nutrient similarities and differences of older lacto-ovo vegetarian and omnivorous women. *Nutr Rep Int.* 1989;39:19–24.

39. Melby CL, Goldflies DG, Hyner GC, Lyle RM. Relation between vegetarian/nonvegetarian diets and blood pressure in black and white adults. *Am J Publ Health.* 1989;79:1283–1288.

40. Millet P, Guilland JC, Fuchs F, Klepping J. Nutrient intake and vitamin status of healthy French vegetarians and nonvegetarians. *Am J Clin Nutr.* 1989;50:718–722.

41. Nieman DC, Underwood BC, Sherman KM, et al. Dietary status of Seventh-Day Adventist vegetarian and nonvegetarian elderly women. *J Am Diet Assoc.* 1989;89:1763–1769.

42. Barbosa JC, Shultz TD, Filley SJ, Nieman DC. The relationship among adiposity, diet and hormone concentrations in vegetarian and nonvegetarian postmenopausal women. *Am J Clin Nutr.* 1990;51: 798–803.

43. Brants HAM, Löwik MRH, Westenbrink S, Hulshof KFAM, Kistemaker C. Adequacy of a vegetarian diet at old age (Dutch Nutrition Surveillance System). *J Am College Nutr.* 1990;9:292–302. *Note:* Values for NV from a separate nationwide survey.

44. Löwik MRH, Schrijver J, van den Berg H, Julshof KFAM, Wedel M, Ockhuizen T. Effect of dietary fiber on the vitamin B_6 status among vegetarian and nonvegetarian elderly (Dutch Nutrition Surveillance System). *J Am College Nutr.* 1990;9:241–249.

45. Oberlin P, Melby CL, Poehlman ET. Resting energy expenditure in young vegetarian and nonvegetarian women. *Nutr Res.* 1990;10:39–49.

46. Pusateri DJ, Roth WT, Ross JK, Schultz TD. Dietary and hormonal evaluation of men at different risks for prostate cancer: plasma and fecal hormone–nutrient interrelationships. *Am J Clin Nutr.* 1990; 51:371–377.

47. Reddy S, Sanders TAB. Haematological studies on premenopausal Indian and Caucasian vegetarians compared with Caucasian omnivores. *Br J Nutr.* 1990;64:331–338.

48. Thorogood M, Roe L, McPherson K, Mann J. Dietary intake and plasma lipid levels: lessons from a study of the diet of health conscious groups. *Br Med J.* 1990;300:1297–1301.
49. Lloyd T, Schaeffer JM, Walker MA, Demers L. Urinary hormonal concentrations and spinal bone densities of premenopausal vegetarian and nonvegetarian women. *Am J Clin Nutr.* 1991;54:1005–1010.
50. Pedersen AB, Bartholomew MJ, Dolence LA, Aljadir LP, Netteburg KL, Lloyd T. Menstrual differences due to vegetarian and nonvegetarian diets. *Am J Clin Nutr.* 1991;53:879–885.
51. Slattery ML, Jacobs DR, Hilner JE Jr, et al. Meat consumption and its association with other diet and health factors in young adults: the CARDIA study. *Am J Clin Nutr.* 1991;54:930–935.
52. Tesar R, Notelovitz M, Shim E, Kauwell G, Brown J. Axial and peripheral bone density and nutrient intakes of postmenopausal vegetarian and omnivorous women. *Am J Clin Nutr.* 1992;56:699–704.
53. Ball D. Robertson JD, Maughan RJ. Acid-based status of premenopausal vegetarian and omnivorous women. *Proc Nutr Soc.* 1992;51:32A [abstr].
54. Draper A, Lewis J, Malhotra N, Wheeler E. The energy and nutrient intakes of different types of vegetarian: a case for supplements. *Br J Nutr.* 1993;69:3–19. *Note:* Approximately 70% and 75% of the vegetarians and nonvegetarians were between 21 and 40 years of age. NV data taken from a separate nationwide survey.
55. Lamberg-Allardt C, Kärkkäinen M, Seppänen R, Biström H. Low serum 25-hydroxyvitamin D concentrations and secondary hyperparathyroidism in middle-aged white strict vegetarians. *Am J Clin Nutr.* 1993;58:684–689.
56. Melby CL, Goldflies DG, Toohey ML. Blood pressure differences in older black and white long-term vegetarians and nonvegetarians. *J Am Coll Nutr.* 1993;12:262–269. *Note:* Subjects in this study may consist of a subset of older individuals included in reference 39.
57. Pan W-H, Chin C-J, Sheu C-T, Lee M-H. Hemostatic factors and blood lipids in young Buddhist vegetarians and omnivores. *Am J Clin Nutr.* 1993;58:354–359. *Note:* The vegetarian diet was described as including no flesh foods, and although milk was allowed, large amounts of milk were reportedly not consumed. No mention was made regarding egg use but the cholesterol intake indicates eggs were not consumed.
58. Alexander D, Ball MJ, Mann J. Nutrient intake and haematological status of vegetarians and age-sex matched omnivores. *Eur J Clin Nutr.* 1994;48:538–546. *Note:* Of the 50 LOV, 5 were vegans. Data for vegans are also reported separately.
59. Toth MJ, Poehlman ET. Sympathetic nervous system activity and resting metabolism rate in vegetarians. *Metabolism.* 1994;43:621–625.
60. Vuoristo M, Miettinen TA. Absorption, metabolism, and serum concentrations of cholesterol in vegetarians: effects of cholesterol feedings. *Am J Clin Nutr.* 1994;59:1326–1331.
61. Melby CL, Toohey M, Cebrick J. Blood pressure and blood lipids among vegetarian, semivegetarian, and nonvegetarian African Americans. *Am J Clin Nutr.* 1994;59:103–109. *Note:* All subjects were black; of the initial 66 vegetarians, 16 were vegans, and 50 were lacto-ovo vegetarians, there were 46 women and 20 men. Of the nonvegetarians, 34 were women and 11 were men.
62. Janelle KC, Barr SI. Nutrient intakes and eating behavior scores of vegetarian and nonvegetarian women. *J Am Diet Assoc.* 1995;95:180–189. *Note:* Eleven of the 15 vegetarians ate eggs.
63. Berk LS, Hubbard RW, Haddad E, et al. Basal fasting cytokine levels in vegans and omnivores. *Am J Clin Nutr.* 1995;61:904 (abstr 74).
64. Thomas EL, Frost G, Barnard ML, et al. An *in vivo* $_{13}C$ *magnetic resonance spectroscopic study of the relationship between diet and adipose tissue composition.* Lipids. 1996;31:145–151. *Note:* Six males and 5 females were LOV, 21 males and 17 females were VEG, 20 males and 19 females were NV.
65. Ball D, Maughan RJ. Blood and urine acid-base status of premenopausal omnivorous and vegetarian women. *Br J Nutr.* 1997;78:683–693. *Note:* Two vegetarians occasionally ate fish.
66. Harman SK, Parnell WR. The nutritional health of New Zealand vegetarian and nonvegetarian Seventh-Day Adventists: selected vitamin, mineral and lipid levels. *NZ Med J.* 1998;111:91–94. *Note:* Of the 24 vegetarians, an unspecified number were lacto vegetarians or vegans. Some nonvegetarians only occasionally ate red meat.
67. Appleby PN, Thorogood M, Mann JI, Key TJ. Low body mass index in non-meat eaters: the possible roles of animal fat, dietary fibre and alcohol. *Int J Obesity.* 1998;22:454–460. *Note:* A total of 480 of the 2847 LOV ate fish; 201 were vegan.
68. Lakin V, Haggarty P, Abramovich DR, et al. Dietary intake and tissue concentration of fatty acids in omnivore, vegetarian and diabetic pregnancy. *Prost Leuk Essent Fat Acids.* 1998;59:209–220. *Note:* All subjects were pregnant.

69. Reddy S, Sanders TAB, Owen RW, Thompson MH. Faecal pH, bile acid and sterol concentrations in premenopausal Indian and white vegetarians compared with white omnivores. *Br J Nutr.* 1998;79:495–500.

70. Toohey ML, Harris MA, Williams D, Foster G, Schmidt WD, Melby CL. Cardiovascular disease risk factors are lower in African-American vegans compared to lacto-ovo vegetarians. *J Am Coll Nutr.* 1998;17:425–434.

71. Ball MJ, Bartlett MA. Dietary intake and iron status of Australian vegetarian women. *Am J Clin Nutr.* 1999;70:353–358. *Note:* Two of the 50 LOV were vegan; vegetarians consumed red meat no more than once a month and consumed fish or chicken no more than once a week.

72. Hebbelinck M, Clarys P, DeMalsche A. Growth, development, and physical fitness of Flemish vegetarian children, adolescents, and young adults. *Am J Clin Nutr.* 1999;70(suppl):579S–585S.

73. Haddad EH, Berk LS, Kettering JD, Hubbard RW, Peters WR. Dietary intake and biochemical, hematologic, and immune status of vegans compared with nonvegetarians. *Am J Clin Nutr.* 1999;70 (suppl):586S–593S.

74. Li D, Sinclair A, Wilson A, et al. Effect of dietary α-linolenic acid on thrombotic risk factors in vegetarian men. *Am J Clin Nutr.* 1999;69:878–882. *Note:* Vegetarian subjects were divided into two groups for study purposes. Only baseline data are reported here.

75. Li D, Sinclair A, Mann N, et al. The association of diet and thrombotic risk factors in healthy male vegetarians and meat-eaters. *Eur J Clin Nutr.* 1999;53:612–619. *Note:* Nonvegetarians are described as "moderate-meat-eaters" (285 g meat/d). Ten LOV and 3 VEG consumed fish occasionally.

76. Allen NE, Appleby PN, Davey GK, Key TJ. Hormones and diet: low insulin-like growth factor-I but normal bioavailable androgens in vegan men. *Br J Cancer.* 2000;83:95–97.

77. Leblanc JC, Yoon H, Kombadjian A, Verger P. Nutritional intakes of vegetarian populations in France. *Eur J Clin Nutr.* 2000;54:443–449. *Note:* Thirty-one of the 94 LOV ate fish or meat at least once a week; 11 were lacto vegetarians and 3 were lacto ovo vegetarians. Thirteen of the 17 VEG ate fish once a week.

78. Ball MJ, Ackland ML. Zinc intake and status in Australian vegetarians. *Br J Nutr.* 2000;83:27–33. *Note:* Two of the 50 LOV females were vegans.

79. Lu S-C, Wu W-H, Lee C-A, et al. LDL of Taiwanese vegetarians are less oxidizable than those of omnivores. *J Nutr.* 2000;130:1591–1596. *Note:* About one third of the LV were vegans.

80. Donaldson MS. Food and nutrient intake of Hallelujah vegetarians. *Nutr Food Sci.* 2001;31:293–303. *Note:* VEG subjects ate a mostly raw diet; 58% consumed some animal product during their week of food intake records.

81. Hung C-J, Huang P-C, Lu S-c, et al. Plasma homocysteine levels in Taiwanese vegetarians are higher than those of omnivores. *J Nutr.* 2002;132:152–158. *Note:* Six of the 45 LV were vegans.

82. Allen NE, Appleby PN, Davey GK, et al. The associations of diet with serum insulin-like growth factor I and its main binding proteins in 292 women meat-eaters, vegetarians, and vegans. *Cancer Epidemiol Biomark Prevent.* 2002;11:1441–1448.

83. Appleby PN, Davey GK, Key TJ. Hypertension and blood pressure among meat eaters, fish eaters, vegetarians, and vegans in EPIC-Oxford. *Public Health Nutr.* 2002;5:645–654.

84. Bissoli L, Di Francesco V, Ballarin A, et al. Effect of vegetarian diet on homocysteine levels. *Ann Nutr Metab.* 2002;46:73–79.

85. Davey GK, Spencer EA, Appleby PN, et al. EPIC-Oxford lifestyle characteristics and nutrient intakes in a cohort of 33883 meat-eaters and 31546 non-meat-eaters in the UK. *Public Health Nutr.* 2003;6:259–268.

86. Spencer EA, Appleby PN, Davey GK, Key TJ. Diet and body mass index in 38000 EPIC-Oxford meat-eaters, fish-eaters, vegetarians and vegans. *Int J Obesity Res.* 2003;27: 728–734. *Note:* Subjects are a subset of those in reference 86.

87. Waldmann A, Koschizke JW, Leitzmann C, Hahn A. Dietary intake and lifestyle factors of a vegan population in Germany: results from the German Vegan Study. *Eur J Clin Nutr.* 2003;57:947–955. *Note:* Ninety-eight subjects did not use animal products for 1 year prior to study; 56 subjects consumed small amounts of dairy products and eggs. The first listing for each gender is for strict vegans, the second listing is for those who consumed small amounts of dairy and eggs.

88. Huang YC, Chang SJ, Chiu YT, et al. The status of plasma homocysteine and related B-vitamins in healthy young vegetarians and nonvegetarians. *Eur J Nutr.* 2003;42:84–90. *Note:* LOV group includes 3 VEG, 18 LV, 16 LOV.

89. Waldmann A, Koschizke JW, Leitzmann C, et al. Dietary iron intake and iron status of German female vegans: results of the German Vegan Study. *Ann Nutr Metab.* 2004;48:103–108. *Note:* Subjects are a subset of those in reference 87.

90. Waldmann A, Koschizke JW, Leitzmann C, et al. Homocysteine and cobalamin status in German vegans. *Public Health Nutr.* 2004;7:467–472. *Note:* The first listing is for strict vegans (42 males and 44 females); the second listing is for those who consumed small amounts of dairy and eggs but were primarily vegan (16 males and 29 females). Subjects are a subset of those in reference 87.

91. Phillips F, Hackett AF, Stratton G, et al. Effect of changing to a self-selected vegetarian diet on anthropometric measurements in UK adults. *J Hum Nutr Dietet.* 2004;17:249–255. *Note:* Results represent intakes before and 6 months after becoming vegetarian. Six subjects identified as vegetarian ate fish. Seven males and 26 females were in each group.

92. Chiplonkar SA, Agte V, Tarwadik V, et al. Micronutrient deficiencies as predisposing factors for hypertension in lacto-vegetarian Indian adults. *J Am Coll Nutr.* 2004;23:239–247.

93. Cade JE, Burley VJ, Greenwood DC, et al. The UK Women's Cohort Study: comparisons of vegetarians, fish-eaters, and meat-eaters. *Public Health Nutr.* 2004;7:871–878. *Note:* Vegetarians ate meat or fish less than once a week.

94. Goff LM, Bell JD, So PW, et al. Veganism and its relationship with insulin resistance and intramyocellular lipid. *Eur J Clin Nutr.* 2005;59:291–298. *Note:* Gender distribution of VEG group not specified; 11 males and 14 females were NV.

95. Fontana L, Shew JL, Holloszy JO, et al. Low bone mass in subjects on a long-term raw vegetarian diet. *Arch Intern Med.* 2005;165:684–689. *Note:* Study subjects ate a raw foods diet. Seven males and 11 females were VEG; 7 males and 11 females were NV.

96. Bedford JL, Barr SI. Diets and selected lifestyle practices of self-defined adult vegetarians from a population-based sample suggest they are more health conscious. *Int J Behav Nutr Phys Act.* 2005;2:4. *Note:* Seventy-five percent of those self-identified as vegetarian consumed fish and/or seafood, 58% consumed poultry; 22% consumed red meat.

97. Newby PK, Tucker KL, Wolk A. Risk of overweight and obesity among semivegetarians, lactovegetarians and vegan women. *Am J Clin Nutr.* 2005;81:1267–1274.

98. Geppert J, Kraft V, Demmelmair H, et al. Docosahexaenoic acid supplementation in vegetarians effectively increases omega-3 index: a randomized trial. *Lipids.* 2005;40:807–814. *Note:* Subjects were divided into two groups.

99. Waldmann A, Koschizke JW, Leitzmann C, et al. German vegan study: diet, lifestyle factors, and cardiovascular risk profile. *Ann Nutr Metab.* 2005;49:366–372. *Note:* The first listing is for strict vegans (48 males and 50 females); the second listing is for those who consumed small amounts of dairy and eggs but were primarily vegan (19 males and 37 females). Subjects are a subset of those in reference 87.

100. Koebnick C, Garcia AL, Dagnelie PC, et al. Long-term consumption of a raw food diet is associated with favorable serum LDL cholesterol and triglycerides but also with elevated plasma homocysteine and low serum HDL cholesterol in humans. *J Nutr.* 2005;135:2372–2378. *Note:* Subjects ate a raw foods diet; no information provided on gender distribution in groups.

101. Valachovicova M, Krajcovicova-Kudlackova M, Blazicek P, et al. No evidence of insulin resistance in normal weight vegetarians. A case study. *Eur J Nutr.* 2006;45:52–54. *Note:* Thirty-nine males and 56 females were LOV; 45 males and 62 females were NV.

102. Hung CJ, Huang PC, Li YH, et al. Taiwanese vegetarians have higher insulin sensitivity than omnivores. *Br J Nutr.* 2006;95:129–135. *Note:* Seven subjects were vegan, 42 were lactovegetarians.

103. Sebekova K, Boor P, Valachovicova M, et al. Association of metabolic syndrome risk factors with selected markers of oxidative status and microinflammation in healthy omnivores and vegetarians. *Mol Nutr Food Res.* 2006;50:858–868. *Note:* Thirty males and 60 females were LOV; 19 males and 27 females were NV.

104. Haldar S, Rowland IR, Barnett RA, et al. Influence of habitual diet on antioxidant status: a study in a population of vegetarians and omnivores. *Eur J Clin Nutr.* 2007;61:1011–1022. *Note:* Vegetarian subjects ate flesh foods no more than six times a year. The vegetarian group included six vegans.

105. Teixeira Rde C, Molina Mdel C, Zandonade E, Mill JG. Cardiovascular risk in vegetarians and omnivores: a comparative study. *Arq Bras Cardiol.* 2007;89:237–244. *Note:* Seventy-three percent LOV, 14% vegan, 3% LV, 10% ate fish. No information on gender distribution.

106. Karabudak E, Kiziltan G, Cigerim N. A comparison of some of the cardiovascular risk factors in vegetarian and omnivorous Turkish females. *J Hum Nutr Diet.* 2008;21:13–22. *Note:* Subjects include 9 LOV, 10 LV, and 7 occasional fish and/or chicken eaters.

107. Yen CE, Yen CH, Huang MC, et al. Dietary intake and nutritional status of vegetarian and omnivorous preschool children and their parents in Taiwan. *Nutr Res.* 2008;28:430–436. *Note:* Adult vegetarians consisted of 16 LOV,

2 ovo-vegetarians, 1 LV, 2 vegans. Four male adults and 17 females were vegetarian; 9 male adults and 19 females were NV. Children consisted of 18 LOV and 3 ovo-vegetarians. Fourteen male children and 7 female children were vegetarians; 15 male children and 13 female children were NV.

108. Kornsteiner M, Singer I, Elmadfa I. Very low n-3 long-chain polyunsaturated fatty acid status in Austrian vegetarians and vegans. *Ann Nutr Metab.* 2008;52:37–47. *Note:* Seven males and 18 females were LOV; 19 males and 18 females were VEG; 8 males and 15 females were NV.

109. Nakamato K, Watanabe S, Kudo H, et al. Nutritional characteristics of middle-aged Japanese vegetarians. *J Atherosclero Throm.* 2008;15:122–129. *Note:* Nine men and 18 women were LOV; 11 men and 37 women in the vegetarian group occasionally ate chicken and meat.

110. Ho-Pham LT, Nguyen PL, Le TT, et al. Veganism, bone density, and body composition: a study in Buddhist nuns. *Osteoporosis Int.* 2009;20:2087–2093.

111. Aubertin-Leheudre M, Adlercreutz H. Relationship between animal protein intake and muscle mass index in healthy women. *Br J Nutr.* 2009;102:1803–1810. *Note:* The vegetarian group included 8 LOV, 10 LV, and 1 vegan.

112. Deriemaeker P, Aerenhouts D, Hebbelinck M, Clarys P. Nutrient based estimation of acid-base balance in vegetarians and non-vegetarians. *Plant Foods Hum Nutr.* 2010;65:77–82. *Note:* Eight men and 22 women were in each group.

Appendix B Lipid Levels in Adult Vegetarians and Nonvegetarians

(REF)/year	Group[1]/Gender (N)	Age (years)[2]	Serum TC[3]	Serum LDL[3]	Serum HDL[3]	Serum TC:HDL[4]	Serum TAG[3]
(1) 1954	LOV M (15)	55	243				
	VEG M (14)	51	206				
	NV M (15)	57	288				
	LOV F (15)	58	269				
	VEG F (11)	49	206				
	NV F (15)	57	295				
(2) 1966	VEG M/F (249)	13–87	159				62.0
	NV M/F (157)	NI	180				73.0
(3) 1970	VEG M (12)	22–80	181				
	NV M (12)	NI	240				
	VEG M (14)	18–68	NDR				
	NV M (14)	NI	NDR				
(4) 1975	LV/LOV (115)	16–62	126	73.0	43	2.93	59.0
	NV (115)	16–62	184	118	49	3.76	86.0
(5) 1978	LOV M/F (20)	39	175				80.0
	NV M/F (39)	37	229				102
(6) 1978	VEG M (17)	20–30	125	79.0	37	3.38	
	NV M (28)	20–30	184	118	48	3.83	
	VEG M (8)	30–40	137	78	37	3.70	
	NV M (7)	30–40	196	130	48	4.08	
	VEG F (24)	20–30	133	81.0	43	3.09	
	NV F (32)	20–30	174	114	50	3.48	
	VEG F (7)	30–40	147	94.0	43	3.42	
	NV F (11)	30–40	193	128	50	3.86	
(7) 1979	LOV M/F (8)	21–66	6.30				1.19
	NV M/F (8)	21–66	6.70				1.51
	VEG M/F (22)	21–66	4.10				0.95
	NV M/F (22)	21–66	6.10				1.35

(Appendix B continued)

Appendix B Lipid Levels in Adult Vegetarians and Nonvegetarians

(REF)/year	Group[1]/Gender (N)	Age (years)[2]	Serum TC[3]	Serum LDL[3]	Serum HDL[3]	Serum TC:HDL[4]	Serum TAG[3]
(8) 1979	LOV M (45)	18–35	4.25		1.04	4.09	
	NV M (48)	18–35	5.28		1.19	4.44	
	LOV F (52)	18–35	4.42		1.17	3.78	
	NV F (22)	18–35	5.26		1.42	3.70	
(9) 1979	LOV M/F (104)	NI	6.00				
	NV M/F (104)		6.60				
(10) 1980	LOV/VEG M (25)	40	4.70				1.20
	NV M (211)	50	6.00				1.68
	LOV/VEG F (25)	44	5.20				0.92
	NV F (71)	52	6.70				1.22
(11) 1980	LOV M (7)	20–26	4.31	2.64	1.34	3.22	1.06
	NV M (7)	18–25	4.84	2.87	1.52	3.18	1.20
(12) 1980	LOV M/F (91)	30–69	5.50		1.70		1.20
	NV M/F (264)	30–69	6.50		1.70		1.40
(13) 1981	LOV M (8)	40	4.70	1.14			
	NV M (50)	44	5.87	1.09			
	LOV M (21)	69	5.49	1.27			
	NV M (32)	69	5.65	1.20			
	LOV F (28)	43	5.41	1.40			
	NV F (85)	45	5.90	1.41			
	LOV F (28)	68	5.93	1.45			
	NV F (48)	68	6.52	1.47			
(14) 1981	LOV F (46)	67	6.80		1.61	4.22	1.70
	NV F (47)	66	7.20		1.54	4.68	1.60
(15) 1982	LOV M (56)	34	4.7		1.40	3.36	0.45
	NV M (52)	35	5.5		1.20	4.58	0.38
(16) 1982	VEG M (8)	30	135	85.0	42.0	3.21	57.0
	NV M (10)	33	185	NI	NI	NI	154
	VEG F (28)	29	137	77.0	49.0	2.80	53.0
	NV F (26)	31	178	NI	NI	NI	82.0

	Group						
(17) 1983	VEG M (86)	61	167		43.0	4.26	79.0
	NV M (86)	61	193		45.0	4.33	98.0
	VEG F (353)	60	173				
	NV F (353)	60	201				
(18) 1983	LOV M (36)	31	183	117			
	NV M (18)	31	195	126			
(19) 1984	LOV M (12)	52	177		37.1	4.77	166
	VEG M (9)	55	136		32.8	4.15	154
	NV M (13)	51	220		53.5	4.11	128
	LOV F (9)	51	205		56.0	3.66	120
	VEG F (13)	60	163		40.3	4.04	193
	NV F (13)	52	211		56.3	3.75	76
(20) 1984	VEG M (11)	NI	3.57	1.91	1.33	3.33	0.72
	NV M (12)	NI	4.62	3.01	1.32	3.50	0.64
	VEG F (12)	NI	3.74	2.02	1.45	2.58	0.60
	NV F (12)	NI	4.03	2.21	1.49	2.70	0.73
(21) 1980	LOV MF (15)	20–47	150	100	45.0	3.33	95.0
	NV MF (10)	20–47	170	114	46.0	3.70	103
	VEG MF (10)	20–47	135	89.0	36.0	3.75	103
	NV MF (15)	20–47	177	117	55.0	3.22	79
(22) 1986	LOV M (14)	29	185		53.0	3.49	153
	NV M (10)	27	180		53.0	3.40	162
	LOV F (12)	29	191		66.0	2.89	139
	NV F (19)	27	193		71.0	2.72	132
(23) 1987	VEG M (11)	21	4.40				
	NV M (11)	22	5.30				
	VEG F (11)	21	4.60				
	NV F (11)	21	4.90				
(24) 1987	LOV MF (1550)	37–39	4.88	2.74	1.50	3.25	
	VEG MF (114)	36–37	4.29	2.28	1.49	2.88	
	NV MF (1198)	40–41	5.31	3.17	1.49	3.56	

(Appendix B continued)

Appendix B Lipid Levels in Adult Vegetarians and Nonvegetarians

(REF)/year	Group[1]/Gender (N)	Age (years)[2]	Serum TC[3]	Serum LDL[3]	Serum HDL[3]	Serum TC:HDL[4]	Serum TAG[3]
(25) 1989	LOV F (23)	72	5.62	3.34	1.62	3.47	1.43
	NV F (13)	71	6.46	4.08	1.76	3.67	1.33
(26) 1989	LOV M/F (17)	37	5.26		1.18	4.46	1.07
	NV M/F (11)	31	5.66		1.32	4.29	0.92
(27) 1990	LOV M (26)	41	5.30	3.14	1.57	3.38	
	VEG M (26)	41	5.00	2.89	1.56	3.21	
	NV M (26)	41	5.90	3.52	1.56	3.78	
	LOV F (26)	45	5.38	3.19	1.68	3.20	
	VEG F (26)	44	4.84	2.72	1.62	2.99	
	NV F (26)	44	5.95	3.79	1.73	3.44	
(28) 1990	LV M/F (25)	29	189				81.0
	NV M/F (100)	28	192				80.0
(29) 1991	LOV M/F (79)	18–30	4.09	2.38	1.40	2.92	6.20
	NV M/F (4821)	18–30	4.58	2.83	1.37	3.34	7.22
(30) 1992	LOV M (18)	20–35	121				
	NV M (18)	20–35	206				
	LOV M (10)	36–50	122				
	NV M (10)	36–50	207				
	LOV F (34)	20–35	136				
	NV F (34)	20–35	183				
	LOV F (17)	36–50	143				
	NV F (17)	36–50	196				
(31) 1992	VEG M (10)	32	3.52	1.85	1.31	2.69	0.76
	NV M (10)	33	4.77	3.14	1.34	3.56	0.65
	VEG F (10)	32	3.74	2.02	1.45	2.58	0.60
	NV F (10)	32	4.21	2.34	1.53	2.75	0.76
(32) 1992	LOV F (18)	30	4.44	2.25	1.83	2.43	0.80
	NV F (22)	34	5.19	3.19	1.66	3.13	0.98

(33) 1993	VEG M (23)	23	3.52				0.57
	NV M (20)	21	4.16				0.62
	VEG F (32)	25	3.50				0.77
	NV F (38)	20	4.43				0.75
(34) 1994	LV/LOV M (31)	19–30	4.34	2.61	1.30	3.34	0.94
	NV M (24)	19–30	5.39	3.41	1.33	4.05	1.44
	LV/LOV F (28)	19–30	4.11	2.39	1.32	3.11	0.89
	NV F (26)	19–30	5.26	3.30	1.36	3.87	1.32
(35) 1994	LOV M/F (12)	36	4.50	2.76	1.35	3.33	0.91
	NV M (14)	50	6.14	4.38	1.47	4.18	1.42
(36) 1994	LOV M/F (64)	47	4.70	3.10	1.20	3.92	1.10
	NV M/F (44)	48	5.40	3.60	1.30	4.15	1.50
(37) 1996	LOV M/F (11)	34	4.57	2.65	1.38	3.31	1.02
	VEG M/F (38)	35	4.41	2.46	1.35	3.27	0.94
	NV M/F (39)	44	5.31	3.41	1.44	3.69	1.04
(38) 1997	LOV F (13)	24	4.54		1.63	2.79	
	NV F (20)	23	4.03		1.58	2.55	
(39) 1997	LOV M (199)	45	4.91	3.08	1.26	4.13	1.26
	NV M (7054)	46	5.08	3.22	1.34	4.03	1.16
	LOV F (152)	39	4.71	2.67	1.61	3.07	0.93
	NV F (1837)	40	4.84	2.79	1.64	3.08	0.92
(40) 1998	LOV M (12)	49	5.0	3.2	1.2	4.17	1.2
	NV M (11)	40	5.2	3.5	1.2	4.33	1.2
	LOV F (12)	43	4.8	3.0	1.4	3.42	1.0
	NV F (12)	39	5.3	3.5	1.3	4.08	1.1
(41) 1998	B-LOV M (49)	50	4.23	2.43	1.20	3.8	1.25
	B-VEG M (14)	46	3.52	2.04	1.12	3.2	0.94
	B-LOV F (94)	52	4.68	2.79	1.37	3.7	1.14
	B-VEG F (31)	51	3.85	2.07	1.39	2.9	0.94
(42) 1999	VEG M/F (25)	36	4.30		1.20	3.58	1.00
	NV M/F (20)	34	4.80		1.50	3.20	1.20

(Appendix B continued)

Appendix B Lipid Levels in Adult Vegetarians and Nonvegetarians

(REF)/year	Group/Gender (N)	Age (years)[2]	Serum TC[3]	Serum LDL[3]	Serum HDL[3]	Serum TC:HDL[4]	Serum TAG[3]
(43) 1999	LOV M (10)	20–50	4.48	2.81	1.13	3.96	1.43
	LOV M (10)	20–50	4.29	2.64	1.26	3.41	1.01
(44) 1999	LOV M (46)	35	3.60	2.11	1.03	3.66	1.20
	VEG M (18)	33	3.52	2.14	0.96	3.69	1.08
	NV M (65)	38	4.50	2.93	1.09	4.34	1.27
(45) 1999	LOV M (18)	42	4.88	2.99	1.22	4.0	1.17
	NV M (19)	42	5.70	3.71	1.18	5.0	1.76
	LOV F (28)	33	4.76	2.76	1.47	3.3	1.01
	NV F (30)	33	5.44	3.51	1.39	4.2	1.17
(46) 2000	LOV M (237)	46	4.55				
	VEG M (233)	43	4.08				
	NV M (226)	53	4.94				
(47) 2000	LV F (29)	38.2	3.79	2.09	1.38	2.75	0.80
	NV F (27)	40.4	5.13	3.33	1.56	3.29	0.95
	LV M (26)	37.7	3.91	2.40	1.13	3.46	0.98
	NV M (26)	38.3	5.00	3.56	1.16	4.31	1.06
	LV F (55)	36.6	3.54	1.97	1.17	3.03	0.75
	NV F (60)	36.9	4.17	2.62	1.19	3.50	1.09
(48) 2001	LOV F (111)	25–65	5.40	3.31	1.66	3.25	1.84
	NV F (138)	25–65	5.53	3.52	1.50	3.69	2.12
(49) 2001	LOV (10M/10F)	58.6	4.20	3.00	1.24	3.39	1.06
	NV (10M/10F)	56.4	4.30	3.11	1.19	3.61	1.11
(50) 2002	LV F (45)	31–45	3.89				0.74
	NV F (45)	31–45	4.40				1.11
(51) 2002	LOV M/F (14)	48.5	193.1		47.3	4.08	103.0
	VEG M/F (31)	45.8	165.9		44.3	3.74	90.5
(52) 2003	LOV M/F (20)	34.8	181.0		62.2	2.91	92.9
	NV M/F (10)	38.4	222.5		56.3	3.95	170.6

(53) 2004	LOV M/F (19)	58.6	160.5	118.5	48.5	3.31	91.4
	NV M/F (17)	55.7	166.9	116.2	45.6	3.66	105.9
(54) 2004	LOV M (32)	18–30				3.7	
	NV M (456)	18–30				3.9	
	LOV M (54)	51–70				4.7	
	NV M (2102)	51–70				5.6	
(55) 2004	LV F (30)	49.5	161		51	3.16	78
	LV F htn (26)	48.7	158		55	2.87	104
	LV M (85)	46.1	163		46	3.54	85
	LV M htn (83)	47.1	182		53	3.43	102
(56) 2004	LOV M/F (30)	44.2	4.8				1.06
	NV M/F (30)	44.0	4.9				1.35
(57) 2005	VEG M/F (21)	35	3.73	2.25	1.22	3.06	0.56
	NV M/F (25)	36	4.18	2.30	1.32	3.17	1.18
(58) 2005	VEG M/F (98)	43.4	4.31	2.41	1.31	3.27	0.81
	VEG M/F (56)	45.7	4.44	2.53	1.40	3.38	0.81
(59) 2006	VEG F (57)	59.2	4.9	2.8	1.5	3.27	1.4
	NV F (61)	57.7	5.5	3.2	1.7	3.24	1.3
(60) 2006	LOV/VEG F (11)	52.3	4.15	2.49	1.06	3.92	1.51
	LOV/VEG F (14)	52.6	4.09	2.32	1.09	3.75	1.40
(61) 2006	LOV M/F (53)	25.7	4.58	2.45	1.65	2.92	1.08
	LOV M/F (53)	26.1	4.72	2.56	1.67	2.92	1.07
(62) 2006	LOV F (35)	55	174	112	50	3.48	63
	NV F (35)	55	204	136	49	4.16	93
(63) 2006	LOV M/F (90)	37.7	4.5	2.5	1.5	3.0	1.2
	NV M/F (46)	37.1	4.6	2.4	1.7	2.71	1.2
(64) 2007	LOV M/F (19)	37.1	175.3	101.5	55.5	3.12	94.0
	LV M/F (17)	35.8	164.8	87.7	57.7	2.70	94.7
	VEG M/F (18)	29.9	141.1	69.3	55.7	2.44	81.3
	NV M/F (22)	38.0	208.1	123.4	56.2	3.45	155.7

(Appendix B continued)

Appendix B Lipid Levels in Adult Vegetarians and Nonvegetarians

(REF)/year	Group¹/Gender (N)	Age (years)²	Serum TC³	Serum LDL³	Serum HDL³	Serum TC:HDL⁴	Serum TAG³
(65) 2007	LOV M (34)	50.9	183.8	120.4	48.0	3.83	127.6
	NV M (53)	49.2	201.4	139.0	49.3	4.08	127.0
	LOV F (65)	51.4	185.2	119.2	60.4	3.06	79.4
	NV F (46)	49.5	202.8	132.3	62.9	3.23	74.7
(66) 2007	LOV M/F (67)	47	173	106	45.2	3.83	113
	NV M/F (134)	47	225	151	45.7	4.92	156
(67) 2008	LO/LSV F (26)	29.0	4.1	2.2	1.3	3.15	1.1
	NV F (26)	27.4	4.4	2.4	1.5	2.93	0.9
(68) 2008	LOV M/F (21)	34.8	159.4		49.1	3.25	103.7
	NV M/F (28)	35.9	187.2		53.3	3.51	165.0
(69) 2008	LO/SV M (19)	45.2	189.4				119.6
	NV M (24)	43.4	213.0				228.8
	LO/SV F (45)	45.9	193.7				85.9
	NV F (18)	43.8	195.5				133.7

Notes: [1]Abbreviations: LV, lacto vegetarian; LOV, lacto-ovo vegetarian; VEG, vegan; NV, nonvegetarian; SV, eats chicken and/or fish; B, black; htn, subjects identified as having hypertension; NI, not indicated; NDR, no difference reported between vegetarians and nonvegetarians, although no data were reported. Only one type of vegetarian was listed in cases where a small percentage of the vegetarians in that group may have been of a different type.

[2]In some cases, only data on age was specifically provided for vegetarians, but generally it was similar to or matched with vegetarians. In addition, vegetarians were often matched for body mass index (BMI), and generally only healthy subjects were eligible for recruitment.

[3]Values for TC, total cholesterol; LDL, low-density lipoprotein cholesterol; HDL, high-density lipoprotein cholesterol; and TAG, triacylglycerol listed as either mg/dl or mmol/L. To convert serum cholesterol values from mg/dL to mmol/L, multiply by 0.0259. To convert serum cholesterol values from mmol/L to mg/dL, multiply by 38.6. To convert serum triacylglycerol from mg/dL to mmol/L, multiply by 0.0113. To convert mmol/L to mg/dL, multiply by 88.5.

[4]TC levels of 200 to 239 mg/dl (5.18 to 6.19 mmol/L) and are considered to be borderline high; TC levels ≥240 mg/dl (6.22 mmol/L) are high. LDL levels of 130–159 mg/dl (3.37–4.12 mmol/L) are considered borderline high; LDL levels ≥160 mg/dl (4.14 mmol/L) are high. HDL levels <40 mg/dl are considered low. Treatment recommendations depend on risk factors. NCEP: Detection, Evaluation, and Treatment of High Cholesterol in Adults (Adult Treatment Panel III). September 2002. http://www.nhlbi.nih.gov/guidelines/cholesterol/atp3full.pdf.

ANNOTATED REFERENCES APPENDIX B

1. Hardinge MG, Stare FJ. Nutritional studies of vegetarians. 2. Dietary and serum levels of cholesterol. *J Clin Nutr.* 1954;2:83–88.
2. Chen J-S. The effect of long-term vegetable diet on serum lipid and lipoprotein levels in man. *J Formosan Med Assoc.* 1966;65:65–77. *Note:* Vegetarians consisted of nuns and monks of 59 temples and hermitages in Taiwan, but the dietary habits of the vegetarians were not described. Of the 249 vegetarians, 62 were male and 187 were female. Of the 157 nonvegetarians, 114 were male and 43 were female.
3. Ellis FR, Path MRC, Montegriffo VME. Veganism, clinical findings and investigations. *Am J Clin Nutr.* 1970;23:249–255.
4. Sacks FM, Castelli WP, Donner A, Kass EH. Plasma lipid and lipoproteins in vegetarians and controls. *N Engl J Med.* 1975;292:1148–1151. *Note:* Vegetarians consisted of macrobiotics 40% of whom consumed fish once per week or more, 28% consumed dairy products and 11% consumed eggs.
5. Simons LA, Gibson JC, Paino C, Hosking M, Bullock J, Trim J. The influence of a wide range of absorbed cholesterol on plasma cholesterol levels in man. *Am J Clin Nutr.* 1978;31:1334–1339. *Note:* There were 8 male and 12 female LOV and 21 male and 17 female NV.
6. Burslem J, Schonfeld G, Hawald MA, Weidman SW, Miller JP. Plasma apoprotein and lipoprotein lipid levels in vegetarians. *Metabol.* 1978;27:711–719.
7. Dickerson JWT, Sanders TAB, Ellis FR. The effects of a vegetarian and vegan diet on plasma and erythrocyte lipids. *Plant Fds Hum Nutr.* 1979;XXIX:85–94.
8. Simons L, Gibson J, Jones A, Bain D. Health status of Seventh-Day Adventists. *Med J Aust.* 1979;2:148.
9. Armstrong B, Clarke H, Martin C, Ward W, Norman N, Masarei J. Urinary sodium and blood pressure in vegetarians. *Am J Clin Nutr.* 1979;32:2472–2476.
10. Haines AP, Chakrabarti R, Fisher D, Meade TW, North WRS, Stirling Y. Haemostatic variables in vegetarians and nonvegetarians. *Thrombosis Res.* 1980;19:139–148.
11. Huijbregts AWM, Schaik AV, Van Berge-Henegouwen GP, Van Der Werf SDJ. Serum lipids, biliary lipid composition, and bile acid metabolism in vegetarians as compared to normal controls. *Eur J Clin Invest.* 1980;10:443–449.
12. Gear JS, Mann JI, Thorogood M, Carter R, Jelfs R. Biochemical and haematological variables in vegetarians. *Br Med J.* 1980;280:1415.
13. Burr ML, Bates CJ, Fehily AM, Leger AS ST. Plasma cholesterol and blood pressure in vegetarians. *J Human Nutr.* 1981;35:437–441.
14. Armstrong BK, Brown JB, Clarke HT, et al. Diet and reproductive hormones: a study of vegetarian and nonvegetarian postmenopausal women. *J Natl Cancer Inst.* 1981;67:761–767.
15. Knuiman JT, West CE. The concentration of cholesterol in serum and in various serum lipoproteins in macrobiotic, vegetarian and nonvegetarian men and boys. *Atherosclerosis.* 1982;43:71–82. *Note:* Values for TAG are for very low density lipoprotein cholesterol (VLDL).
16. Lock DR, Varhol A, Grimes S, Patsch W, Schonfeld G. Apolipoprotein E levels in vegetarians. *Metabol.* 1982;31:917–921.
17. Ko YC. Blood pressure in Buddhist vegetarians. *Nutr Rep Int.* 1983;28:1375–1383.
18. Liebman M, Bazzarre TL. Plasma lipids of vegetarian and nonvegetarian males: effects of egg consumption. *Am J Clin Nutr.* 1983;38:612–619.
19. Kritchevsky D, Tepper SA, Goodman G. Diet, nutrition intake, and metabolism in populations at high and low risk for colon cancer. *Am J Clin Nutr.* 1984;40:921–926.
20. Roshanai F, Sanders TAB. Assessment of fatty acid intakes in vegans and omnivores. *Hum Nutr Appl Nutr.* 1984;38a:345–354.
21. Fisher M, Levine PH, Weiner B, et al. The effect of vegetarian diets on plasma lipid and platelet levels. *Arch Intern Med.* 1986;146:1193–1197.
22. Faber M, Gouws E, Benade AJS, Labadarios D. Anthropometric measurements, dietary intake and biochemical data of South African lacto-ovo vegetarians. *S Afr Med J.* 1986;89:723–738.

23. Sanders TAB, Key TJA. Blood pressure, plasma renin activity and aldosterone concentrations in vegans and omnivore controls. *Human Nutr Appl Nutr.* 1987;41A:204–211.

24. Thorogood M, Carter R, Benfield I, McPherson K, Mann J. Plasma lipids and lipoprotein cholesterol concentrations in people with different diets in Britain. *Br Med J.* 1987;295:351–353. *Note:* Among the LOV, VEG, and NV, there were 501, 45, and 486 males, respectively, and 1049, 969, and 712 females, respectively.

25. Nieman DC, Underwood BC, Sherman KM, Arabatzis K, Barbosa JC, Johnson M, Shultz TD. Dietary status of Seventh-Day Adventist vegetarian and nonvegetarian elderly women. *J Am Diet Assoc.* 1989;89:1763–1769.

26. Kumpusalo E, Karinpää A, Jauhiainen M, Laitinen M, Lappeteläinen R, Mäenpää PH. Multivitamin supplementation of adult omnivores and lacto vegetarians: circulating levels of vitamin A, D, and E, lipids, apolipoproteins and selenium. *Intern J Vit Nutr Res.* 1989;60:58–66. *Note:* Values represent the average of 4 different measures taken at 4 different times during the year.

27. Thorogood M, Roe L, McPherson K, Mann J. Dietary intake and plasma lipid levels: lessons from a study of the diet of health conscious groups. *Br Med J.* 1990;300:1297–1301.

28. Phinney SD, Odin RS, Johnson SB, Holman RT. Reduced arachidonate in serum phospholipids and cholesteryl esters associated with vegetarian diets in humans. *Am J Clin Nutr.* 1990;51:385–392.

29. Slattery ML, Jacobs DR, Hilner JE Jr, Caan BJ, Van Horn L, Bragg C, Manolio TA, Kushi LH, Liu K. Meat consumption and its association with other diet and health factors in young adults: the CARDIA study. *Am J Clin Nutr.* 1991;54:930–935.

30. Pronczuk A, Kipervarg Y, Hayes KC. Vegetarians have higher plasma alpha-tocopherol relative to cholesterol than do nonvegetarians. *J Am Coll Nutr.* 1992;11:50–55.

31. Sanders TAB, Roshanai F. Platelet phospholipid fatty acid composition and function in vegans compared with age- and sex-matched omnivore controls. *Eur J Clin Nutr.* 1992;46:823–831.

32. Reddy S, Sanders TAB. Lipoprotein risk factors in vegetarian women of Indian descent are unrelated to dietary intake. *Atherosclerosis.* 1992;95:223–229.

33. Pan W-H, Chin C-J, Sheu C-T, Lee M-H. Homostatic factors and blood lipids in young Buddhist vegetarians and omnivores. *Am J Clin Nutr.* 1993;58:354–359.

34. Krajcovicová-Kudláčková M, Simoncic R, Béderová A, Ondreicka R, Klvanová J. Selected parameters of lipid metabolism in young vegetarians. *Ann Nutr Metab.* 1994;38:331–335.

35. Vuoristo M, Miettinen TA. Absorption, metabolism, and serum concentrations of cholesterol in vegetarians: effects of cholesterol feedings. *Am J Clin Nutr.* 1994;59:1325–1331. *Note:* There were 8 male and 4 female LOV.

36. Melby CL, Toohey M, Cebrick J. Blood pressure and blood lipids among vegetarian, semivegetarian, and nonvegetarian African Americans. *Am J Clin Nutr.* 1994;59:103–109. *Note:* All subjects were black Seventh-day Adventists. Of the 66 vegetarians, 16 were vegans, and 50 were lacto-ovo vegetarians, there were 46 women and 20 men. Of the nonvegetarians, 34 were women and 11 men.

37. Thomas EL, Frost G, Barnard ML, Bryant DJ, Taylor-Robinson SD, Simbrunner J, et al. An *in vivo* ^{13}C magnetic resonance spectroscopic study of the relationship between diet and adipose tissue composition. *Lipids.* 1996;31:145–151. *Note:* Six males and 5 females were LOV, 21 males and 17 females were VEG, 20 males and 19 females were NV.

38. Ball D, Maughan RJ. Blood and urine acid-base status of premenopausal omnivorous and vegetarian women. *Br J Nutr.* 1997;78:683–693. *Note:* Two vegetarians occasionally ate fish.

39. Williams PT. Interactive effects of exercise, alcohol, and vegetarian diet on coronary artery disease risk factors in 9242 runners: The National Runners' Health Study. *Am J Clin Nutr.* 1997; 66:1197–1206. *Note:* Male vegetarian group includes 32 vegans. Female vegetarian group includes 30 vegans.

40. Harman SK, Parnell WR. The nutritional health of New Zealand vegetarian and nonvegetarian Seventh-Day Adventists: selected vitamin, mineral and lipid levels. *NZ Med J.* 1998;111:91–94. *Note:* Of the 24 vegetarians, an unspecified number were lacto vegetarians or vegans. Some nonvegetarians only occasionally ate red meat.

41. Toohey ML, Harris MA, Williams D, Foster G, Schmidt WD, Melby CL. Cardiovascular disease risk factors are lower in African-American vegans compared to lacto-ovo vegetarians. *J Am Coll Nutr.* 1998;17:425–434.

42. Haddad EH, Berk LS, Kettering JD, Hubbard RW, Peters WR. Dietary intake and biochemical, hematologic, and immune status of vegans compared with nonvegetarians. *Am J Clin Nutr.* 1999;70 (suppl): 586S–593S.

43. Li D, Sinclair A, Wilson A, et al. Effect of dietary α-linolenic acid on thrombotic risk factors in vegetarian men. *Am J Clin Nutr.* 1999;69:878–882. *Note:* Vegetarian subjects were divided into two groups for study purposes. Only baseline data are reported here.

44. Li D, Sinclair A, Mann N, et al. The association of diet and thrombotic risk factors in healthy male vegetarians and meat-eaters. *Eur J Clin Nutr.* 1999;53:612–619. *Note:* Nonvegetarians are described as "moderate-meat-eaters" (<285 g meat/d); 10 LOV and 3 VEG consumed fish occasionally.

45. Richter V, Purschwitz K, Bohusch A, et al. Lipoproteins and other clinical-chemistry parameters under the conditions of lacto-ovo vegetarian nutrition. *Nutr Res.* 1999;19:545–554.

46. Allen NE, Appleby PN, Davey GK, Key TJ. Hormones and diet: low insulin-like growth factor-I but normal bioavailable androgens in vean men. *Br J Cancer.* 2000;83:95–97.

47. Lu S-C, Wu W-H, Lee C-A, et al. LDL of Taiwanese vegetarians are less oxidizable than those of omnivores. *J Nutr.* 2000;130:1591–1596. *Note:* About one third of the LV were vegans.

48. Hoffmann I, Groeneveld MJ, Boeing H, et al. Giessen Wholesome Nutrition Study: relation between a health-conscious diet and blood lipids. *Eur J Clin Nutr.* 2001;55:887–895.

49. Lin CL, Fang TC, Gueng MK. Vascular dilatory functions of ovo-lacto vegetarians compared with omnivores. *Atherosclerosis.* 2001;158:247–251.

50. Hung C-J, Huang P-C, Lu S-c, et al. Plasma homocysteine levels in Taiwanese vegetarians are higher than those of omnivores. *J Nutr.* 2002;132:152–158. *Note:* Six of the 45 LV were vegans.

51. Bissoli L, Di Francesco V, Ballarin A, et al. Effect of vegetarian diet on homocysteine levels. *Ann Nutr Metab.* 2002;46:73–79.

52. Siani V, Mohamed EI, Maiolo C, et al. Body composition analysis for healthy Italian vegetarians. *Acta Diabetol.* 2003;40:S297–S298. *Note:* No information was provided on gender distribution.

53. Kuo CS, Lai NS, Ho LT, et al. Insulin sensitivity in Chinese ovo-lactovegetarians compared with omnivores. *Eur J Clin Nutr.* 2004;58:312–316. *Note:* Nine males and 10 females were LOV; 10 males and 7 females were NV.

54. Richter V, Rassoul F, Hentschel B, et al. Age-dependence of lipid parameters in the general population and vegetarians. *Z Gerontol Geriat.* 2004;37:207–213. *Note:* Vegetarians include vegans, lactovegetarians, and lacto-ovo vegetarians.

55. Chiplonkar SA, Agte V, Tarwadik V, et al. Micronutrient deficiencies as predisposing factors for hypertension in lacto-vegetarian Indian adults. *J Am Coll Nutr.* 2004;23:239–247.

56. Szeto YT, Kwok TC, Benzie IF. Effects of a long-term vegetarian diet on biomarkers of antioxidant status and cardiovascular disease risk. *Nutrition.* 2004;20:863–866. *Note:* Three males and 27 females were LOV; 3 males and 27 females were NV.

57. Goff LM, Bell JD, So PW, et al. Veganism and its relationship with insulin resistance and intramyocellular lipid. *Eur J Clin Nutr.* 2005;59:291–298. *Note:* Gender distribution of VEG group not specified; 11 males and 14 females were NV.

58. Waldmann A, Koschizke JW, Leitzmann C, et al. German vegan study: diet, lifestyle factors, and cardiovascular risk profile. *Ann Nutr Metab.* 2005;49:366–372. *Note:* The first listing is for strict vegans (48 males and 50 females); the second listing is for those who consumed small amounts of dairy and eggs but were primarily vegan (19 males and 37 females).

59. Su TC, Jeng JS, Wang JD, et al. Homocysteine, circulating vascular cell adhesion molecule and carotid atherosclerosis in postmenopausal vegetarian women and omnivores. *Atherosclerosis.* 2006;184:356–362. *Note:* Fifty-one subjects were vegan; 16 were lacto vegetarians.

60. Wu WH, Lu SC, Wang TF, et al. Effects of docosahexaenoic acid supplementation on blood lipids, estrogen metabolism, and in vivo oxidative stress in postmenopausal vegetarian women. *Eur J Clin Nutr.* 2006;60:386–392. *Note:* Subjects were a mixture of LOV and vegans.

61. Geppert J, Kraft V, Demmelmair H, et al. Microalgal docosahexaenoic acid decreases plasma triacylglycerol in normolipidaemic vegetarians: a randomized trial. *Br J Nutr.* 2006;95:779–786. *Note:* Fifteen males and 44 females were in the first group; 12 males and 43 females were in the second group.

62. Fu CH, Yang CC, Lin CL, et al. Effects of long-term vegetarian diets on cardiovascular autonomic functions in healthy post-menopausal women. *Am J Clin Nutr.* 2006;97:380–383.

63. Sebekova K, Boor P, Valachovicova M, et al. Association of metabolic syndrome risk factors with selected markers of oxidative status and microinflammation in healthy omnivores and vegetarians. *Mol Nutr Food Res.* 2006;50:858–868. *Note:* Thirty males and 60 females were LOV; 19 males and 27 females were NV.

64. DeBlase SG, Fernandes SF, Gianini RJ, et al. Vegetarian diet and cholesterol and triglyceride levels. *Arq Bras Cardiol.* 2007;88:35–39.

65. Chen CW, Lin YL, Lin TK, et al. Total cardiovascular risk profile of Taiwanese vegetarians. *Eur J Clin Nutr.* 2008;62:138–144.

66. Teixeira RdeC, Molina MdelC, Zandonade E, et al. Cardiovascular risk in vegetarians and omnivores: a comparative study. *Arq Bras Cardiol.* 2007;89:237–244. *Note*: 73% LOV, 14% vegan, 3% LV, 10% ate fish. No information was provided on gender distribution.

67. Karabudak E, Kiziltan G, Cigerim N. A comparison of some of the cardiovascular risk factors in vegetarian and omnivorous Turkish females. *J Hum Nutr Diet.* 2008;21:13–22. *Note*: Subjects include 9 LOV, 10 LV, and 7 occasional fish and/or chicken eaters.

68. Yen CE, Yen CH, Huang MC, et al. Dietary intake and nutritional status of vegetarian and omnivorous preschool children and their parents in Taiwan. *Nutr Res.* 2008;28:430–436. *Note*: Adult vegetarians consisted of 16 LOV, 2 ovo-vegetarians, 1 LV, 2 vegans. Four male adults and 17 females were vegetarian; 9 male adults and 19 females were NV. Children consisted of 18 LOV and 3 ovo-vegetarians. Fourteen male children and 7 female children were vegetarians; 15 male children and 13 female children were NV.

69. Nakamato K, Watanabe S, Kudo H, et al. Nutritional characteristics of middle-aged Japanese vegetarians. *J Atherosclero Throm.* 2008;15:122–129. *Note*: Nine men and 18 women were LOV; 11 men and 37 women in the vegetarian group occasionally ate chicken and meat.

Appendix C Blood Pressure of Adult Vegetarians and Nonvegetarians

(REF)/year	Adjustments[1]	Group[2]/Gender (N)	Age	SDA/NSDA[3]	Systolic Blood Pressure (mm Hg)	Diastolic Blood Pressure (mm Hg)
(1) 1975	Age/Sex	LOV M/F (115)	16–62	NSDA	119	77
		NV M/F (115)	16–62	NSDA	108	63
(2) 1977	Age/Sex/BMI	LOV M (177)	30–79	SDA	126	76
		NV M (103)	30–79	NSDA	136	86
		LOV F (241)	30–79	SDA	130	76
		NV F (187)	30–79	NSDA	142	85
(3) 1978	NI	LOV M (86)	25–29	SDA	117	73
		NV M (86)	25–29	NSDA	119	77
		LOV M (86)	55–59	SDA	125	79
		NV M (86)	55–59	NSDA	137	86
		LOV F (86)	25–29	SDA	109	66
		NV F (86)	25–29	NSDA	113	71
		LOV F (86)	55–59	SDA	121	76
		NV F (86)	55–59	NSDA	138	81
(4) 1979	Age/Sex	LOV M/F (102)	20–69	SDA	142	89
		NV M/F (102)	20–69	SDA/NSDA	148	91
(5) 1980	None	LOV/VEG M (25)	40	NSDA	128	79
		NV M (211)	50	NSDA	146	93
		LOV/VEG F (25)	44	NSDA	134	81
		NV F (71)	52	NSDA	147	92
	Age/Sex/Skinfold thickness	LOV/VEG M (25)	40	NSDA	128	79
		NV M (211)	50	NSDA	139	88
		LOV/VEG F (25)	44	NSDA	134	81
		NV F (71)	52	NSDA	139	88

(Appendix C continued)

Appendix C Blood Pressure of Adult Vegetarians and Nonvegetarians

(REF)/year	Adjustments[1]	Group[2]/Gender (N)	Age	SDA/NSDA[3]	Systolic Blood Pressure (mm Hg)	Diastolic Blood Pressure (mm Hg)
(6) 1981		LOV M (8)	40	NSDA	124	84
		NV M (50)	44	NSDA	129	83
		LOV M (21)	69	NSDA	147	87
		NV M (32)	69	NSDA	148	86
		LOV F (28)	43	NSDA	131	82
		NV F (55)	45	NSDA	129	80
		LOV F (28)	68	NSDA	156	89
		NV F (48)	68	NSDA	148	91
(7) 1982	None	LOV M (47)	33	SDA	114	67
		NV M (59)	34	NSDA	122	73
		LOV F (51)	34	SDA	109	67
		NV F (54)	33	NSDA	117	75
	Age/BMI	LOV M (47)	33	SDA	116	69
		NV M (59)	34	NSDA	121	72
		LOV F (51)	34	SDA	109	67
		NV F (54)	33	NSDA	115	73
(8) 1983	Age/Sex/BMI	VEG M (86)	61	NSDA	128	81
		NV M (86)	61	NSDA	134	83
		VEG F (353)	60	NSDA	129	79
		NV F (353)	60	NSDA	134	82
(9) 1983	Age/Sex	OV M/F (98)	60	NSDA	126	77
		NV M/F (98)	62	NSDA	147	88
(10) 1985	None	LOV M (41)	59	SDA	119	74
		NV M (12)	51	SDA	129	77
		LOV F (93)	51	SDA	112	69
		NV F (41)	51	SDA	120	73

Ref/Year	Adjustment	Subgroup	Age	Diet	Value 1	Value 2
	Age/Sex/BMI	LOV M (41)	51	SDA	119	74
		NV M (12)	51	SDA	128	76
		LOV F (93)	51	SDA	114	70
		NV F (41)	51	SDA	116	70
(11) 1986		LOV M/F (48)	29	NSDA	110	73
		NV M/F (41)	31	NSDA	126	80
(12) 1987	Age/Sex/BMI	VEG M (11)	32	NSDA	116	75
		NV M (11)	31	NSDA	114	66
		VEG F (11)	28	NSDA	115	70
		NV F (11)	24	NSDA	107	67
(13) 1988	Age/Sex/BMI	LOV M (14)	23	NSDA	118	59
		NV M (22)	23	NSDA	120	61
(14) 1988	None	LOV M (14)	70	SDA	129	72
		NV M (5)	70	SDA	152	82
		LOV F (34)	70	SDA	120	71
		NV F (17)	70	SDA	131	71
	Age/Sex/BMI	LOV M/F (48)	70	SDA	126	NDR
		NV M/F (22)	70	SDA	128	NDR
(15) 1988	Age/Sex/BMI	LV M/F (63)	16–65	NSDA	112	69
		VEG M/F (226)	16–65	NSDA	113	65
		NV M/F (458)	16–65	NSDA	121	76
		NV M/F (63)	16–65	NSDA	119	79
(16) 1989	Age/Sex	B-LOV M/F (55)	55	SDA	123	74
		B-NV M/F (59)	59	SDA	132	76
		W-LOV M/F (164)	52	SDA	114	66
		W-NV M/F (100)	53	SDA	116	68
	Age/Sex/BMI	B-LOV M/F (55)	55	SDA	123	74
		B-NV M/F (59)	59	SDA	130	75
		W-LOV M/F (164)	52	SDA	115	67
		W-NV M/F (100)	53	SDA	115	67

(Appendix C continued)

Appendix C Blood Pressure of Adult Vegetarians and Nonvegetarians

(REF)/year	Adjustments[1]	Group[2]/Gender (N)	Age	SDA/NSDA[3]	Systolic Blood Pressure (mm Hg)	Diastolic Blood Pressure (mm Hg)
(17) 1991	Age/Sex	LOV MF (79)	18–30	NSDA	109	68
		NV MF (4821)	18–30	NSDA	111	69
(18) 1993	None	B-LOV M (27)	69	SDA	133	76
		B-NV M (37)	65	NSDA	141	67
		W-LOV M (85)	67	SDA	121	76
		W-NV M (54)	65	NSDA	122	68
	Age/Sex/BMI	B-LOV M (27)	69	SDA	131	76
		B-NV M (37)	65	NSDA	138	75
		W-LOV M (85)	67	SDA	123	67
		W-NV M (54)	65	NSDA	123	67
(19) 1994	NI	LV/LOV M (17)	25	NI	111	72
		NV M (40)	24	NI	117	68
(20) 1994	None	LOV MF (64)	47	SDA	117	77
		NV MF (44)	47	SDA	120	79
	Age/Sex	LOV MF (64)	47	SDA	118	78
		NV MF (44)	47	SDA	120	79
(21) 1997	None	LOV M (199)	45	NSDA	122	77
		NV M (7054)	46		122	77
		LOV F (152)	39		112	73
		NV F (1837)	40		113	72
(22) 1998	None	LOV M (12)	49	SDA	119	74
		NV M (11)	40		128	82
		LOV F (12)	43		117	71
		NV F (12)	39		113	75
(23) 1998	None	B-LOV M (49)	50	SDA	127	79
		B-VEG M (14)	46		122	78
		B-LOV F (94)	52		127	78
		B-VEG F(31)	51		129	81

(24) 1999	None	LOV M (10)	20–50	NI	117	70
		LOV M (10)	20–50	NI	112	74
(25) 1999	None	LOV M (43)	35	NI	124	78
		VEG M (18)	33		122	78
		NV M (60)	38		126	82
(26) 2000	None	LV F (30)	38.2	NSDA	93	62
		NV F (26)	40.4		107	68
		LV M (26)	37.7		102	69
		NV M (27)	38.3		110	71
		LV F (53)	36.6		102	67
		NV F (54)	36.9		107	71
(27) 2001	None	LOV (10M/10F)	58.6	NSDA	123	77
		NV (10M/10F)	56.4		121	78
(28) 2002	Age	LOV M (786)	45	NSDA	125.5	77.1
		VEG M (272)	40		122.4	75.3
		NV M (996)	54		126.6	78.1
		LOV F (3014)	41		120.0	73.8
		VEG F (467)	37		117.6	72.2
		NV F (3741)	51		120.1	74.0
	Age/BMI	LOV M (786)	45		125.8	77.3
		VEG M (272)	40		123.5	76.1
		NV M (996)	54		126.0	77.6
		LOV F (3014)	41		120.2	74.0
		VEG F (467)	37		118.4	72.7
		NV F (3741)	51		126.0	77.6
(29) 2004	None	LOV M/F (19)	58.6	NSDA	124.1	76.9
		NV M/F (17)	55.7		122.2	78.8
(30) 2004	None	LV F (30)	49.5	NSDA	114.0	75.2
		LV F htn (26)	48.7		149.4	88.7
		LV M (85)	46.1		119.1	76.4
		LV M htn (83)	47.1		150.3	93.9

(Appendix C continued)

Appendix C Blood Pressure of Adult Vegetarians and Nonvegetarians

(REF)/year	Adjustments[1]	Group[2]/Gender (N)	Age	SDA/NSDA[3]	Systolic Blood Pressure (mm Hg)	Diastolic Blood Pressure (mm Hg)
(31) 2005	None	VEG M/F (21)	35.0	NSDA	112.7	66.9
		NV M/F (25)	36.0		123.7	70.1
(32) 2005	None	VEG M/F (98)	43.4	NI	122	74.6
		VEG M/F (56)	45.7		117	75.9
(33) 2006	None	VEG F (57)	59.2	NSDA	127.8	71.1
		NV F (61)	57.7		126.7	73.0
(34) 2006	None	LOV M/F (59)	25.7	NI	98	67
		LOV M/F (55)	26.1		96	67
(35) 2006	None	LOV F (35)	55	NSDA	121	72
		NV F (35)	55		133	82
(36) 2006	None	LOV M/F (90)	37.7	NI	110.9	70.4
		NV M/F (46)	37.1		115	71.9
(37) 2008	None	LOV M (34)	50.9	NI	123.2	79.7
		NV M (53)	49.2		126.9	81.4
		LOV F (65)	51.4		119.1	72.6
		NV F (46)	49.5		124.0	75.7
(38) 2008	None	LOV M/F (21)	34.8	NI	106.9	70.8
		NV M/F (28)	35.9		115.9	72.8
(39) 2008	None	LO/SV M (20)	45.2	NI	118.3	71.7
		NV M (29)	43.4		129.4	83.3
		LO/SV F (55)	45.9		111.7	67.0
		NV F (18)	43.8		118.4	72.8

Notes: [1]Adjustments indicate factors controlled for when analyzing blood pressure difference.

[2]Abbreviations: LV, lacto vegetarian; LOV, lacto-ovo vegetarian; VEG, vegan; OV, ovo vegetarian; NV, nonvegetarian; SV, eats chicken and/or fish; htn, subjects identified as having hypertension; BMI, body mass index; NI, not indicated; NDR, no difference between vegetarians and nonvegetarians, although data were not provided; B, black; W, white.

[3]SDA indicates the vegetarians were specifically identified as Seventh-day Adventists, whereas NSDA indicates the vegetarians were not exclusively SDAs, although some SDAs may have been included in the vegetarian group. NI indicates the process by which subjects were recruited for the study was not indicated or the extent to which SDAs composed the vegetarian groups was not possible to determine by the information provided.

ANNOTATED REFERENCES APPENDIX C

1. Sacks FM, Castelli WP, Donner A, Kass EH. Plasma lipids and lipoproteins in vegetarians and controls. *New Engl J Med.* 1975;292:1148–1151. *Note:* Vegetarians consisted of macrobiotics 40% of whom consumed fish once per week or more, 28% consumed dairy products and 11% consumed eggs.
2. Armstrong B, Van Merwyk AJ, Coates H. Blood pressure in Seventh-Day Adventist vegetarians. *Am J Epidemiol.* 1977;105:444–449.
3. Anholm AC. The relationship of a vegetarian diet to blood pressure. *Prev Med.* 1978;7:35 (abstr a-6). *Note:* The authors indicated that more older nonvegetarians were overweight than vegetarians, but even after controlling for this difference, vegetarians still had significantly lower blood pressure.
4. Armstrong B, Clarke H, Martin C, Ward W, Norman N, Masarei J. Urinary sodium and blood pressure in vegetarians. *Am J Clin Nutr.* 1979;32:2472–2476. *Note:* Vegetarians were lighter but the authors considered this an insufficient explanation for the blood pressure differences between groups.
5. Haines AP, Chakrabarti R, Fisher D, Meade TW, North WRS, Stirling Y. Haemostatic variables in vegetarians and nonvegetarians. *Thrombosis Res.* 1980;19:139–148.
6. Burr ML, Bates CJ, Fehily AM, Leger AS. Plasma cholesterol and blood pressure in vegetarians. *J Human Nutr.* 1981;35:437–441. *Note:* For all age/gender groups with the exception of women under 60, the BMI of the LOV was lower than that of the NV.
7. Rouse IL, Armstrong BK, Beilin LJ. Vegetarian diet, lifestyle and blood pressure in two religious populations. *Clin Exp Parmacol Physiol.* 1982;9:327–330. *Note:* The NV group consisted of Mormons.
8. Ko YC. Blood pressure in Buddhist vegetarians. *Nutr Rep Int.* 1983;28:1375–1383. *Note:* Vegetarian classification was based on data showing that at least 97% of calories was derived from plant products.
9. Ophir O, Peer G, Giland J, Blum M, Aviram A. Low blood pressure in vegetarians: the possible role of potassium. *Am J Clin Nutr.* 1983;37:755–762. *Note:* OV rarely used milk or milk products and consumed no more than 3 eggs per week. The OV and NV groups consisted of 48 women and 50 men each. When subjects within the OV and NV groups were compared according to weight within the range of −20% to +20% of the ideal body weight, vegetarians still had lower blood pressure.
10. Melby CL, Hyner GC, Zoog B. Blood pressure in vegetarians and nonvegetarians: a cross-sectional analysis. *Nutr Res.* 1985;5:1077–1082. *Note:* Of LOV and NV, 14% and 37%, respectively, reported a history of being informed by their doctor they had high blood pressure. Of the LOV and NV, 10% and 18.5%, respectively, were taking hypertensive medications and were excluded from analysis.
11. Ernst E, Pietsch L, Matrai A, Eisenberg J. Blood rheology in vegetarians. *Br J Nutr.* 1986;56: 555–560. *Note:* The LOV were equally divided between males and females, there were 29 male and 12 female NV. The LOV weighed slightly less than the NV (Broca index 0.9 vs. 1.0).
12. Sanders TAB, Key TJA. Blood pressure, plasma renin activity and aldosterone concentrations in vegans and omnivore controls. *Human Nutr Appl Nutr.* 1987;41A:204–211.
13. Aalberts JS, Weegels PL, van der Heijden L, Borst MH, Burema J, Hautvast J GAT, Kouwenhoven T. Calcium supplementation: effect on blood pressure and urinary mineral excretion in normotensive male lacto-ovo vegetarians and omnivores. *Am J Clin Nutr.* 1988;48:131–138.
14. Melby CL, Lyle RM, Poehlman ET. Blood pressure and body mass index in elderly long-term vegetarians and nonvegetarians. *Nutr Rep Int.* 1988;37:47–55. *Note:* Of the LOV and NV, 32% and 62.1%, respectively, were either using hypertensive medication or exhibited medication-free blood pressure ≥240/90 mm Hg and were excluded from the analysis.
15. Sacks FM, Kass EH. Low blood pressure in vegetarians: effects of specific foods and nutrients. *Am J Clin Nutr.* 1988;48:795–800. *Note:* Vegetarians consisted of macrobiotics. See reference 1 for a description of dietary habits.
16. Melby CL, Goldflies DG, Hyner GC, Lyle RM. Relation between vegetarian/nonvegetarian diets and blood pressure in black and white adults. *Am J Public Health.* 1989;79:1283–1288.
17. Slattery ML, Jacobs DR, Hilner JE Jr. Meat consumption and its association with other diet and health factors in young adults: the CARDIA study. *Am J Clin Nutr.* 1991;54:930–935.

18. Melby CL, Goldflies DG, Toohey ML. Blood pressure differences in older black and white long-term vegetarians and nonvegetarians. *J Am Coll Nutr.* 1993;12:262–269.

19. Toth MJ, Poehlman ET. Sympathetic nervous system activity and resting metabolic rate in vegetarians. *Metabolism.* 1994;43:621–625. *Note:* Among the vegetarians, 10 were LV, and 7 were VEG.

20. Melby CL, Toohey M, Cebrick J. Blood pressure and blood lipids among vegetarian, semivegetarian, and nonvegetarian African Americans. *Am J Clin Nutr.* 1994;59:103–109. *Note:* All subjects were black; of the initial 66 vegetarians, 50 were LOV and 16 were VEG, there were 46 women and 20 men. Of the initial 45 NV, 11 were male and 44 were female.

21. Williams PT. Interactive effects of exercise, alcohol, and vegetarian diet on coronary artery disease risk factors in 9242 runners: The National Runners' Health Study. *Am J Clin Nutr.* 1997;66: 1197–1206. *Note:* Male vegetarian group includes 32 vegans; female vegetarian group includes 30 vegans.

22. Harman SK, Parnell WR. The nutritional health of New Zealand vegetarian and nonvegetarian Seventh-Day Adventists: selected vitamin, mineral and lipid levels. *NZ Med J.* 1996;111:91–94. *Note:* Of the 24 vegetarians, an unspecified number were lacto vegetarians or vegans. Some nonvegetarians only occasionally ate red meat.

23. Toohey ML, Harris MA, Williams D, Foster G, Schmidt WD, Melby CL. Cardiovascular disease risk factors are lower in African-American vegans compared to lacto-ovo vegetarians. *J Am Coll Nutr.* 1998;17:425–434.

24. Li D, Sinclair A, Wilson A, et al. Effect of dietary α-linolenic acid on thrombotic risk factors in vegetarian men. *Am J Clin Nutr.* 1999;69:878–882. *Note:* Vegetarian subjects were divided into two groups for study purposes. Only baseline data are reported here.

25. Li D, Sinclair A, Mann N, et al. The association of diet and thrombotic risk factors in healthy male vegetarians and meat-eaters. *Eur J Clin Nutr.* 1999;53:612–619. *Note:* Nonvegetarians are described as "moderate-meat-eaters (<285 g meat/d). 10 LOV and 3 VEG consumed fish occasionally.

26. Lu S-C, Wu W-H, Lee C-A, et al. LDL of Taiwanese vegetarians are less oxidizable than those of omnivores. *J Nutr.* 2000;130:1591–1596. *Note:* About one third of the LV were vegans.

27. Lin CL, Fang TC, Gueng MK. Vascular dilatory functions of ovo-lacto vegetarians compared with omnivores. *Atherosclerosis.* 2001;158:247–251.

28. Appleby PN, Davey GK, Key TJ. Hypertension and blood pressure among meat eaters, fish eaters, vegetarians, and vegans in EPIC-Oxford. *Public Health Nutr.* 2002;5:645–654.

29. Kuo CS, Lai NS, Ho LT, et al. Insulin sensitivity in Chinese ovo-lactovegetarians compared with omnivores. *Eur J Clin Nutr.* 2004;58:312–316. *Note:* Nine males and 10 females were LOV; 10 males and 7 females were NV.

30. Chiplonkar SA, Agte V, Tarwadik V, et al. Micronutrient deficiencies as predisposing factors for hypertension in lacto-vegetarian Indian adults. *J Am Coll Nutr.* 2004;23:239–247.

31. Goff LM, Bell JD, So PW, et al. Veganism and its relationship with insulin resistance and intramyocellular lipid. *Eur J Clin Nutr.* 2005;59:291–298. *Note:* Gender distribution of VEG group not specified; 11 males and 14 females were NV.

32. Waldmann A, Koschizke JW, Leitzmann C, et al. German vegan study: diet, lifestyle factors, and cardiovascular risk profile. *Ann Nutr Metab.* 2005;49:36–372. *Note:* The first listing is for strict vegans (48 males and 50 females); the second listing is for those who consumed small amounts of dairy and eggs but were primarily vegan (19 males and 37 females).

33. Su TC, Jeng JS, Wang JD, et al. Homocysteine, circulating vascular cell adhesion molecule and carotid atherosclerosis in postmenopausal vegetarian women and omnivores. *Atherosclerosis.* 2006;184:356–362. *Note:* 51 subjects were vegan; 6 were lacto vegetarians.

34. Geppert J, Kraft V, Demmelmair H, et al. Microalgal docosahexaenoic acid decreases plasma triacylglycerol in normolipidaemic vegetarians: a randomized trial. *Br J Nutr.* 2006;95:779–786. *Note:* Fifteen males and 44 females were in the first group; 12 males and 43 females were in the second group.

35. Fu CH, Yang CC, Lin CL, et al. Effects of long-term vegetarian diets on cardiovascular autonomic functions in healthy post-menopausal women. *Am J Clin Nutr.* 2006;97:380–383.

36. Sebekova K, Boor P, Valachovicova M, et al. Association of metabolic syndrome risk factors with selected markers of oxidative status and microinflammation in healthy omnivores and vegetarians. *Mol Nutr Food Res.* 2006;50:858–868. *Note:* Thirty males and 60 females were LOV; 19 males and 27 females were NV.

37. Chen CW, Lin YC, Lin TK, et al. Total cardiovascular risk profile of Taiwanese vegetarians. *Eur J Clin Nutr.* 2008;62:138–144.
38. Yen CE, Yen CH, Huang MC, et al. Dietary intake and nutritional status of vegetarian and omnivorous preschool children and their parents in Taiwan. *Nutr Res.* 2008;28:430–436. *Note:* Adult vegetarians consisted of 16 LOV, 2 ovo-vegetarians, 1 LV, 2 vegans. Four male adults and 17 females were vegetarian; 9 male adults and 19 females were NV. Children consisted of 18 LOV and 3 ovo-vegetarians. Fourteen male children and 7 female children were vegetarians; 15 male children and 13 female children were NV.
39. Nakamato K, Watanabe S, Kudo H, et al. Nutritional characteristics of middle-aged Japanese vegetarians. *J Atherosclero Throm.* 2008;15:122–129. *Note:* Nine men and 18 women were LOV; 11 men and 37 women in the vegetarian group occasionally ate chicken and meat.

Appendix D Anthropometric Data of Female Adult Vegetarians and Nonvegetarians and of Mixed (Male and Female) Groups

(REF)/year	Group[1]/(N)	SDA/NSDA[2]	Age	Height (cm)	Weight (kg)	Body Mass Index (kg/m²)	Body fat[3]
(1) 1954	LOV (15)	SDA/NSDA	58	158.8	62.7	24.9	
	NV (15)	SDA/NSDA	57	162.6	64.5	24.4	
(2) 1975	LOV (42)	NSDA	16–40		58.0		6.0
	NV (42)	NSDA	16–40		73.0		17.0
(3) 1978	LOV (42)	SDA	57	161.3	62.6	24.1	
	NV (36)	NSDA	59	161.3	64.4	24.8	
(4) 1980	LOV/VEG (25)	NSDA	44				53.8
	NV (71)	NSDA	52				67.0
(5) 1980	LOV (13)	NSDA	26	164.6	59.8	22.1	22.4
	OMN (24)	NSDA	26	166.6	60.1	21.7	23.8
(6) 1981	LOV (28)	NSDA	43			22.4	
	NV (85)	NSDA	45			23.0	
	LOV (28)	NSDA	68			22.3	
	NV (48)	NSDA	68			24.9	
(7) 1981	LOV (46)	SDA	67	159.2	58.6	23.1	19.2
	NV (47)	SDA/NSDA	66	158.4	60.2	24.0	18.8
(8) 1982	LOV (101)	SDA/NSDA	57	161.0	61.9	23.9	27.0
	NV (107)	SDA/NSDA	62	161.5	65.3	25.0	32.1
(9) 1982	LOV (10)	NI	27	163.7	59.9	22.6	
	NV (10)	NI	26	166.8	63.8	22.7	
(10) 1983	LOV (51)	SDA	34	160.8	60.3	23.3	18.7
	NV (54)	NSDA	33	161.1	68.2	26.3	24.1
(11) 1983	LOV (14)	SDA	33	167.7	61.8	22.0	
	NV (9)	NSDA	36	164.2	63.0	23.3	
(12) 1985	LOV (93)	SDA	51			23.9	
	NV (41)	SDA	51			28.1	

No.	Year	Group (n)	Diet	Age	Height	Weight		
(13)	1985	LOV (5)	NSDA	27–49			22.0	
		VEG (5)	NSDA	27–49			23.0	
		NV (5)	NSDA	27–49			22.0	
(14)	1986	VEG (10)	NSDA	18–40			21.0	
		NV (10)	NSDA	18–40			21.0	
(15)	1986	LOV (32)	NSDA	51	159.5	53.2	20.9	
		NV (60)	NSDA	52	161.9	63.8	24.3	
(16)	1986	LOV (19)	SDA/NSDA	18–40	163.5	57.7	21.5	26.6
		NV (12)	NSDA	18–40	167.8	59.7	21.1	25.4
(17)	1986	LOV (22)	NSDA	26	160.0	53.4	20.9	
		NV (18)	NSDA	22	160.0	52.9	20.7	
(18)	1987	VEG (11)	NSDA	28			20.6	13.5
		NV (11)	NSDA	24			20.6	17.3
(19)	1988	LOV (25)	NSDA	36	164.8	58.7	21.6	
		NV (21)	NSDA	38	163.3	61.5	23.1	
(20)	1988	LOV (10)	NSDA	58	160.5	57.5	22.3	
		NV (10)	NSDA	57	162.0	67.2	25.6	
(21)	1988	LOV (88)	SDA	73	159.0	62.9	31.5	39.6
		NV (278)	NSDA	79	158.3	60.1	30.1	38.4
(22)	1988	LOV (20)	NSDA	31	165.9	57.9	21.0	
		NV (16)	NSDA	29	163.6	59.8	22.1	
(23)	1988	LOV (15)	SDA/NSDA	34	164.6	61.2	22.6	
		NV (16)	SDA/NSDA	34	160.5	60.5	23.5	
(24)	1989	LOV (144)	SDA	67	161.0	64.8	25.0	
		NV (146)	NSDA	66	163.0	63.6	23.9	
(25)	1989	LV/LOV (11)	NSDA	36	167.0	59.6	21.1	
		NV (12)	NSDA	32	168.0	60.0	21.5	
(26)	1989	LOV (10)	SDA/NSDA	67	163.0	69.8	26.3	
		NV (10)	SDA/NSDA	64	163.0	67.1	25.3	

(Appendix D continued)

Appendix D Anthropometric Data of Female Adult Vegetarians and Nonvegetarians and of Mixed (Male and Female) Groups

(REF)/year	Group[1]/(N)	SDA/NSDA[2]	Age	Height (cm)	Weight (kg)	Body Mass Index (kg/m²)	Body fat[3]
(27) 1989	LOV (23)	SDA	72	162.0	60.0	22.8	71.8
	NV (14)	SDA	71	160.0	62.5	24.2	82.8
(28) 1989	LOV (26)	NSDA	35	164.0	53.8	20.0	
	NV (36)	NSDA	49	163.0	60.5	23.3	
(29) 1989	LOV (9)	SDA	58	161.0	70.2	27.2	
	NV (10)	NI	57	161.0	58.6	22.8	
(30) 1990	LOV (12)	SDA	76	159.6	57.4	22.5	67.2
	NV (12)	SDA	72	160.4	63.9	24.7	85.0
(31) 1990	LOV (17)	NSDA	82		62.0	24.5	
	NV (216)	NSDA	72		70.0	27.3	
(32) 1990	VEG (18)	NSDA	30	161.0	59.4	22.5	
	NV (22)	NSDA	34	164.0	64.6	24.1	
(33) 1990	LOV (26)	NSDA	45			21.8	
	VEG (26)	NSDA	44			21.7	
	NV (26)	NSDA	44			22.7	
(34) 1990	LOV (8)	NSDA	27	167.0	57.0	21.1	20.6
	NV (8)	NSDA	23	164.0	60.5	21.6	21.1
(35) 1991	LOV (34)	SDA/NSDA	36	165.1	58.5	21.5	
	NV (41)	SDA/NSDA	29	164.1	59.6	22.0	
(36) 1994	LV/LOV (28)	NSDA	22	168.5	56.4	19.9	
	NV (26)	NSDA	25	167.1	60.2	21.6	
(37) 1994	LOV M/F (66)	SDA	47	167.6	74.7	26.8	31.7
	NV M/F (45)	SDA	47	166.6	79.4	28.6	36.3
(38) 1995	LV (15)	NSDA	26	166.4	58.8	21.2	24.1
	VEG (8)	NSDA	28	168.2	58.6	20.7	23.7
	NV (22)	NSDA	28	165.0	61.9	22.7	27.4

(39) 1995	LOV (22) NV (22)	NSDA	20–57 20–57			21.7 21.3	
(40) 1996	LOV M/F (11) VEG M/F (38) NV M/F (39)	NI	34 35 44			22.6 21.8 23.6	22.5 21.9 24.0
(41) 1997	LOV (13) NV (20)	NI	24 23	164 166	57.7 60.9	21.5 22.1	25.0 25.9
(42) 1997	LOV (152) NV (1837)	NSDA	39 40			20.8 21.3	
(43) 1998	LOV (12) NV (12)	SDA	43 39			23.6 25.8	
(44) 1998	LOV (1908) NV (1470)	NI	38 38			21.3[4] 22.3[4]	
(45) 1998	LOV (18) NV (22)	NSDA	30 34	161 164	58.3 64.8	22.5 24.1	26.2 30.7
(46) 1998	B-LOV (94) B-NV (31)	SDA	52 51	161.4 162.1	69.6 66.5	26.7 25.3	
(47) 1999	LOV (50) NV (24)	NSDA	25 25			22.5 22.4	
(48) 1999	LOV (31)	NI	16–30	164.7	59.3	21.8	
(49) 2000	LOV (6) VEG (6) NV (16)	NSDA	33 37 33	166 169 166	58 57 63	21 20 23	
(50) 2000	LV (30) NV (26) LV (53) NV (54)	NSDA	38.2 40.4 36.6 36.9	155.9 158.5 157.0 158.6	48.8 56.6 51.1 55.4	20.0 22.5 20.7 22.0	
(51) 2001	VEG (87)	NSDA	53			21.5	

(Appendix D continued)

Appendix D Anthropometric Data of Female Adult Vegetarians and Nonvegetarians and of Mixed (Male and Female) Groups

(REF)/year	Group[1]/(N)	SDA/NSDA[2]	Age	Height (cm)	Weight (kg)	Body Mass Index (kg/m²)	Body fat[3]
(52) 2001	LOV (10M/10F)	NSDA	58.6			23.1	
	NV (10M/10F)		56.4			24.8	
(53) 2002	LOV (101)	NSDA	44	163	59.7	22.5	
	VEG (94)		44	163	58.6	22.0	
	NV (99)		45	164	62.2	23.1	
(54) 2002	LOV (3014)	NSDA	41			22.8	
	VEG (467)		37			22.0	
	NV (3741)		51			24.1	
(55) 2002	VEG (15)	NSDA	40.1	162	55.6	21.1	
(56) 2002	LOV M/F (14)	NSDA	48.5		65.1	23.2	
	VEG M/F (31)		45.8		64.4	21.8	
(57) 2003	LOV (14669)	NSDA	35			22.7	
	VEG (1659)		32			21.9	
	NV (26116)		48			24.3	
(58) 2003	LOV (62)	SDA	25–74	162.2	71.7	27.3	
	NV (191)		25–74	161.0	71.2	27.5	
(59) 2003	LOV (9419)	NSDA	34			22.5	
	VEG (983)		32			21.8	
	NV (13506)		45			23.7	
(60) 2003	VEG (50)	NSDA	42.4			20.5	27.0
	VEG (37)		44.5				
(61) 2003	LOV M/F (37)	NI	28.9	161.7	54.3	20.7	
	NV M/F (32)		22.9	163.1	55.9	20.9	
(62) 2003	LOV M/F (20)	NI	34.8	167	62.5	22.4	15.6
	NV M/F (10)		38.4	170	68.1	23.4	13.4

(63) 2004	LOV M/F (17) NV M/F (14)	NSDA	58.6 55.7			23.4 24.5	
(64) 2004	VEG (50) VEG (25)	NI	35.4 62.0			20.4 21.9	
(65) 2004	VEG M/F (86) VEG M/F (45)	NI	43.8 44.6			21.5 21.3	
(66) 2004	LOV M/F (33) NV M/F (33)	NI	18–42 18–42	167.4 167.4	69.3 69.5	24.6 24.7	27.9 29.0
(67) 2004	LV (30) LV htn (26)	NSDA	49.5 48.7		48.6 59.5	21.9 27.3	
(68) 2004	LOV (6478) NC (24738)	NI	49 54			23.3 25.0	
(69) 2005	VEG M/F (21) NV M/F (25)	NSDA	35.0 36.0		66.6 68.4	22.7 23.4	21.8 22.8
(70) 2005	VEG (11) NV (11)	NSDA	56.5 53.2	160 161	53.9 66.5	20.1 25.4	24.1 33.5
(71) 2005	LOV (75) NV (842)	NI	NI NI		62.5 67.9	23.1 25.7	
(72) 2005	LV (159) VEG (83) NV (54257)	NI	51.1 54.8 52.5	165 164 164	64.0 62.4 66.6	23.4 23.3 24.7	
(73) 2005	VEG M/F (98) VEG M/F (56)	NI	43.4 45.7			21.3 21.3	
(74) 2005	LOV (30) NV (30) NV (30)	NI	31 32 34	166 165 166	64.8 66.4 66.2	23 24 24	
(75) 2005	LOV (206) NV (4793)	NI	37.0 49.8			22.1 24.6	

(Appendix D continued)

Appendix D Anthropometric Data of Female Adult Vegetarians and Nonvegetarians and of Mixed (Male and Female) Groups

(REF)/year	Group¹/(N)	SDA/NSDA²	Age	Height (cm)	Weight (kg)	Body Mass Index (kg/m²)	Body fat³
(76) 2005	LOV (257)⁵	NI	≥20	163.1	63.1	23.7	
	LOV (257)		≥20	164.2	64.3	23.9	
	LOV (1042)		≥20	163.6	63.8	23.8	
	LOV (2226)		≥20	163.6	63.1	23.6	
	LOV (7880)		≥20	163.5	62.9	23.5	
	NV (23148)		≥20	163.8	65.0	24.2	
(77) 2006	VEG (57)	NSDA	59.2			23.0	
	NV (61)		57.7			23.5	
(78) 2006	LOV M/F (95)	NI	37.8			22.1	
	NV M/F (107)		38.7			22.5	
(79) 2006	LOV/VEG (11)	NI	52.3	154.7	54.9	22.9	
	LOV/VEG (14)		52.6	153.4	54.9	23.3	
(80) 2006	LV (49)	NSDA	36.6	156.9	51.5	20.9	
	NV (49)		36.9	158.7	55.4	22.0	
(81) 2006	LOV M/F (36)	NI	34.2			22.5	
	VEG M/F (42)		30.7			21.8	
	NV M/F (40)		38.4			23.1	
(82) 2007	LOV (20)	NI	33.8			24.2	
	NV (41)		36.6			23.9	
(83) 2008	LOV (65)	NI	51.4	155.2	54.2	22.5	
	NV (46)		49.5	156.5	55.1	22.8	
(84) 2008	LO/L/SV (26)	NI	29.0	166.6	60.6	21.7	24.1
	NV (26)		27.4	169.2	61.9	21.6	24.4
(85) 2008	LOV M/F (21)	NI	34.8	160.1	58.2	22.6	24.6
	NV M/F (28)		35.9	163.4	62.3	23.2	23.8
(86) 2008	LO/SV (55)	NI	45.9	154.0	50.4	21.3	
	NV (18)		43.8	157.1	54.1	21.9	

(87) 2009	LOV (17)	NI	27.6	163	59.5	22	
(88) 2009	LOV MF (20408)	SDA	58.1			23.6	
	VEG MF (2731)		58.1			25.7	
	NV MF (28761)		54.9			28.8	
(89) 2009	VEG (105)	NSDA	62	148	53	24	34.9
	NV (105)		62	149	54	24	35.1
(90) 2009	LO/LV (19)	NI	48	164	60	22.1	
	NV (21)		43	164	63	23.5	
(91) 2010	LOV (30)	NI	23	172	64.1	21.6	
	NV (30)		24	172	64.5	21.8	

Notes: [1]Abbreviations: LV, lacto vegetarian; LOV, lacto-ovo vegetarian; VEG, vegan; NV, nonvegetarian; SV, eats chicken and/or fish; htn, subjects identified as having hypertension; B, black.

[2]SDA indicates the vegetarians were specifically identified as Seventh-day Adventists, whereas NSDA indicates the vegetarians were not exclusively SDAs, although some SDAs may have been included in the vegetarian group. NI indicates the process by which subjects were recruited for the study was not indicated or the extent to which SDAs composed the vegetarian groups was not possible to determine by the information provided.

[3]Reference 2, body fat calculated from subscapular thickness (mm), references 4 and 16, from sum of skinfold thickness (mm) at triceps, forearm, subscapular and suprailiac sites, references 5, 7, 10, 18, and 37 from triceps skinfold thickness (mm), references 27 and 30 from sum of triceps, suprailiac, and thigh skinfolds (mm), reference 66, percentage body fat based on biceps and triceps skinfolds, reference 34, from hydrostatic weighing, reference 38, percentage body fat based on skinfold measurements at the triceps, abdominal, suprailiac, and thigh sites, and references 40, 41, and 44, percentage body fat based on skinfold measurements at the triceps, biceps, suprailiac, and subscapular sites; Reference 60, percentage body fat measured by the infrared method, lean body mass was calculated from the following equation $18.23 + 0.01014 \times ([14.6 \times weight] + (22.07 \times height) - (9.05 \times age) - 1669)$. Reference 62 (kg) and Reference 70 (percentage) body fat measured using DEXA total body scan. Reference 69, 84, 85, body fat (%) measured with bioelectrical impedance. Reference 88, body fat (percentage) method not reported. Reference 8 measured in mm but no details provided. Reference 22, no data provided, but no difference was reported.

[4]Age-adjusted BMI.

[5]The first listing is for lifelong vegetarians, second listing is for those who became vegetarian at age 1 to 9 years, third listing is for those who became vegetarian at 10 to 14 years, fourth listing at 15 to 18 years, fifth listing at ≥20 years of age.

ANNOTATED REFERENCES APPENDIX D

1. Hardinge MG, Stare FJ. Nutritional studies of vegetarians. 1. Nutritional, physical, and laboratory studies. *J Clin Nutr.* 1954;2:73–82.

2. Sacks FM, Castelli WP, Donner A, Kass EH. Plasma lipids and lipoproteins in vegetarians and controls. *N Engl J Med.* 1975;292:1148–1151. *Note:* Vegetarians consisted of macrobiotics 40% of whom consumed fish once per week or more, 28% consumed dairy products and 11% consumed eggs. Values presented for females actually include 73 males in both the vegetarian and nonvegetarin groups.

3. Mason RL, Kunkel ME, Davis TA, Beauchene RE. Nutrient intakes of vegetarian and nonvegetarian women. *Tenn Farm Home Sci.* 1978;1:18–20.

4. Haines AP, Chakrabarti R, Fisher D, Meade TW, North WRS, Stirling Y. Haemostatic variables in vegetarians and nonvegetarians. *Thrombosois Res.* 1980;19:139–148.

5. Taber LAL, Cook RA. Dietary and anthropometic assessment of adult omnivores, fish-eaters, and lacto-ovo vegetarians. *J Am Diet Assoc.* 1980;76:21–29. *Note:* Differences in BMI between LOV and NV were not statistically significant, but it was reported that 10 NV (42%) but only two LOV (15%) were considered obese.

6. Burr ML, Bates CJ, Fehily AM, Leger AS. Plasma cholesterol and blood pressure in vegetarians. *J Human Nutr.* 1981; 35:437–441.

7. Armstrong BK, Brown JB, Clarke HT, et al. Diet and reproductive hormones: a study of vegetarian and nonvegetarian postmenopausal women. *J Natl Cancer Inst.* 1981;67:761–767.

8. Beauchene RE, Kunkel ME, Bredderman SH, Mason RL. Nutrient intake and physical measurements of aging vegetarian and nonvegetarian women. *J Am Coll Nutr.* 1982;1:131.

9. Goldin BR, Adlercreutz H, Gorbach SL, et al. Estrogen excretion patterns and plasma levels in vegetarian and omnivorous women. *N Engl J Med.* 1982;307:1542–1547.

10. Rouse IL, Armstrong BK, Beilin LJ. The relationship of blood pressure to diet and lifestyle in two religious populations. *J Hypertension.* 1983;1:65–71. *Note:* The NV consisted of Mormons.

11. Shultz TD, Leklem JE. Nutrient intake and hormonal status of premenopausal vegetarian Seventh-Day Adventists and premenopausal nonvegetarins. *Nutr Cancer.* 1983;4:247–259.

12. Melby CL, Hyner GC, Zoog B. Blood pressure in vegetarians and nonvegetarians: a cross section analysis. *Nutr Res.* 1985;5:1077–1082. *Note:* The age of each group included data for males.

13. Carlson E, Kips M, Lockie A, Thomson J. A comparative evaluation of vegan, vegetarian and omnivore diets. *J Plant Foods.* 1985;6:89–100.

14. Rana SK, Sanders TAB. Taurine concentrations in the diet, plasma, urine and breast milk of vegans compared omnivores. *Br J Nutr.* 1986;56:17–27.

15. Levin N, Ratton J, Gilat T. Energy intake and body weight in ovo-lacto vegetarians. *J Clin Gastroenterol.* 1986; 8:451–453.

16. Faber M, Gouws E, Benade AJS, Labadarios D. Anthropometric measurements, dietary intake and biochemical data of South African lacto-ovo vegetarians. *S Afr Med J.* 1986;69:733–738.

17. Locong A. Nutritional status and dietary intake of a selected sample of young adult vegetarians. *Can Diet Assoc J.* 1986;47:101–106.

18. Sanders TAB, Key TJA. Blood pressure, plasma renin activity and aldosterone concentrations in vegans and omnivores. *Human Nutr: Appl Nutr.* 1987;41A:204–211.

19. Fentiman IS, Caleffi M, Wang DY, et al. The binding of blood-borne estrogens in normal vegetarian and omnivorous women and risk of breast cancer. *Nutr Cancer.* 1988;11:101–106.

20. Korpela JT, Adlercreutz H, Turunen MJ. Fecal free and conjugated bile acids and neutral sterols in vegetarians, omnivores and patients with colorectal cancer. *Scand J Gastroenterol.* 1988:23:277–283.

21. Tylavsky FA, Anderson JJB. Dietary factors in bone health of elderly lacto-ovo vegetarians and omnivorous women. *Am J Clin Nutr.* 1988;48:842–849.

22. Worthington-Roberts BS, Breskin MW, Monsen ER. Iron status of premenopausal women in a university community and its relationship to habitual dietary sources of protein. *Am J Clin Nutr.* 1988;47:275–279.

23. Kelsay JL, Frazier CW, Prather E, Canary JJ, Clark WM, Powell AS. Impact of variations in carbohydrate intake on mineral utilization by vegetarians. *Am J Clin Nutr.* 1988;48:875–879.

24. Hunt IF, Murphy NJ, Henderson C, et al. Bone mineral content in postmenopausal women: comparison of omnivores and vegetarians. *Am J Clin Nutr.* 1989;50:517–523.

25. Adlercreutz H, Fotsis T, Hockerstedt K, et al. Diet and urinary estrogen profile in premenopausal omnivorous and vegetarian women and in premenopausal women with breast cancer. *J Steroid Biochem.* 1989;34:527–530.

26. Marsh AG, Christensen DK, Sanchez TV, Mickelson O, Chaffee FL. Nutrient similarities and differences of older lacto-ovo vegetarian and omnivorous women. *Nutr Rep Int.* 1989;39:19–24.

27. Neiman DC, Underwood BC, Sherman KM, Arabatizis K, Barbosa JC, Johnson M, Shulz TD. Dietary status of Seventh-Day Adventist vegetarian and nonvegetarian elderly women. *J Am Diet Assoc.* 1989;89:1763–1769.

28. Millet P, Guilland JC, Fuchs F, Klepping J. Nutrient intake and vitamin status of healthy French vegetarians and nonvegetarians. *Am J Clin Nutr.* 1989;50:718–727.

29. Adlercreutz H, Hamalainen E, Gorbach SL, Goldin BR, Woods MN, Dwyer JT. Diet and plasma androgens in postmenopausal vegetarian and omnivorous women and postmenopausal women with breast cancer. *Am J Clin Nutr.* 1989;49:433–432.

30. Barbosa JC, Shultz TD, Filley SJ, Nieman DC. The relationship among adiposity, diet, and hormone concentrations in vegetarian and nonvegetarian postmenopausal women. *Am J Clin Nutr.* 1990;51: 798–803. *Note:* Among the vegetarians, 6 were LV and 6 were LOV, two of whom ate fish.

31. Löwik MRH, Schrijver J, van den Berg H, Hulsof KFAM, Wedel M, Ockhuizen T. Effect of dietary fiber on the vitamin B6 status among vegetarian and nonvegetarin elderly (Dutch Nutrition Surveillance System). *J Am College Nutr.* 1990;9:241–249.

32. Reddy S, Sanders TAB. Haematological studies on premenopausal Indian and Caucasian vegetarians compared with Caucasian omnivores. *Br J Nutr.* 1990;64:331–338.

33. Thorogood M, Roe L, McPherson K, Mann J. Dietary intake and plasma lipid levels: lessons from a study of the diet of health conscious groups. *Br Med J.* 1990;300:1297–1301.

34. Oberlin P, Melby CL, Poehlman ET. Resting energy expenditures in young vegetarian and nonvegetarian women. *Nutr Res.* 1990:10:39–49.

35. Pedersen AB, Bartholomew MJ, Dolence LA, Aljadir LP, Netteburg KL, Lloyd T. Mental differences due to vegetarian and nonvegetarian diets. *Am J Clin Nutr.* 1991;53:879–885.

36. Krajcovicová-Kudlackova M, Simoncic R, Béderová A, Ondreicka R, Klvanová J. Selected parameters of lipid metabolism in young vegetarians. *Ann Nutr Metab.* 1994;38:331–335. *Note:* One-half of the vegetarians were LV, one-half were LOV.

37. Melby CL, Toohey M, Cebrick J. Blood pressure and blood lipids among vegetarian, semivegetarian, and nonvegetarian African Americans. *Am J Clin Nutr.* 1994;59:103–109. *Note:* All subjects were black Seventh-day Adventists, of the the 66 vegetarians, 16 were vegans, and 50 were lacto-ovo vegetarians, there were 46 women and 20 men. Of the nonvegetarians, 34 were women and 11 were men.

38. Janelle KC, Barr SI. Nutrient intakes and eating behavior scores of vegetarian and nonvegetarian women. *J Am Dir Assoc.* 1995;95:180–189.

39. Kadrabova J, Madaric A, Kovácikova Z, Ginter E. Selenium status, plasma zinc, copper and magnesium in vegetarians. *Biological Trace Elem Res.* 1995;50:13–24.

40. Thomas EL, Frost G, Barnard ML, et al. An *in vivo* ^{13}C magnetic resonance spectroscopic study of the relationship between diet and adipose tissue composition. *Lipids.* 1996;31:145–151. *Note:* Six males and 5 females were LOV, 21 males and 17 females were VEG, 20 males and 19 females were NV.

41. Ball D, Maughan RJ. Blood and urine acid-base status of premenopausal omnivorous and vegetarian women. *Br J Nutr.* 1997;78:683–693. *Note:* Two vegetarians occasionally ate fish.

42. Williams PT. Interactive effects of exercise, alcohol, and vegetarian diet on coronary artery disease risk factors in 9242 runners: The National Runners' Health Study. *Am J Clin Nutr.* 1997;66:1197–1206. *Note:* Male vegetarian group includes 32 vegans. Female vegetarian group includes 30 vegans.

43. Harman SK, Parnell WR. The nutritional health of New Zealand vegetarian and nonvegetarian Seventh-day Adventists: selected vitamin, mineral and lipid levels. *NZ Med J.* 1998;111:91–94. *Note:* Of the 24 vegetarians, an unspecified number were lacto vegetarians or vegans. Some nonvegetarians only occasionally ate red meat.

44. Appleby PN, Thorogood M, Mann JI, Key TJ. Low body mass index in non-meat eaters: the possible roles of animal fat, dietary fibre and alcohol. *Int J Obesity.* 1998;22:454–460. *Note:* A total of 480 of the 2847 LOV ate fish; 201 were vegan.

45. Reddy S, Sanders TAB, Owen RW, Thompson MH. Faecal pH, bile acid and sterol concentrations in premenopausal Indian and white vegetarians compared with white omnivores. *Br J Nutr.* 1998;79:495–500.

46. Toohey ML, Harris MA, Williams D, Foster G, Schmidt WD, Melby CL. Cardiovascular disease risk factors are lower in African-American vegans compared to lacto-ovo vegetarians. *J Am Coll Nutr.* 1998;17:425–434. *Note:* All subjects were black.

47. Ball MJ, Bartlett MA. Dietary intake and iron status of Australian vegetarian women. *Am J Clin Nutr.* 1999;70:353–358. *Note:* Two of the 50 LOV were vegan; vegetarians consumed red meat no more than once a month and consumed fish or chicken no more than once a week.

48. Hebbelinck M, Clarys P, DeMalsche A. Growth, development, and physical fitness of Flemish vegetarian children, adolescents, and young adults. *Am J Clin Nutr.* 1999;70 (suppl):579S–585S.

49. Outila TA, Karkkainen MUM, Seppanen RH, Lamberg-Allardt JE. Dietary intake of vitamin D in premenopausal healthy vegans was insufficient to maintain concentrations of serum 25-hydroxyvitamin D and intact parathyroid hormone within normal ranges during the winter in Finland. *J Am Diet Assoc.* 2000;100:434–441.

50. Lu S-C, Wu W-H, Lee C-A, et al. LDL of Taiwanese vegetarians are less oxidizable than those of omnivores. *J Nutr.* 2000;130:1591–1596. *Note:* About one third of the LV were vegans.

51. Donaldson MS. Food and nutrient intake of Hallelujah vegetarians. *Nutr Food Sci.* 2001;31:293–303. *Note:* VEG subjects ate a mostly raw diet; 58% consumed some animal product during their week of food intake records.

52. Lin CL, Fang TC, Gueng MK. Vascular dilatory functions of ovo-lacto vegetarians compared with omnivores. *Atherosclerosis.* 2001;158:247–251.

53. Allen NE, Appleby PN, Davey GK, et al. The associations of diet with serum insulin-like growth factor I and its main binding proteins in 292 women meat-eaters, vegetarians, and vegans. *Cancer Epidemiol Biomark Prevent.* 2002; 11:1441–1448.

54. Appleby PN, Davey GK, Key TJ. Hypertension and blood pressure among meat eaters, fish eaters, vegetarians, and vegans in EPIC-Oxford. *Public Health Nutr.* 2002;5:645–654.

55. Lightowler HJ, Davies GJ. Assessment of iodine intake in vegans: weighted dietary record vs duplicate portion technique. *Eur J Clin Nutr.* 2002;56:765–770.

56. Bissoli L, Di Francesco V, Ballarin A, et al. Effect of vegetarian diet on homocysteine levels. *Ann Nutr Metab.* 2002; 46:73–79. *Note:* The LOV group consisted of 8 females and 6 males; the VEG group had 12 females and 19 males.

57. Davey GK, Spencer EA, Appleby PN, et al. EPIC-Oxford lifestyle characteristics and nutrient intakes in a cohort of 33,883 meat-eaters and 31,546 non meat-eaters in the UK. *Public Health Nutr.* 2003;6:259–268

58. Braithwaite N, Fraser HS, Modeste N, et al. Obesity, diabetes, hypertension, and vegetarian status among Seventh-day Adventists in Barbados: preliminary results. *Eth Dis.* 2003;13:34–39. *Note:* Vegetarian status was ascertained by self-report.

59. Spencer EA, Appleby PN, Davey GK, Key TJ. Diet and body mass index in 38000 EPIC-Oxford meat-eaters, fish-eaters, vegetarians and vegans. *Int J Obesity Res.* 2003;27:728–734. *Note:* Subjects are a subset of those in reference 54.

60. Waldmann A, Koschizke JW, Leitzmann C, Hahn A. Dietary intake and lifestyle factors of a vegan population in Germany: results from the German Vegan Study. *Eur J Clin Nutr.* 2003;57:947–955. *Note:* Fifty subjects did not use animal products for 1 year prior to study; 37 subjects consumed small amounts of dairy products and eggs. The first listing is for strict vegans, the second listing is for those who consumed small amounts of dairy and eggs.

61. Huang YC, Chang SJ, Chiu YT, et al. The status of plasma homocysteine and related B-vitamins in healthy young vegetarians and nonvegetarians. *Eur J Nutr.* 2003;42:84–90. *Note:* The LOV group actually includes 3 vegans, 18 lacto vegetarians and 16 lacto-ovo vegetarians.

62. Siani V, Mohamed EI, Maiolo C, et al. Body composition analysis for healthy Italian vegetarians. *Acta Diabetol.* 2003;40:S297–S298. *Note:* No information was provided on gender distribution.

63. Kuo CS, Lai NS, Ho LT, et al. Insulin sensitivity in Chinese ovo-lactovegetarians compared with omnivores. *Eur J Clin Nutr.* 2004;58:312–316. *Note:* Nine males and 10 females were LOV; 10 males and 7 females were NV.

64. Waldmann A, Koschizke JW, Leitzmann C, et al. Dietary iron intake and iron status of German female vegans: results of the German Vegan Study. *Ann Nutr Metab.* 2004;48:103–108. *Note:* Subjects are a subset of those in reference 60.

65. Waldmann A, Koschizke JW, Leitzmann C, et al. Homocysteine and cobalamin status in German vegans. *Public Health Nutr.* 2004;7:467–472. *Note:* The first listing is for strict vegans (42 males and 44 females); the second listing

is for those who consumed small amounts of dairy and eggs but were primarily vegan (16 males and 29 females). Subjects are a subset of those in reference 60.

66. Phillips F, Hackett AF, Stratton G, et al. Effect of changing to a self-selected vegetarian diet on anthropometric measurements in UK adults. *J Hum Nutr Dietet.* 2004;17:249–255. *Note:* Results represent intakes before and 6 months after becoming vegetarian. Six subjects identified as vegetarian ate fish. Seven males and 26 females were in each group.

67. Chiplonkar SA, Agte V, Tarwadik V, et al. Micronutrient deficiencies as predisposing factors for hypertension in lacto-vegetarian Indian adults. *J Am Coll Nutr.* 2004;23:239–247.

68. Cade JE, Burley VJ, Greenwood DC, et al. The UK Women's Cohort Study: comparisons of vegetarians, fish-eaters, and meat-eaters. *Public Health Nutr.* 2004;7:871–878. *Note:* Vegetarians ate meat or fish less than once a week.

69. Goff LM, Bell JD, So PW, et al. Veganism and its relationship with insulin resistance and intramyocellular lipid. *Eur J Clin Nutr.* 2005;59:291–298. *Note:* Gender distribution of VEG group not specified; 11 males and 14 females were NV.

70. Fontana L, Shew JL, Holloszy JO, et al. Low bone mass in subjects on a long-term raw vegetarian diet. *Arch Intern Med.* 2005;165:684–689. *Note:* Study subjects ate a raw foods diet. Seven males and 11 females were VEG; 7 males and 11 females were NV.

71. Bedford JL, Barr SI. Diets and selected lifestyle practices of self-defined adult vegetarians from a population-based sample suggest they are more health conscious. *Int J Behav Nutr Phys Act.* 2005;2:4. *Note:* Seventy-five percent of those self-identified as vegetarian consumed fish and/or seafood, 58% consumed poultry; 22% consumed red meat.

72. Newby PK, Tucker KL, Wolk A. Risk of overweight and obesity among semivegetarians, lactovegetarians and vegan women. *Am J Clin Nutr.* 2005;81:1267–1274.

73. Waldmann A, Koschizke JW, Leitzmann C, et al. German vegan study: diet, lifestyle factors, and cardiovascular risk profile. *Ann Nutr Metab.* 2005;49:366–372. *Note:* The first listing is for strict vegans (48 males and 50 females); the second listing is for those who consumed small amounts of dairy and eggs but were primarily vegan (19 males and 37 females). Subjects are a subset of those in reference 60.

74. Harvey LJ, Arman CN, Dainly JR, et al. Impact of menstrual blood loss and diet on iron deficiency among women in the UK. *Br J Nutr.* 2005;94:557–564. *Note:* The first NV group consists of poultry and fish eaters; the second NV group is red meat eaters.

75. Alewaeters K, Clarys P, Hebbelinck M, et al. Cross-sectional analysis of BMI and some life style variables in Flemish vegetarians compared to non-vegetarians. *Ergonomics.* 2005;48:1433–1444. *Note:* In the study, 8% were ovo vegetarians, 2.1% were LV, and 15% were VEG.

76. Rosell M, Appleby P, Key T. Height, age at menarche, body weight, and body mass index in life-long vegetarians. *Public Health Nutr.* 2005;8:870–875. *Note:* The LOV group included 695 male vegans and 1188 female vegans.

77. Su TC, Jeng JS, Wang JD, et al. Homocysteine, circulating vascular cell adhesion molecule and carotid atherosclerosis in postmenopausal vegetarian women and omnivores. *Atherosclerosis.* 2006;184:356–362. *Note:* Fifty-one subjects were vegan; six were lacto vegetarians.

78. Valachovicova M, Krajcovicova-Kudlackova M, Blazicek P, et al. No evidence of insulin resistance in normal weight vegetarians. A case study. *Eur J Nutr.* 2006;45:52–54. *Note:* Thirty-nine males and 56 females were LOV; 45 males and 62 females were NV.

79. Wu WH, Lu SC, Wang TF, et al. Effects of docosahexaenoic acid supplementation on blood lipids, estrogen metabolism, and in vivo oxidative stress in postmenopausal vegetarian women. *Eur J Clin Nutr.* 2006;60:386–392. *Note:* Subjects were a mixture of LOV and vegans.

80. Hung CJ, Huang PC, Li YH, et al. Taiwanese vegetarians have higher insulin sensitivity than omnivores. *Br J Nutr.* 2006;95:129–135. *Note:* Seven subjects were vegan, 42 were lactovegetarians.

81. Majchrzak D, Singer I, Manner M, et al. B-vitamin status and concentrations of homocysteine in Austrian omnivores, vegetarians, and vegans. *Ann Nutr Metab.* 2006;50:485–491. *Note:* Ten males and 26 females were LOV; 21 males and 21 females were VEG; 11 males and 29 females were NV.

82. Haldar S, Rowland IR, Barnett RA, et al. Influence of habitual diet on antioxidant status: a study in a population of vegetarians and omnivores. *Eur J Clin Nutr.* 2007;61:1011–1022. *Note:* Vegetarian subjects ate flesh foods no more than six times a year. The vegetarian group included six vegans.

83. Chen CW, Lin YL, Lin TK, et al. Total cardiovascular risk profile of Taiwanese vegetarians. *Eur J Clin Nutr.* 2008;62:138–144.

84. Karabudak E, Kiziltan G, Cigerim N. A comparison of some of the cardiovascular risk factors in vegetarian and omnivorous Turkish females. *J Hum Nutr Diet.* 2008;21:13–22. *Note:* Subjects include 9 LOV, 10 LV, and 7 occasional fish and/or chicken eaters.

85. Yen CE, Yen CH, Huang MC, et al. Dietary intake and nutritional status of vegetarian and omnivorous preschool children and their parents in Taiwan. *Nutr Res.* 2008;28:430–436. *Note:* Adult vegetarians consisted of 16 LOV, 2 ovo-vegetarians, 1 LV, 2 vegans. Four male adults and 17 females were vegetarian; 9 male adults and 19 females were NV. Children consisted of 18 LOV and 3 ovo-vegetarians. Fourteen male children and 7 female children were vegetarians; 15 male children and 13 female children were NV.

86. Nakamato K, Watanabe S, Kudo H, et al. Nutritional characteristics of middle-aged Japanese vegetarians. *J Atherosclero Throm.* 2008;15:122–129. *Note:* Nine men and 18 women were LOV; 11 men and 37 women in the vegetarian group occasionally ate chicken and meat.

87. deBertoli MC, Cozzolini SM. Zinc and selenium nutritional status in vegetarians. *Biol Trace Elem Res.* 2009; 127:228–233. *Note:* Type of vegetarian was not specified.

88. Tonstad S, Butler T, Yan R, et al. Type of vegetarian diet, body weight, and prevalence of type 2 diabetes. *Diabetes Care;* 2009;32:791–796. *Note:* In the study, 7694 males and 12,714 females were LOV; 1090 males and 1641 females were VEG; 10,584 males and 18,177 females were NV.

89. Ho-Pham LT, Nguyen PL, Le TT, et al. Veganism, bone density, and body composition: a study in Buddhist nuns. *Osteoporosis Int.* 2009;20:2087–2093.

90. Aubertin-Leheudre M, Adlercreutz H. Relationship between animal protein intake and muscle mass index in healthy women. *Br J Nutr.* 2009;102:1803–1810. *Note:* The vegetarian group included 8 LOV, 10 LV, and 1 vegan.

91. Deriemaeker P, Aerenhouts D, Hebbelinck M, Clarys P. Nutrient based estimation of acid-base balance in vegetarians and non-vegetarians. *Plant Foods Hum Nutr.* 2010;65:77–82. *Note:* Eight men and 22 women were in each group.

Appendix E Anthropometric Data of Male Adult Vegetarians and Nonvegetarians

(REF)/year	Group[1]/(N)	SDA/NSDA[2]	Age	Height (cm)	Weight (kg)	Body Mass Index (kg/m²)	Body fat[3]
(1) 1954	LOV (15)	SDA/NSDA	55	172.7	73.6	24.7	
	NV (15)	SDA/NSDA	57	176.5	77.3	24.8	
(2) 1975	LOV (73)	NSDA	16–40		58.0		6.0
	NV (73)		16–40		73.0		17.0
(3) 1980	LOV (25)	NSDA	40				39.2
	NV (211)		50				49.3
(4) 1980	LOV (15)	NSDA	28	179.2	72.6	22.6	14.4
	NV (25)		27	179.0	78.4	24.5	17.8
(5) 1981	LOV (8)	NSDA	40			20.5	
	NV (50)		44			24.5	
	LOV (21)		69			22.7	
	NV (32)		69			24.9	
(6) 1982	LOV (52)	NSDA	35	180.0	69.0	21.4	
	NV (56)		33	178.0	77.0	24.4	
(7) 1983	LOV (47)	SDA	33	173.2	68.8	22.9	9.2
	NV (59)	NSDA	34	175.3	77.3	25.1	10.3
(8) 1984	LOV (36)	NSDA	31	179.0	74.2	23.1	24.6
	NV (18)		31	179.0	75.8	23.7	27.2
(9) 1985	LOV (41)	SDA	51			25.3	
	NV (12)		51			27.1	
(10) 1985	LOV (4)	NSDA	27–49			22.0	
	VEG (5)		27–49			23.0	
	NV (5)		27–49			24.0	
(11) 1985	LOV (12)	SDA	57	180.8	84.0	25.7	21.6
	NV (8)	NSDA	56	180.6	84.4	25.8	20.9
(12) 1986	LOV (14)	NSDA	28	173.0	63.7	21.3	
	NV (14)		21	175.0	66.4	21.7	

(Appendix E continued)

Appendix E Anthropometric Data of Male Adult Vegetarians and Nonvegetarians

(REF)/year	Group¹/(N)	SDA/NSDA²	Age	Height (cm)	Weight (kg)	Body Mass Index (kg/m²)	Body fat³
(13) 1986	LOV (60)	NSDA	55	169.0	64.9	22.7	
	NV (53)	NSDA	50	172.1	75.1	25.4	
(14) 1986	VEG (8)	NSDA	18–40			21.0	
	NV (8)		18–40			23.0	
(15) 1986	LOV (14)	SDA/NSDA	18–40	178.0	75.7	23.9	18.5
	NV (10)	NSDA	18–40	177.8	77.8	24.6	15.4
(16) 1987	VEG (11)	NSDA	32			21.1	8.8
	NV (11)		31			21.8	10.7
(17) 1988	LOV (14)	NI	23	181.0	69.7	20.9	
	NV (22)	NI	23	184.0	74.5	22.0	
(18) 1988	LOV (14)	SDA/NSDA	34	175.7	73.2	23.7	
	NV (13)	NSDA	35	174.3	76.6	25.2	
(19) 1989	LOV (11)	NSDA	37	173.0	63.4	21.2	
	NV (33)		40	175.0	76.0	24.7	
(20) 1989	LOV (15)	NSDA	29	174.0	64	20.9	
	NV (14)		27	177.0	74	23.4	
(21) 1990	LOV (20)	SDA	26	186.0	73.9	21.3	8.6
	VEG (15)	SDA	30	179.3	67.2	20.8	8.0
	NV (18)	SDA	26	178.2	75.2	23.6	14.0
(22) 1990	LOV (15)	NSDA	82		67.7	23.8	
	NV (225)		72		76.3	25.6	
(23) 1990	LOV (26)	NSDA	41			23.1	
	VEG (26)	NSDA	41			22.3	
	NV (26)	NSDA	41			23.1	
(24) 1994	LOV (31)	NSDA	23	180.3	71.6	22.0	
	NV (24)	NSDA	26	178.4	74.3	23.3	
(25) 1994	LV/VEG (17)	NI	25	178.0	75.0	23.7	85.0
	NV (40)	NI	24	178.0	76.0	24.0	93.0

No. / Year	Group (n)		Age	Height	Weight	BMI
(26) 1995	LOV (22)	NSDA	20–57			22.3
	NV (22)		20–57			25.2
(27) 1997	LOV (199)	NSDA	45			22.9
	NV (7054)		46			23.8
(28) 1998	LOV (12)	SDA	49			24.1
	NV (11)		40			26.4
(29) 1998	LOV (931)	NI	39			22.0[4]
	NV (975)		38			23.2[4]
(30) 1998	B-LOV (49)	SDA	50	174.0	79.2	26.1
	B-VEG (14)		46	174.3	71.8	23.6
(31) 1999	LOV (13)	NI	18–30	176.9	69.2	22.1
(32) 1999	LOV (43)	NI	35			23.6
	VEG (18)		33			23.3
	NV (60)		38			26.4
(33) 2000	LOV (237)	NI	46	178	74.4	23.4
	VEG (233)		43	178	71.8	22.7
	NV (226)		53	178	82.4	26.1
(34) 2000	LV (26)	NSDA	37.7	169.2	59.4	20.8
	NV (27)		38.3	169.5	66.0	22.9
(35) 2001	VEG (54)	NSDA	57			22.9
(36) 2002	LOV (786)	NSDA	45			23.4
	VEG (272)		40			22.6
	NV (996)		54			24.6
(37) 2002	VEG (11)	NSDA	40.2	179	70.5	22.0
(38) 2003	LOV (4171)	NSDA	39			23.5
	VEG (937)		35			22.5
	NV (7767)		51			24.9

(Appendix E continued)

Appendix E Anthropometric Data of Male Adult Vegetarians and Nonvegetarians

(REF)/year	Group[1]/(N)	SDA/NSDA[2]	Age	Height (cm)	Weight (kg)	Body Mass Index (kg/m²)	Body fat[3]
(39) 2003	LOV (49) NV (100)	SDA	25–74 25–74	171.7 173.5	71.6 74.9	24.4 24.9	
(40) 2003	LOV (2888) VEG (570) NV (4318)	NSDA	38 35 48			23.3 22.3 24.5	
(41) 2003	VEG (48) VEG (19)		42.4 45.2			22.2 21.2	16.3 16.6
(42) 2004	LV (85) LV htn (83)	NSDA	46.1 47.1		58.8 63.0	21.7 23.9	
(43) 2005	VEG (7) NV (7)	NSDA	52.7 52.3	180 180	65.0 82.5	20.7 25.5	13.9 20.8
(44) 2005	LOV (31) NV (869)	NI	NI NI		82.2 83.1	25.9 26.7	
(45) 2005	LOV (120) NV (4666)	NI	42.3 48.0			22.6 25.7	
(46) 2005	LOV (122)[5] LOV (71) LOV (118) LOV (538) LOV (3012) NV (6103)	NI	≥20 ≥20 ≥20 ≥20 ≥20 ≥20	176.3 176.1 176.9 176.2 176.5 176.8	75.5 79.0 76.4 75.3 75.7 78.8	24.2 25.4 24.4 24.2 24.3 25.2	
(47) 2007	LOV (11) NV (17)	NI	37.8 42.2			24.8 26.7	
(48) 2008	LOV (34) NV (53)	NI	50.9 49.2	166.7 167.8	67.1 69.6	24.0 24.7	

| (49) 2008 | LO/SV (20) NV (29) | NI | 45.2 43.4 | 164.5 169.2 | 58.1 66.3 | 21.4 23.2 |
| (50) 2009 | LOV (13) | NI | 26.5 | 176 | 66.4 | 21.4 |

Notes: [1]Abbreviations: LV, lacto vegetarian; LOV, lacto-ovo vegetarian; VEG, vegan; NV, nonvegetarian; SV, eats chicken and/or fish; htn, subjects identified as having hypertension; NI, not indicated; B, black.

[2]SDA indicates the vegetarians were specifically identified as Seventh-day Adventists, whereas NSDA indicates the vegetarians were not exclusively SDAs, although some SDAs may have been included in the vegetarian group. NI indicates the process by which subjects were recruited for the study was not indicated or the extent to which SDAs composed the vegetarian groups was not possible to determine by the information provided.

[3]Reference 2, body fat calculated from subscapular thickness (mm), references 3, 15, and 16, from sum of skinfold thickness (mm) at triceps, forearm, subscapular and suprailiac sites (data for nonvegetarians for reference 16 came from the Ten-State Nutrition Survey, 1968–1970: III Clinical, Anthropometry, Dental. DHEW Publication No. (HSM) 72:8131, 1972), references 4 and 7, from triceps skinfold thickness (mm), reference 8 from sum of triceps and subscapular skinfolds (mm), references 11 and 21 from skinfold thickness (mm) at chest, abdomen, and thigh, reference 24, from abdomen, axilla, biceps, calf, chest, subscapula, suprailiac, thigh and triceps skinfolds (mm), reference 41, percentage of body fat measured by the infrared method, reference 43 body fat (percentage) measured using DEXA total body scan.

[4]Age-adjusted BMI.

[5]The first listing is for lifelong vegetarians, second listing is for those who became vegetarian at age 1 to 9 years, third listing is for those who became vegetarian at 10 to 14 years, fourth listing at 15 to 18 years, fifth listing at ≥20 years of age.

ANNOTATED REFERENCES APPENDIX E

1. Hardinge MG, Stare FJ. Nutritional studies of vegetarians. 1. Nutritional, physical, and laboratory studies. *J Clin Nutr.* 1954;2:73–82.
2. Sacks FM, Castelli WP, Donner A, Kass EH. Plasma lipids and lipoproteins in vegetarians and controls. *N Engl J Med.* 1975;292:1148–1151. *Note:* Vegetarians consisted of macrobiotics 40% of whom consumed fish once per week or more, 28% consumed dairy products and 11% consumed eggs. Values presented for males actually include 42 females in both the LOV and NV groups.
3. Haines AP, Chakrabarti R, Fisher D, Meade TW, North WRS, Stirling Y. Haemostatic variables in vegetarians and nonvegetarians. *Thrombosis Res.* 1980;19:139–148.
4. Taber LAL, Cook RA. Dietary and anthropometric assessment of adult omnivores, fish-eaters, and lacto-ovo vegetarians. *J Am Diet Assoc.* 1980;76:21–29.
5. Burr ML, Bates CJ, Fehily AM, Leger AS. Plasma cholesterol and blood pressure in vegetarians. *Am J Human Nutr.* 1981;35:437–441.
6. Knuiman JT, West CE. The concentration of cholesterol in serum and in various serum lipoproteins in macrobiotic, vegetarian and nonvegetarian men and boys. *Atherosclerosis.* 1982;43:71–82.
7. Rouse IL, Armstrong BK, Beilin LJ. The relationship of blood pressure to diet and lifestyle in two religious populations. *J Hypertension.* 1983;1:65–71.
8. Latta D, Liebman M. Iron and zinc status of vegetarian and nonvegetarian males. *Nutr Rep Int.* 1984;30:141–149.
9. Melby CL, Hyner CG, Zoog B. Blood pressure in vegetarians and nonvegetarians: a cross sectional analysis. *Nutr Res.* 1985;5:1077–1082.
10. Carlson E, Kipps M, Lockie A, Thomson J. A comparative evaluation of vegan, vegetarian and omnivore diets. *J Plant Foods.* 1985;6:89–100.
11. Howie BJ, Shultz TD. Dietary and hormonal interrelationships among vegetarian Seventh-Day Adventists and nonvegetarian men. *Am J Clin Nutr.* 1985;42:127–134.
12. Locong A. Nutritional status and dietary intake of a selected sample of young adult vegetarians. *Can Diet Assoc J.* 1986;47:101–106.
13. Levin N, Ratton J, Gilat T. Energy intake and body weight in ovo-lacto vegetarians. *J Clin Gastroenterol.* 1986; 8:451–453.
14. Rana SK, Sanders TAB. Taurine concentrations in the diet, plasma, urine and breast milk of vegans compared with omnivores. *Br J Nutr.* 1986;56:17–27.
15. Faber M, Gouws E, Benade AJS, Labadarios D. Anthropometric measurements, dietary intake and biochemical data of South African lacto-ovo vegetarians. *S Afr Med J.* 1986;69:733–738.
16. Sanders TAB, Key TJA. Blood pressure, plasma renin activity and aldosterone concentrations in vegans and omnivores. *Human Nutr: Appl Nutr.* 1987;41A:204–211.
17. Aalberts JS, Weegels PL, van der Hijden L, et al. Calcium supplementation: effect on blood pressure and urinary mineral excretion in normotensive male lacto-ovo vegetarians and omnivores. *Am J Clin Nutr.* 1988;48:131–138.
18. Kelsay JL, Frazier CW, Prather E, Canary JJ, Clark WM, Powell AS. Impact of variation in carbohydrate intake on mineral utilization by vegetarians. *Am J Clin Nutr.* 1988;48:875–879.
19. Millet P., Guilland JC, Fuchs F, Klepping J. Nutrient intake and vitamin status of healthy French vegetarians and nonvegetarians. *Am J Clin Nutr.* 1989;50:718–727.
20. Bélanger A, Locong A, Noel C, Cusan L, Dupont A, Prévost J, Caron S, Sévigny J. Influence of diet on plasma steroid and sex plasma binding globulin levels in adult men. *J Steroid Biochem.* 1989;32:829–833.
21. Ross JK, Pusateri DJ, Shultz TD. Dietary and hormonal evaluation of men at different risks for prostate cancer: fiber intake, excretion, and composition, with in vitro evidence for an association between steroid hormones and specific components. *Am J Clin Nutr.* 1990;51:365–370.
22. Löwik MRH, Schrijver J, van den Berg H, Hulshof KFAM, Wedel M, Ockhuizen T. Effect of dietary fiber on the vitamin B6 status among vegetarian and nonvegetarian elderly (Dutch Nutrition Surveillance System). *J Am College Nutr.* 1990;9:241–249.

23. Thorogood M, Roe L, McPherson K, Mann J. Dietary intake and plasma lipid levels: lessons from a study of the diet of health conscious groups. *Br Med J*. 1990;300:1297–1301.
24. Krajcovicová-Kudlackova M, Simoncic R, Béderová A, Ondreicka R, Klvanová J. Selected parameters of lipid metabolism in young vegetarians. *Ann Nutr Metab*. 1994;38:331–335. *Notes:* One-third of the vegetarians were LV, 2/3 were LOV.
25. Toth MJ, Poehlman ET. Sympathetic nervous system activity and resting metabolic rate in vegetarians. *Metabolism*. 1994;43:621–625. *Note:* Among the vegetarians, 10 were LV, and 7 were VEG.
26. Kadrabova J, Madaric A, Kovácíková Z. Ginter E. Selenium status, plasma zinc, copper, and magnesium in vegetarians. *Biolo Trace Elem Res*. 1995;50:13–24.
27. Williams PT. Interactive effects of exercise, alcohol, and vegetarian diet on coronary artery disease risk factors in 9242 runners: The National Runners' Health Study. *Am J Clin Nutr*. 1997;66:1197–1206. *Note:* Male vegetarian group includes 32 vegans. Female vegetarian group includes 30 vegans.
28. Harman SK, Parnell WR. The nutritional health of New Zealand vegetarian and nonvegetarian Seventh-Day Adventists: selected vitamin, mineral and lipid levels. *NZ Med J*. 1998;111:91–94. *Note:* Of the 24 vegetarians, an unspecified number were lacto vegetarians or vegans. Some nonvegetarians only occasionally ate red meat.
29. Appleby PN, Thorogood M, Mann JI, Key TJ. Low body mass index in non-meat eaters: the possible roles of animal fat, dietary fibre and alcohol. *Int J Obesity*. 1998;22:454–460. *Note:* A total of 480 of the 2847 LOV ate fish; 201 were vegan.
30. Toohey ML, Harris MA, Williams D, Foster G, Schmidt WD, Melby CL. Cardiovascular disease risk factors are lower in African-American vegans compared to lacto-ovo vegetarians. *J Am Coll Nutr*. 1998;17:425–434. *Note:* All subjects were black.
31. Hebbelinck M, Clarys P, DeMalsche A. Growth, development, and physical fitness of Flemish vegetarian children, adolescents, and young adults. *Am J Clin Nutr*. 1999;70(suppl):579S–585S. 31 LOV and 3 VEG consumed fish occasionally.
32. Li D, Sinclair A, Mann N, et al. The association of diet and thrombotic risk factors in healthy male vegetarians and meat-eaters. *Eur J Clin Nutr*. 1999;53:612–619. *Note:* Nonvegetarians are described as "moderate-meat-eaters" (<285 g meat/d).
33. Allen NE, Appleby PN, Davey GK, Key TJ. Hormones and diet: low insulin-like growth factor-I but normal bioavailable androgens in vegan men. *Br J Cancer*. 2000;83:95–97.
34. Lu S-C, Wu W-H, Lee C-A, et al. LDL of Taiwanese vegetarians are less oxidizable than those of omnivores. *J Nutr*. 2000;130:1591–1596. *Note:* About one third of the LV were vegans.
35. Donaldson MS. Food and nutrient intake of Hallelujah vegetarians. *Nutr Food Sci*. 2001;31:293–303. *Note:* VEG subjects ate a mostly raw diet; 58% consumed some animal product during their week of food intake records.
36. Appleby PN, Davey GK, Key TJ. Hypertension and blood pressure among meat eaters, fish eaters, vegetarians, and vegans in EPIC-Oxford. *Public Health Nutr*. 2002;5:645–654.
37. Lightowler HJ, Davies GJ. Assessment of iodine intake in vegans: weighted dietary record vs duplicate portion technique. *Eur J Clin Nutr*. 2002;56:765–770.
38. Davey GK, Spencer EA, Appleby PN, et al. EPIC-Oxford lifestyle characteristics and nutrient intakes in a cohort of 33883 meat-eaters and 31546 non-meat-eaters in the UK. *Public Health Nutr*. 2003; 6:259–268
39. Braithwaite N, Fraser HS, Modeste N, et al. Obesity, diabetes, hypertension, and vegetarian status among Seventh-Day Adventists in Barbados: preliminary results. *Eth Dis*. 2003;13:34–39. *Note:* Vegetarian status was ascertained by self-report.
40. Spencer EA, Appleby PN, Davey GK, Key TJ. Diet and body mass index in 38000 EPIC-Oxford meat-eaters, fish-eaters, vegetarians and vegans. *Int J Obesity Res*. 2003;27: 728–734. *Note:* Subjects are a subset of those in reference 36.
41. Waldmann A, Koschizke JW, Leitzmann C, Hahn A. Dietary intake and lifestyle factors of a vegan population in Germany: results from the German Vegan Study. *Eur J Clin Nutr*. 2003;57:947–955. *Note:* Forty-eight subjects did not use animal products for 1 year prior to study; 19 subjects consumed small amounts of dairy products and eggs. The first listing is for strict vegans; the second listing is for those who consumed small amounts of dairy and eggs.
42. Chiplonkar SA, Agte V, Tarwadik V, et al. Micronutrient deficiencies as predisposing factors for hypertension in lacto-vegetarian Indian adults. *J Am Coll Nutr*. 2004;23:239–247.

43. Fontana L, Shew JL, Holloszy JO, et al. Low bone mass in subjects on a long-term raw vegetarian diet. *Arch Intern Med*. 2005;165:684–689. *Note*: Study subjects ate a raw foods diet. Seven males and 11 females were VEG; 7 males and 11 females were NV.
44. Bedford JL, Barr SI. Diets and selected lifestyle practices of self-defined adult vegetarians from a population-based sample suggest they are more health conscious. *Int J Behav Nutr Phys Act*. 2005;2:4. *Note*: Seventy-five percent of those self-identified as vegetarian consumed fish and/or seafood, 58% consumed poultry; 22% consumed red meat.
45. Alewaeters K, Clarys P, Hebbelinck M, et al. Cross-sectional analysis of BMI and some life style variables in Flemish vegetarians compared to non-vegetarians. *Ergonomics*. 2005;48:14333–1444. *Note*: In the study, 1.8% were ovo vegetarians, 2.1% were LV, and 15% were VEG.
46. Rosell M, Appleby P, Key T. Height, age at menarche, body weight, and body mass index in life-long vegetarians. *Public Health Nutr*. 2005;8:870–875. *Note*: The LOV group included 695 male vegans and 1188 female vegans.
47. Haldar S, Rowland IR, Barnett RA, et al. Influence of habitual diet on antioxidant status: a study in a population of vegetarians and omnivores. *Eur J Clin Nutr*. 2007;61:1011–1022. *Note*: Vegetarian subjects ate flesh foods no more than six times a year. The vegetarian group included six vegans.
48. Chen CW, Lin YL, Lin TK, et al. Total cardiovascular risk profile of Taiwanese vegetarians. *Eur J Clin Nutr*. 2008; 62:138–144.
49. Nakamato K, Watanabe S, Kudo H, et al. Nutritional characteristics of middle-aged Japanese vegetarians. *J Atherosclero Throm*. 2008;15:122–129. *Note*: Nine men and 18 women were LOV; 11 men and 37 women in the vegetarian group occasionally ate chicken and meat.
50. deBertoli MC, Cozzolini SM. Zinc and selenium nutritional status in vegetarians. *Biol Trace Elem Res*. 2009;127: 228–233. *Note*: Type of vegetarian was not specified.

Appendix F Dietary Intake Ratios of N-6 (Linoleic acid) to N-3 (α-Linolenic acid) Fatty Acids among Vegetarians and Nonvegetarians

(REF)/year	Group¹/Gender (N)	Country	Age (years)	Linoleic acid (grams)	α-Linolenic acid (grams)	Linoleic: α-Linolenic acid (g:g)
(1) 1962	LOV F (15)	United States	NI	10.5	0.2	52.5
	NV F (15)			11.2	0.5	22.4
	LOV M (15)			14.8	0.4	37.0
	NV M (15)			26.3	0.7	37.6
(2) 1984	VEG M (10)	Great Britain	NI	31.9	1.8	17.7
	NV M (12)			10.7	1.0	10.7
	VEG F (10)			21.4	1.2	17.8
	NV F (12)			9.10	1.1	8.3
(3) 1992	VEG M/F (18)	Great Britain	5.8–12.8	16.8	0.38	44.2
(4) 1993	LV M (23)	Taiwan	22.6	25.1	3.6	7.0
	NV M (20)		20.6	33.2	2.7	12.3
	LV F (32)		24.8	29.5	3.7	8.0
	NV F (39)		20.3	37.2	2.3	16.2
(5) 1993	LOV M (16)	Great Britain	21–40	19.2	2.1	9.1
	VEG M (18)		21–40	28.6	2.0	14.3
	NV M (386)		NI	14.5	2.0	7.3
	LOV F (36)		21–40	18.5	1.7	10.9
	VEG F (20)		21–40	22.4	1.5	14.9
	NV F (377)		NI	10.4	1.4	7.4
(6) 1998	LOV F (4)	Scotland	27	10.4	1.5	7.0
	NV F (10)		28	9.6	1.2	7.8
(7) 1999	LOV M (10)	Australia	20–50	16.2	1.9	8.5
	LOV M (10)		20–50	30.5	1.9	16.1

(Appendix F continued)

Appendix F Dietary Intake Ratios of N-6 (Linoleic acid) to N-3 (α-Linolenic acid) Fatty Acids among Vegetarians and Nonvegetarians

(REF)/year	Group[1]/Gender (N)	Country	Age (years)	Linoleic acid (grams)	α-Linolenic acid (grams)	Linoleic: α-Linolenic acid (g:g)
(8) 2000	LOV M/F (54)	Slovak Republic	37.3	21.0	2.06	10.2
	VEG M/F (32)		41.5	21.1	1.99	10.6
	NV/ M/F (59)		40.9	18.4	1.33	13.8
(9) 2005	LOV M/F (55)	Germany	18–43[2]	10.6	1.53	6.9
	NV M/F (53)			12.4	1.56	8.4
(10) 2006	LOV M (43)	Australia	34.9	18.4	1.4	13.0
	VEG M (18)		33.0	21.6	1.2	18.8
	NV M (60)		38.3	10.9	1.3	8.6
(11) 2008	LOV M/F (25)	Austria	36.4	14.96	1.73	8.6
	VEG M/F (37)		29.5	22.52	2.63	8.6
	NV M/F (23)		38.5	7.86	1.19	6.6
(12) 2009	VEG M (57)	United Kingdom	NI	24.8	2.2	2.1
	NV M (138)		NI	12.0	1.3	9.2

Note: [1]Abbreviations: LV, lacto vegetarian, LOV, lacto-ovo vegetarian, VEG, vegan, and NV, nonvegetarian, NI, not indicated.
[2]Age range of all study subjects.

ANNOTATED REFERENCES APPENDIX F

1. Hardinge MG, Crooks H, Stare FJ. Nutritional studies of vegetarians. IV. Dietary fatty acids and serum cholesterol levels. *Am J Clin Nutr.* 1962;10:516–524.
2. Roshanai F, Sanders TAB. Assessment of fatty acid intakes in vegans and omnivores. *Hum Nutr: Appl Nutr.* 1984;(A)38:345–354.
3. Sanders TAB, Manning J. The growth and development of vegan children. *J Human Nutr Diet.* 1992; 5:11–21. *Note:* Values for linoleic and linolenic acid were converted from percentage of calories to grams per day.
4. Pan W-H, Chin C-J, Sheu C-T, Lee M-H. Hemostatic factors and blood lipids in young Buddhist vegetarians and omnivores. *Am J Clin Nutr.* 1993;58:354–359.
5. Draper A, Lewis J, Malhotra N, Wheeler E. The energy and nutrient intakes of different types of vegetarian: a case for supplements? *Br J Nutr.* 1993;69(1):3–19.
6. Lakin V, Haggarty P, Abramovich DR, et al. Dietary intake and tissue concentration of fatty acids in omnivore, vegetarian and diabetic pregnancy. *Prostaglandins Leukot Essent Fatty Acids.* 1998;59(3):209–220. *Note:* All subjects were pregnant.
7. Li D, Sinclair A, Wilson A, et al. Effect of dietary alpha-linolenic acid on thrombotic risk factors in vegetarian men. *Am J Clin Nutr.* 1999;69(5):872–882.
8. Krajcovicova-Kudlackova M, Blazicek P, Babinska K, et al. Traditional and alternative nutrition—levels of homo-cysteine and lipid parameters in adults. *Scand J Clin Lab Invest.* 2000;60(8):657–664.
9. Geppert J, Kraft V, Demmelmair H, et al. Docosahexaenoic acid supplementation in vegetarians effectively increases omega-3 index: a randomized trial. *Lipids.* 2005;40:807–814. *Note:* Subjects were divided into two groups.
10. Mann N, Pirotta Y, O'Vonnell S, et al. Fatty acid composition of habitual omnivore and vegetarian diets. *Lipids.* 2006;41:637–646. *Note:* Nonvegetarians are described as "moderate-meat-eaters" (<285 g meat/d). Ten LOV and three VEG consumed fish occasionally.
11. Kornsteiner M, Singer I, Elmadfa I. Very low n-3 long-chain polyunsaturated fatty acid status in Austrian vegetarians and vegans. *Ann Nutr Metab.* 2008;52:37–47. *Note:* Seven males and 18 females were LOV; 19 males and 18 females were VEG; 8 males and 15 females were NV.
12. Sanders TAB. DHA status of vegetarians. *Prostaglandins Leukot Essent Fatty Acids.*2009;2009;81(2–3):137–141. *Note:* NV data from Sanders TA, Lewis F, Slaughter S, et al. Effect of varying the ratio of n-6 to n-3 fatty acids by increasing the dietary intake of alpha-linolenic acid, eicosapentaenoic and docosahexaenoic acid, or both on fibrinogen and clotting factors VII and XII in persons aged 45–70 y: the OPTILIP study, *Am J Clin Nutr.* 2006;84:513–522.

Appendix G Protein, Calcium, Phosphorus, Sodium, and Potassium Intakes of Adult Vegetarians and Nonvegetarians

(Ref)/ year	Group/ Gender(N)	Country	Kcal	Protein (grams)	Protein %Kcal	Calcium (mg)	Calcium (mg): Protein (g)	Phosphorus (mg)	Calcium: Phosphorus	Sodium (mg)	Potassium (mg)
(1) 1954	LOV M (15)	United States	3020	98.0	13.0	1700	17.3	2200	0.77		
	VEG M (14)		3260	83.0	10.2	1100	13.3	1900	0.58		
	NV M (15)		3720	125.0	13.4	1400	11.2	2200	0.64		
	LOV F (15)		2450	82.0	13.4	1600	19.5	1800	0.89		
	VEG F (11)		2400	61.0	10.2	900	14.8	1400	0.64		
	NV F (15)		2690	94.0	14.0	1000	10.6	1600	0.63		
(2) 1963	LOV F (26)	Australia	1980	52.8	10.7	813	15.4				
	NV F (25)		2115	64.6	12.2	661	10.2				
(3) 1978	LOV F (42)	United States	1600	65.0	16.3	1017	15.6	1325	0.77	2221	2817
	NV F (36)		1579	67.0	17.0	784	11.7	1114	0.70	2083	2467
(4) 1980	LOV M/F (57)	United States	2270	69.0	12.2	1200	17.4	1564	0.77	1755	3643
	LV M/F (14)		1830	56.0	12.2	856	15.3	1311	0.65	1203	4203
	VEG M/F (8)		1665	34.0	8.2	535	15.7	827	0.64	251	4127
	NV F (41)		2072	84.0	16.2	1099	13.1	1444	0.76	2289	2650
(5) 1980	LOV M (15)	United States	2624	90.0	13.7	1481	16.5	2078	0.71		
	NV M (25)		2684	112.0	16.7	1154	10.3	1889	0.61		
	LOV F (13)		2174	79.0	14.5	1386	17.5	1855	0.75		
	NV F (24)		1859	76.0	16.4	898	11.8	1240	0.72		
(6) 1981	LOV F (5)	United States	1329	51.0	15.3	723	14.2	962	0.75	1656	2356
(7) 1982	LOV F (101)	United States	1565	59.4	15.2	825	13.9	1188	0.69		
	NV F (107)		1573	68.4	17.4	782	11.4	1153	0.68		
(8) 1983	LOV M (18)	United States		79.1		1409	17.8	1536	0.92		
(9) 1983	LOV M (20)	United States	2324	74.0	12.7	993	13.4				
	NV M (17)		2652	97.0	14.6	1244	12.8				
	LOV F (31)		1776	60.0	13.5	782	13.0				
	NV F (36)		1754	62.0	14.1	841	13.6				

(10) 1984	United States	LOV M (25)	2128	70.0	13.2	1188	17.0	1463	0.81		
		VEG M (9)	2259	66.0	11.7	762	11.5	1314	0.58		
		NV M (25)	2335	102.0	17.5	875	8.60	1406	0.62		
		LOV F (25)	1615	52.0	12.9	921	17.7	1076	0.86		
		VEG F (9)	1497	48.0	12.8	541	11.3	860	0.63		
		NV F (25)	1821	67.0	14.7	803	12.0	1117	0.72		
(11) 1985	Great Britain	LOV M/F (9)	91.8	123.7		1207				2688	4676
		VEG M/F (10)	98.0	110.2		493				2935	4855
		NV M/F (10)	100.9	134.7		937				3186	3362
(12) 1985	Great Britain	LOV M (17)	2290	66.0	11.5	1109	16.8				
		VEG M (17)	2381	61.0	10.2	577	9.50				
		NV M (17)	2313	84.0	14.5	1118	13.30				
(13) 1986	South Africa	LOV M (14)	2717	77.6	11.4	1264	16.3	1714			4092
		NV M (10)	3167	111.6	14.1	997	8.90	1756			3798
		LOV F (19)	1916	57.8	12.1	1003	17.4	1235			2911
		NV F (12)	1890	68.9	14.6	749	10.9	1152			2449
(14/15) 1986	Israel	LOV M (60)	3290	99.5	12.1	1374	13.8				
		NV M (53)	2896	121.0	16.7	1198	9.90				
		LOV F (32)	2544	74.0	11.6	1162	15.7				
		NV F (60)	2389	112.3	18.8	1142	10.2				
(16) 1986	Canada	LOV M (14)	2401	71.0	11.8	1207	17.0			3023	3656
		NV M (14)	2809	99.0	14.1	1320	13.3			3116	3588
		LOV F (22)	1760	64.0	14.5	1179	18.4			1999	3182
		NV F (18)	2097	80.0	15.3	956	12.0			2747	2691
(17) 1987	Great Britain	VEG M (11)	2643	73.0	11.0	671	9.2			2806	5382
		NV M (11)	2381	92.0	15.4	1089	11.8			3197	4056
		VEG F (11)	1881	55.0	11.6	437	7.9			1817	3666
		NV F (11)	1833	69.0	15.1	976	14.1			2461	3276
(18) 1988	Australia	LOV M (47)	2610	91.7	14.1					3726	4368
		NV M (59)	2767	103.6	15.0					3565	3588
		LOV F (51)	2036	72.1	14.2					3013	3432
		NV F (54)	2008	79.4	15.8					2507	2964

(Appendix G continued)

Appendix G Protein, Calcium, Phosphorus, Sodium, and Potassium Intakes of Adult Vegetarians and Nonvegetarians

(Ref)/ year	Group/ Gender/(N)	Country	Kcal	Protein (grams)	Protein %Kcal	Calcium (mg)	Calcium (mg): Protein (g)	Phosphorus (mg)	Calcium: Phosphorus	Sodium (mg)	Potassium (mg)
(19) 1988	LOV F (88)	United States	1533	54.6	14.2	823	15.1	1112	0.74	1923	2622
	NV F (278)		1633	69.9	17.1	902	12.9	1233	0.73	1897	2554
(20) 1988	LOV M (14)	United States	2444	78.2	12.8	1294	16.5				
	NV M (13)		2329	81.1	13.9	879	10.8				
	LOV F (15)		1742	53.9	12.4	860	16.0				
	NV F (16)		1656	59.2	14.3	641	10.8				
(21) 1989	LOV F (144)	United States	1474	51.8	14.1	748	14.4	1050	0.71		
	NV F (146)		1563	63.2	16.2	772	12.2	1147	0.67		
(22) 1989	LOV F (10)	United States	1612	56.0	13.9	898	16.0	1109			
	NV F (10)		1641	68.0	16.6	712	10.5	1079			
(23) 1989	LOV-B M/F (51)	United States	2406	66.8	11.1	820	12.3	1219	0.67	2385	3721
	NV-B M/F (49)		2504	97.1	15.5	960	9.9	1534	0.63	2833	3938
	LOV-W M/F (163)		2340	79.9	13.7	1113	13.9	1646	0.68	2815	4553
	NV-W M/F (89)		2225	80.8	14.5	1103	13.7	1526	0.72	2841	3945
(24) 1989	LOV F (23)	United States	1452	46.8	12.9	628	13.4	889	0.70	1930	2628
	NV F (14)		1363	55.0	16.1	633	11.5	892	0.71	1936	2342
(25) 1990	LOV M (18)	Netherlands	1960	59.8	12.2	1219	20.4				
	NV M		2412	82.2	13.6	1128	13.7				
	LOV F (26)		1667	54.4	13.1	1141	21.0				
	NV F		1879	70.1	14.9	1013	14.5				
(26) 1991	LOV F (23)	United States	1939	62.0	12.8	973	15.7	1318	0.74	2462	3221
	NV F (36)		1835	76.0	16.6	770	10.1	1219	0.63	2815	2747
(27) 1991	LOV F (34)	United States	1819	63.0	13.9	931	14.8	1159	0.80	2304	2803
	NV F (41)		1700	75.0	17.6	873	11.6	1138	0.77	2649	2664
(28) 1991	LOV M/F (79)	United States	2800	95.9	13.7	1521	15.9				
	NV M/F (4821)		2980	111.0	14.9	1310	11.8				

Study / Year	Group	Country									
(29) 1992	LOV F (28)	United States	1652	62.6	15.2	821	13.1	1155	0.71	2202	3012
	NV F (28)		1657	76.5	18.5	863	11.3	1250	0.69	2285	2687
(30) 1993	LOV M (16)	Great Britain	2238	66.0	11.8	995	15.1				
	VEG M (18)		2190	65.0	11.9	582	9.0				
	NV M (387)		2452	87.0	14.2	1006	11.6				
	LOV F (36)		1826	56.0	12.3	891	15.9				
	VEG F (20)		1750	47.0	10.7	497	10.6				
	NV F (377)		1733	66.0	15.2	790	12.0				
(31) 1993	LOV M/F (14)	Finland	2029			925		1339			
	LV M/F (6)		1913			800		1235			
	VEG M/F (10)		1927			480		1207			
	NV F (12)		1778			980		1351			
(32) 1994	LOV M/F (50)	New Zealand	2272	69.7	12.3	906	13.0			2800	
	VEG F (5)		1842	55.2	12.0	507	9.2			2400	
	NV M/F (50)		2608	83.2	12.8	954	11.5			3600	
(33) 1994	LV/VEG M (17)	United States	3005	100.0	13.3					3359	
	NV M (40)		2906	106.0	14.6					3575	
(34) 1994	LOV M/F (64)	United States	2272	72.7	12.8	720	9.9			2841	3661
	NV M/F (44)		2603	95.6	14.7	879	9.2			2833	3903
(35) 1995	LV F (15)	Canada	2024	57.1	11.3	875	15.3	1125	0.78	2175	2884
	VEG F (8)		1923	51.9	10.8	578	11.1	1217	0.47	2275	3587
	NV F (22)		2086	77.1	14.8	950	12.3	1409	0.67	2789	3042
(36) 1997	LOV F (13)	Scotland	1728	55.1	12.8	1018	18.5	1251	0.81	2139	3042
	NV F (20)		2184	69.9	12.9	978	14.0	1251	0.78	2691	2808
(37) 1998	LOV M (12)	New Zealand	2280	69.0	12.1	721	10.4				
	NV M (11)		2688	90.7	13.5	943	10.4				
	LOV F (12)		1872	57.1	12.2	690	12.1				
	NV F (12)		2016	72.1	14.3	672	9.3				
(38) 1998	B-LOV M (49)	United States	2356	75.1	12.1	696	9.3	1292	0.54	2870	3904
	B-VEG M (14)		1869	62.3	12.0	407	6.5	1194	0.34	2268	3619
	B-LOV F (94)		1922	61.5	11.7	633	10.3	1119	0.57	2307	3470
	B-VEG F (31)		1865	55.8	11.3	449	8.0	1083	0.41	1613	4073

(Appendix G continued)

Appendix G Protein, Calcium, Phosphorus, Sodium, and Potassium Intakes of Adult Vegetarians and Nonvegetarians

(Ref)/ year	Group/ Gender/(N)	Country	Kcal	Protein (grams)	Protein %Kcal	Calcium (mg)	Calcium (mg): Protein (g)	Phosphorus (mg)	Calcium: Phosphorus	Sodium (mg)	Potassium (mg)
(39) 1999	VEG M (10)2	United States	2230	75	13	840	11.2				
	NV M (10)2		2170	85	16	720	8.5				
	VEG F (15)2		1702	52	12	710	13.7				
	NV F (10)2		1978	74	15	855	11.6				
(40) 1999	LOV M (10)	Australia	2143	76	14	957	12.6			2502	3448
	LOV M (10)		2877	89	12	997	11.2			2606	5491
(41) 2000	LOV M(34)	France	1951	60	12	863	14.4				
	VEG M (6)		2051	77	15	758	9.8				
	LOV F (55)		1675	50	13	863	17.3				
	VEG F (11)		1302	46	15	501	10.9				
(42) 2001	VEG M (54)	United States	1830	47.2	10.3	687	14.6	1100	0.62	1510	6400
	VEG F (87)		1460	37.3	10.2	577	15.5	857	0.67	1220	5420
(43) 2002	LOV M (786)	Great Britain	2121	69.5	13.1	1091	15.7			2979	3972
	VEG M(272)		1919	61.4	12.8	589	9.6			2792	4061
	NV M (996)		2171	87.4	16.1	1064	12.2			2986	4033
	LOV F (3014)		1835	63.8	13.9	1021	16.0			2632	3773
	VEG F (467)		1696	56.8	13.4	580	10.2			2539	3836
	NV F (3741)		1906	82.9	17.4	998	12.0			2713	3927
(44) 2003	LOV M (3748)	United Kingdom	2090	68.4	13.1	1067	15.6				3867
	VEG M (770)		1907	61.5	12.9	610	9.9				4029
	NV M (6951)		2186	87.4	16.0	1057	12.1				3965
	LOV F (12347)		1810	62.4	13.8	1012	16.2				3656
	VEG F (1342)		1660	56.0	13.5	582	10.4				3817
	NV F (22962)		1910	82.6	17.3	989	12.0				3839

No.	Year	Group	Country									
(45)	2003	VEG M (48)	Germany	2381	67.9	11.4	915	13.5	1601	0.57	2310	5460
		VEG M (19)		2186	62.3	11.4	889	14.3	1450	0.61	2030	5250
		VEG F (50)		1721	53.4	12.4	790	14.8	1251	0.63	2020	4460
		VEG F (37)		1617	43.7	10.8	784	17.9	1079	0.73	1600	4540
(46)	2004	LV F (30)	India	1618	36.6	9.1	439	12.0			1945	920
		LV F htn (26)		1737	38.5	8.9	473	12.3			2122	819
		LV M (85)		2166	52.5	9.3	585	11.1			2065	1261
		LV M htn (83)		2260	49.5	9.1	549	11.1			1991	1142
(47)	2004	LOV F (6478)	United Kingdom	2303	75	13.1	1134	15.1				
		NV F (24738)		2370	95	15.7	1133	11.9				
(48)	2005	VEG M/F (18)	United States	1285–2432	54.2	9.1	579					
		NV M/F (18)		1976–3537	NI	17.9	1093					
(49)	2005	LOV M (31)	United States	2605	86	13.0	1559	18.1	1886	0.83	3241	4189
		NV M (869)		2605	107	16.5	980	9.2	1641	0.60	3719	3604
		LOV F (75)		1840	71	15.3	830	11.7	1339	0.62	2206	3060
		NV F (842)		1793	70	16.0	777	11.1	1155	0.67	2545	2741
(50)	2007	LOV M (2148)	United Kingdom	2103			1085					
		VEG M (426)		1912			603					
		NV M (4528)		2199			1062					
		LOV F (7272)		1840			1018					
		VEG F (700)		1697			586					
		NV F (14726)		1936			995					
(51)	2008	LO/LSV F (26)	Turkey	1832	58.5	13.4	946	16.2				
		NV F (26)		1849	68.2	15.7	796	11.7				
(52)	2008	LOV M/F (21)	Taiwan	1884	53.5	11.3	418.7	7.8				
		NV M/F (28)		1944	61.6	12.6	330.7	5.4				
(53)	2008	LO/SV M (20)	Japan	1983	65.4	13.2	630	9.6	1076	0.59	2750	2782
		NV M (32)		1843	69.5	15.1	381	5.5	971	0.39	2900	2061
		LO/SV F (50)		1675	61.3	14.6	555	9.1	992	0.56		2719

(Appendix G continued)

Appendix G Protein, Calcium, Phosphorus, Sodium, and Potassium Intakes of Adult Vegetarians and Nonvegetarians

(Ref)/ year	Group[1]/ Gender/(N)	Country	Kcal	Protein (grams)	Protein %Kcal	Calcium (mg)	Calcium (mg): Protein (g)	Phosphorus (mg)	Calcium: Phosphorus	Sodium (mg)	Potassium (mg)
(54) 2009	VEG F (105)	Vietnam	1130	35.4	12.5	375	10.6	465	0.81	2819	1328
	NV F (105)		1486	62.6	16.9	483	7.7	865	0.56	2147	1916
(55) 2010	LOV M/F (30)	Belgium	2110	71	13.8	989	13.9	1376	0.72	2733	3479
	NV M/F (30)		2215	89	16.5	871	9.8	1473	0.59	3210	2868

Notes: [1]Abbreviations: LV, lacto vegetarian; LOV, lacto-ovo vegetarian; VEG, vegan; SV, eats chicken and/or fish; NV, nonvegetarian; htn, subjects identified as having hypertension; B, black; W, white.

[2]Data include nutrient supplements.

ANNOTATED REFERENCES APPENDIX G

1. Hardinge MG, Stare FJ. Nutritional studies of vegetarians. *Am J Clin Nutr.* 1954;2:73–82.
2. Hitchcock NE, English RM. A comparison of food consumption in lacto-ovo vegetarians and nonvegetarians. *Food Nutr Notes Rev.* 1963;20:141–146.
3. Mason RL, Kunkel ME, Davis TA, Beauchene RE. Nutrient intakes of vegetarian and nonvegetarian women. *Tenn Farm Home Sci.* 1978;1:18–20.
4. Freeland-Graves JH, Bodzy PW, Eppright MA. Zinc status of vegetarians. *J Am Diet Assoc.* 1980;77:655–661. *Notes:* Of the 79 total vegetarians, 44 were reportedly male, but data for the individual vegetarian groups were not provided.
5. Taber LAL, Cook RA. Dietary and anthropometric assessment of adult omnivores, fish-eaters, and lacto-ovo vegetarian. *J Am Diet Assoc.* 1980;76:21–29.
6. King JC, Stein T, Doyle M. Effect of vegetarianism on the zinc status of pregnant women. *Am J Clin Nutr.* 1981;34:1049–1055.
7. Beauchene RE, Kunkel ME, Bredderman SH, Mason RL. Nutrient intake and physical measurements of aging vegetarian and nonvegetarian women. *J Am Coll Nutr.* 1982;1:131.
8. Read MH, Thomas DC. Nutrient and food supplement practices of lacto-ovo vegetarians. *J Am Diet Assoc.* 1983; 82:401–404.
9. Schultz TD, Leklem JE. Dietary status of Seventh-day Adventists and nonvegetarians. *J Am Diet Assoc.* 1983;83:27–33.
10. Calkins BM, Whittaker DJ, Nair PP, Rider AA, Turjman N. Diet, nutrition intake, and metabolism in populations at high and low risk for colon cancer. *Am J Clin Nutr.* 1984;40:896–905.
11. Carlson E, Kipps M, Lockie A, Thomson J. A comparative evaluation of vegan, vegetarian, and omnivore diets. *J Plant Foods.* 1985;6:89–100. *Note:* The LOV, VEG, and NV groups contained 4, 5, and 5 males, respectively. Values for protein and calories are expressed as a percentage of the recommended intake for Great Britain. Calcium intake is based on the percentage of the recommended intake value of 500 mg indicated in the text. Sodium and phosphorus intakes are taken directly from the text.
12. Davies GJ, Crowder M, Dickerson JWT. Dietary fibre intakes of individuals with different eating patterns. *Human Nutr: Appl Nutr.* 1985;39A:139–148.
13. Faber M, Gouws E, Benadé AJS, Labadarios D. Anthropometric measurements, dietary intake and biochemical data of South African lacto-ovo vegetarians. *S Afr Med J.* 1986;69:733–738.
14. Levin N, Rattan J, Gilat T. Mineral intake and blood levels in vegetarians. *Isr J Med Sci.* 1986;22:105–108.
15. Levin N, Rattan J, Gilat T. Energy intake and body weight in ovo-lacto vegetarians. *J Clin Gastroenterol.* 1986; 8:451–453.
16. Locong A. Nutritional status and dietary intake of a selected sample of young adult vegetarians. *Can Med Assoc J.* 1986;47:101–106.
17. Sanders TAB, Key TJA. Blood pressure, plasma renin activity and aldosterone concentrations in vegans and omnivore controls. *Human Nutr: Appl Nutr.* 1987;41A:204–211.
18. Rouse IL, Armstrong BK, Beilin LJ. The relationship of blood pressure to diet and lifestyle in two religious populations. *J Hypertension.* 1983;1:65–71.
19. Tylavsky FA, Anderson JJB. Dietary factors in bone health of elderly lacto-ovo vegetarian and omnivorous women. *Am J Clin Nutr.* 1988;48:842–849.
20. Kelsay JL, Frazier CW, Prather E, Canary JJ, Clark WM, Powell AS. Impact of variation in carbohydrate intake on mineral utilization by vegetarians. *Am J Clin Nutr.* 1988;48:875–879.
21. Hunt IF, Murphy NJ, Henderson C, et al. Bone mineral content in postmenopausal women: comparison of omnivores and vegetarians. *Am J Clin Nutr.* 1989;50:517–523.
22. Marsh AG, Christensen DK, Sanchez TV, Mickelsen O, Chaffee FL. Nutrient similarities and differences of older lacto-ovo vegetarian and omnivorous women. *Nutr Rep Int.* 1989;39:19–24.
23. Melby CL, Goldflies DG, Hyner GC, Lyle RM. Relation between vegetarian/nonvegetarian diets and blood pressure in black and white adults. *Am J Public Health.* 1989;79:1283–1288. *Note:* Of the initial 114 Black subjects, 89 were females and 25 were males. Of the initial 264 white subjects, 222 were female and 42 were male.

24. Nieman DC, Underwood BC, Sherman KM, et al. Dietary status of Seventh-day Adventist vegetarian and nonvegetarian elderly women. *J Am Diet Assoc.* 1989;89:1763–1769.

25. Brants HAM, Löwik MRH, Westenbrink S, Hulshof KFAM, Kistemaker C. Adequacy of a vegetarian diet at old age (Dutch Nutrition Surveillance System). *J Am Coll Nutr.* 1990;9:292–302.

26. Lloyd T, Schaeffer JM, Walker MA, Demers LM. Urinary hormonal concentrations and spinal bone densities of premenopausal vegetarian and nonvegetarian women. *Am J Clin Nutr.* 1991;54:1005–1010.

27. Pedersen AB, Bartholomew MJ, Dolence LA, Aljadir LP, Netteburg KL, Lloyd T. Menstrual differences due to vegetarian and nonvegetarian diets. *Am J Clin Nutr.* 1991;53:879–885.

28. Slattery ML, Jacobs DR, Hilner JE Jr, et al. Meat consumption and its association with other diet and health factors in young adults: the CARDIA study. *Am J Clin Nutr.* 1991;54:930–935. *Note:* Of the 79 vegetarians, 57 (72%) were females and of the 4821 nonvegetarians, 2577 (53%) were females.

29. Tesar R, Notelovitz M, Shim E, Kauwell G, Brown J. Axial and peripheral bone density and nutrient intakes of postmenopausal vegetarian and omnivorous women. *Am J Clin Nutr.* 1992;56:699–704.

30. Draper A, Lewis J, Malhotra N, Wheeler E. The energy and nutrient intakes of different types of vegetarian: a case for supplements? *Br J Nutr.* 1993;69:3–19. *Note:* Data for nonvegetarians was taken from a separate nationwide survey.

31. Lamberg-Allardt C, Kärkkäinen M, Seppänen R, Biström H. Low serum 25-hydroxyvitamin D concentrations and secondary hyperparathyroidism in middle-aged white strict vegetarians. *Am J Clin Nutr.* 1993;58:684–689. *Note:* The LOV, LV, and VEG groups each contained 8, 3, and 10 females. Calcium intake estimate from figure in references.

32. Alexander D, Ball MJ, Mann J. Nutrient intake and haematological status of vegetarians and age-sex matched omnivores. *Eur J Clin Nutr.* 1994;48:538–546. *Note:* Data for the LOV group includes data for the VEG group, which are also listed separately. There were 36 females each in the LOV and NV groups.

33. Toth MJ, Poehlman ET. Sympathetic nervous system activity and resting metabolic rate in vegetarians. *Metabolism.* 1994;43:621–625. *Note:* Of the 17 vegetarians, 10 were LV and 7 were VEG.

34. Melby CL, Toohey M, Cebrick J. Blood pressure and blood lipids among vegetarian, semivegetarian, and nonvegetarian African Americans. *Am J Clin Nutr.* 1994;59:103–109. *Note:* All subjects were black Seventh-day Adventists. Of the 66 vegetarians, 16 were vegans, and 50 were lacto-ovo vegetarians, there were 46 women and 20 men. Of the nonvegetarians, 34 were women and 11 were men.

35. Janelle KC, Barr SI. Nutrient intakes and eating behavior scores of vegetarian and nonvegetarian women. *J Am Diet Assoc.* 1995;95:180–185. *Note:* Of the 15 LV, 11 ate eggs.

36. Ball D, Maughan RJ. Blood and urine acid-base status of premenopausal omnivorous and vegetarian women. *Br J Nutr.* 1997;78:683–693. *Note:* Two vegetarians occasionally ate fish.

37. Harman SK, Parnell WR. The nutritional health of New Zealand vegetarian and nonvegetarian Seventh-day Adventists: selected vitamin, mineral and lipid levels. *NZ Med J.* 1998;111:91–94. *Note:* Of the 24 vegetarians, an unspecified number were lacto vegetarians or vegans. Some nonvegetarians only occasionally ate red meat.

38. Toohey ML, Harris MA, Williams D, Foster G, Schmidt WD, Melby CL. Cardiovascular disease risk factors are lower in African-American vegans compared to lacto-ovo vegetarians. *J Am Coll Nutr.* 1998;17:425–434. *Note:* All subjects were black.

39. Haddad EH, Berk LS, Kettering JD, Hubbard RW, Peters WR. Dietary intake and biochemical, hematologic, and immune status of vegans compared with nonvegetarians. *Am J Clin Nutr.* 1999;70 (suppl):586S–593S.

40. Li D, Sinclair A, Wilson A, et al. Effect of dietary α-linolenic acid on thrombotic risk factors in vegetarian men. *Am J Clin Nutr.* 1999;69:878–882. *Note:* Vegetarian subjects were divided into 2 groups for study purposes. Only baseline data are reported here.

41. Leblanc JC, Yoon H, Kombadjian A, Verger P. Nutritional intakes of vegetarian populations in France. *Eur J Clin Nutr.* 2000;54:443–449. *Note:* Thirty-one of the 96 LOV ate fish or meat at least once a week; 11 were lacto vegetarians and 3 were ovo vegetarians; 13 of the 17 VEG ate fish once a week.

42. Donaldson MS. Food and nutrient intake of Hallelujah vegetarians. *Nutr Food Sci.* 2001;31:293–303. *Note:* VEG subjects ate a mostly raw diet; 58% consumed some animal product during their week of food intake records.

43. Appleby PN, Davey GK, Key TJ. Hypertension and blood pressure among meat eaters, fish eaters, vegetarians, and vegans in EPIC-Oxford. *Public Health Nutr.* 2002;5:645–654.

44. Davey GK, Spencer EA, Appleby PN, et al. EPIC-Oxford lifestyle characteristics and nutrient intakes in a cohort of 33,883 meat-eaters and 31,546 non-meat-eaters in the UK. *Public Health Nutr.* 2003;6:259–268.

45. Waldmann A, Koschizke JW, Leitzmann C, Hahn A. Dietary intake and lifestyle factors of a vegan population in Germany: results from the German Vegan Study. *Eur J Clin Nutr.* 2003;57:947–955. *Note:* Ninety-eight subjects did not use animal products for 1 year prior to study; 56 subjects consumed small amounts of dairy products and eggs. The first listing for each gender is for strict vegans, the second listing is for those who consumed small amounts of dairy and eggs.

46. Chiplonkar SA, Agte V, Tarwadik V, et al. Micronutrient deficiencies as predisposing factors for hypertension in lacto-vegetarian Indian adults. *J Am Coll Nutr.* 2004;23:239–247.

47. Cade JE, Burley VJ, Greenwood DC, et al. The UK Women's Cohort Study: comparisons of vegetarians, fish-eaters, and meat-eaters. *Public Health Nutr.* 2004;7:871–878. *Note:* Vegetarians ate meat or fish less than once a week.

48. Fontana L, Shew JL, Holloszy JO, et al. Low bone mass in subjects on a long-term raw vegetarian diet. *Arch Intern Med.* 2005;165:684–689. *Note:* Study subjects ate a raw foods diet. Seven males and 11 females were VEG; 7 males and 11 females were NV.

49. Bedford JL, Barr SI. Diets and selected lifestyle practices of self-defined adult vegetarians from a population-based sample suggest they are more health conscious. *Int J Behav Nutr Phys Act.* 2005;2:4. *Note:* Seventy-five percent of those self-identified as vegetarian consumed fish and/or seafood, 58% consumed poultry; 22% consumed red meat.

50. Appleby P, Roddam A, Allen N, et al. Comparative fracture risk in vegetarians and nonvegetarians in EPIC-Oxford. *Eur J Clin Nutr.* 2007;61:1400–1406.

51. Karabudak E, Kiziltan G, Cigerim N. A comparison of some of the cardiovascular risk factors in vegetarian and omnivorous Turkish females. *J Hum Nutr Diet.* 2008;21:13–22. *Note:* Subjects include 9 LOV, 10 LV, and 7 occasional fish and/or chicken eaters.

52. Yen CE, Yen CH, Huang MC, et al. Dietary intake and nutritional status of vegetarian and omnivorous preschool children and their parents in Taiwan. *Nutr Res.* 2008;28:430–436. *Note:* Adult vegetarians consisted of 16 LOV, 2 ovo-vegetarians, 1 LV, 2 vegans. Four male adults and 17 females were vegetarian; 9 male adults and 19 females were NV. Children consisted of 18 LOV and 3 ovo-vegetarians. Fourteen male children and 7 female children were vegetarians; 15 male children and 13 female children were NV.

53. Nakamato K, Watanabe S, Kudo H, et al. Nutritional characteristics of middle-aged Japanese vegetarians. *J Atherosclero Throm.* 2008;15:122–129. *Note:* Nine men and 18 women were LOV; 11 men and 37 women in the vegetarian group occasionally ate chicken and meat.

54. Ho-Pham LT, Nguyen PL, Le TT, et al. Veganism, bone density, and body composition: a study in Buddhist nuns. *Osteoporosis Int.* 2009;20:2087–2093.

55. Deriemaeker P, Aerenhouts D, Hebbelinck M, Clarys P. Nutrient based estimation of acid-base balance in vegetarians and non-vegetarians. *Plant Foods Hum Nutr.* 2010;65:77–82. *Note:* Eight men and 22 women were in each group.

Appendix H Iron Intake and Status of Adult Vegetarians and Nonvegetarians

(Ref)/ year	Group[1]/ Gender(N)	Country	Age	Iron Intake (mg)	Serum Ferritin (ng/ml)[2]	Total Iron Binding Capacity[3]	Hemoglobin (g/dl)[4]	Hematocrit (%)	Plasma or Serum Iron[5]
(1) 1974	LOV M (187)	Australia	50				14.5	46.0	
	NV M (879)		49				14.6	46.4	
	LOV F (244)		51				13.1	41.9	
	NV F (1339)		49				13.2	42.4	
(2) 1981	LOV F (39)[6]	Canada	53	12.5		312.0	13.2		107.0
	LOV F (10)[6]		53			346.0	12.9		135.0
(3) 1984	LOV M (36)	United States	31	17.0		393.0		46.0	116.0
	NV M (18)		31	18.0		373.0		45.0	104.0
(4) 1986	LOV M (24)	Germany	29		537.0		14.9		89.3
	LOV F (24)		29		537.0		12.9		89.3
(5) 1986	LOV M (14)	South Africa	29	17.9	60.7				
	NV M (10)		29	17.9	146.8				
	NV F (19)		27	11.5	16.1				
	NV F (12)		27	11.7	47.3				
(6) 1986	LOV M (60)	Israel	55	37.0		351.6			103.9
	NV M (53)		50	25.8		393.3			93.8
	LOV F (32)		51	29.7		361.8			90.6
	NV F (60)		52	21.7		409.1			96.7
(7) 1986	LOV M (14)	Canada	28	16.5	88.0				
	NV M (14)		21	16.9	107.0				
	LOV F (22)		26	14.1	33.0				
	NV (18)		22	14.9	45.0				
(8) 1987	LOV M/F (93)	Australia	29		45.0				
	NV M/F (37)		31		70.0				
(9) 1988	LOV F (20)	United States	29	11.8	21.0	360.0	13.3	39.0	
	NV F (16)		31	12.7	30.0	345.0	13.9	41.5	

(10)	LV/VEG M/F (13)	Sweden	47–74		52.5		13.5		15.2
1989	NV M/F (6)		45–69		85.7		14.5		16.8
(11)	LOV M (39)	Germany	45		56.2		14.3	42.6	76.9
1989	NV M (52)		38		93.0		14.2	42.5	83.6
	LOV F (11)		47		19.0		13.6	41.0	102.4
	NV F (8)		49		67.4		13.7	40.8	96.0
(12)	LOV F (18)	Great		13.8	10.4				
1990	NV F (20)	Britain		12.1	18.0				
(13)	LOV M (17)	Netherlands	65–97	13.7	18%		35%		12%
1990	NV M (54)		65+	13.1	2%		4%		9%
	LOV F (23)		65–97	12.2	9%		4%		13%
	NV F (54)		65+	11.4	11%		1%		0%
(14)	LV M (64)	Thailand	36				16.4		
1992	NV M (20)		33				16.6		
	LV F (68)		33				13.7		
	NV F (270)		32				14.3		
(15)	LOV M (14)	New	26–30	18.7	36.6				
1994	NV M (14)	Zealand	26–30	15.5	105.4				
	LOV F (36)		26–30	14.4	13.6				
	NV F (36)		26–30	13.7	33.6				
(16)	LOV M (23)	Taiwan	23	18.4	47.0	69.0	9.2		23
1995	NV M (20)		21	16.1	91.0	64.0	9.4		16
	LOV F (32)		25	15.6	12.0	72.0	7.6		17
	NV F (39)		20	11.7	27.0	69.0	7.9		17
(17)	LOV F (79)	Canada	18	11.2	18.2	77.0	13.8	41.0	13.5
1995	NV F (29)		18	11.3	20.0	78.5	13.8	41.0	14.1
(18)	LOV F (13)	Scotland	24				11.6		
1997	NV F (20)		23				11.5		

(Appendix H continued)

Appendix H Iron Intake and Status of Adult Vegetarians and Nonvegetarians

(Ref)/ year	Group/ Gender/(N)	Country	Age	Iron Intake (mg)	Serum Ferritin (ng/ml)[2]	Total Iron Binding Capacity[3]	Hemoglobin (g/dl)[4]	Hematocrit (%)	Plasma or Serum Iron[5]
(19) 1998	LOV M (12)	New Zealand	49	15.5	79.8		15.1		
	NV M (11)	Zealand	40	16.2	148.0		14.2		
	LOV F (12)		43	14.7	50.4		12.4		
	NV F (12)		39	12.8	59.6		12.9		
(20) 1999	LOV F (50)	Australia	25	10.7	25.0				
	NV F (24)		25	9.9	45.5				
(21) 1999	VEG M (10)[7]	United States	20–60	43.4	72.0		15.4	45	
	NV M (10)[7]	States	20–60	20.9	141.0		15.6	45	
	VEG F (15)[7]		20–60	22.6	27.0		13.2	39	
	NV F (10)[7]		20–60	20.2	22.0		13.3	40	
(22) 1999	LOV M (10)	Australia	20–50	16.8			14.9		
	LOV M (10)		20–50	22.1			14.8		
(23) 2001	LOV M/F (30)	United States	41		35				
	NV M/F (30)	States	40		72				
(24) 2002	LOV F (23)	Hong Kong	78.1				13.0		
	LOV F (28)		80.2				12.1		
	LOV F (45)		78.0				12.4		
(25) 2002	LOV M/F (14)	Italy	48.5				13.6		
	VEG M/F (31)		45.8				13.5		
(26) 2002	LOV/LV (M28/F36)	Germany	46		30F/36M		13.5		91
	VEG M/F (29)		46		21F/30M		13.9		80
	NV M/F (20)		46		20F/76M		13.2		93
(27) 2004	VEG F (50)	Germany	35.4	20.0	14.0		13.2		
	VEG F (25)		62.0	19.6	28.0		13.4		
(28) 2004	VEG M/F (86)	Germany	43.8				14.0		
	VEG M/F (45)		44.6				13.5		

(29) 2005	LOV F (30)	United Kingdom	31		11.1	387	13.5	85.5
	NV F (30)	Kingdom	32		17.5	381	13.7	90.1
	NV F (30)		34		6.8	391	13.4	80.1
(30) 2008	LOV M/F (21)	Taiwan	34.8	16.1	45.6		13.0	38.4	101.7
	NV M/F (28)		35.9	10.0	103.5		13.9	41.6	99.0

Notes: [1]Abbreviations: LV, lacto vegetarian; LOV, lacto-ovo vegetarian; VEG, vegan; NV, nonvegetarian.

[2]Values for reference 13 represent the percentage of each group considered deficient.

[3]Total iron binding capacity, references 2, 3, 6, 9, and 29 (μg/dL); references 16 and 17 (μmol/L).

[4]Values for reference 13 represent the percentage of each group considered deficient and for reference 16, hemoglobin is expressed as μmol/L.

[5]Plasma or serum iron; references 2–4, 6, 11, 26, 29, and 30 (μg/dL); references 10, 16, and 17 (μmol/L) and reference 13, the percentage of each group considered deficient.

[6]The first group of LOV are individuals who did not take iron supplements. The second group consists of supplement users.

[7]Data include nutrient supplements.

ANNOTATED REFERENCES APPENDIX H

1. Armstrong BK, Davis RE, Nicol DJ, van Merwyk AJ, Larwood CJ. Hematological, vitamin B12, and folate studies on Seventh-day Adventist vegetarians. *Am J Clin Nutr.* 1974;27:712–718. *Note:* Data for nonvegetarians from a separate survey.

2. Anderson BM, Gibson RS, Sabry JH. The iron and zinc status of long-term vegetarian women. *Am J Clin Nutr.* 1981; 34:1042–1048.

3. Latta D, Liebman M. Iron and zinc status of vegetarian and nonvegetarian males. *Nutr Rep Int.* 1984;30:141–149.

4. Ernst E, Pietsch L, Matrai A, Eisenberg J. Blood rheology in vegetarians. *Br J Nutr.* 1986;56:555–560. *Note:* There were equal numbers of men and women, values for serum ferritin, and plasma iron were reported for the entire group, not according to gender. The normal range for ferritin was indicated to be 300–3,000 μg/l; for hemoglobin (g/l), 140–180 (men) and 120–160 (women) and for plasma iron, 800–1800 μg/l. Thus, although all values were within the normal range for ferritin and plasma iron, they were at the very low end of the range.

5. Faber M, Gouws E, Benadé AJS, Labadarios D. Anthropometric measurements, dietary intake and biochemical data of South African lacto-ovo vegetarians. *S Afr Med J.* 1986;69:733–738.

6. Levin N, Rattan J, Gilat T. Mineral intake and blood levels in vegetarians. *Israel J Med Sci.* 1986;22:105–108.

7. Locong A. Nutritional status and dietary intake of a selected sample of young adult vegetarians. *Can Med Assoc J.* 1986:101–108.

8. Helman AD, Darnton-Hill I. Vitamin and iron status in new vegetarians. *Am J Clin Nutr.* 1987;45:785–789. *Note:* There were initially a total of 120 LOV equally divided between men and women but ferritin values were reported for only 93 LOV, the proportion of men and women was not reported specifically for this subset. The nonvegetarian group initially consisted of 53 subjects, 40 women and 13 men but ferritin values were reported for only 37 nonvegetarians, the proportion of men and women was not reported specifically for this subset. Given that ferritin values are generally lower in women, and the LOV group likely contained a greater proportion of women, differences between LOV and NV are actually underestimated.

9. Worthington-Roberts BS, Breskin MW, Monsen ER. Iron status of premenopausal women in a university community and its relationship to habitual dietary sources of protein. *Am J Clin Nutr.* 1988;47:275–279. *Note:* Values were estimated from figures in reference. Approximately 43% and 30% of the LOV and NV, respectively, had serum ferritin levels (15 μg/L) considered deficient by laboratory standards.

10. Brune M, Rossander L, Hallberg L. Iron absorption: no intestinal adaptation to a high phytate diet. *Am J Clin Nutr.* 1989;49:542–545. *Note:* Among the 13 vegetarians, there were 4 VEG and 9 LV, there were 4 male vegetarians, one of which was vegan. Among the NV, there were 3 males and 3 females, 3 of the 6 nonvegetarians were blood donors.

11. Seiler D, Nagel D, Franz H, et al. Effects of long-distance running on iron metabolism and hematological parameters. *In J Sports Med.* 1989;10:357–362. *Note:* All subjects were long-distance runners.

12. Reddy S, Sanders TAB. Haematological studies on premenopausal Indian and Caucasian vegetarians compared with Caucasian omnivores. *Br J Nutr.* 1990;64:331–338.

13. Brants HAM, Löwik MRH, Westenbrink S, Hulshof KFAM, Kistemaker C. Adequacy of a vegetarian diet at old age (Dutch Nutrition Surveillance System). *J Am College Nutr.* 1990;9:292–302. *Note:* Values refer to the percentage of individuals in each group that were below the cutoff points considered to be within the normal range; for serum ferritin, hemoglobin, and serum iron, cutoff points were 12 μg/L, 8.1 mmol/L, and 9.0 umol/l, respectively.

14. Tungtrongchitr R, Pongpaew P, Prayurahong B, et al. Vitamin B12, folic acid, and haematological status of 132 Thai vegetarians. *Inter J Vit Nutr Res.* 1993;63:201–207.

15. Alexander D, Ball MJ, Mann J. Nutrient intake and haematological status of vegetarians and age-sex matched omnivores. *Eur J Clin Nutr.* 1994;48:538–546. *Note:* Data for female LOV included 5 VEG.

16. Shaw N-S, Chin C-J, Pan W-H. A vegetarian diet rich in soybean products compromises iron status in young students. *J Nutr.* 1995;125:212–219. *Note:* The extent to which eggs and dairy were consumed by vegetarians could not be determined from the text.

17. Donovan UM, Gibson RS. Iron and zinc status of young women aged 14 to 19 years consuming vegetarian and omnivorous diets. *J Am Coll Nutr.* 1995;14:463–472. *Note:* Twenty-nine percent of the LOV and 17.2% of the NV had ferritin levels below the cutoff point (12 μg/L) considered to be deficient.

18. Ball D, Maughan RJ. Blood and urine acid-base status of premenopausal omnivorous and vegetarian women. *Br J Nutr.* 1997;78:683–693. *Note:* Two vegetarians occasionally ate fish.

19. Harman SK, Parnell WR. The nutritional health of New Zealand vegetarian and nonvegetarian Seventh-Day Adventists: selected vitamin, mineral and lipid levels. *NZ Med J.* 1998;111:91–94. *Note:* Of the 24 vegetarians, an unspecified number were lacto vegetarians or vegans. Some nonvegetarians only occasionally ate red meat.

20. Ball MJ, Bartlett MA. Dietary intake and iron status of Australian vegetarian women. *Am J Clin Nutr.* 1999;70:353–358. *Note:* Two of the 50 LOV were vegan; vegetarians consumed red meat no more than once a month and consumed fish or chicken no more than once a week. Seven LOV used iron supplements more than three times a week. No NV used iron supplements regularly.

21. Haddad EH, Berk LS, Kettering JD, Hubbard RW, Peters WR. Dietary intake and biochemical, hematologic, and immune status of vegans compared with nonvegetarians. *Am J Clin Nutr.* 1999;70 (suppl): 586S–593S.

22. Li D, Sinclair A, Wilson A, et al. Effect of dietary α-linolenic acid on thrombotic risk factors in vegetarian men. *Am J Clin Nutr.* 1999;69:878–882. *Note:* Vegetarian subjects were divided into two groups for study purposes. Only baseline data are reported here.

23. Hua NW, Stoohs RA, Facchini FS. Low iron status and enhanced insulin sensitivity in lacto-ovo vegetarians. *Br J Nutr.* 2001;86:515–519.

24. Kwok T, Cheng G, Woo J, et al. Independent effect of vitamin B12 deficiency on hematological status in older Chinese vegetarian women. *Am J Hematol.* 2002;70:186–190. *Note:* Subjects were divided into three groups based on no, possible, and definite vitamin B12 deficiency.

25. Bissoli L, Di Francesco V, Ballarin A, et al. Effect of vegetarian diet on homocysteine levels. *Ann Nutr Metab.* 2002;46:73–79.

26. Obeid R, Geisel J, Schorr H, et al. The impact of vegetarianism on some haematological parameters. *Eur J Haematol.* 2002;69:275–279. *Note:* Nonvegetarian subjects had a reduced intake of meat (once weekly).

27. Waldmann A, Koschizke JW, Leitzmann C, et al. Dietary iron intake and iron status of German female vegans: results of the German Vegan Study. *Ann Nutr Metab.* 2004;48:103–108.

28. Waldmann A, Koschizke JW, Leitzmann C, et al. Homocysteine and cobalamin status in German vegans. *Public Health Nutr.* 2004;7:467–472. *Note:* The first listing is for strict vegans (42 males and 44 females); the second listing is for those who consumed small amounts of dairy and eggs but were primarily vegan (16 males and 29 females).

29. Harvey LJ, Arman CN, Dainly JR, et al. Impact of menstrual blood loss and diet on iron deficiency among women in the UK. *Br J Nutr.* 2005;94:557–564. *Note:* The first NV group consists of poultry and fish eaters; the second NV group consists of red meat eaters.

30. Yen CE, Yen CH, Huang MC, et al. Dietary intake and nutritional status of vegetarian and omnivorous preschool children and their parents in Taiwan. *Nutr Res.* 2008;28:430–436. *Note:* Adult vegetarians consisted of 16 LOV, 2 ovo-vegetarians, 1 LV, 2 vegans. Four male adults and 17 females were vegetarian; 9 male adults and 19 females were NV. Children consisted of 18 LOV and 3 ovo-vegetarians. Fourteen male children and 7 female children were vegetarians; 15 male children and 13 female children were NV.

Appendix I Mineral Intake of Adult Vegetarians and Nonvegetarians

(Ref)/ year	Group/ Gender/(N)	Country	Age	Kcal	Iron (mg)	Zinc (mg)	Magnesium (mg)	Copper[1] (mg)	Manganese (mg)	Selenium (µg)
(1) 1954	LOV M (15)	United States	55	3020	22.0					
	VEG M (14)		51	3260	30.0					
	NV M (15)		57	3720	22.0					
	LOV F (15)		58	2450	16.0					
	VEG F (11)		49	2400	25.0					
	NV F (15)		57	2690	17.0					
(2) 1963	LOV F (26)	Australia	18–40	1980	10.1					
	NV F (25)		18–40	2115	10.5					
(3) 1978	LOV F (42)	United States	57	1600	11.2					
	NV F (36)		59	1579	10.8					
(4) 1980	LOV M/F (57)	United States	18–40	2270	17.2	11.2		3.9		
	LV M/F (14)		18–40	1830	18.1	11.3		3.4		
	VEG M/F (8)		18–40	1665	17.1	7.9		3.7		
	NV F (41)		18–40	2072	12.7	12.7		3.4		
	LOV M (32)	United States	18–40			13.3				
	LV M (8)		18–40			13.5				
	VEG M (4)		18–40			14.1				
	NV M (1)		18–40			16.8				
	LOV F (25)	United States	18–40			8.5				
	LV F (6)		18–40			8.2				
	VEG F (4)		18–40			1.5				
	NV F (40)		18–40			10.1				
(5) 1980	LOV M (15)	United States	28	2624	21.0					
	NV M (25)		27	2684	16.0					
	LOV F (13)		26	2174	18.0					
	NV F (24)		26	1859	11.0					
(6) 1980	LOV	India	NI							92.7
	NV		NI							84.8

	Group (n)	Country	Age						
(7) 1981	LOV (49)	Canada	52	1630	12.5	9.2			113.0
					9.2				109.0
(8) 1981	LOV (5)	United States	22	1329		6.4	262	1.3	
(9) 1983	LOV M (20)	United	36	2324	16.0				
	NV M (17)	States	44	2652	16.0				
	LOV F (31)		31	1776	12.0				
	NV F (36)		36	1754	11.0				
(10) 1983	LOV F (36)	Canada	69	1615				2.1	4.4
	NV F (30)		60	1727				1.6	2.6
(11) 1984	LOV M (25)	United	39–65	2128	21.3				
	VEG M (9)	States	39–65	2259	22.6				
	NV M (25)		39–65	2335	15.9				
	LOV F (25)		39–65	1615	21.5				
	VEG F (9)		39–65	1497	14.9				
	NV F (25)		39–65	1821	16.3				
(12) 1984	LOV M (36)	United	31	2532	17.0				
	NV M (18)	States	31	2836	18.0				
(13) 1985	LOV M/F (17)	Great	34	2290	14.8	9.2			
	VEG M/F (17)	Britain	31	2381	18.5	8.8			
	NV M/F (17)		35	2313	15.9	11.4			
(14) 1986	LOV M (14)	Canada	28	2401	16.5				
	NV M (14)		21	2809	16.9				
	LOV F (22)		26	1760	14.1				
	NV F (18)		22	2097	14.9				
(15) 1986	LOV M (14)	South	18–40	2717	17.9	11.1	467	2.4	
	NV M (10)	Africa	18–40	3167	17.9	16.2	376	2.1	
	LOV F (19)		18–40	1916	11.5	7.4	282	1.5	
	NV F (12)		18–40	1890	11.7	9.7	244	1.4	

(Appendix I continued)

Appendix I Mineral Intake of Adult Vegetarians and Nonvegetarians

(Ref)/year	Group/Gender(N)	Country	Age	Kcal	Iron (mg)	Zinc (mg)	Magnesium (mg)	Copper¹ (mg)	Manganese (mg)	Selenium (µg)
(16) 1986	LOV M (60)	Israel	55	3290	37.0	15.2	690			
	NV M (53)		50	2896	25.8	14.7	443			
	LOV F (32)		51	2544	29.7	11.9	533			
	NV F (60)		52	2389	21.7	12.5	358			
(17) 1987	VEG M (11)	Great Britain	32	2643	25.0		571			
	NV M (11)		31	2381	16.0		424			
	VEG F (11)		28	1881	16.0		462			
	NV F (11)		24	1833	14.0		371			
(18) 1988	LOV F (88)	United States	73	1533	10.7					
	NV F (278)		79	1633	10.2					
(19) 1988	LOV M (47)	Australia	33	2619			527			
	NV M (59)		34	2777			366			
	LOV F (51)		34	2040			396			
	NV F (54)		33	2010			289			
(20) 1988	LOV F (20)	United States	29	1814	11.8					
	NV F (16)		31	1788	12.7					
(21) 1988	LOV M (14)	United States	34	2444	17.9	12.7	382	1.8	5.1	
	NV M (13)		35	2329	14.8	11.6	309	1.3	3.3	
	LOV F (15)		34	1742	13.9	8.8	316	1.4	4.1	
	NV F (16)		34	1656	11.0	9.0	231	1.1	2.6	
(22) 1989	LOV F (23)	United States	72	1452	12.3	6.3	283	1.4	2.2	
	NV F (14)		71	1363	11.4	6.3	226	1.0	1.3	
(23) 1989	LOV F (10)	United States	67	1612	12.3					
	NV F (10)		64	1641	13.3					
(24) 1989	LOV F (144)	United States	67	1474		7.2	312	1.4		
	NV F (146)		66	1563		8.8	294	1.4		

Group	Country	Age						
(25) 1989								
B-LOV M/F (51)	United States	55				368		
B-NV M/F (49)	States	56				379		
W-LOV M/F (163)		52				468		101.0
W-NV (89)		53				364		106.0
(26) 1989								
LOV F (26)[2]	United States	29						
NV F (12)2	States	29						
(27) 1990								
LOV M (18)	Netherlands	65–97	1960	13.7	8.5[3]			
NV M		65+		13.1	10.3[3]			
LOV F (26)		65–97	1667	12.2	7.6[3]			
NV F		65+		11.4	9.3[3]			
(28) 1990								
LOV F (22)	Great Britain	30	1826	13.8			1.5	
NV F (18)	Britain	34	1779	12.1			1.4	
(29) 1991								
LOV F (18)	United States	35	1939	17.5	8.2	370		2.6
NV F (36)	States	36	1835	13.4	11.3	267		1.4
(30) 1991								
LOV F (34)	United States	36	1819	20.0	13.0	323		
NV F (41)	States	29	1700	22.0	10.0	250		
(31) 1992								
LOV F (28)	United States	63	1652	13.0	7.2	318	1.4	
NV F (28)	States	63	1657	15.5	7.9	266	1.0	
(32) 1993								
LOV M (16)[4]	Great Britain	21–40	2238	15.4	9.4	412	1.8	
VEG M (18)[4]	Britain	21–40	2190	18.9	10.1	939	3.4	
NV M (386)[4]		21–40	2452	15.0	11.8	342	1.7	
LOV F (36)[4]		21–40	1826	15.0	8.8	423	2.1	
VEG F (20)[4]		21–40	1750	14.8	7.0	538	2.4	
NV F (377)[4]		21–40	1733	12.9	9.0	261	1.4	
(33) 1994								
LOV M/F (50)	New Zealand	27	2272	16.6	11.1			39.1
VEG F (5)		27	1842	18.7	9.3			47.8
NV M/F (50)		27	2608	14.6	11.9			35.5
LOV M (14)				20.2				
NV M (14)				17.4				
LOV F (36)				15.5				
VEG F (5)				18.7				
NV F (36)				13.5				

(Appendix I continued)

Appendix I Mineral Intake of Adult Vegetarians and Nonvegetarians

(Ref)/ year	Group/ Gender(N)	Country	Age	Kcal	Iron (mg)	Zinc (mg)	Magnesium (mg)	Copper[1] (mg)	Manganese (mg)	Selenium (µg)
(34) 1995	LV F (15)	Canada	26	2024	13.7	8.2	337	1.6		
	VEG F (8)		28	1923	17.7	8.5	396	2.2		
	NV F (22)		28	2086	15.3	11.1	303	1.4		
(35) 1997	LOV F (13)	Scotland	24	1728			614			
	NV F (20)		23	2184			526			
(36) 1997	LOV M (12)	New Zealand	49	2280	15.5	9.8				
	NV M (11)		40	2688	16.2	11.1				
	LOV F (12)		43	1872	14.7	8.9				
	NV F (12)		39	2016	12.8	8.9				
(37) 1998	B-LOV M (49)	United States	50	2356	21.4	10.6	436			
	B-VEG M (14)		46	1869	17.5	11.4	477			
	B-LOV F (94)		52	1922	24.7	8.7	369			
	B-VEG F (31)		51	1865	18.1	8.7	446			
(38) 1999	VEG M/F (30)[5]	Great Britain	39	NI	16.4	12.4				64
(39) 1999	LOV F (50)	Australia	25	1652	10.7					
	NV F (24)		25	1655	9.9					
(40) 1999	VEG M (10)[5]	United States	20–60	2230	43.4	12.2	605	3.1	5.6	
	NV M (10)[5]		20–60	2170	20.9	15.0	365	2.0	3.6	
	VEG F (15)[5]		20–60	1702	22.6	10.8	440	2.6	4.7	
	NV F (10)[5]		20–60	1978	20.2	13.2	315	1.8	2.7	
(41) 1999	LOV M (10)	Australia	20–50	2143	16.8	9.2				
	LOV M (10)		20–50	2877	22.1	12.7				
(42) 2000	LOV M (37)	France	50	1951	13.2		372			
	VEG M (6)		31	2051	22.6		656			
	LOV F (57)		53	1675	14.6		334			
	VEG F (11)		46	1302	16.9		456			

(43) 2000	LOV M (39)	Australia	20–50	2520	20.4	11.1				
	VEG M (10)		20–50	2784	22.9	11.9				
	NV M (25)		20–50	2640	15.8	12.7				
	LOV F (50)		20–50	1656	10.7	6.8				
	NV F (24)		20–50	1656	9.9	8.4				
(44) 2001	VEG M (54)	United States	57	1830	17.0	8.3	483	2.4	6.3	54.3
	VEG F (87)		53	1460	14.0	6.7	392	2.0	5.0	67.0
(45) 2001	LOV F (101)	Great Britain	44	1855		9.5[5]				
	VEG F (94)		44	1767		10.0[5]				
	NV F (99)		45	1974		10.6[5]				
(46) 2003	LOV M (3748)	United Kingdom	39	2090	13.9	8.4	396			
	VEG M (770)		35	1907	15.3	8.0	440			
	NV M (6951)		51	2186	13.4	9.8	366			
	LOV F (12347)		35	1810	12.6	7.7	352			
	VEG F (1342)		32	1660	14.1	7.2	391			
	NV F (22962)		48	1910	12.6	9.2	341			
(47) 2003	VEG M (48)	Germany	42.4	2381	24.8	13.5	706	3.7	10.4	
	VEG M (19)		45.2	2186	23.0	12.0	666	3.4	8.9	
	VEG F (50)		42.4	1721	20.1	10.5	585	3.0	8.0	
	VEG F (37)		44.5	1617	18.5	9.3	525	2.7	7.2	
(48) 2004	LV F (30)	India	49.5	1618	13.4	5.3	339	1.6		
	LV F htn (26)		48.7	1737	13.2	5.2	366	1.4		
	LV M (85)		46.1	2166	19.6	7.7	493	2.3		
	LV M htn (83)		47.1	2260	18.5	7.3	485	1.8		
(49) 2004	LOV F (6478)	United Kingdom	49	2303	18.9	10.2				
	NV F (24738)		54	2370	18.8	12.0				
(50) 2005	LOV M (31)	United States	19–84[6]	2605	19.1	12.3	492			
	NV M (869)			2605	18.1	15.1	393			
	LOV F (75)			1840	14.1	9.5	359			
	NV F (842)			1793	12.8	10.1	296			

(Appendix I continued)

542   Appendixes

Appendix I Mineral Intake of Adult Vegetarians and Nonvegetarians

(Ref)/ year	Group[1]/ Gender/(N)	Country	Age	Kcal	Iron (mg)	Zinc (mg)	Magnesium (mg)	Copper[1] (mg)	Manganese (mg)	Selenium (µg)
(51) 2007	LOV M (11)	Ireland	37.8	2486		10.7				52
	NV M (17)		42.2	2366		10.4				62
	LOV F (20)		33.8	1888		7.8				35
	NV F (41)		36.6	1936		8.0				46
(52) 2008	LOV M/F (21)	Taiwan	34.8	1884	16.1	8.3				
	NV M/F (28)		35.9	1944	10.0	7.7				
(53) 2008	LO/SV M (20)	Japan	45.2	1983	10.9	8.1	381	1.5	4.2	
	NV M (32)		44.2	1843	6.3	9.2	217	1.2	2.5	
	LO/SV F (50)		45.9	1675	9.5	7.0	306	1.2	3.0	

Notes: [1]Abbreviations: LV, lacto vegetarian; LOV, lacto-ovo vegetarian; VEG, vegan; NV, nonvegetarian; SV, eats chicken and/or fish; NI, not indicated; htn, subjects identified as having hypertension.
[2]All subjects were lactating women.
[3]Data for NV from a separate nationwide survey, data for zinc not calculated at the individual levels but based on the average consumption of food products.
[4]Data include nutrient supplements. Data for NV are from a separate nationwide survey.
[5]Data include nutrient supplements.
[6]Age range of all subjects.

ANNOTATED REFERENCES APPENDIX I

1. Hardinge MG, Stare FJ. Nutritional studies of vegetarians. *Am J Clin Nutr.* 1954;2:73–82.
2. Hitchcock NE, English RM. A comparison of food consumption in lacto-ovo vegetarians and nonvegetarians. *Food Nutr Notes Rev.* 1963;20:141–146.
3. Mason RL, Kunkel ME, Ann Davis T, Beauchene RE. Nutrient intakes of vegetarian and nonvegetarian women. *Tenn Farm Home Science.* 1978;1:18–20.
4. Freeland-Graves JH, Bodzy PW, Eppright MA. Zinc status of vegetarians. *J Am Diet Assoc.* 1980;77:655–661. *Note:* Zinc values for the individual male and female groups are subsets of the combined male/female groups.
5. Taber LAL, Cook RA. Dietary and anthropometric assessment of adult omnivores, fish-eaters, and lacto-ovo vegetarians. *J Am Diet Assoc.* 1980;76:21–29.
6. Ganapathy SN, Dhanda R. Selenium content of omnivorous and vegetarian diets. *In J Nutr Dietet.* 1980;17:53–59.
7. Anderson BM, Gibson RS, Sabry JH. The iron and zinc status of long-term vegetarian women. *Am J Clin Nutr.* 1981;34:1042–1048.
8. King JC, Stein NC, Doyle M. Effect of vegetarianism on the zinc status of pregnant women. *Am J Clin Nutr.* 1981;34:1049–1055.
9. Shultz TD, Leklem JE. Dietary status of Seventh-day Adventists and nonvegetarians. *J Am Diet Assoc.* 1983;83:27–33.
10. Gibson RS, Anderson BM, Sabry JH. The trace metal status of a group of post-menopausal vegetarians. *J Am Diet Assoc.* 1983;82:246–250.
11. Calkins BM, Whittaker DJ, Nair PP, Rider AA, Turjman N. Diet, nutrition intake, and metabolism in populations at high and low risk for colon cancer. *Am J Clin Nutr.* 1984;40:896–905.
12. Latta D, Liebman M. Iron and zinc status of vegetarian and nonvegetarian males. *Nutr Rep Int.* 1984;30:141–149.
13. Davies GJ, Crowder M, Dickerson JWT. Dietary fibre intakes of individuals with different eating patterns. *Human Nutr: Appl Nutr.* 1985;39A:139–148.
14. Locong A. Nutritional status and dietary intake of a selected sample of young adult vegetarians. *Can Diet Assoc J.* 1986;47:101–106.
15. Faber M, Gouws E, Benadé AJS, Labadarios D. Anthropometric measurements, dietary intake and biochemical data of South African lacto-ovo vegetarians. *S Afr Med J.* 1986;69:733–738.
16. Levin N, Rattan J, Gilat T. Mineral intake and blood levels in vegetarians. *Israel J Med Sci.* 1986;22:105–108.
17. Sanders TAB, Key TJA. Blood pressure, plasma renin activity and aldosterone concentrations in vegans and omnivores. *Human Nutr: Appl Nutr.* 1987;41A:204–211.
18. Tylavsky FA, Anderson JJB. Dietary factors in bone health of elderly lacto-ovo vegetarian and omnivorous women. *Am J Clin Nutr.* 1988;48:842–849.
19. Rouse IL, Armstrong BK, Beilin LJ. The relationship of blood pressure to diet and lifestyle in two religious populations. *J Hypertension.* 1983;65–71.
20. Worthington-Roberts BS, Breskin MW, Monsen ER. Iron status of premenopausal women in a university community and its relationship to habitual dietary sources of protein. *Am J Clin Nutr.* 1988;47:275–279.
21. Kelsay JL, Frazier CW, Prather E, Canary JJ, Clark WM, Powell AS. Impact of variation in carbohydrate intake on mineral utilization by vegetarians. *Am J Clin Nutr.* 1988;48:875–879.
22. Nieman DC, Underwood BC, Sherman KM, Arabatzis K, Barbosa JC, Johnson M, Shultz TD. Dietary status of Seventh-day Adventist vegetarian and nonvegetarian elderly women. *J Am Diet Assoc.* 1989;89:1763–1769.
23. Marsh AG, Christensen DK, Sanchez TV, Mickelsen O, Chaffee FL. Nutrient similarities and differences of older lacto-ovo vegetarian and omnivorous women. *Nutr Rep Int.* 1989;39:19–24.
24. Hunt I-F, Murphy NJ, Henderson C, Clark VA, Jacobs RM, Johnston PK, Coulson AH. Bone mineral content in postmenopausal women: Comparison of omnivores and vegetarians. *Am J Clin Nutr.* 1989;50:517–523.
25. Melby CL, Goldflies DG, Hyner GC, Lyle RM. Relation between vegetarian/nonvegetarian diets and blood pressure in black and white adults. *Am J Public Health.* 1989;79:1283–1288.
26. Debski B, Finley DA, Picciano MF, Lönnerdal B, Milner J. Selenium content and glutathione peroxidase activity of milk from vegetarian and nonvegetarian women. *J Nutr.* 1989;119:215–220.

27. Brants HAM, Löwik MRH, Westenbrink S, Hulshof KFAM, Kistemaker C. Adequacy of a vegetarian diet at old age (Dutch Nutrition Surveillance System). *J Am College Nutr.* 1990;9:292–302.
28. Reddy S, Sanders TAB. Haematological studies on premenopausal Indian and Caucasian vegetarians compared with Caucasian omnivores. *Br J Nutr.* 1990;64:331–338.
29. Lloyd T, Schaeffer JM, Walker MA, Demers L. Urinary hormonal concentrations and spinal bone densities of premenopausal vegetarian and nonvegetarian women. *Am J Clin Nutr.* 1991;54:1005–1010.
30. Pedersen AB, Bartholomew MJ, Dolence LA, Aljadir LP, Netteburg KL, Lloyd T. Menstrual differences due to vegetarian and nonvegetarian diets. *Am J Clin Nutr.* 1991;53:879–885.
31. Tesar R, Notelovitz M, Shim E, Kauwell G, Brown J. Axial and peripheral bone density and nutrient intakes of postmenopausal vegetarian and omnivorous women. *Am J Clin Nutr.* 1992;56:699–704.
32. Draper A, Lewis J, Malhotra N, Wheeler E. The energy and nutrient intakes of different types of vegetarian: A case for supplements. *Br J Nutr.* 1993;69:3–19.
33. Alexander D, Ball MJ, Mann J. Nutrient intake and haematological status of vegetarians and age-sex matched omnivores. *Eur J Clin Nutr.* 1994;48:538–546. *Note:* Iron values for the individual male and female groups are subsets of the combined male/female groups.
34. Janelle KC, Barr SI. Nutrient intakes and eating behavior scores of vegetarian and nonvegetarian women. *J Am Diet Assoc.* 1995;95:180–189.
35. Ball D, Maughan RJ. Blood and urine acid-base status of premenopausal omnivorous and vegetarian women. *Br J Nutr.* 1997;78:683–693. *Note:* Two vegetarians occasionally ate fish.
36. Harman SK, Parnell WR. The nutritional health of New Zealand vegetarian and nonvegetarian Seventh-Day Adventists: selected vitamin, mineral and lipid levels. *NZ Med J.* 1998;111:91–94. *Note:* Of the 24 vegetarians, an unspecified number were lacto vegetarians or vegans. Some nonvegetarians only occasionally ate red meat.
37. Toohey ML, Harris MA, Williams D, Foster G, Schmidt WD, Melby CL. Cardiovascular disease risk factors are lower in African-American vegans compared to lacto-ovo vegetarians. *J Am Coll Nutr.* 1998;17:425–434.
38. Lightowler HJ, Davies GJ. The effect of self-selected dietary supplements on micronutrient intakes in vegans. *Proc Nutr Soc.* 1999;58;35A *Note:* Subjects were 11 males and 19 females.
39. Ball MJ, Bartlett MA. Dietary intake and iron status of Australian vegetarian women. *Am J Clin Nutr.* 1999;70:353–358. *Note:* Two of the 50 LOV were vegan; vegetarians consumed red meat no more than once a month and consumed fish or chicken no more than once a week.
40. Haddad EH, Berk LS, Kettering JD, Hubbard RW, Peters WR. Dietary intake and biochemical, hematologic, and immune status of vegans compared with nonvegetarians. *Am J Clin Nutr.* 1999;70 (suppl): 586S–593S.
41. Li D, Sinclair A, Wilson A, et al. Effect of dietary α-linolenic acid on thrombotic risk factors in vegetarian men. *Am J Clin Nutr.* 1999;69:878–882. *Note:* Vegetarian subjects were divided into two groups for study purposes. Only baseline data are reported here.
42. Leblanc JC, Yoon H, Kombadjian A, Verger P. Nutritional intakes of vegetarian populations in France. *Eur J Clin Nutr.* 2000;54:443–449. *Note:* Thirty-one of the 94 LOV ate fish or meat at least once a week; 11 were lacto vegetarians and 3 were ovo vegetarians; 13 of the 17 VEG ate fish once a week.
43. Ball MJ, Ackland ML. Zinc intake and status in Australian vegetarians. *Br J Nutr.* 2000;83:27–33. *Note:* Two of the 50 LOV females were vegans.
44. Donaldson MS. Food and nutrient intake of Hallelujah vegetarians. *Nutr Food Sci.* 2001;31:293–303. *Note:* VEG subjects ate a mostly raw diet; 58% consumed some animal product during their week of food intake records.
45. Allen NE, Appleby PN, Davey GK, et al. The associations of diet with serum insulin-like growth factor I and its main binding proteins in 292 women meat-eaters, vegetarians, and vegans. *Cancer Epidemiol Biomark Prevent.* 2002; 11:1441–1448.
46. Davey GK, Spencer EA, Appleby PN, et al. EPIC-Oxford lifestyle characteristics and nutrient intakes in a cohort of 33883 meat-eaters and 31546 non-meat-eaters in the UK. *Public Health Nutr.* 2003;6:259–268.
47. Waldmann A, Koschizke JW, Leitzmann C, Hahn A. Dietary intake and lifestyle factors of a vegan population in Germany: results from the German Vegan Study. *Eur J Clin Nutr.* 2003;57:947–955. *Note:* Ninety-eight subjects did not use animal products for 1 year prior to study; 56 subjects consumed small amounts of dairy products and eggs. The first listing for each gender is for strict vegans; the second listing is for those who consumed small amounts of dairy and eggs. Data exclude vitamin and mineral supplements.

48. Chiplonkar SA, Agte V, Tarwadik V, et al. Micronutrient deficiencies as predisposing factors for hypertension in lacto-vegetarian Indian adults. *J Am Coll Nutr.* 2004;23:239–247.

49. Cade JE, Burley VJ, Greenwood DC, et al. The UK Women's Cohort Study: comparisons of vegetarians, fish-eaters, and meat-eaters. *Public Health Nutr.* 2004;7:871–878. *Note:* Vegetarians ate meat or fish less than once a week.

50. Bedford JL, Barr SI. Diets and selected lifestyle practices of self-defined adult vegetarians from a population-based sample suggest they are more health conscious. *Int J Behav Nutr Phys Act.* 2005;2:4. *Note:* Seventy-five percent of those self-identified as vegetarian consumed fish and/or seafood, 58% consumed poultry, and 22% consumed red meat.

51. Haldar S, Rowland IR, Barnett RA, et al. Influence of habitual diet on antioxidant status: a study in a population of vegetarians and omnivores. *Eur J Clin Nutr.* 2007;61:1011–1022. *Note:* Vegetarian subjects ate flesh foods no more than six times a year. The vegetarian group included six vegans.

52. Yen CE, Yen CH, Huang MC, et al. Dietary intake and nutritional status of vegetarian and omnivorous preschool children and their parents in Taiwan. *Nutr Res.* 2008;28:430–436. *Note:* Adult vegetarians consisted of 16 LOV, 2 ovo-vegetarians, 1 LV, 2 vegans. Four male adults and 17 females were vegetarian; 9 male adults and 19 females were NV. Children consisted of 18 LOV and 3 ovo-vegetarians. Fourteen male children and 7 female children were vegetarians; 15 male children and 13 female children were NV.

53. Nakamato K, Watanabe S, Kudo H, et al. Nutritional characteristics of middle-aged Japanese vegetarians. *J Athero-sclero Throm.* 2008;15:122–129. *Note:* Nine men and 18 women were LOV; 11 men and 37 women in the vegetarian group occasionally ate chicken and meat.

Appendix J Water-Soluble Vitamin Intake of Adult Vegetarians and Nonvegetarians

(Ref)/ year	Group/ Gender(N)	Country	Age	Kcal	Vit. C (mg)	Thiamin (mg)	Riboflavin (mg)	Niacin (mg)	Vit. B_6 (mg)	Folate (µg)	Pantothenic acid (mg)	Vit. B_{12} (µg)
(1) 1954	LOV M (15)	United States	55	3020	250	2.3	2.8	19.0				
	VEG M (14)		51	3260	355	2.7	1.8	26.0				
	NV M (15)		57	3720	185	2.0	2.8	23.0				
	LOV F (15)		58	2450	220	1.7	2.6	13.0				
	VEG F (11)		49	2400	280	2.1	1.5	16.0				
	NV F (15)		57	2690	185	1.5	2.1	18.0				
(2) 1963	LOV F (26)	Australia	18-40	1980	107	1.0	1.3	11.0				
	NV F (25)		18-40	2115	72	0.8	1.6	11.4				
(3) 1978	LOV F (42)	United States	57	1600	141	1.2	1.7					
	NV F (36)		59	1579	119	0.9	1.6					
(4) 1980	LOV M/F (57)	United States	18-40	2270	196	3.7	3.9	15.9				
	LV M/F (14)		18-40	1830	226	5.2	4.6	13.1				
	VEG M/F (8)		18-40	1665	584	1.8	1.5	13.9				
	NV F (41)		18-40	2072	151	2.3	2.9	15.8				
(5) 1980	LOV M (15)	United States	28	2624	217	2.7	2.3	22.0				
	NV M (25)		27	2684	121	1.4	2.2	24.0				
	LOV F (13)		26	2174	194	2.3	2.0	17.0				
	NV F (24)		26	1859	110	1.0	1.5	19.0				
(6) 1981	LOV M (11)	Great Britain	28-80	2015	94							
	NV M (18)		28-80	2300	77							
	LOV F (14)		28-80	1737	76							
	NV F (28)		28-80	1656	69							
(7) 1981	LOV F (5)	United States	22	1329	135	0.9	1.2	8.6	1.8	247		2.6
(8) 1983	LOV M (20)	United States	36	2324	182	2.0	2.0	17.6	2.0			
	NV M (17)		44	2652	141	1.6	2.4	23.9	2.0			
	LOV F (31)		31	1776	183	1.8	1.8	14.8	1.8			
	NV F (36)		36	1754	158	1.2	1.7	17.9	1.6			

(9) 1984	United States	LOV M (25)	39–65	2128	193	2.2	2.0	21.8			
		VEG M (9)	39–65	2259	313	2.4	2.0	22.4			
		NV M (25)	39–65	2335	196	3.6	3.8	33.1			
		LOV F (25)	39–65	1615	194	2.4	1.6	14.8			
		VEG F (9)	39–65	1497	131	1.2	5.1	15.0			
		NV F (25)	39–65	1821	137	1.2	1.5	18.1			
(10) 1985	Great Britain	LOV M/F (17)	34	2290	112						2.7
		VEG M/F (17)	31	2381	156						3.0²
		NV M/F (17)	35	2313	117						9.2
(11) 1986	Canada	LOV M (14)	28	2401	171	2.0	2.0	27.9³		327	
		NV M (14)	21	2809	158	1.9	2.9	38.4³		252	
		LOV F (22)	26	1760	166	1.7	2.0	25.3³		273	
		NV F (18)	22	2097	143	1.9	2.6	30.7³		215	
(12) 1986	South Africa	LOV M (14)	18–40	2717	212	1.8	2.0	20.3	1.6	342	2.2
		NV M (10)	18–40	3167	115	1.5	1.9	35.4	1.9	251	7.0
		LOV F (19)	18–40	1916	178	1.2	1.4	12.1	1.1	214	1.7
		NV F (12)	18–40	1890	85	1.0	1.4	15.5	1.2	177	3.4
(13) 1987	Great Britain	VEG M (11)	32	2643	161	2.1	2.1	28.0		304	1.2
		NV M (11)	31	2381	168	1.5	2.3	26.0		233	6.5
		VEG F (11)	28	1881	115	1.6	1.7	21.0		288	1.1
		NV F (11)	24	1833	139	1.3	1.5	18.0		201	2.5
(14) 1988	United States	LOV F (88)	73	1533	184	1.0	1.3	11.3			
		NV F (278)	79	1633	157	0.9	1.5	13.8			
(15) 1988	United States	LOV F (20)	29	1814	169						
		NV F (16)	31	1788	144						
(16) 1989	France	LOV M (11)	37	2100	133	2.7	2.0		1.5		
		NV M (33)	40	2600	89	1.3	1.7		1.4		
		LOV F (26)	26	1700	142	2.5	1.8		1.3		
		NV F (36)	36	1800	91	1.2	1.6		1.1		
(17) 1989	United States	LOV F (23)	72	1452	155	1.4	1.5	14.3	1.6	273	2.3
		NV F (14)	71	1363	114	1.1	1.4	14.2	1.3	215	2.6

(Appendix J continued)

Appendix J Water-Soluble Vitamin Intake of Adult Vegetarians and Nonvegetarians

(Ref)/ year	Group/ Gender(N)	Country	Age	Kcal	Vit. C (mg)	Thiamin (mg)	Riboflavin (mg)	Niacin (mg)	Vit. B6 (mg)	Folate (µg)	Pantothenic acid (mg)	Vit. B12 (µg)
(18) 1990	LOV M (18)	Netherlands	65–97	1960	136	1.3	1.9		1.3			
	NV M[4]		65+	2412	94	1.1	1.7		1.4			
	LOV F (26)		65–97	1667	149	1.1	1.7		1.1			
	NV F[4]		65+	1879	101	0.9	1.5		1.2			
(19) 1990	LOV F (22)	Great Britain	30	1826	114					262		1.5
	NV F (18)		34	1779	69					170		5.5
(20) 1991	LOV F (23)	United States	35	1939	200	1.7		17.9	1.7	355	3.6	2.1
	NV F (36)		36	1835	134	1.4		20.1	1.5	235	3.5	4.9
(21) 1991	LOV F (34)	United States	36	1819	316				2.0	374		
	NV F (41)		29	1700	184				2.0	385		
(22) 1991	LOV M/F (79)	United States	18–30	2800	264							
	NV M/F (4821)		18–30	2980	197							
(23) 1992	LOV F (28)	United States	63	1652	143	1.4	1.7	14.4	1.8	255	3.6	2.5
	NV F (28)		63	1657	118	1.4	1.9	20.0	1.6	249	3.5	4.2
(24) 1992	VEG M (10)	Great Britain	32	2548	136							
	NV M (10)		33	2524	84							
	VEG F (10)		32	2214	151							
	NV F (10)		32	1976	82							
(25) 1993	LOV M (16)[5]	Great Britain	21–40	2238	119	1.9	2.1	33.0	2.2	366		2.7
	VEG M (18)[5]		21–40	2190	172	2.1	1.4	33.2	3.2	448		0.7
	NV M (386)[4]		21–40	2452	97	2.5	2.7	43.0	3.0	321		7.4
	LOV F (36)[5]		21–40	1826	131	1.6	1.7	27.7	2.3	354		1.8
	VEG F (20)[5]		21–40	1750	124	1.6	1.0	24.5	3.3	298		0.6
	NV F (377)[4]		21–40	1733	96	1.6	2.0	33.0	3.3	235		6.0
(26) 1994	LOV M/F (50)	New Zealand	27	2272	145					455		1.9
	VEG F (5)		27	1842	155					471		0.5
	NV M/F (50)		27	2608	149					343		4.2

No./Year	Diet (n)	Country										
(27) 1995	LV F (15)	Canada	26	2024	141	1.3	1.5	12.0	1.4	310	3.9	1.5
	VEG F (8)		28	1923	186	1.8	1.3	15.9	1.9	416	5.3	0.5
	NV F (22)		28	2086	116	1.6	1.7	18.7	1.6	269	5.0	3.8
(28) 1998	LOV M (12)	New Zealand	49	2280	208	2.5				354		
	NV M (11)		40	2688	203	2.3				334		
	LOV F (12)		43	1872	288	2.0				387		
	NV F (12)		39	2016	163	2.3				247		
(29) 1998	VEG M/F (30)[5]	Great Britain	39	NI	219		2.8					7.7
(30) 1998	B-LOV M (49)	United States	50	2356	222	2.5	2.1	24.8	2.7	511		4.3
	B-VEG M (14)		46	1869	189	2.3	1.9	26.4	3.2	564		3.3
	B-LOV F (94)		52	1922	176	2.0	1.7	18.9	2.4	447		3.0
	B-VEG F (31)		51	1865	224	2.3	1.4	18.6	2.5	525		1.6
(31) 1999	LOV F (50)	Australia	25	1652	150							
	NV F (24)		25	1655	111							
(32) 1999	VEG M (10)[5]	United States	20–60	2230	240	3.5	1.8	26.3	3.2	640		5.0
	NV M (10)[5]		20–60	2170	140	2.1	2.2	30.7	2.4	400		5.3
	VEG F (15)[5]		20–60	1702	275	2.3	1.7	21.5	2.6	520		6.0
	NV F (10)[5]		20–60	1978	125	1.6	1.9	25.8	2.0	300		5.7
(33) 1999	LOV M (10)	Australia	20–50	2143	189							
	LOV M (10)		20–50	2877	347							
(34) 2000	LOV M (37)	France	50	1951	150							1.0
	VEG M (6)		31	2051	76							0.6
	LOV F (57)		53	1675	109							1.4
	VEG F (11)		46	1302	58							0.2
(35) 2000	LV F (28)	Taiwan	38.2	1333	195							
	NV F (25)		40.4	1619	162							
	LV M (21)		37.7	2000	190							
	NV M (21)		38.3	2000	141							
	LV F (51)		36.6	1524	123							
	NV F (53)		36.9	1738	112							

(Appendix J continued)

Appendix J Water-Soluble Vitamin Intake of Adult Vegetarians and Nonvegetarians

(Ref)/year	Group'l Gender(N)	Country	Age	Kcal	Vit. C (mg)	Thiamin (mg)	Riboflavin (mg)	Niacin (mg)	Vit. B₆ (mg)	Folate (µg)	Pantothenic acid (mg)	Vit. B₁₂ (µg)
(36) 2001	VEG M (54)	United States	57	1830	481	2.4	2.0	18.0	3.9	594	6.4	0.6
	VEG F (87)		53	1460	442	2.0	1.7	14.8	3.2	487	5.2	0.5
(37) 2002	LV F (45)	Taiwan	31–45	1524		1.0	0.7	10.1				
	NV F (45)		31–45	1738		0.8	1.2	13.1				
(38) 2002	LOV M/F (14)	Italy	48.5	2002					2.5	521.9		
	VEG M/F (31)		45.8	1930					4.1	623.3		
(39) 2003	LOV M (3748)	United Kingdom	39	2090	123	1.9	2.2	20.8	2.0	367		2.6
	VEG M (770)		35	1907	155	2.3	2.3	23.9	2.2	431		0.4
	NV M (6951)		51	2186	119	1.7	2.3	24.7	2.3	329		7.2
	LOV F (12347)		35	1810	147	1.8	2.1	18.3	1.9	350		2.5
	VEG F (1342)		32	1660	169	2.1	2.1	21.1	2.1	412		0.5
	NV F (22962)		48	1810	138	1.6	2.2	23.2	2.2	321		7.0
(40) 2003	LOV M/F (37)	Taiwan	28.9	2125					0.9			0.7
	NV M/F (32)		22.9	1873					1.0			3.3
(41) 2003	VEG M (48)	Germany	42.4	2381	353	2.2	1.5	29.7	3.0	571		0.8
	VEG M (19)		45.2	2186	318	2.0	1.4	28.0	3.0	527		0.9
	VEG F (50)		42.4	1721	274	1.8	1.3	23.7	2.6	482		0.8
	VEG F (37)		44.5	1617	358	1.4	1.2	20.3	2.4	467		0.2
(42) 2004	LV F (30)	India	49.5	1618	77	1.0	0.7	10.3		116		
	LV F htn (26)		48.7	1737	51	1.0	0.6	9.8		98		
	LV M (85)		46.1	2166	59	1.4	0.8	14.8		159		
	LV M htn (83)		47.1	2260	47	1.4	0.7	14.4		140		
(43) 2004	LOV F (6478)	United Kingdom	49	2303	129					416		
	NV F (24738)		54	2370	168					397		
(44) 2005	LOV M (31)	United States	19–84[6]	2605	197	2.1	2.6	38.4	2.2	608	6.2	3.5
	NV M (869)			2605	130	2.1	2.3	49.0	2.3	556	6.2	5.0
	LOV F (75)			1840	125	1.7	1.7	34.2	1.7	460	5.1	2.9
	NV F (842)			1793	109	1.4	1.7	31.2	1.5	372	4.2	3.2

Reference / Year	Group (n)	Country	Age	Energy							
(45) 2005	LOV M/F (43)	Germany	25–64[6]	1792					3.0	458	0.2
	VEG M/F (43)			1888					3.3	518	0.2
	NV M/F (115)			2055					3.0	477	0.4
(46) 2006	VEG M/F (93)	Germany	43.7						2.83		
(47) 2006	LOV M/F (90)	Slovak Republic	37.7	1945	141.8						
	NV M/F (46)		37.1	2438	103.6						
(48) 2006	LOV M/F (36)	Austria	34.2			1.27	1.63		1.88	322	2.28
	VEG M/F (42)		30.7			2.14	1.27		2.88	455	0.39
	NV M/F (40)		38.4			1.17	1.51		1.72	253	4.29
(49) 2007	LOV M (11)	Ireland	37.8	2486	206					310	
	NV M (17)		42.2	2366	103					295	
	LOV F (20)		33.8	1888	123					270	
	NV F (41)		36.6	1936	111					226	
(50) 2008	LO/LSV F (26)	Turkey	29.0	1832	179.2	0.97	1.36	10.1	1.53	374.8	1.49
	NV F (26)		27.4	1849	131.6	0.88	1.44	12.4	1.47	322.4	3.73
(51) 2008	LOV M/F (21)	Taiwan	34.8	1884	182.6	1.3	0.9				
	NV M/F (28)		35.9	1944	180.4	1.1	1.3				
(52) 2008	LO/SV M (20)	Japan	45.2	1983	105	1.3	1.2	13.4	1.2	455	1.9
	NV M (32)		44.2	1843	87	0.9	1.0	14.6	1.1	276	11.3
	LO/SV F (50)		45.9	1675	119	1.0	1.1	12.5	1.2	365	3.7

Notes: [1]Abbreviations: LV, lacto vegetarian; LOV, lacto-ovo vegetarian; VEG, vegan; SV, eats chicken and/or fish; NV, nonvegetarian; htn, subjects identified as having hypertension; B, black; NI, not indicated.

[2]Vegan vitamin B_{12} intake was due to the consumption of vitamin B_{12}-fortified foods.

[3]Niacin as niacin equivalents (NE). The convention is to consider 60 mg of tryptophan as equivalent to 1 mg of niacin.

[4]Data for NV from a separate nationwide survey.

[5]Data include nutrient supplements.

[6]Age range of all subjects.

ANNOTATED REFERENCES APPENDIX J

1. Hardinge MG, Stare FJ. Nutritional studies of vegetarians. *Am J Clin Nutr.* 1954;2:73–82.

2. Hitchcock NE, English RM. A comparison of food consumption in lacto-ovo vegetarians and nonvegetarians. *Food Nutr Notes Rev.* 1963;20:141–146.

3. Mason RL, Kunkel ME, Ann Davis T, Beauchene RE. Nutrient intakes of vegetarian and nonvegetarian women. *Tenn Farm Home Science.* 1978;1:18–20.

4. Freeland-Graves JH, Bodzy PW, Eppright MA. Zinc status of vegetarians. *J Am Diet Assoc.* 1980;77:655–661.

5. Taber LAL, Cook RA. Dietary and anthropometric assessment of adult omnivores, fish-eaters, and lacto-ovo vegetarians. *J Am Diet Assoc.* 1980;76:21–29.

6. Burr ML, Bates CJ, Fehily AM, Leger AS ST. Plasma cholesterol and blood pressure in vegetarians. *J Human Nutr.* 1981;35:437–441.

7. King JC, Stein JC, Doyle M. Effect of vegetarianism on the zinc status of pregnant women. *Am J Clin Nutr.* 1981; 34:1049–1055.

8. Shultz TD, Leklem JE. Dietary status of Seventh-day Adventists and nonvegetarians. *J Am Diet Assoc.* 1983;83:27–33.

9. Calkins BM, Whittaker DJ, Nair PP, Rider AA, Turjman N. Diet, nutrition intake, and metabolism in populations at high and low risk for colon cancer. *Am J Clin Nutr.* 1984;40:896–905.

10. Davies GJ, Crowder M, Dickerson JWT. Dietary fibre intakes of individuals with different eating patterns. *Human Nutr: Appl Nutr.* 1985;39A:139–148.

11. Locong A. Nutritional status and dietary intake of a selected sample of young adult vegetarians. *Can Diet Assoc J.* 1986;47:101–106.

12. Faber M, Gouws E, Benadé AJS, Labadarios D. Anthropometric measurements, dietary intake and biochemical data of South African lacto-ovo vegetarians. *S Afr Med J.* 1986;69:733–738.

13. Sanders TAB, Key TJA. Blood pressure, plasma renin activity and aldosterone concentrations in vegans and omnivores. *Human Nutr: Appl Nutr.* 1987;41A:204–211.

14. Tylavsky FA, Anderson JJB. Dietary factors in bone health of elderly lacto-ovo vegetarian and omnivorous women. *Am J Clin Nutr.* 1988;48:842–849.

15. Worthington-Roberts BS, Breskin MW, Monsen ER. Iron status of premenopausal women in a university community and its relationship to habitual dietary sources of protein. *Am J Clin Nutr.* 1988; 47:275–279.

16. Millet P, Guilland JC, Fuchs F, Klepping J. Nutrient intake and vitamin status of healthy French vegetarians and nonvegetarians. *Am J Clin Nutr.* 1989;50:718–722.

17. Nieman DC, Underwood BC, Sherman KM, et al. Dietary status of Seventh-day Adventist vegetarian and nonvegetarian elderly women. *J Am Diet Assoc.* 1989;89:1763–1769.

18. Brants Ham, Löwik MRH, Westenbrink S, Hulshof KFAM, Kistemaker C. Adequacy of a vegetarian diet at old age (Dutch Nutrition Surveillance System). *J Am College Nutr.* 1990;9:292–302.

19. Reddy S, Sanders TAB. Haematological studies on premenopausal Indian and Caucasian vegetarians compared with Caucasian omnivores. *Br J Nutr.* 1990;64:331–338.

20. Lloyd T, Schaeffer JM, Walker MA, Demers L. Urinary hormonal concentrations and spinal bone densities of premenopausal vegetarian and nonvegetarian women. *Am J Clin Nutr.* 1991;54:1005–1010.

21. Pedersen AB, Bartholomew MJ, Dolence LA, Aljadir LP, Netteburg KL, Lloyd T. Menstrual differences due to vegetarian and nonvegetarian diets. *Am J Clin Nutr.* 1991;53:879–885.

22. Slattery ML, Jacobs DR, Hilner JE, et al. Meat consumption and its association with other diet and health factors in young adults: the CARDIA study. *Am J Clin Nutr.* 1991;54:930–935.

23. Tesar R, Notelovitz M, Shim E, Kauwell G, Brown J. Axial and peripheral bone density and nutrient intakes of postmenopausal vegetarian and omnivorous women. *Am J Clin Nutr.* 1992;56:699–704.

24. Sanders TAB, Roshanai F. Platelet phospholipid fatty acid composition and function in vegans compared with age- and sex-matched omnivorous controls. *Eur J Clin Nutr.* 1992;46:823–831.

25. Draper A, Lewis J, Malhotra N, Wheeler E. The energy and nutrient intakes of different types of vegetarian: a case for supplements. *Br J Nutr.* 1993;69:3–19.

26. Alexander D, Ball MJ, Mann J. Nutrient intake and haematological status of vegetarians and age-sex matched omnivores. *Eur J Clin Nutr.* 1994;48:538–546.

27. Janelle KC, Barr SI. Nutrient intakes and eating behavior scores of vegetarian and nonvegetarian women. *J Am Diet Assoc.* 1995;95:180–189.

28. Harman SK, Parnell WR. The nutritional health of New Zealand vegetarian and nonvegetarian Seventh-Day Adventists: selected vitamin, mineral and lipid levels. *NZ Med J.* 1998;111:91–94. *Note:* Of the 24 vegetarians, an unspecified number were lacto vegetarians or vegans. Some nonvegetarians only occasionally ate red meat.

29. Lightowler HJ, Davies GJ. The effect of self-selected dietary supplements on micronutrient intakes in vegans. *Proc Nutr Soc.* 1999;58;35A *Note:* Subjects were 11 males and 19 females.

30. Toohey ML, Harris MA, Williams D, Foster G, Schmidt WD, Melby CL. Cardiovascular disease risk factors are lower in African-American vegans compared to lacto-ovo vegetarians. *J Am Coll Nutr.* 1998;17:425–434.

31. Ball MJ, Bartlett MA. Dietary intake and iron status of Australian vegetarian women. *Am J Clin Nutr.* 1999;70:353–358. *Note:* Two of the 50 LOV were vegan; vegetarians consumed red meat no more than once a month and consumed fish or chicken no more than once a week.

32. Haddad EH, Berk LS, Kettering JD, Hubbard RW, Peters WR. Dietary intake and biochemical, hematologic, and immune status of vegans compared with nonvegetarians. *Am J Clin Nutr.* 1999;70 (suppl): 586S–593S.

33. Li D, Sinclair A, Wilson A, et al. Effect of dietary α-linolenic acid on thrombotic risk factors in vegetarian men. *Am J Clin Nutr.* 1999;69:878–882. *Note:* Vegetarian subjects were divided into two groups for study purposes. Only baseline data are reported here.

34. Leblanc JC, Yoon H, Kombadjian A, Verger P. Nutritional intakes of vegetarian populations in France. *Eur J Clin Nutr.* 2000;54:443–449. *Note:* Thirty-one of the 96 LOV ate fish or meat at least once a week; 11 were lacto vegetarians and 3 were ovo vegetarians. 13 of the 17 VEG ate fish once a week.

35. Lu SC, Wu WH, Lee CA, et al. LDL of Taiwanese vegetarians are less oxidizable than those of omnivores. *J Nutr.* 2000;130:1591–1596. *Note:* About one third of the LV were vegans.

36. Donaldson MS. Food and nutrient intake of Hallelujah vegetarians. *Nutr Food Sci.* 2001;31:293–303. *Note:* VEG subjects ate a mostly raw diet; 58% consumed some animal product during their week of food intake records.

37. Hung CJ, Huang PC, Lu SC, et al. Plasma homocysteine levels in Taiwanese vegetarians are higher than those of omnivores. *J Nutr.* 2002;132:152–158. *Note:* Six of the 45 LV were vegans.

38. Bissoli L, Di Francesco V, Ballarin A, et al. Effect of vegetarian diet on homocysteine levels. *Ann Nutr Metab.* 2002;46:73–79.

39. Davey GK, Spencer EA, Appleby PN, et al. EPIC-Oxford lifestyle characteristics and nutrient intakes in a cohort of 33883 meat-eaters and 31546 non-meat-eaters in the UK. *Public Health Nutr.* 2003; 6:259–268.

40. Huang YC, Chang SJ, Chiu YT, et al. The status of plasma homocysteine and related B-vitamins in healthy young vegetarians and nonvegetarians. *Eur J Nutr.* 2003;42:84–90. *Note:* LOV group includes 3 VEG, 18 LV, 16 LOV.

41. Waldmann A, Koschizke JW, Leitzmann C, Hahn A. Dietary intake and lifestyle factors of a vegan population in Germany: results from the German Vegan Study. *Eur J Clin Nutr.* 2003;57:947–955. *Note:* Ninety-eight subjects did not use animal products for 1 year prior to study; 56 subjects consumed small amounts of dairy products and eggs. The first listing for each gender is for strict vegans; the second listing is for those who consumed small amounts of dairy and eggs. Data exclude vitamin and mineral supplements.

42. Chiplonkar SA, Agte V, Tarwadik V, et al. Micronutrient deficiencies as predisposing factors for hypertension in lacto-vegetarian Indian adults. *J Am Coll Nutr.* 2004;23:239–247.

43. Cade JE, Burley VJ, Greenwood DC, et al. The UK Women's Cohort Study: comparisons of vegetarians, fish-eaters, and meat-eaters. *Public Health Nutr.* 2004;7:871–878. *Note:* Vegetarians ate meat or fish less than once a week.

44. Bedford JL, Barr SI. Diets and selected lifestyle practices of self-defined adult vegetarians from a population-based sample suggest they are more health conscious. *Int J Behav Nutr Phys Act.* 2005;2:4. *Note:* Seventy-five percent of those self-identified as vegetarian consumed fish and/or seafood, 58% consumed poultry; 22% consumed red meat.

45. Koebnick C, Garcia AL, Dagnelie PC, et al. Long-term consumption of a raw food diet is associated with favorable serum LDL cholesterol and triglycerides but also with elevated plasma homocysteine and low serum HDL cholesterol in humans. *J Nutr.* 2005;135:2372–2378. *Note:* Subjects ate a raw foods diet; no information provided on gender distribution in groups.

46. Waldmann A, Dorr B, Koschizke JW, et al. Dietary intake of vitamin B6 and concentration of vitamin B6 in blood samples of German vegans. *Public Health Nutr.* 2006;9:779–784. *Note:* Forty-three males and 50 females were VEG. Subjects are a subset of those in reference 41.

47. Sebekova K, Boor P, Valachovicova M, et al. Association of metabolic syndrome risk factors with selected markers of oxidative status and microinflammation in healthy omnivores and vegetarians. *Mol Nutr Food Res.* 2006;50:858–868. *Note:* Thirty males and 60 females were LOV; 19 males and 27 females were NV.

48. Majchrzak D, Singer I, Manner M, et al. B-vitamin status and concentrations of homocysteine in Austrian omnivores, vegetarians, and vegans. *Ann Nutr Metab.* 2006;50:485–491. *Note:* Ten males and 26 females were LOV; 21 males and 21 females were VEG; 11 males and 29 females were NV.

49. Haldar S, Rowland IR, Barnett RA, et al. Influence of habitual diet on antioxidant status: a study in a population of vegetarians and omnivores. *Eur J Clin Nutr.* 2007;61:1011–1022. *Note:* Vegetarian subjects ate flesh foods no more than six times a year. The vegetarian group included six vegans.

50. Karabudak E, Kiziltan G, Cigerim N. A comparison of some of the cardiovascular risk factors in vegetarian and omnivorous Turkish females. *J Hum Nutr Diet.* 2008;21:13–22. *Note:* Subjects include 9 LOV, 10 LV, and 7 occasional fish and/or chicken eaters.

51. Yen CE, Yen CH, Huang MC, et al. Dietary intake and nutritional status of vegetarian and omnivorous preschool children and their parents in Taiwan. *Nutr Res.* 2008;28:430–436. *Note:* Adult vegetarians consisted of 16 LOV, 2 ovo-vegetarians, 1 LV, 2 vegans. Four male adults and 17 females were vegetarian; 9 male adults and 19 females were NV. Children consisted of 18 LOV and 3 ovo-vegetarians. Fourteen male children and 7 female children were vegetarians; 15 male children and 13 female children were NV.

52. Nakamato K, Watanabe S, Kudo H, et al. Nutritional characteristics of middle-aged Japanese vegetarians. *J Atherosclero Throm.* 2008;15:122–129. *Note:* Nine men and 18 women were LOV; 11 men and 37 women in the vegetarian group occasionally ate chicken and meat.

Appendix K Fat-Soluble Vitamin Intake of Adult Vegetarians and Nonvegetarians

(Ref)/ year	Group[1]/ Gender/(N)	Country	Age	Kcal	Vitamin A[2]	Carotene[3]	Vitamin D[4]	Vitamin E[5]	Vitamin K (μg)
(1) 1954	LOV M (15)	United States	55	3020	15400				
	VEG M (14)		51	3260	25570				
	NV M (15)		57	3720	14420				
	LOV F (15)		58	2450	13470				
	VEG F (11)		49	2400	19510				
	NV F (15)		57	2690	13730				
(2) 1963	LOV F (26)	Australia	18–40	1980	6800				
	NV F (25)		18–40	2115	9530				
(3) 1978	LOV F (42)	United States	57	1600	7601				
	NV F (36)		59	1579	6528				
(4) 1980	LOV M/F (57)	United States	18–40	2270	14678				
	LV M/F (14)		18–40	1830	33378				
	VEG M/F (8)		18–40	1665	19246				
	NV F (41)		18–40	2072	8069				
(5) 1980	LOV M (15)	United States	28	2624	13802				
	NV M (25)		27	2684	8189				
	LOV F (13)		26	2174	11516				
	NV F (24)		26	1859	5937				
(6) 1981	LOV F (5)	United States	22	1329	12930		92	7.4	
(7) 1983	LOV M (20)	United States	36	2324	1794				
	NV M (17)		44	2652	1806				
	LOV F (31)		31	1776	1646				
	NV F (36)		36	1754	1824				
(8) 1984	LOV M (25)	United States	39–65	2128	7249				
	VEG M (9)		39–65	2259	18115				
	NV M (25)		39–65	2335	6683				
	LOV F (25)		39–65	1615	6212				
	VEG F (9)		39–65	1497	7332				
	NV F (25)		39–65	1821	4937				

(Appendix K continued)

Appendix K Fat-Soluble Vitamin Intake of Adult Vegetarians and Nonvegetarians

(Ref)/year	Group/Gender/(N)	Country	Age	Kcal	Vitamin A²	Carotene³	Vitamin D⁴	Vitamin E⁵	Vitamin K (µg)
(9) 1986	LOV M (14)	Canada	28	2401	1606				
	NV M (14)		21	2809	1147				
	LOV F (22)		26	1760	994				
	NV F (18)		22	2097	1197				
(10) 1986	LOV M (14)	South Africa	18–40	2717	10554				
	NV M (10)		18–40	3167	8009				
	NV F (19)		18–40	1916	9114				
	NV F (12)		18–40	1890	6667				
(11) 1987	VEG M (11)	Great Britain	32	2643	204	2446		11.3	
	NV M (11)		31	2381	470	1439		6.9	
	VEG F (11)		28	1881	225	4725		12.0	
	NV F (11)		24	1833	354	3801		6.3	
(12) 1988	LOV F (88)	United States	73	1533	922				
	NV F (278)		79	1633	875				
(13) 1989	LOV M (11)	France	37	2100	1900	8.0	1.1	14	
	NV M (33)		40	2600	1400	3.6	2.6	13	
	LOV F (26)		26	1700	1500	6.8	0.9	15	
	NV F (36)		36	1800	1400	3.9	1.8	10	
(14) 1989	LOV F (23)	United States	72	1452	11081		89	6.5	
	NV F (14)		71	1363	7915		106	4.3	
(15) 1990	LOV M (18)	Netherlands	65–97	1960	1270				
	NV M		65+	2412	1070				
	LOV F (26)		65–97	1667	1270				
	NV F		65+	1879	950				
(16) 1991	LOV F (23)	United States	35	1939	3838		104	9.0	275
	NV F (36)		36	1835	1306		127	4.1	205
(17) 1991	LOV F (34)	United States	36	1819	3760		5.3		
	NV F (41)		29	1700	2980		5.6		

	Group (n)	Country	Age					
(18) 1991	LOV M/F (79)	United States	18–30	2800	24674			
	NV M/F (4821)	States	18–30	2980	10549			
(19) 1992	LOV F (28)	United States	63	1652	2842			
	NV F (28)	States	63	1657	3015			
(20) 1992	VEG M (10)	Great Britain	32	2548				14.0
	NV M (10)		33	2524				6.0
	VEG F (10)		32	2214				11.0
	NV F (10)		32	1976				5.0
(21) 1993	LOV M (16)[6]	Great Britain	21–40	2238	538	6010	3.0	15.8
	VEG M (18)[6]		21–40	2190	181	6710	1.9	23.1
	NV M (386)[7]		21–40	2452	1735	2730	4.2	12.4
	LOV F (36)[6]		21–40	1826	374	5420	2.2	16.1
	VEG F (20)[6]		21–40	1750	172	4280	1.6	16.5
	NV F (377)[7]		21–40	1733	1722	2530	3.3	8.7
(22) 1993	LV M/F (14)	Finland	44	2029			2.2[8]	
	VEG M/F (10)		42	1927			0.3[8]	
	NV M/F (12)		33	1778			4.5[8]	
(23) 1994	LOV M/F (50)[9]	New Zealand	27	2272	5.4	5400	2.2	
	VEG F (5)		27	1842	5.2	5200	1.9	
	NV M/F (50)		27	2608	4.7	4700	3.4	
(24) 1998	B-LOV M (49)	United States	50	2356	2052		2.3	33.5
	B-VEG M (14)		46	1869	1966		1.5	28.5
	B-LOV F (94)		52	1922	1964		1.7	28.0
	B-VEG F (31)		51	1865	2934		0.6	33.0
(25) 1999	VEG M/F (30)[6]	Great Britain	39	NI	734		1.1	
(26) 1999	VEG M (10)[6]	United States	20–60	2230	2041			21
	NV M (10)[6]		20–60	2170	1200			21
	VEG F (15)[6]		20–60	1702	2430			19
	NV F (10)[6]		20–60	1978	1475			25
(27) 1999	LOV M (10)	Australia	20–50	2143	3704			
	LOV M (10)		20–50	2877	6017			

(Appendix K continued)

Appendix K Fat-Soluble Vitamin Intake of Adult Vegetarians and Nonvegetarians

(Ref)/year	Group[1]/Gender/(N)	Country	Age	Kcal	Vitamin A[2]	Carotene[3]	Vitamin D[4]	Vitamin E[5]	Vitamin K (μg)
(28) 2000	LV F (6)	Finland	33	NI			0.7		
	VEG F (6)		37	NI			0.09		
	NV F (16)		33	NI			4.0		
(29) 2000	LV F (28)	Taiwan	38.2	1333				5.6	
	NV F (25)		40.4	1619				7.2	
	LV M (21)		37.7	2000				7.0	
	NV M (21)		38.3	2000				5.7	
	LV F (51)		36.6	1524				5.7	
	NV F (53)		36.9	1738				5.8	
(30) 2001	VEG M (54)	United States	57	1830	8110	4080	0.46	17.0	406
	VEG F (87)		53	1460	6740	3390	0.28	14.9	326
(31) 2003	LOV M (3748)	United Kingdom	39	2090	306		1.56	13.7	
	VEG M (770)		35	1907	74.2		0.88	16.1	
	NV M (6951)		51	2186	740		3.39	11.8	
	LOV F (12347)		35	1810	277		1.51	11.6	
	VEG F (1342)		32	1660	76.6		0.88	14.0	
	NV F (22962)		48	1910	654		3.32	10.7	
(32) 2003	VEG M (48)	Germany	42.4	2381	2000		0.78	31.8	
	VEG M (19)		45.2	2186	1940		0.89	23.6	
	VEG F (50)		42.4	1721	1820		0.50	19.8	
	VEG F (37)		44.5	1617	2090		0.56	19.0	
(33) 2004	LV F (30)	India	49.5	1618		1327			
	LV F htn (26)		48.7	1737		1194			
	LV M (85)		46.1	2166		1234			
	LV M htn (83)		47.1	2260		1082			
(34) 2004	LOV F (6478)	United Kingdom	49	2303	1075				
	NV F (24738)		54	2370	1318				
(35) 2005	VEG M/F (18)	United States	54.2	1285–2432			16		
	NV M/F (18)		NI	1976–3537			348		

Ref / Year	Group	Country	Age						
(36) 2005	LOV M (31)	United States	19–84[10]	2605	1772				
	NV M (869)			2605	1314				
	LOV F (75)			1840	1208				
	NV F (842)			1793	1186				
(37) 2006	LOV M/F (90)	Slovak Republic	37.7	1945		6200			
	NV M/F (46)		37.1	2438		4800			
(38) 2007	LOV M (11)	Ireland	37.8	2486	1109	4300		11.1	
	NV M (17)		42.2	2366	687	2200		7.5	
	LOV F (20)		33.8	1888	850	3200		8.2	
	NV F (41)		36.6	1936	798	2500		6.8	
(39) 2008	LO/LSV F (26)	Turkey	29.0	1832	1380			15.3	
	NV F (26)		27.4	1849	1321			14.4	
(40) 2008	LOV M/F (21)	Taiwan	34.8	1884	4149.8			7.9	
	NV M/F (28)		35.9	1944	2130.1			8.3	
(41) 2008	LO/SV M (20)	Japan	45.2	1983	966			11.0	355
	NV M (32)		44.2	1843	877			8.0	204
	LO/SVF (50)		45.9	1675	876			9.1	246
(42) 2009	LOV W M/F (93)	United States	63				351[6]		
	LOV B M/F (43)		58.3				403[6]		
	NV W M/F (88)		63				375[6]		
	NV B M/F (103)		58.3				326[6]		

Notes: [1]Abbreviations: LV, lacto vegetarian; LOV, lacto-ovo vegetarian; VEG, vegan; NV, nonvegetarian; SV, eats chicken and/or fish; htn, subjects identified as having hypertension; NI, not indicated; B, black; W, white.

[2]Vitamin A as IU for references 1–6, 10, and 14. Vitamin A as RE for references 7, 9, 12, 13, 15, 16, 19, 30, 32, 36, and 38. Vitamin A as µg for references 11, 17, 21, 24, 31, 34, 39, 40, and 41. No information was provided for reference 18.

[3]Carotene as µg carotene for references 11, 21, 23, and 38, and as µg β-carotene for references 18, 27, 30, 33, and 37.

[4]Vitamin D as µg for references 13, 16, 17, 21, 22, 24, 25, 28, 30–32, and 41 and as IU for references 6, 13, 35, and 42.

[5]Vitamin E as mg for references 6, 11, 16, 20, 24, 30–32, 38, 39, 40, and 41, as mg RRR-α-tocopherol (represented as the sum of the weight of RRR-α-tocopherol plus the weights of other tocopherols or tocotrienols after their equivalency as RRR-α-tocopherol), reference 14 and 29 as mg of RRR-α-tocopherol, reference 26 as tocopherol equivalents.

[6]Data include use of supplements.

[7]Values for NV were from a separate nationwide survey.

[8]Vitamin D values were estimated from figure in reference.

[9]Values of LOV include data for the VEG that were also listed separately.

[10]Age range of all subjects.

ANNOTATED REFERENCES APPENDIX K

1. Hardinge MG, Stare FJ. Nutritional studies of vegetarians. *Am J Clin Nutr.* 1954;2:73–82.
2. Hitchcock NE, English RM. A comparison of food consumption in lacto-ovo vegetarians and nonvegetarians. *Food Nutr Notes Rev.* 1963;20:141–146.
3. Mason RL, Kunkel ME, Ann Davis T, Beauchene RE. Nutrient intakes of vegetarian and nonvegetarian women. *Tenn Farm Home Science.* 1978;1:18–20.
4. Freeland-Graves JH, Bodzy PW, Eppright MA. Zinc status of vegetarians. *J Am Diet Assoc.* 1980;77:655–661.
5. Taber LAL, Cook RA. Dietary and anthropometric assessment of adult omnivores, fish-eaters, and lacto-ovo vegetarians. *J Am Diet Assoc.* 1980;76:21–29.
6. King JC, Stein JC, Doyle M. Effect of vegetarianism on the zinc status of pregnant women. *Am J Clin Nutr.* 1981;34:1049–1055.
7. Shultz TD, Leklem JE. Dietary status of Seventh-day Adventists and nonvegetarians. *J Am Diet Assoc.* 1983;83:27–33.
8. Calkins BM, Whittaker DJ, Nair PP, Rider AA, Turjman N. Diet, nutrition intake, and metabolism in populations at high and low risk for colon cancer. *Am J Clin Nutr.* 1984;40:896–905.
9. Locong A. Nutritional status and dietary intake of a selected sample of young adult vegetarians. *Can Diet Assoc J.* 1986;47:101–106.
10. Faber M, Gouws E, Benadé AJS, Labadarios D. Anthropometric measurements, dietary intake and biochemical data of South African lacto-ovo vegetarians. *S Afr Med J.* 1986;69:733–738.
11. Sanders TAB, Key TJA. Blood pressure, plasma renin activity and aldosterone concentrations in vegans and omnivores. *Human Nutr: Appl Nutr.* 1987;41A:204–211.
12. Tylavsky FA, Anderson JJB. Dietary factors in bone health of elderly lacto-ovo vegetarian and omnivorous women. *Am J Clin Nutr.* 1988;48:842–849.
13. Millet P, Guilland JC, Fuchs F, Klepping J. Nutrient intake and vitamin status of healthy French vegetarians and nonvegetarians. *Am J Clin Nutr.* 1989;50:718–722.
14. Nieman DC, Underwood BC, Sherman KM, et al. Dietary status of Seventh-day Adventist vegetarian and nonvegetarian elderly women. *J Am Diet Assoc.* 1989;89:1763–1769.
15. Brants Ham, Löwik MRH, Westenbrink S, Hulshof KFAM, Kistemaker C. Adequacy of a vegetarian diet at old age (Dutch Nutrition Surveillance System). *J Am College Nutr.* 1990;9:292–302.
16. Lloyd T, Schaeffer JM, Walker MA, Demers L. Urinary hormonal concentrations and spinal bone densities of premenopausal vegetarian and nonvegetarian women. *Am J Clin Nutr.* 1991;54:1005–1010.
17. Pedersen AB, Bartholomew MJ, Dolence LA, Aljadir LP, Netteburg KL, Lloyd T. Menstrual differences due to vegetarian and nonvegetarian diets. *Am J Clin Nutr.* 1991;53:879–885.
18. Slattery ML, Jacobs DR, Hilner JE, et al. Meat consumption and its association with other diet and health factors in young adults: The CARDIA study. *Am J Clin Nutr.* 1991;54:930–935.
19. Tesar R, Notelovitz M, Shim E, Kauwell G, Brown J. Axial and peripheral bone density and nutrient intakes of postmenopausal vegetarian and omnivorous women. *Am J Clin Nutr.* 1992;56:699–704.
20. Sanders TAB, Roshanai F. Platelet phospholipid fatty acid composition and function in vegans compared with age- and sex-matched omnivore controls. *Eur J Clin Nutr.* 1992;46:823–831.
21. Draper A, Lewis J, Malhotra N, Wheeler E. The energy and nutrient intakes of different types of vegetarian: a case for supplements. *Br J Nutr.* 1993;69:3–19.
22. Lamberg-Allardt C, Kärkkäinen M, Seppänen R, Biström H. Low serum 25-hydroxyvitamin D concentrations and secondary hyperparathyroidism in middle-aged white strict vegetarians. *Am J Clin Nutr.* 1993;58:684–689.
23. Alexander D, Ball MJ, Mann J. Nutrient intake and haematological status of vegetarians and age-sex matched omnivores. *Eur J Clin Nutr.* 1994;48:538–546.
24. Toohey ML, Harris MA, Williams D, Foster G, Schmidt WD, Melby CL. Cardiovascular disease risk factors are lower in African-American vegans compared to lacto-ovo vegetarians. *J Am Coll Nutr.* 1998;17:425–434.
25. Lightowler HJ, Davies GJ. The effect of self-selected dietary supplements on micronutrient intakes in vegans. *Proc Nutr Soc.* 1999;58;35A. *Note:* Subjects were 11 males and 19 females.

26. Haddad EH, Berk LS, Kettering JD, Hubbard RW, Peters WR. Dietary intake and biochemical, hematologic, and immune status of vegans compared with nonvegetarians. *Am J Clin Nutr.* 1999;70 (suppl):586S–593S.

27. Li D, Sinclair A, Wilson A, et al. Effect of dietary α-linolenic acid on thrombotic risk factors in vegetarian men. *Am J Clin Nutr.* 1999;69:878–882. *Note:* Vegetarian subjects were divided into two groups for study purposes. Only baseline data are reported here.

28. Outila TA, Karkkainen MUM, Seppanen RH, Lamberg-Allardt JE. Dietary intake of vitamin D in premenopausal healthy vegans was insufficient to maintain concentrations of serum 25-hydroxyvitamin D and intact parathyroid hormone within normal ranges during the winter in Finland. *J Am Diet Assoc.* 2000;100:434–441.

29. Lu S-C, Wu W-H, Lee C-A, et al. LDL of Taiwanese vegetarians are less oxidizable than those of omnivores. *J Nutr.* 2000;130:1591–1596. *Note:* About one third of the LV were vegans.

30. Donaldson MS. Food and nutrient intake of Hallelujah vegetarians. *Nutr Food Sci.* 2001;31:293–303. *Note:* VEG subjects ate a mostly raw diet; 58% consumed some animal product during their week of food intake records.

31. Davey GK, Spencer EA, Appleby PN, et al. EPIC-Oxford lifestyle characteristics and nutrient intakes in a cohort of 33,883 meat-eaters and 31,546 non meat-eaters in the UK. *Public Health Nutr.* 2003;6:259–268.

32. Waldmann A, Koschizke JW, Leitzmann C, Hahn A. Dietary intake and lifestyle factors of a vegan population in Germany: results from the German Vegan Study. *Eur J Clin Nutr.* 2003;57:947–955. *Note:* Ninety-eight subjects did not use animal products for 1 year prior to study; 56 subjects consumed small amounts of dairy products and eggs. The first listing for each gender is for strict vegans; the second listing is for those who consumed small amounts of dairy and eggs. Data exclude vitamin and mineral supplements.

33. Chiplonkar SA, Agte V, Tarwadik V, et al. Micronutrient deficiencies as predisposing factors for hypertension in lacto-vegetarian Indian adults. *J Am Coll Nutr.* 2004;23:239–247.

34. Cade JE, Burley VJ, Greenwood DC, et al. The UK Women's Cohort Study: comparisons of vegetarians, fish-eaters, and meat-eaters. *Public Health Nutr.* 2004;7:871–878. *Note:* Vegetarians ate meat or fish less than once a week.

35. Fontana L, Shew JL, Holloszy JO, et al. Low bone mass in subjects on a long-term raw vegetarian diet. *Arch Intern Med.* 2005;165:684–689. *Note:* Study subjects ate a raw foods diet. Seven males and 11 females were VEG; 7 males and 11 females were NV.

36. Bedford JL, Barr SI. Diets and selected lifestyle practices of self-defined adult vegetarians from a population-based sample suggest they are more health conscious. *Int J Behav Nutr Phys Act.* 2005;2:4. *Note:* Seventy-five percent of those self-identified as vegetarian consumed fish and/or seafood, 58% consumed poultry; 22% consumed red meat.

37. Sebekova K, Boor P, Valachovicova M, et al. Association of metabolic syndrome risk factors with selected markers of oxidative status and microinflammation in healthy omnivores and vegetarians. *Mol Nutr Food Res.* 2006;50:858–868. *Note:* Thirty males and 60 females were LOV; 19 males and 27 females were NV.

38. Haldar S, Rowland IR, Barnett RA, et al. Influence of habitual diet on antioxidant status: a study in a population of vegetarians and omnivores. *Eur J Clin Nutr.* 2007;61:1011–1022. *Note:* Vegetarian subjects ate flesh foods no more than six times a year. The vegetarian group included six vegans.

39. Karabudak E, Kiziltan G, Cigerim N. A comparison of some of the cardiovascular risk factors in vegetarian and omnivorous Turkish females. *J Hum Nutr Diet.* 2008;21:13–22. *Note:* Subjects include 9 LOV, 10 LV, and 7 occasional fish and/or chicken eaters.

40. Yen CE, Yen CH, Huang MC, et al. Dietary intake and nutritional status of vegetarian and omnivorous preschool children and their parents in Taiwan. *Nutr Res.* 2008;28:430–436. *Note:* Adult vegetarians consisted of 16 LOV, 2 ovo-vegetarians, 1 LV, 2 vegans. Four male adults and 17 females were vegetarian; 9 male adults and 19 females were NV. Children consisted of 18 LOV and 3 ovo-vegetarians. Fourteen male children and 7 female children were vegetarians; 15 male children and 13 female children were NV.

41. Nakamato K, Watanabe S, Kudo H, et al. Nutritional characteristics of middle-aged Japanese vegetarians. *J Atherosclero Throm.* 2008;15:122–129. *Note:* Nine men and 18 women were LOV; 11 men and 37 women in the vegetarian group occasionally ate chicken and meat.

42. Chan J, Jaceldo-Siegl K, Fraser GE. Serum 25-hydroxyvitamin D status of vegetarians, partial vegetarians, and non-vegetarians: The Adventist Health Study 2. *Am J Clin Nutr.* 2009;89(suppl):1686S–1692S. *Note:* Gender distribution of subjects not indicated.

Appendix L Fiber, Cholesterol, and Macronutrient Intakes of Vegetarian and Nonvegetarian School-Aged Children and Teenagers

(Ref)/ year	Group/ Gender(N)	Country	Age (years)	SDA/ NSDA[2]	Kcal[3]	Protein[3] % Kcal	Fat[3] % Kcal	CHO[3] % Kcal	SF (g)	PUFA or LA (g)	PUFA: SF[4]	Cholesterol (mg)	Fiber[5]
(1) 1954	LOV F (15)	United States	14.0	NSDA	3030	13.2			39.3	13.6	0.35	408	12.9
	NV F (15)		14.0		4100	14.7			75.4	18.5	0.25	829	10.6
	LOV M (15)		15.5		4450	12.7			56.4	19.0	0.34	599	17.8
	NV M (15)		15.5		5350	13.4			95.4	25.0	0.26	1046	12.2
(2) 1982	LOV M/F (15)[6]	Great Britain	10–16	NSDA	1900								31.1
	NV M/F (12)[6]		10–16		1898								16.2
(3) 1984	LOV M/F (34)	United States	15–17	SDA	1947	15.4	35.7	48.9	21.1	18.3	0.87	192	5.1
	NV M/F[7]		13–15	NSDA	2302	13.9	37.9	45.7	41.0	14.0	0.34	295	
(4) 1989	LOV F (9)	United States	11.4	SDA	1650	13.7	31.5	57.6				183	4.5
	NV F (10)		11.1	NSDA	2106	14.8	38.5	48.6				273	4.0
	LOV M (8)		11.8	SDA	2316	11.6	27.6	63.4				188	5.0
	NV M (12)		11.3	NSDA	2074	16.0	35.6	49.8				278	4.0
(5) 1992	LOV F (32)	United States	16.2	SDA	1895	12.5	33.3				0.65	302	3.2
	NV F (35)		16.7	NSDA	1742	14.9	39.3				0.43	204	2.2
(6) 1992	VEG M/F (18)	Great Britain	9.5	NSDA	1720	12.4	31.5	59.2	9.2	16.8	1.83		37.5
	NV M/F (194)[8]		7–12	NSDA	1700	12.3	37.0	54.0					15.6
(7) 1995	LOV F (78)	Canada	18	NSDA	1663	12.3							14.0
	NV F (29)		18	NSDA	1688	14.5							10.0
(8) 1996	LOV F (78)	Canada	17.7	NSDA	1705	12	33	58					
	NV F (29)		18.2		1735	13	32	55					
(9) 1996	LOV M/F (50)	Great Britain	9.1	NSDA	1824	11.1	36.4	52.5	27.2	16.2	0.7	132	
	NV M/F (50)		9.4		1920	12.6	36.5	51.0	27.1	14.1	0.5	184	
(10) 1997	LOV F (88)	Canada	14–20	NSDA	1783	11.9	31.8	58.5					14.6
	NV F (111)		14–20		1685	13.6	31.0	55.9					10.0
(11) 1999	LOV M (9)	Belgium	6–11	NI	1517								
	LOV F (9)		6–9		1369								
	LOV M (6)		12–17		1907								
	LOV F (10)		10–15		1397								

Ref / Year	Group	Country	Type										
(12) 2000	LOV M/F (25)	Great		1.5–<3	1040	12.0	35.6	52.4	19.0	5.7	0.3	91	6.4
	NV M/F (668)	Britain		1.5–<3	1100	13.3	36.3	50.4	20.4	5.4	0.3	127	5.7
	LOV M/F (19)			3–4.5	1162	11.4	33.6	55.0	19.2	6.7	0.3	116	7.1
	NV M/F (639)			3–4.5	1238	12.6	35.6	51.8	21.6	6.6	0.3	137	6.6
(13) 2001	LOV (5M/5F)	Hong	NSDA	5.9	1376	12.3	23.2	64.8	9.8	8.7	1.0	116	5.8
	LOV (12M/12F)	Kong		9.3	1423	13.7	23.1	62.2	10.9	10.9	1.0	154	8.5
	LOV (7M/7F)			12.3	1991	11.8	19.6	68.8	12.2	23.9	1.1	135	8.7
(14) 2002	LOV M/F (262)	United	NSDA	14.9	1973	13.7	26.9	60.9	20.4	11.8	0.6	186	18.8
	NV M/F (4259)	States		14.9	2092	14.3	30.1	56.4	24.9	13.2	0.5	222	16.1
(15) 2002	VEG M (15)	Sweden	NSDA	17.5	2904	10	27	63	25	21	0.8	2	44
	NV M (15)			17.5	3143	15	29	55	45	12	0.3	326	25
	VEG F (15)			17.5	2126	10	24	66	15	15	1.0	2	34
	NV F (15)			17.5	2267	14	29	56	34	8.6	0.3	230	21
(16) 2006	LOV M/F (32)	Poland	NI	6.5	1426	11.9	32.3	55.8					
(17) 2007	LOV M/F (50)	Poland	NI	2–10	1468	13.1	30.1	56.2					
	NV M/F (50)			2–10	1591	14.2	30.5	55.3					
(18) 2008	LOV M/F (21)	Taiwan	NI	5.2	1647	10.5	34.7	55.3					3.7
	NV M/F (28)			5.0	1698	12.8	38.8	48.9					2.8
(19) 2010	LV F (630)	India	NSDA	12.2	1373	8.8							

Notes: [1]Abbreviations: LOV, lacto-ovo vegetarian; VEG, vegan; NV, nonvegetarian; CHO, carbohydrate; SF, saturated fat; PUFA, polyunsaturated fat; and LA, linoleic acid.

[2]SDA indicates the vegetarians were specifically identified as Seventh-day Adventists, whereas NSDA indicates the vegetarians were not exclusively SDAs, although some SDAs may have been included in the vegetarian group.

[3]When energy intake was listed as kilojoules, a factor of 4.2 was used to convert kilojoules into kilocalories. Values for protein, fat, and carbohydrate are the percentage of calories contributed by each nutrient. The percentage of calories contributed by protein, fat, and carbohydrate was determined by multiplying the number of grams consumed per day, by 4, 9, and 4 calories per gram, respectively, and then dividing the calories provided by each macronutrient by the total number of calories listed in the reference. In some cases, this led to differences between the calculated percentage of calories contributed by each nutrient and the percentage listed in the reference and often resulted in the total percentage not equaling 100. In cases where only the percentage of calories for each nutrient was listed and not grams, those percentages were used.

(Appendix L continued)

[4]PUFA (polyunsaturated fat): Saturated fat ratios represent values as listed in the reference or were determined by dividing the number of grams of PUFA or LA (linoleic acid) by the number of grams of saturated fat.

[5]Values for fiber are listed as either grams of dietary fiber (references 2, 6, 10, 11, 14, 15, 18), crude fiber (references 1, 3–5, 13), or nonstarch polysaccharide (references 7 and 12). Typically, 1 g of crude fiber represents between 3 and 4 g of dietary fiber.

[6]The entire study initially consisted of 12 males and 22 females. Each nonvegetarian was matched for age, sex, race, and socioeconomic status to a vegetarian.

[7]Data for nonvegetarians are from a separate study of adolescents residing in Cincinnati, Ohio.

[8]Data for nonvegetarians are from a separate survey of British children presented in the reference.

ANNOTATED REFERENCES APPENDIX L

1. Hardinge MG, Stare FJ. Nutritional studies of vegetarians. Nutritional, physcial, and laboratory studies. *Am J Clin Nutr.* 1954;2:73–82.
2. Treuherz J. Possible inter-relationship between zinc and dietary fibre in a group of lacto-ovo vegetarian adolescents. *J Plant Foods.* 1982;4:89–95.
3. Cooper R, Allen A, Goldberg R, et al. Seventh-Day Adventist adolescents—life-style patterns and cardiovascular risk factors. *West J Med.* 1984;140:471–477.
4. Tayter M, Stanek KL. Anthropometric and dietary assessment of omnivore and lacto-ovo vegetarian children. *J Am Diet Assoc.* 1989;89:1861–1863.
5. Persky VW, Chatterton RT, Van Horn LV, Grant MD, Langenberg P, Marvin J. Hormone levels in vegetarian and nonvegetarian teenage girls: potential implications for breast cancer risk. *Cancer Res.* 1992;50:578–583.
6. Sanders TAB, Manning J. The growth and development of vegan children. *J Human Nutr Diet.* 1992;5:11–21.
7. Donovan UM, Gibson RS. Iron and zinc status of young women aged 14 to 19 years consuming vegetarian and omnivorous diets. *J Am Coll Nutr.* 1995;14:463–472.
8. Donovan UM, Gibson RS. Dietary intakes of adolescent females consuming vegetarian, semi-vegetarian, and omnivorous diets. *J Adol Health.* 1996;18:292–300. *Note:* Two adolescents in the LOV group did not use dairy products.
9. Nathan I, Hackett AF, Kirby S. The dietary intake of a group of vegetarian children aged 7–11 years compared with matched omnivores. *Br J Nutr.* 1996;75:533–544. *Note:* Two vegetarians ate fish; mean consumption was 10.3 g/person/d. Each group had 29 females and 21 males.
10. Houghton LA, Green TJ, Donovan UM, Gibson RS, Stephen AM, O'Connor DL. Association between dietary fiber intake and the folate status of a group of female adolescents. *Am J Clin Nutr.* 1997;66:1414–1421.
11. Hebbelinck M, Clarys P, DeMalsche A. Growth, development, and physical fitness of Flemish vegetarian children, adolescents, and young adults. *Am J Clin Nutr.* 1999;70 (suppl):579S–585S.
12. Thane CW, Bates CJ. Dietary intakes and nutrient status of vegetarian preschool children from a British national survey. *J Hum Nutr Dietet.* 2000;13:149–162. *Note:* Subjects identified as "vegetarians" appear to have consumed fish "although generally in smaller amounts than did omnivores."
13. Leung SS, Lee RH, Sung RY, et al. Growth and nutrition of Chinese vegetarian children in Hong Kong. *J Paediatr Child Health.* 2001;37:247–253.
14. Perry CL, McGuire MT, Neumark-Sztainer D, Story M. Adolescent vegetarians. How well do their dietary patterns meet the Healthy People 2010 objectives? *Arch Pediatr Adolesc Med.* 2002;156:431–437. *Note:* A total of 62% of vegetarians reported eating chicken and/or fish; 32% ate eggs and/or dairy products but not chicken or fish; 6% were vegan.
15. Larsson CL, Johansson GK. Dietary intake and nutritional status of young vegans and omnivores in Sweden. *Am J Clin Nutr.* 2002;76:100–106.
16. Ambroszkiewicz J, Klemarczyk W, Chelchowska M, et al. Serum homocysteine, folate, vitamin B12 and total antioxidant status in vegetarian children. *Adv Med Sci.* 2006;51:265–268. *Note:* Sample includes 21 LOV, 1 LV, 5 OV, 5 VEG. Eighteen males and 14 females were in the vegetarian group.
17. Ambroszkiewicz J, Klemarczyk W, Gajewska J, et al. Serum concentration of biochemical bone turnover markers in vegetarian children. *Adv Med Sci.* 2007;52:279–282. *Note:* Sample includes 28 LOV, 4 LV, 5 OV, 13 VEG. Twenty-seven males and 23 females were vegetarian; 25 males and 25 females were NV.
18. Yen CE, Yen CH, Huang MC, et al. Dietary intake and nutritional status of vegetarian and omnivorous preschool children and their parents in Taiwan. *Nutr Res.* 2008;28:430–436. *Note:* Adult vegetarians consisted of 16 LOV, 2 ovo-vegetarians, 1 LV, 2 vegans. Four male adults and 17 females were vegetarian; 9 male adults and 19 females were NV. Children consisted of 18 LOV and 3 ovo-vegetarians. Fourteen male children and 7 female children were vegetarians; 15 male children and 13 female children were NV.
19. Tupe R, Chiplonkar SA. Diet patterns of lactovegetarian adolescent girls: need for devising recipes with high zinc bioavailability. *Nutrition.* 2010;26:390–398.

Appendix M Water-Soluble Vitamin Intake of Vegetarian and Nonvegetarian School-Aged Children and Teenagers

(Ref)/year	Group[1]/Gender/(N)	Country	Age	Kcal[2]	Vit. C (mg)	Thiamin (mg)	Riboflavin (mg)	Niacin (mg)	Vit. B_6 (mg)	Folate (µg)	Biotin (µg)	Vit. B_{12} (µg)
(1) 1954	LOV F (15)	United States	14.0	3030	185	1.7	2.6	13.0				
	NV F (15)	States	14.0	4100	210	1.5	2.1	18.0				
	LOV M (15)		15.5	4450	210	2.3	2.8	19.0				
	NV M (15)		15.5	5350	185	2.0	2.8	23.0				
(2) 1984	LOV M/F (34)	United States	15–17	1947	126	1.4	2.1	19.0				
(3) 1989	LOV F (9)	United States	11.4	1650	76	1.1	1.7	9.2				
	NV F (10)	States	11.1	2106	55	1.3	1.8	17.5				
	LOV M (8)		11.8	2316	125	1.5	3.1	13.2				
	NV M (12)		11.3	2074	92	1.5	2.7	18.8				
(4) 1992	LOV F (32)	United States	16.2	1895	132	1.6	2.1	13.8				
	NV F (35)	States	16.7	1742	105	1.2	1.6	15.9				
(5) 1992	VEG M/F (18)	Great	9.5	1720	93	1.7	1.7	24.1	1.4	251	18.7	2.2
	NV M/F (194)[3]	Britain	7–12	1700	65	1.1	1.4	24.0	1.1	131	13.4	2.8
(6) 1995	LOV F (78)	Canada	18	1663	119							
	NV F (29)		18	1688	85							
(7) 1996	LOV F (78)	Canada	17.7	1705	144	1.3	1.3	21.5[4]				
	NV F (29)		18.2	1735	110	1.4	1.7	27.3[4]				
(8) 1996	LOV M/F (50)	Great	9.1	1824	66	1.7	1.7	14.9		238		2.5
	NV M/F (50)	Britain	9.4	1920	64	1.4	1.6	16.9		214		3.4
(9) 1997	LOV F (88)	Canada	14–20	1783	122	1.3	1.3			228		
	NV F (111)		14–20	1685	104	1.3	1.4			164		
(10) 2000	LOV M/F (25)	Great	1.5–<3	1040	51	0.7	1.1	13.2				2.3
	NV M/F (668)	Britain	1.5–<3	1100	38	0.8	1.2	15.7				2.6
	LOV M/F (19)		3–4.5	1162	34	0.8	1.3	15.6				2.3
	NV M/F (639)		3–4.5	1238	40	0.9	1.2	17.7				2.6

	Country	Group									
(11) 2001	Hong Kong	LOV (5M/5F)	5.9	1376	64.6	0.5	0.7	5.7			
		LOV (12M/12F)	9.3	1423	67.7	0.5	0.7	5.9			
		LOV (7M/7F)	12.3	1991	84.0	0.7	0.7	8.2			
(12) 2002	United States	LOV M/F (262)	14.9	1973	157				1.7	349	6.3
		NV M/F (4259)	14.9	2092	149				1.7	308	7.2
(13) 2002	Sweden	VEG M (15)	17.5	2904	203	1.9	1.2	34	2.7	551	0.1
		NV M (15)	17.5	3143	96	2.2	2.8	48	2.8	263	5.9
		VEG F (15)	17.5	2126	178	1.5	1.1	26	2.1	473	0
		NV F (15)	17.5	2267	104	1.5	1.9	32	2.0	226	5.0
(14) 2006	Poland	LOV M/F (32)	6.5	1426						195.7	1.6
(15) 2008	Taiwan	LOV M/F (21)	5.2	1647	212.6	1.5	1.0				
		NV M/F (28)	5.0	1698	63.2	0.7	1.2				
(16) 2009	New Zealand	LV F (6)	9–11								1.79
		NV F (6)	9–11								2.53

Notes: [1]Abbreviations: LOV, lacto-ovo vegetarian; VEG, vegan; NV, nonvegetarian.

[2]When energy intake was listed as kilojoules, a factor of 4.2 was used to convert kilojoules into kilocalories.

[3]Values for NV are from a separate survey of British children presented in the reference.

[4]Niacin as niacin equivalents (NE). The convention is to consider 60 mg of tryptophan as equivalent to 1 mg of niacin.

ANNOTATED REFERENCES APPENDIX M

1. Hardinge MG, Stare FJ. Nutritional studies of vegetarians. 1. Nutritional, physical, and laboratory studies. *J Clin Nutr.* 1954;2:73–82.
2. Cooper R, Allen A, Goldberg R, Trevisan M, Van Horn L, Liu K, Steinhauer M, Rubenstein A, Stamler J. Seventh-day Adventist adolescents—life-style patterns and cardiovascular risk factors. *West J Med.* 1984;140:471–477.
3. Tayter M, Stanek KL. Anthropometric and dietary assessment of omnivore and lacto-ovo vegetarian children. *J Am Diet Assoc.* 1989;89:1861–1863.
4. Persky VW, Chatterton RT, Van Horn LV, Grant MD, Langenberg P, Marvin J. Hormone levels in vegetarian and nonvegetarian teenage girls: potential implications for breast cancer risk. *Cancer Res.* 1992;50:578–583.
5. Sanders TAB, Manning J. The growth and development of vegan children. *J Human Nutr Diet.* 1992;5:11–21.
6. Donovan UM, Gibson RS. Iron and zinc status of young women aged 14 to 19 years consuming vegetarian and omnivorous diets. *J Am Coll Nutr.* 1995;14:463–472.
7. Donovan UM, Gibson RS. Dietary intakes of adolescent females consuming vegetarian, semi-vegetarian, and omnivorous diets. *J Adol Health.* 1996;18:292–300. *Note:* Two adolescents in the LOV group did not use dairy products.
8. Nathan I, Hackett AF, Kirby S. The dietary intake of a group of vegetarian children aged 7–11 years compared with matched omnivores. *Br J Nutr.* 1996;75:533–544. *Note:* Two vegetarians ate fish; mean consumption was 10.3 g/person/d. Each group had 29 females and 21 males.
9. Houghton LA, Green TJ, Donovan UM, Gibson RS, Stephen AM, O'Connor DL. Association between dietary fiber intake and the folate status of a group of female adolescents. *Am J Clin Nutr.* 1997;66:1414–1421.
10. Thane CW, Bates CJ. Dietary intakes and nutrient status of vegetarian preschool children from a British national survey. *J Hum Nutr Dietet.* 2000;13:149–162. *Note:* Subjects identified as "vegetarians" appear to have consumed fish "although generally in smaller amounts than did omnivores."
11. Leung SS, Lee RH, Sung RY, et al. Growth and nutrition of Chinese vegetarian children in Hong Kong. *J Paediatr Child Health.* 2001;37:247–253.
12. Perry CL, McGuire MT, Neumark-Sztainer D, Story M. Adolescent vegetarians. How well do their dietary patterns meet the Healthy People 2010 objectives? *Arch Pediatr Adolesc Med.* 2002;156:431–437. *Note:* A total of 62% of vegetarians reported eating chicken and/or fish; 32% ate eggs and/or dairy products but not chicken or fish; 6% were vegan.
13. Larsson CL, Johansson GK. Dietary intake and nutritional status of young vegans and omnivores in Sweden. *Am J Clin Nutr.* 2002;76:100–106.
14. Ambroszkiewicz J, Klemarczyk W, Chelchowska M, et al. Serum homocysteine, folate, vitamin B12 and total antioxidant status in vegetarian children. *Adv Med Sci.* 2006;51:265–268. *Note:* Sample includes 21 LOV, 1 LV, 5 OV, 5 VEG. Eighteen males and 14 females were in the vegetarian group.
15. Yen CE, Yen CH, Huang MC, et al. Dietary intake and nutritional status of vegetarian and omnivorous preschool children and their parents in Taiwan. *Nutr Res.* 2008;28:430–436. *Note:* Adult vegetarians consisted of 16 LOV, 2 ovo-vegetarians, 1 LV, 2 vegans. Four male adults and 17 females were vegetarian; 9 male adults and 19 females were NV. Children consisted of 18 LOV and 3 ovo-vegetarians. Fourteen male children and 7 female children were vegetarians; 15 male children and 13 female children were NV.
16. Rush EC, Chhichhia P, Hinckson E, et al. Dietary patterns and vitamin B12 status of migrant Indian preadolescent girls. *Eur J Clin Nutr.* 2009;63:585–587.

Appendix N Fat-Soluble Vitamin Intake of Vegetarian and Nonvegetarian School-Aged Children and Teenagers

(Ref)/year	Group¹/Gender (N)	Country	Age	Kcal	Vitamin A²	Vitamin D (µg)	Vitamin E³ (mg)
(1) 1954	LOV F (15)	United States	14.0	3030	16380		
	NV F (15)	States	14.0	4100	16820		
	LOV M (15)		15.5	4450	17920		
	NV M (15)		15.5	5350	17230		
(2) 1984	LOV M/F (34)	United States	15–17	1947	1421		
(3) 1989	LOV F (9)	United States	11.4	1650	3724		
	NV F (10)	States	11.1	2106	7082		
	LOV M (8)		11.8	2316	8078		
	NV M (12)		11.3	2074	5544		
(4) 1992	LOV F (32)	United States	16.2	1895	4394		
	NV F (35)	States	16.7	1742	3922		
(5) 1992	VEG M/F (18)	Great Britain	9.5	1720	939	1.9	7.6
	NV M/F (194)		7–12	1700	629	1.5	4.3
(6) 1996	LOV M/F (50)	Great Britain	9.1	1824	684	2.6	5.6
	VEG M/F (50)		9.4	1920	602	2.2	4.4
(7) 1997	LOV F (88)	Canada	14–20	1783	648		
	NV F (111)		14–20	1685	596		
(8) 2000	LOV M/F (25)	Great Britain	1.5–<3	1040	389	1.0	4.2
	NV M/F (668)		1.5–<3	1100	430	1.0	3.8
	LOV M/F (19)		3–4.5	1162	407	1.1	4.9
	NV M/F (639)		3–4.5	1238	419	1.1	4.6
(9) 2001	LOV (5M/5F)	Hong Kong	5.9	1376	1308		
	LOV (12M/12F)		9.3	1423	1782		
	LOV (7M/7F)		12.3	1991	1978		
(10) 2002	LOV M/F (262)	United States	14.9	1973	9931		
	NV M/F (4259)	States	14.9	2092	8480		

Appendix N Fat-Soluble Vitamin Intake of Vegetarian and Nonvegetarian School-Aged Children and Teenagers

(Ref)/year	Group[1]/Gender (N)	Country	Age	Kcal	Vitamin A[2]	Vitamin D (µg)	Vitamin E[3] (mg)
(11)	VEG M (15)	Sweden	17.5	2904	1045	3.7	18[3]
2002	NV M (15)		17.5	3143	1226	7.7	9.2[3]
	VEG F (15)		17.5	2126	966	2.0	13[3]
	NV F (15)		17.5	2267	1169	5.1	7.3[3]
(12)	LOV M/F (50)	Poland	2–10	1468		1.37	
2007	NV M/F (50)		2–10	1591		2.43	
(13)	LOV M/F (21)	Taiwan	5.2	1647	2207		8.8
2008	NV M/F (28)		5.0	1698	1929		6.9

Notes: [1]Abbreviations: LOV, lacto-ovo vegetarian; VEG, vegan; and NV, nonvegetarian.

[2]Vitamin A as IU (includes carotene) for reference 1; vitamin A as mg RE for references 2, 5, and 11; vitamin A as IU for references 3 and 4; vitamin A as µg RE for references 6, 7, 8, 9, and 13, and vitamin A as Units (not further specified) for reference 10.

[3]Vitamin E as β-tocopherol equivalents.

ANNOTATED REFERENCES APPENDIX N

1. Hardinge MG, Stare FJ. Nutritional studies of vegetarians. 1. Nutritional, physical, and laboratory studies. *J Clin Nutr.* 1954;2:73–82.

2. Cooper R, Allen A, Goldberg R, Trevisan M, Van Horn L, Liu K, Steinhauer M, Rubenstein A, Stamler J. Seventh-Day Adventist adolescents—life-style patterns and cardiovascular risk factors. *West J Med.* 1984;140:471–477.

3. Tayter M, Stanek KL. Anthropometric and dietary assessment of omnivore and lacto-ovo vegetarian children. *J Am Diet Assoc.* 1989;89:1861–1863.

4. Persky VW, Chatterton RT, Van Horn LV, Grant MD, Langenberg P, Marvin J. Hormone levels in vegetarian and nonvegetarian teenage girls: potential implications for breast cancer risk. *Cancer Res.* 1992;50:578–583.

5. Sanders TAB, Manning J. The growth and development of vegan children. *J Human Nutr Diet.* 1992;5:11–21.

6. Nathan I, Hackett AF, Kirby S. The dietary intake of a group of vegetarian children aged 7–11 years compared with matched omnivores. *Br J Nutr.* 1996;75:533–544. *Note:* Two vegetarians ate fish; mean consumption was 10.3 g/person/d. Each group had 29 females and 21 males.

7. Houghton LA, Green TJ, Donovan UM, Gibson RS, Stephen AM, O'Connor DL. Association between dietary fiber intake and the folate status of a group of female adolescents. *Am J Clin Nutr.* 1997;66:1414–1421.

8. Thane CW, Bates CJ. Dietary intakes and nutrient status of vegetarian preschool children from a British national survey. *J Hum Nutr Dietet.* 2000;13:149–162. *Note:* Subjects identified as "vegetarians" appear to have consumed fish "although generally in smaller amounts than did omnivores."

9. Leung SS, Lee RH, Sung RY, et al. Growth and nutrition of Chinese vegetarian children in Hong Kong. *J Paediatr Child Health.* 2001;37:247–253.

10. Perry CL, McGuire MT, Neumark-Sztainer D, Story M. Adolescent vegetarians. How well do their dietary patterns meet the Healthy People 2010 objectives? *Arch Pediatr Adolesc Med.* 2002;156: 431–437. *Note:* A total of 62% of vegetarians reported eating chicken and/or fish; 32% ate eggs and/or dairy products but not chicken or fish; 6% were vegan.

11. Larsson CL, Johansson GK. Dietary intake and nutritional status of young vegans and omnivores in Sweden. *Am J Clin Nutr.* 2002;76:100–106.

12. Ambroszkiewicz J, Klemarczyk W, Gajewska J, et al. Serum concentration of biochemical bone turnover markers in vegetarian children. *Adv Med Sci.* 2007;52:279–282. *Note:* Sample includes 28 LOV, 4 LV, 5 OV, 13 VEG. Twenty-seven males and 23 females were vegetarian; 25 males and 25 females were NV.

13. Yen CE, Yen CH, Huang MC, et al. Dietary intake and nutritional status of vegetarian and omnivorous preschool children and their parents in Taiwan. *Nutr Res.* 2008;28:430–436. *Note:* Adult vegetarians consisted of 16 LOV, 2 ovo-vegetarians, 1 LV, 2 vegans. Four male adults and 17 females were vegetarian; 9 male adults and 19 females were NV. Children consisted of 18 LOV and 3 ovo-vegetarians. Fourteen male children and 7 female children were vegetarians; 15 male children and 13 female children were NV.

Appendix O Mineral Intake of Vegetarian and Nonvegetarian School-Aged Children and Teenagers

(Ref)/ year	Group/ Gender/(N)	Country	Age	Kcal	Calcium (mg)	Iron (mg)	Zinc (mg)	Copper (mg)	Phosphorus (mg)	Sodium (mg)	Potassium (mg)
(1) 1954	LOV F (15)	United	14.0	3030	1700	18.0			2000		
	NV F (15)	States	14.0	4100	2200	23.0			2800		
	LOV M (15)		15.5	4450	2600	25.0			3100		
	NV M (15)		15.5	5350	2400	28.0			3300		
(2) 1982	LOV M/F (15)[2]	Great	10–15	1900			9.3				
	NV M/F (12)	Britain	10–16	1898			7.6				
(3) 1984	LOV M/F (34)	United States	15–17	1947	998	12.4			1263	2400	2800
(4) 1989	LOV F (9)	United	11.4	1650	1041	10.7					
	NV F (10)	States	11.1	2106	1028	13.0					
	LOV M (8)		11.8	2316	1399	17.0					
	NV M (12)		11.3	2074	1163	13.0					
(5) 1992	LOV F (32)	United	16.2	1895	881	11.4					
	NV F (35)	States	16.7	1742	700	9.5					
(6) 1992	VEG M/F (18)	Great	9.5	1720	464	21.7	7.4	1.7			
	NV M/F (194)[3]	Britain	7–12	1700	680	9.7	6.6	1.6			
(7) 1995	LOV F (78)	Canada	17.7	1663	707	11.2	6.6				
	NV F (29)		18.2	1688	771	11.3	7.9				
(8) 1996	LOV M/F (50)	Great	9.1	1824	825	11.2	5.9				
	NV M/F (50)	Britain	9.4	1920	737	10.6	6.8				
(9) 1996	LOV F (78)	Canada	17.7	1705	733	11.0	6.7		1186		
	NV F (29)		18.2	1735	747	11.7	7.8		1283		
(10) 1997	LOV F (88)	Canada	14–20	1783	709	11.5	7.0				
	NV F (11)		14–20	1685	687	11.2	7.0				
(11) 2000	LOV M/F (25)	Great	1.5–<3	1040	679	5.0	3.8			1165	1585
	NV M/F (668)	Britain	1.5–<3	1100	674	5.2	4.4			1480	1526
	LOV M/F (19)		3–4.5	1162	675	6.0	4.1			1336	1583
	NV M/F (639)		3–4.5	1238	629	6.0	4.6			1663	1579

			Age							
(12) 2001	LOV (5M/5F)	Hong Kong	5.9	1376	470	10.3	6.0			
	LOV (12M/12F)		9.3	1423	466	11.5	5.9			
	LOV (7M/7F)		12.3	1991	471	12.1	7.1			
(13) 2002	LOV M/F (262)	United	14.9	1973	1070	16.1	11.4			
	NV M/F (4259)	States	14.9	2092	1090	14.7	11.7			
(14) 2002	VEG M (15)	Sweden	17.5	2904	517	18	10.0	1361	3797	4200
	NV M (15)		17.5	3143	1697	18	16	2176	4656	4100
	VEG F (15)		17.5	2126	538	14	7.8	1025	2580	3460
	NV F (15)		17.5	2267	1328	11	11	1536	3040	3160
(15) 2005	LO/LV M (139)	Netherlands	12.7	665						
	NV M (39)		11.7	1056						
	LO/LV F (37)		11.9	518						
	NV F (55)		11.7	1080						
(16) 2007	LOV M/F (50)	Poland	2–10	1468	559			910		
	NV M/F (50)		2–10	1591	821			949		
(17) 2008	LOV M/F (21)	Taiwan	5.2	1647	388	10.1	6.2			
	NV M/F (28)		5.0	1698	521	8.8	6.6			
(18) 2010	LV F (630)	India	12.1	1373			3.6			

Notes: [1]Abbreviations: LOV, lacto-ovo vegetarian; LV, lacto vegetarian; VEG, vegan; NV, nonvegetarian.
[2]Initially, study consisted of 12 males and 22 females. LOV were matched for age, sex, race, and socioeconomic status to NV.
[3]Data for NV are from a separate survey of British children presented in the reference.

ANNOTATED REFERENCES APPENDIX O

1. Hardinge MG, Stare FJ. Nutritional studies of vegetarians. 1. Nutritional, physical, and laboratory studies. *J Clin Nutr.* 1954;2:73–82.

2. Treuherz J. Possible inter-relationship between zinc and dietary fibre in a group of lacto-ovo vegetarian adolescents. *J Plant Foods.* 1982;4:89–93.

3. Cooper R, Allen A, Goldberg R, Trevisan M, Van Horn L, Liu K, Steinhauer M, Rubenstein A, Stamler J. Seventh-day Adventist adolescents—life-style patterns and cardiovascular risk factors. *West J Med.* 1984;140:471–477.

4. Tayter M, Stanek KL. Anthropometric and dietary assessment of omnivore and lacto-ovo vegetarian children. *J Am Diet Assoc.* 1989;89:1861–1863.

5. Persky VW, Chatterton RT, Van Horn LV, Grant MD, Langenberg P, Marvin J. Hormone levels in vegetarian and nonvegetarian teenage girls: potential implications for breast cancer risk. *Cancer Res.* 1992;50:578–583.

6. Sanders TAB, Manning J. The growth and development of vegan children. *J Human Nutr Diet.* 1992;5:11–21.

7. Donovan UM, Gibson RS. Iron and zinc status of young women aged 14 to 19 years consuming vegetarian and omnivorous diets. *J Am Coll Nutr.* 1995;14:463–472.

8. Nathan I, Hackett AF, Kirby S. The dietary intake of a group of vegetarian children aged 7–11 years compared with matched omnivores. *Br J Nutr.* 1996;75:533–544. *Note:* Two vegetarians ate fish; mean consumption was 10.3 g/person/d. Each group had 29 females and 21 males.

9. Donovan UM, Gibson RS. Dietary intakes of adolescent females consuming vegetarian, semi-vegetarian, and omnivorous diets. *J Adol Health.* 1996;18:292–300. *Note:* Two adolescents in the LOV group did not use dairy products.

10. Houghton LA, Green TJ, Donovan UM, Gibson RS, Stephen AM, O'Connor DL. Association between dietary fiber intake and the folate status of a group of female adolescents. *Am J Clin Nutr.* 1997;66:1414–1421.

11. Thane CW, Bates CJ. Dietary intakes and nutrient status of vegetarian preschool children from a British national survey. *J Hum Nutr Dietet.* 2000;13:149–162. *Note:* Subjects identified as "vegetarians" appear to have consumed fish "although generally in smaller amounts than did omnivores."

12. Leung SS, Lee RH, Sung RY, et al. Growth and nutrition of Chinese vegetarian children in Hong Kong. *J Paediatr Child Health.* 2001;37:247–253.

13. Perry CL, McGuire MT, Neumark-Sztainer D, Story M. Adolescent vegetarians. How well do their dietary patterns meet the Healthy People 2010 objectives? *Arch Pediatr Adolesc Med.* 2002;156:431–437. *Note:* A total of 62% of vegetarians reported eating chicken and/or fish; 32% ate eggs and/or dairy products but not chicken or fish; 6% were vegan.

14. Larsson CL, Johansson GK. Dietary intake and nutritional status of young vegans and omnivores in Sweden. *Am J Clin Nutr.* 2002;76:100–106.

15. Dhonukshe-Rutten RAM, van Dusseldorp M, Schneede J, et al. Low bone mineral density and bone mineral content are associated with low cobalamin status in adolescents. *Eur J Nutr.* 2005;44:341–347.

16. Ambroszkiewicz J, Klemarczyk W, Gajewska J, et al. Serum concentration of biochemical bone turnover markers in vegetarian children. *Adv Med Sci.* 2007;52:279–282. *Note:* Sample includes 28 LOV, 4 LV, 5 OV, 13 VEG. Twenty-seven males and 23 females were vegetarian; 25 males and 25 females were NV.

17. Yen CE, Yen CH, Huang MC, et al. Dietary intake and nutritional status of vegetarian and omnivorous preschool children and their parents in Taiwan. *Nutr Res.* 2008;28:430–436. *Note:* Adult vegetarians consisted of 16 LOV, 2 ovo-vegetarians, 1 LV, 2 vegans. Four male adults and 17 females were vegetarian; 9 male adults and 19 females were NV. Children consisted of 18 LOV and 3 ovo-vegetarians. Fourteen male children and 7 female children were vegetarians; 15 male children and 13 female children were NV.

18. Tupe R, Chiplonkar SA. Diet patterns of lactovegetarian adolescent girls: need for devising recipes with high zinc bioavailability. *Nutrition.* 2010;26:390–398.

Appendix P Fiber, Cholesterol, and Macronutrient Intakes of Elderly Vegetarians and Nonvegetarians

(Ref)/ year	Group/ Gender(N)	Country	Age (years)	SDA/ NSDA[2]	Kcal[3]	Protein[4] % Kcal	Fat[4] % Kcal	CHO[4] % Kcal	SF (g)	PUFA or LA (g)	PUFA: SF[5]	Cholesterol (mg)	Fiber[6]
(1) 1983	LOV F (36)	Canada	69	SDA	1615	14.5							33.2
	NV F (30)		60	NSDA	1727	15.6							20.2
(2) 1988	LOV F (88)	United States	73	SDA	1533	14.2	32.9	56.4				167	5.6
	NV F (278)		79	NSDA	1633	17.1	48.5	46.1				305	4.2
(3) 1989	LOV F (144)	United States	67	SDA	1474	14.1	30.8	58.6	15.0			155	20.0
	NV F (146)		66	NSDA	1563	16.2	34.9	49.1	20.6			243	16.0
(4) 1989	LOV F (10)	United States	67	NI	1612	13.9	36.0				0.75	194	5.2
	NV F (10)		65		1641	16.6	42.0				0.48	294	4.7
(5) 1990	LOV F (23)	United States	72	SDA	1452	12.9	31.7	60.0	12.2	9.2	0.85	89	21.5
	NV F (14)		71	SDA	1363	16.2	35.9	50.2	14.9	7.9	0.51	183	13.0
(6) 1990	LOV F (12)	United States	76	SDA	1425	13.2	31.6	60.6	10.0	7.0		72	24.0
	NV F (12)		72	SDA	1334	16.2	36.4	49.8	17.0	7.0		181	13.0
(7) 1990	LOV M (18)	Netherlands	83	NSDA	1960	12.2	37.2	50.8	15.0	8.5	0.57	200	33.7
	NV M[7]		Elderly		2412	13.6	40.8	41.8	17.3	6.8	0.39	356	27.4
	LOV F (26)		81		1667	13.1	37.3	49.8	15.8	8.3	0.53	216	28.7
	NV F[7]		Elderly		1879	14.9	40.1	43.2	17.2	6.5	0.38	294	23.7
(8) 1990	LOV M (15)	Netherlands	82	NSDA	2014	11.7	39.3	49.5					33.0
	NV M (225)		72		2414	13.6	41.0	41.6					27.0
	LOV F (17)		82		1681	12.8	39.1	48.1					28.0
	NV F (216)		72		1874	14.9	40.3	42.7					23.0
(9) 1992	LOV F (28)	United States	63	SDA/NSDA	1652	15.2	30.5	58.7	16.5	10.1		98	10.3
	NV F (28)		63	SDA/NSDA	1657	18.5	33.6	48.1	19.1	10.9		214	7.6
(10) 1993	B-LOV M (23)	United States	69	SDA	1900	14.0	30.8	59.8	13.5	15.0		84	
	B-NV M (29)	States	65	SDA	2487	14.5	37.1	52.3	25.5	24.7		303	
	W-LOV M (83)		67	SDA	2336	13.6	30.8	61.1	17.8	19.4		137	
	W-NV M (43)		65	SDA	2078	14.1	33.8	56.8	20.1	18.3		183	

(Appendix P continued)

Appendix P Fiber, Cholesterol, and Macronutrient Intakes of Elderly Vegetarians and Nonvegetarians

(Ref)/year	Group¹/Gender/(N)	Country	Age (years)	SDA/NSDA²	Kcal³	Protein⁴ % Kcal	Fat⁴ % Kcal	CHO⁴ % Kcal	SF (g)	PUFA or LA (g)	PUFA: SF⁵	Cholesterol (mg)	Fiber⁶
(11) 2003	VEG/LV F htn (71)	Hong Kong	78.7	NSDA	1181	11.2							9.2
	VEG/LV F (40)		76.7		1225	12.5							9.2

Notes: ¹Abbreviations: LV, lacto vegetarian; LOV, lacto-ovo vegetarian; VEG, vegan; NV, nonvegetarian; NI, not indicated; htn, subjects identified as having hypertension; CHO, carbohydrates; SF, saturated fat; PUFA, polyunsaturated fat; LA, linoleic acid; B, black; W, white.

²SDA indicates the vegetarians were specifically identified as Seventh-day Adventists, whereas NSDA indicates the vegetarians were not exclusively SDAs, although some SDAs may have been included in the vegetarian group. NI indicates the process by which subjects were recruited for the study was not indicated or the extent to which SDAs composed the vegetarian groups was not possible to determine by the information provided.

³When energy intake was listed as kilojoules, a factor of 4.2 was used to convert kilojoules into kilocalories.

⁴Values for protein, fat, and carbohydrate are the percentage of calories contributed by each nutrient. The percentage of calories contributed by protein, fat, and carbohydrate was determined by multiplying the number of grams consumed per day, by 4, 9, and 4 calories per gram, respectively, and then dividing the calories provided by each macronutrient by the total number of calories listed in the reference. In some cases, this led to differences between the calculated percentage of calories contributed by each nutrient and the percentage listed in the reference and often resulted in the total percentage not equaling 100. In cases where only the percentage of calories for each nutrient was listed and not grams, those percentages were used.

⁵PUFA: Saturated fat ratios represent values as listed in the reference or were determined by dividing the number of grams of PUFA or linoleic acid by the number of grams of saturated fat.

⁶Values for fiber are listed as either dietary fiber (g) or crude fiber (g) (references 2 and 4). Typically, 1 g of crude fiber represents between 3 and 4 g of dietary fiber.

⁷Data for NV are from a separate nationwide survey of elderly individuals.

ANNOTATED REFERENCES APPENDIX P

1. Gibson RS, Anderson BM, Sabry JH. The trace metal status of a group of post-menopausal vegetarians. *J Am Diet Assoc.* 1983;82:246–250.
2. Tylavsky FA, Anderson JJB. Dietary factors in bone health of elderly lacto-ovo vegetarian and omnivorous women. *Am J Clin Nutr.* 1988;48:842–849.
3. Hunt I-F, Murphy NJ, Henderson C, Clark VA, Jacobs RM, Johnston PK, Coulson AH. Bone mineral content in postmenopausal women: Comparison of omnivores and vegetarians. *Am J Clin Nutr.* 1989;50:517–523.
4. Marsh AG, Christensen DK, Sanchez TV, Mickelsen O, Chaffee FL. Nutrient similarities and differences of older lacto-ovo vegetarian and omnivorous women. *Nutr Rep Int.* 1989;39:19–24.
5. Nieman DC, Underwood BC, Sherman KM, Arabatzis K, Barbosa JC, Johnson M, Shultz TD. Dietary status of Seventh-Day Adventist vegetarian and nonvegetarian elderly women. *J Am Diet Assoc.* 1989;89:1763–1769.
6. Barbosa JC, Shultz TD, Filley SJ, Nieman DC. The relationship among adiposity, diet and hormone concentrations in vegetarian and nonvegetarian postmenopausal women. *Am J Clin Nutr.* 1990;51:798–803.
7. Brants HAM, Löwik MRH, Westenbrink S, Hulshof KFAM, Kistemaker C. Adequacy of a vegetarian diet at old age (Dutch Nutrition Surveillance System). *J Am College Nutr.* 1990;9:292–302.
8. Löwik MRH, Schrijver J, van den Berg H, Hulshof KFAM, Wedel M, Ockhuizen T. Effect of dietary fiber on the vitamin B6 status among vegetarian and nonvegetarian elderly (Dutch Nutrition Surveillance System). *J Am College Nutr.* 1990;9:241–249.
9. Tesar R, Notelovitz M, Shim E, Kauwell G, Brown J. Axial and peripheral bone density and nutrient intakes of postmenopausal vegetarian and omnivorous women. *Am J Clin Nutr.* 1992;56:699–704.
10. Melby CL, Goldflies DG, Toohey ML. Blood pressure differences in older black and white long-term vegetarians and nonvegetarians. *J Am Coll Nutr.* 1993;12:262–269.
11. Kwok TCY, Chan TYK, Woo J. Relationship of urinary sodium/potassium excretion and calcium intake to blood pressure and prevalence of hypertension among older Chinese vegetarians. *Eur J Clin Nutr.* 2003;57:299–304.

Appendix Q Water-Soluble Vitamin Intake of Elderly Vegetarians and Nonvegetarians

(Ref)/ year	Group[1]/Gen- der/(N)	Country	Age	Kcal	Vit. C (mg)	Thaimin (mg)	Riboflavin (mg)	Niacin (mg)	Vit. B₆ (mg)	Folate (mg)	Pantothenic acid (mg)	Vit. B₁₂ (µg)
(1) 1988	LOV F (88)	United States	73	1533	184	1.0	1.3	11.3				
	NV F (278)		79	1633	157	0.9	1.5	13.8				
(2) 1989	LOV F (23)	United States	72	1452	155	1.4	1.5	14.3	1.6	273	3.6	2.3
	NV F (14)		71	1363	114	1.1	1.4	14.2	1.3	215	2.8	2.6
(3) 1990	LOV F (18)	Netherlands	83	1960	136	1.3	1.9		1.3			
	NV M[2]		Elderly	2412	94	1.1	1.7		1.4			
	LOV F (26)		81	1667	149	1.1	1.7		1.1			
	NV F[2]		Elderly	1879	101	0.9	1.5		1.2			
(4) 1992	LOV F (28)	United States	63	1652	143	1.4	1.7	14.4	1.8	255	3.6	2.5
	NV F (28)		63	1657	118	1.4	1.9	20.0	1.6	249	3.5	4.2
(5) 2003	VEG/LV F htn (71)	Hong Kong	78.7	1181	128	0.5						
	VEG/LV F (40)		76.7	1225	136	0.5						

Notes: [1]Abbreviations: LOV, lacto-ovo vegetarian; LV, lacto vegetarian; VEG, vegan; NV, nonvegetarian; htn, subjects identified as having hypertension.
[2]Data for NV from a separate nationwide survey of elderly individuals.

ANNOTATED REFERENCES APPENDIX Q

1. Tylavsky FA, Anderson JJB. Dietary factors in bone health of elderly lacto-ovo vegetarian and omnivorous women. *Am J Clin Nutr.* 1988;48:842–849.
2. Nieman DC, Underwood BC, Sherman KM, et al. Dietary status of Seventh-day Adventist vegetarian and nonvegetarian elderly women. *J Am Diet Assoc.* 1989;89:1763–1769.
3. Brants HAM, Löwik MRH, Westenbrink S, Hulshof KFAM, Kistemaker C. Adequacy of a vegetarian diet at old age (Dutch Nutrition Surveillance System). *J Am College Nutr.* 1990;9:292–302.
4. Tesar R, Notelovitz M, Shim E, Kauwell G, Brown J. Axial and peripheral bone density and nutrient intakes of postmenopausal vegetarian and omnivorous women. *Am J Clin Nutr.* 1992;56:699–704.
5. Kwok TCY, Chan TYK, Woo J. Relationship of urinary sodium/potassium excretion and calcium intake to blood pressure and prevalence of hypertension among older Chinese vegetarians. *Eur J Clin Nutr.* 2003;57:299–304.

Appendix R Mineral Intake of Elderly Vegetarians and Nonvegetarians

(Ref)/year	Group[1]/Gender(N)	Age	Kcal	Ca (mg)	Fe (mg)	Zn (mg)	Mg (mg)	Cu (mg)	Mn (mg)	Se (μg)	Na (mg)	K (mg)	P (mg)
(1) 1983	LOV F (36)	69	1615					2.1	4.4	113			
	NV F (30)	60	1727					1.6	2.6	109			
(2) 1988	LOV F (88)	73	1533	823	10.7								
	NV F (278)	79	1633	902	10.2								
(3) 1989	LOV F (23)	72	1452	628	12.3	6.3	283	1.4	2.2		1930	2628	889
	NV F (14)	71	1363	633	11.4	6.3	226	1.0	1.3		1936	2342	892
(4) 1989	LOV F (10)	67	1612	898	12.3								1109
	NV F (10)	64	1641	712	13.3								1079
(5) 1989	LOV F (144)	67	1474	748		7.2	312						1050
	NV F (146)	66	1563	772		8.8	294						1147
(6) 1990	LOV M (18)	65–97	1960	1219	13.7	8.5							
	NV M[2]	65+		1128	13.1	10.3							
	LOV F (26)	65–97	1667	1141	12.2	7.6							
	NV F[2]	65+		1013	11.4	9.3							
(7) 1992	LOV F (28)	63	1652	821	13.0	7.2	318	1.4		16.9	2202	3012	1155
	NV F (28)	63	1657	863	15.5	7.9	266	1.0		17.4	2285	2687	1250
(8) 2003	VEG/LV F htn (71)	78.7	1181	411								1160	
	VEG/LV F (40)	71.7	1225	589								1131	
(9) 2005	LOV M (44)	≥65	NI				244						
	VEG M (18)	≥65					196						
	NV M (680)	≥65					263						
	LOV F (211)	≥65					225						
	VEG F (102)	≥65					193						
	NV F (403)	≥65					233						

Notes: [1]Abbreviations: LOV, lacto-ovo vegetarian; LV, lacto vegetarian; VEG, vegan; NV, nonvegetarian; htn, subjects identified as having hypertension; NI, not indicated.
[2]Data for NV from a separate nationwide survey of elderly individuals.

ANNOTATED REFERENCES APPENDIX R

1. Gibson RS, Anderson BM, Sabry JH. The trace metal status of a group of post-menopausal vegetarians. *J Am Diet Assoc.* 1983;82:246–250.
2. Tylavsky FA, Anderson JJB. Dietary factors in bone health of elderly lacto-ovo vegetarian and omnivorous women. *Am J Clin Nutr.* 1988;48:842–849.
3. Nieman DC, Underwood BC, Sherman KM, Arabatzis K, Barbosa JC, Johnson M, Shultz TD. Dietary status of Seventh-day Adventist vegetarian and nonvegetarian elderly women. *J Am Diet Assoc.* 1989;89:1763–1769.
4. Marsh AG, Christensen DK, Sanchez TV, Mickelsen O, Chaffee FL. Nutrient similarities and differences of older lacto-ovo vegetarian and omnivorous women. *Nutr Rep Int.* 1989;39:19–24.
5. Hunt I-F, Murphy NJ, Henderson C, Clark VA, Jacobs RM, Johnston PK, Coulson AH. Bone mineral content in postmenopausal women: Comparison of omnivores and vegetarians. *Am J Clin Nutr.* 1989;50:517–523.
6. Brants HAM, Löwik MRH, Westenbrink S, Hulshof KFAM, Kistemaker C. Adequacy of a vegetarian diet at old age (Dutch Nutrition Surveillance System). *J Am College Nutr.* 1990;9:292–302.
7. Tesar R, Notelovitz M, Shim E, Kauwell G, Brown J. Axial and peripheral bone density and nutrient intakes of postmenopausal vegetarian and omnivorous women. *Am J Clin Nutr.* 1992;56:699–704.
8. Kwok TCY, Chan TYK, Woo J. Relationship of urinary sodium/potassium excretion and calcium intake to blood pressure and prevalence of hypertension among older Chinese vegetarians. *Eur J Clin Nutr.* 2003;57:299–304.
9. Wang JL, Shaw NS, Yeh HY, et al. Magnesium status and association with diabetes in the Taiwanese elderly. *Asia Pac J Clin Nutr.* 2005;14:263–269.

Index